JUDITH McGREGOR, M.D.

An Atlas of Cross-sectional Anatomy

edited by

STEPHEN A. KIEFFER, M.D.

Professor and Chairman, Department of Radiology, State University of New York Upstate Medical Center, Syracuse, New York

E. ROBERT HEITZMAN, M.D.

Professor and Director, Division of Diagnostic Radiology, Department of Radiology, State University of New York Upstate Medical Center, Syracuse, New York

With contributions by

Eugene F. Binet, M.D.
Jerry Brown, M.D.
Patrick J. Bryan, M.B., B.Ch., F.R.C.R.
William N. Cohen, M.D.
W. Martin Dinn, M.D.
Richard L. Goldwin, M.D.
Leo V. Gould, M.D.
E. Mark Levinsohn, M.D.
Anthony V. Proto, M.D.
Frank E. Seidelmann, D.O.

With the technical assistance of

John G. Hodgson, B.S.
Joseph J. Moro, R.T.
Ludwig J. Rimmler

An Atlas of Cross-sectional Anatomy

COMPUTED TOMOGRAPHY, ULTRASOUND, RADIOGRAPHY, GROSS ANATOMY

**From the Department of Radiology,
SUNY Upstate Medical Center**

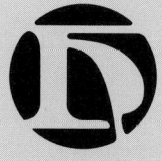

Medical Department
Harper & Row, Publishers
Hagerstown, Maryland
New York, San Francisco, London

79 80 81 82 83 84   10 9 8 7 6 5 4 3 2 1

An Atlas of Cross-sectional Anatomy. Copyright © 1979 by Harper & Row, Publishers, Inc. All rights reserved. No part of this book may be used or reproduced in any manner whatsoever without written permission except in the case of brief quotations embodied in critical articles and reviews. Printed in the United States of America. For information address Medical Department, Harper & Row, Publishers, Inc., 2350 Virginia Avenue, Hagerstown, Maryland 21740.

Library of Congress Cataloging in Publication Data

Kieffer, Stephen A
   An atlas of cross-sectional anatomy.
    Developed by the Division of Diagnostic Radiology, Department of Radiology, State University of New York Upstate Medical Center, Syracuse, N.Y.
   Includes bibliographical references and index.
   1. Anatomy, Human—Atlases. 2. Tomography—Atlases. 3. Diagnosis, Radioscopic—Atlases. 4. Diagnosis, Ultrasonic—Atlases. I. Heitzman, E. Robert, 1927- joint author. II. New York (State). Upstate Medical Center, Syracuse. Division of Diagnostic Radiology. III. Title. [DNLM: 1. Anatomy—Atlases. 2. Tomography, Computerized axial-Atlases. 3. Ultrasonics—Atlases. QS17 K47a]
QM25.K5   611'.022'2   78-18859
ISBN 0-06-141152-3

Contents

Contributors vii
Preface ix
Introduction xi

1 Skull and Brain 2
Stephen A. Kieffer

Anatomic Correlations 4
Normal *In Vivo* Computed Tomographic Studies 24

2 Orbit 39
Stephen A. Kieffer

Anatomic Correlations 40
Normal *In Vivo* Computed Tomographic Studies 48

3 Neck and Face 53
Leo V. Gould

4 Spine 77
Eugene F. Binet

Anatomic Correlations 78
Normal *In Vivo* Computed Tomographic Studies: Metrizamide 98

5 Chest 102
Anthony V. Proto, Richard L. Goldwin, E. Robert Heitzman

Anatomic Correlations 104
Normal *In Vivo* Computed Tomographic Studies 138

6 Abdomen and Pelvis 144
Patrick J. Bryan, William N. Cohen, Jerry Brown, Frank E. Seidelmann, W. Martin Dinn

Anatomic Correlations 146
  Male Pelvis 202
Longitudinal (Sagittal) Sections 208
Normal *In Vivo* Studies 220

7 Extremities 227

E. Mark Levinsohn

    Wrist 228
    Forearm 236
    Elbow 238
    Upper Arm 244
    Shoulder 246
    Ankle 252
    Lower Leg 262
    Knee 264
    Thigh 278

Index 283

Contributors

EUGENE F. BINET, M.D.
Chapter 4
Professor, Department of Radiology, University of Arkansas Medical Center, Little Rock, Arkansas; Formerly Associate Professor, Department of Radiology, State University of New York Upstate Medical Center, Syracuse, New York

JERRY BROWN, M.D.
Chapter 6
Instructor, Department of Radiology, State University of New York Upstate Medical Center, Syracuse, New York

PATRICK J. BRYAN, M.B., B.Ch., F.R.C.R.
Chapter 6
Consultant Radiologist, St. Vincent's Hospital, Dublin, Ireland; Formerly Assistant Professor, Department of Radiology, State University of New York Upstate Medical Center, Syracuse, New York

WILLIAM N. COHEN, M.D.
Chapter 6
Professor, Department of Radiology, State University of New York Upstate Medical Center, Syracuse, New York

W. MARTIN DINN, M.D.
Chapter 6
Radiologist, Boxford, Massachusetts; Formerly Assistant Professor, Department of Radiology, State University of New York Upstate Medical Center, Syracuse, New York

RICHARD L. GOLDWIN, M.D.
Chapter 5
Associate Radiologist, Department of Radiology, Corning Hospital, Corning, New York; Formerly Chief Resident, Department of Radiology, State University of New York Upstate Medical Center, Syracuse, New York

LEO V. GOULD, M.D.
Chapter 3
Associate Professor, Department of Radiology; Associate Professor, Department of Otolaryngology and Communication Sciences, State University of New York Upstate Medical Center, Syracuse, New York

E. ROBERT HEITZMAN, M.D.
Chapter 5
Professor and Director, Division of Diagnostic Radiology, Department of Radiology, State University of New York Upstate Medical Center, Syracuse, New York

STEPHEN A. KIEFFER, M.D.
Chapters 1, 2
Professor and Chairman, Department of Radiology, State University of New York Upstate Medical Center, Syracuse, New York

E. MARK LEVINSOHN, M.D.
Chapter 7
Assistant Professor, Department of Radiology, State University of New York Upstate Medical Center, Syracuse, New York

ANTHONY V. PROTO, M.D.
Chapter 5
Associate Professor, Department of Radiology, University of Cincinnati Medical Center, Cincinnati, Ohio; Formerly Assistant Professor, Department of Radiology, State University of New York Upstate Medical Center, Syracuse, New York

FRANK E. SEIDELMANN, D.O.
Chapter 6
Associate Professor, Department of Radiology, Case Western Reserve University School of Medicine, Cleveland Ohio; Formerly Assistant Professor, Department of Radiology, State University of New York Upstate Medical Center, Syracuse, New York

Preface

The development in recent years of new imaging modalities, particularly computed tomography and diagnostic ultrasound, has revolutionized medical diagnosis. These examinations generate images which are displayed in transverse and sagittal perspectives; their interpretation therefore requires a thorough knowledge of normal anatomic relationships as demonstrated in these planes. Although some treatises of anatomy, notably those of Eyclesheimer and Schoemaker (1) and Pernkopf (2) do provide such information, their value to the diagnostic radiologist is limited since they do not afford direct roentgen-anatomic or sonographic anatomic correlations.

In an effort to provide a comprehensive atlas of the human body, correlating anatomy as shown in transverse sections (and some sagittal sections) with computed tomographic and sonographic images, the Division of Diagnostic Radiology of the Department of Radiology of the Upstate Medical Center undertook the development of such material as a group project. A strong impetus to this effort has been the long history of fruitful cooperation between the departments of Radiology and Anatomy at our institution. The success of past collaborative efforts (leading to many scientific exhibits and publications) led us to feel that a correlative atlas of high quality could be developed.

Our principal aim in this endeavor has been to produce a carefully annotated work directly correlating gross anatomic sections of the body and x-rays of these sections with computed tomographic and sonographic images from the identical cadaver.

This atlas could not have been produced without the untiring efforts and cooperation of a large number of individuals deeply committed to its development. Over 20 members of the Department of Radiology participated in this project.

The cooperation of the Department of Anatomy chaired by Dr. Donald C. Goodman has once again proven to be exceptional. Ludwig J. Rimmler, technical specialist in anatomy, meticulously prepared the gross body sections with the assistance of Charles Carter. Dr. Henry S. DiStefano, professor of anatomy, helped to provide the anatomic materials and was ever ready to provide expertise and guidance.

Computed tomography of the intact cadaver and radiography of the gross sections were performed by Joseph J. Moro, R.T., who also carefully planned and identified the locations and landmarks for the planes of section. Mr. Moro was ably assisted by Kathryn Kimball, R.T., Libnan Astafan, R.T., Gary Litvin, R.T., Marilyn Dibble, R.T., Maureen Seubert, R.T., Thomas Roczen, R.T., and Judy Dromms, R.T. Sonography was performed with the able assistance of Mrs. Florence Champlin, R.T.

The considerable responsibility for photography (both black-and-white and color) for this volume was carried entirely by John G. Hodgson. The clarity and precision of the images displayed on these pages attest to his care and competence.

Allen Ayres, medical illustrator at the Syracuse Veterans Administration Hospital, provided all of the reference level diagrams. Miss Cindy Stevens, Ms. Gladys Russell, Mrs. Linda Markell, and Mrs. Diane Pajak ably performed the secretarial work, and Mrs. Gail Mitchell and Miss Jean Bartlett provided additional clerical assistance.

Dr. Ronald C. Kim of the Department of Pathology (Section of Neuropathology) and Dr. Jorge V. Esguerra of the Department of Radiology assisted in the annotation of the chapter on the skull and brain. Doctors Beverly Spirt and Richard Rozanski assisted in the development of the chapter on the abdomen and pelvis.

Clearly, this atlas could not have been produced without the dedication and skill of those listed above. The high quality of the roentgen–anatomic correlations appearing on every page amply attest to their talent. All of the collaborators extend to them our deep appreciation and admiration.

It is our sincere hope that this volume will become a reference source useful to anatomists and physicians in other clinical fields as well as radiologists. We further hope that it will find daily application as a reliable and helpful reference whenever computed tomographic and sonographic examinations are being interpreted, and that it will lead to more accurate assessment of all sonographic and radiographic images.

S.A.K.
E.R.H.

REFERENCES

1. Eyclesheimer AC, Schoemaker DM: A Cross-Section Anatomy. New York, D. Appleton and Company, 1911. Reissued in 1970 by Appleton-Century-Crofts
2. Pernkopf E: Atlas of Topographical and Applied Human Anatomy (Ferner H, ed). Philadelphia, WB Saunders, 1963

Introduction

This atlas is composed of a series of anatomic cross sections (and some sagittal sections) of the entire human body. On full-color photographs of these sections anatomic structures are identified in considerable detail and are correlated with their appearance on radiographs and computed tomograms of the same section. In the chapter on the abdomen and pelvis, diagnostic ultrasound images of the same sections also were included at some levels.

An important principle which was followed throughout the making of the atlas is that the radiographic, computed tomographic, and sonographic correlations would be carried out at each cross-sectional level with the identical gross section from the same cadaver. However, since not all regions of a single cadaver could be expected to provide ideal comparative material, it was necessary to use several cadavers. Yet, for every level of section, the correlative material is from the same cadaver. With the exception of the chapter on the spine, all of the gross cross sections in a given chapter were taken from the same cadaver.

The fresh cadaver, upon arrival in the Department of Anatomy, was transported unembalmed to the Department of Radiology, where complete computed tomographic and sonographic examinations were performed. Markers were placed on the skin of the cadaver to indicate the precise levels of section. In certain areas, thin metallic markers were introduced through the skin into underlying bone to serve as a check against possible shifting of the skin in relation to deeper structures.

Cross-sectional computed tomographic images were obtained in the transaxial plane at 13-mm intervals in the examination of the neck and face, spine, chest, abdomen and pelvis, and extremities. In the examination of the skull and brain, the plane of section was angled 20° caudad according to the accepted clinical convention. In the study of the orbit, the plane of section was transaxial, but the interval between sections was reduced to 8 mm.

Sonographic images of the abdomen were then recorded at the identical cross-sectional levels, utilizing a Unirad Sono III ultrasound unit with gray scale capability. Most of the images were obtained with a 3.5-mHz transducer.

The cadaver was then returned to the anatomy laboratory, embalmed, and packed in dry ice. Approximately 7 to 10 days later the completely frozen body was sectioned with a commercial band saw; the skin markers were used to establish the position of the cuts. Some slight tissue loss occurred during slicing so that the resulting gross anatomic sections were reduced 1 or 2 mm in thickness.

The frozen gross specimens were allowed to thaw, were fixed in formalin, and were then photographed using a Polaroid MP-3 camera and Kodak

Ektachrome film. This yielded a transparency from which an "inter" negative was made, the negative being used to print the final photograph. The reader will doubtless note a difference in flesh tones on the gross anatomic photographs from one chapter to another. This is due primarily to the fact that in the chapters on the skull and brain and the orbit, and in the upper two levels of the chapter on the spine, the sections were photographed immediately after slicing and thawing, while in the other chapters, the sections were photographed after a period of immersion in formalin.

Immediately following photography, the sections were radiographed using Kodak X-omat TL film, a fine-grain type of nonscreen x-ray film designed for localization of radiation therapy fields. A conventional radiographic apparatus and tube with a 1-mm focal spot were employed. The specimen was carefully positioned on the cassette, the field of exposure was closely collimated, and exposures were made according to the following table:

Area	Kilovoltage	Milliampere-Seconds
Head	27	200
Neck	25	200
Chest	25	150
Abdomen	35	200
Extremities	35	200

This atlas displays all cross-sectional anatomic images according to the convention which has been advocated by *Radiology* (2) and the *American Journal of Roentgenology* (3): the images are presented as though viewed from below (inferior aspect). The left side of the image appears to the viewer's right in a manner identical to the viewing of conventional frontal radiographs.

At any level, the reader may note some lack of correspondence in anatomic detail between the gross anatomic photograph and the radiographic, computed tomographic, or sonographic images. This is because the latter images are two-dimensional representations of a three-dimensional structure (the 13-mm thick "slice"), while the gross photograph displays only one surface of that slice. Structures within the slice or on its opposite surface are not visible on the anatomic photograph, while they can be visualized by radiography, computed tomography, or sonography.

In a few of the gross anatomic sections, the superior aspect of the slice depicted anatomic details much more clearly than the inferior aspect. However, in order to maintain consistency of right and left sides, the color negative was reversed left for right during the photographic process. Because of the presence of bilateral symmetry of the anatomy and the lack of any three-dimensional features on the surface of these specimens, the reversal of the resulting color print does not lead to confusion. The sections on which the reader is viewing the superior aspect of the gross anatomy are clearly identified in the titles by the addition in parenthesis of the words "superior aspect."

In each chapter, the arrangement of the levels of section is from inferior to superior. The first section is the lowest, and the last level is the highest in any chapter. This cephalad numbering system reiterates the conventional sequence of computed tomography in clinical practice in which the levels being scanned are examined in ascending order.

The anatomic terminology used in this volume is based on the nomenclature used in the 29th American edition of *Gray's Anatomy* (4), mainly consisting of the Nomina Anatomica (NA). Because the inclusion of some radiologic terms, e.g., paratracheal line, was felt to be mandatory, some terms and designations are not anatomic in the classical sense. However, only those radiologic terms which are in the standard parlance of the specialty have been included.

The computed tomographic images in this atlas were obtained on a Deltascan 50 unit (1) utilizing scanning times in the range of 2.0 to 2.7 minutes. The scanning times varied with the diameter of the scanning circle, but the relatively long scanning times were, of course, of no consequence in the motionless cadaver. Technical factors for computed tomography were 120 kVp and 30 mA. Ranges of settings for the center and width of the scanning window, as well as the size of the scanning circle, are listed in the Introduction to each chapter. These settings are expressed in terms of Hounsfield units, the generally accepted term for the numerical expression of the linear x-ray attenuation coefficient of tissue relative to that of water. The values listed, although given for the Deltascan unit, should be applicable to other computed tomographic units. However, measurements on different computed tomographic scanners may differ slightly due to variations in effective energy (5).

Several chapters include supplementary computed tomographic images of normal anatomy from living patients. These *"in vivo"* images were obtained with the unit described above and also with a Deltascan 50-FS unit utilizing scanning times in the range of 15 to 18 seconds. This atlas does not include any computed tomographic image reconstructions in either the coronal or sagittal planes. Such reconstructions, obtained from manipulation of data from overlapping transaxial images, in our opinion do not yet produce images of a quality comparable to the basic transaxial image at acceptable radiation exposure levels. However, there seems little doubt that technologic progress will in the future result in reconstructions of improved quality at acceptable radiation exposure levels and that coronal and sagittal anatomic correlations will become of great importance.

REFERENCES

1. Bassano DA, Chamberlain CC, Mozley JM, Kieffer SA: Physical, performance, and dosimetric characteristics of the Deltascan 50 whole body/brain scanner. Radiology 123:455–462, 1977
2. Eyler WR, Figley MM: Computed tomography display. Radiology 119:487, 1976
3. Figley MM, Eyler WR: Orientation of CT images. Am J Roentgenol 127:199, 1976
4. Goss CM (ed): Gray's Anatomy, 29th American Edition. Philadelphia, Lea & Febiger, 1973
5. McCullough EC, Payne JT, Baker HL, Jr, et al: Performance evaluation and quality assurance of computed tomography scanners. Radiology 120: 173–188, 1976

An Atlas of Cross-sectional Anatomy

1
Skull and Brain
STEPHEN A. KIEFFER

In practice, computed "transaxial" tomography of the skull and brain is carried out in a plane which is not truly transaxial, *i.e.*, not truly perpendicular to the vertical axis of the body. In order to obtain a complete examination of the brain and its surrounding bony investment with the least possible number of sections (thus reducing radiation dose and examination time), the plane of section for computed tomography should roughly parallel the longest anteroposterior diameter of the skull. By generally accepted convention, this plane lies at an angle of approximately 20 degrees to the orbitomeatal line (from the external canthus of the eye to the center of the external auditory meatus) or 30 degrees to the anthropologic baseline (from the inferior rim of the anterior margin of the orbit to the superior margin of the external auditory meatus). The computed tomographic images of the cadaver skull for this atlas were obtained in this modified transaxial plane, and metallic markers were then inserted into the bone to assure symmetry and uniformity of thickness without rotation or tilt. Using the metallic markers as guides, the head was sectioned parallel to this plane at levels identical to those of the computed tomographic images. Each section displayed in the color photographs of the gross anatomy and in the radiographs is 13 mm thick, corresponding to the thickness of tissue represented in the computed tomographic image.

In general, the gross anatomic photographs display the inferior aspect of each section. However, when pertinent anatomy was better displayed on the superior aspect, that surface was selected for photography (Levels 1, 3, and 6).

Because the computed tomographic image integrates all the structures lying within its thickness, a structure which lies only partially within the thickness of a given section may be obscured. This "partial-volume effect" is particularly evident when a relatively thin portion of a dense structure overlies a relatively thick portion of a lucent structure; an example is seen in Level 6 where the corpus callosum is obscured on the computed tomographic image by the underlying lateral ventricles.

The width of the window (visible range of x-ray attenuation coefficients) for the computed tomographic images in Levels 3–10 was 120–140 Hounsfield units, with a center setting of 25–35 Hounsfield units. These correspond closely to the settings used in clinical practice for computed tomography of the brain. However, the window setting for the computed tomographic images in Levels 1 and 2 was approximately 500 units, with a center of 80–90 units. The wider window and higher center are necessary to visualize bony detail at these levels, but the reader will note that the contrast and detail in brain tissue are minimal in these images. The diameter of the scanning circle for all computed tomographic studies of the skull and brain was 29 cm.

Artifacts related to the anatomic preparation explain some apparent disparities between the computed tomographic images (obtained prior to slicing the cadaver) and the radiographic and gross anatomic images. Thus, clotted blood in the larger blood vessels (e.g., the dural venous sinuses) appears dense (white) on the computed tomographic images; after sectioning and prior to radiography or photography, these clots were removed and the vessels filled with air so that they appear lucent (black) on the radiographs and clear on the anatomic photographs. Similarly, the ventricles are filled with cerebrospinal fluid on the computed tomographic images but were drained of fluid during sectioning and thus appear collapsed on the radiographs and anatomic photographs.

Following intravenous bolus injection of contrast medium in the living patient, the major blood vessels of the brain can frequently be identified on computed tomography. Dural structures (e.g., the falx and the tentorium) are opacified, and the differential contrast between white and gray matter is enhanced. It is, therefore, not surprising that contrast enhancement has become a valuable and frequently utilized adjunct to the clinical practice of computed tomography of the skull and brain. Intravenous injection of contrast medium was, of course, not possible in the cadaver, but several representative contrast-enhanced computed tomographic images from living patients are presented in the section Normal *In Vivo* Computed Tomographic Studies at the conclusion of this chapter.

With the recent introduction of metrizamide (Amipaque) as a water-soluble contrast medium for myelography, the intracranial cisterns and sulci can be opacified and identified on both conventional tomograms and computed tomograms. Representative images of the skull and brain with the cisterns, sulci, and ventricles opacified by metrizamide are included in the section Normal *In Vivo* Computed Tomographic Studies.

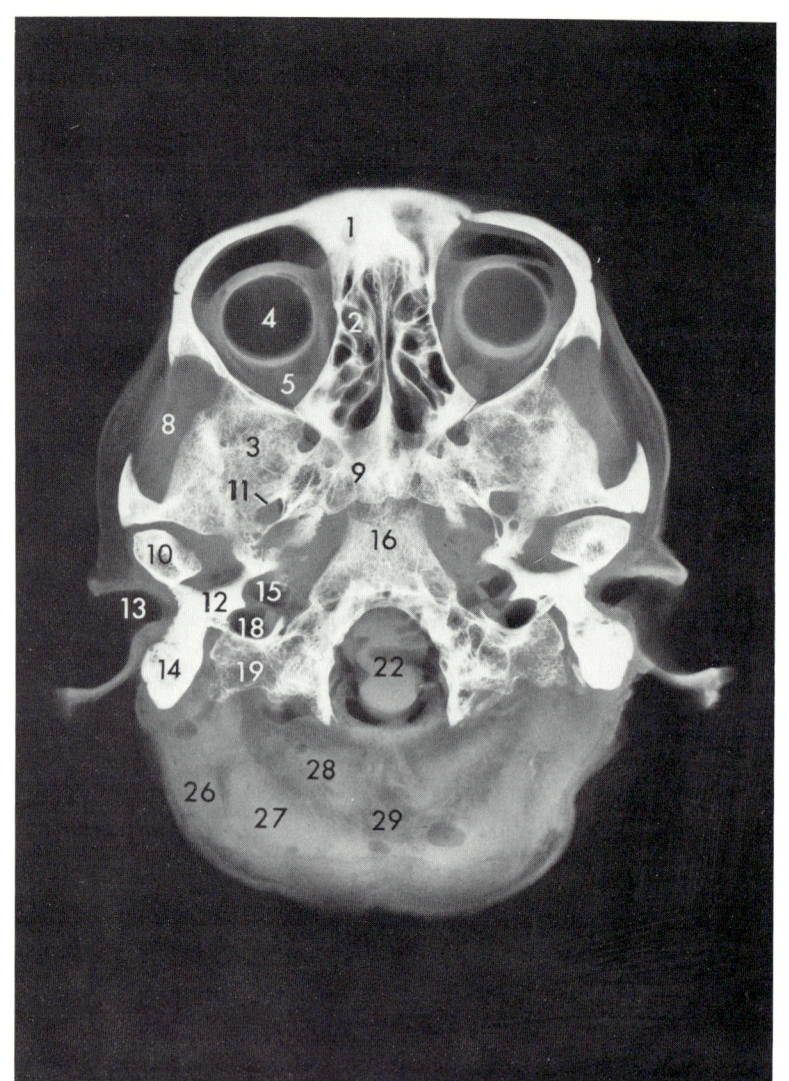
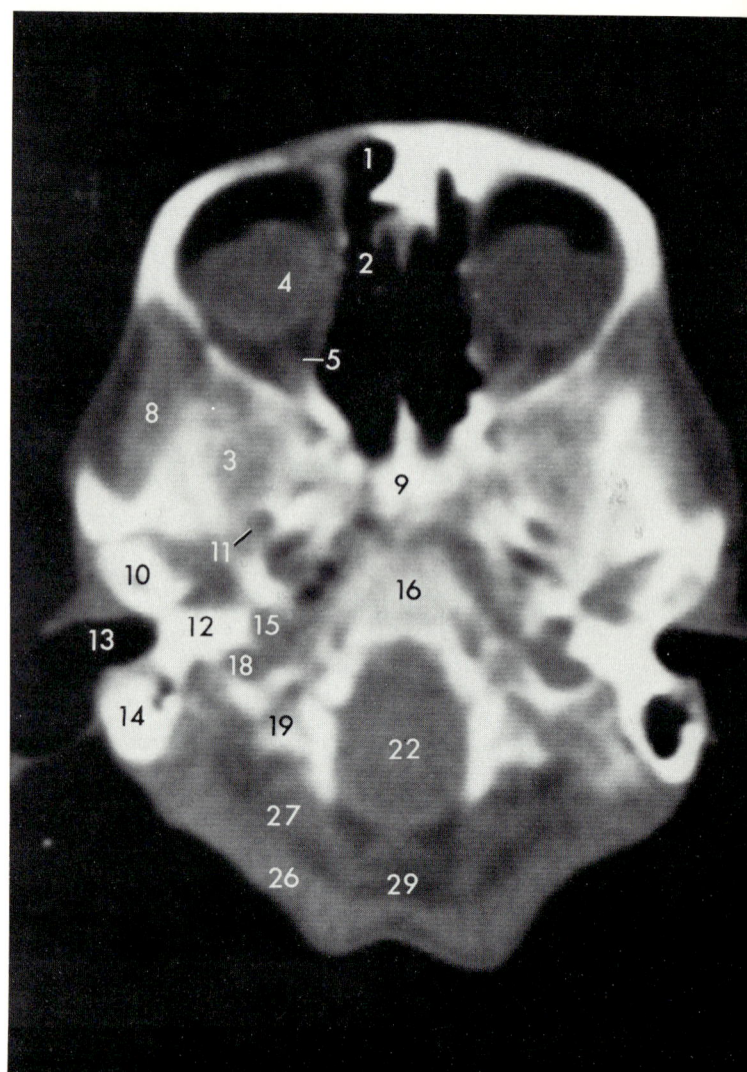
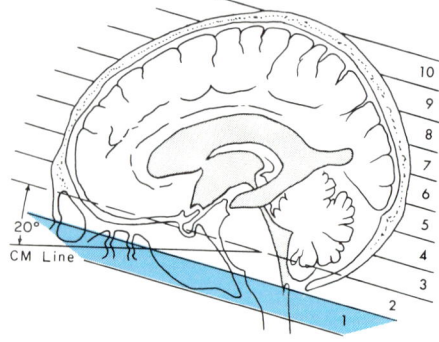

SKULL AND BRAIN

Level 1
(Superior aspect)

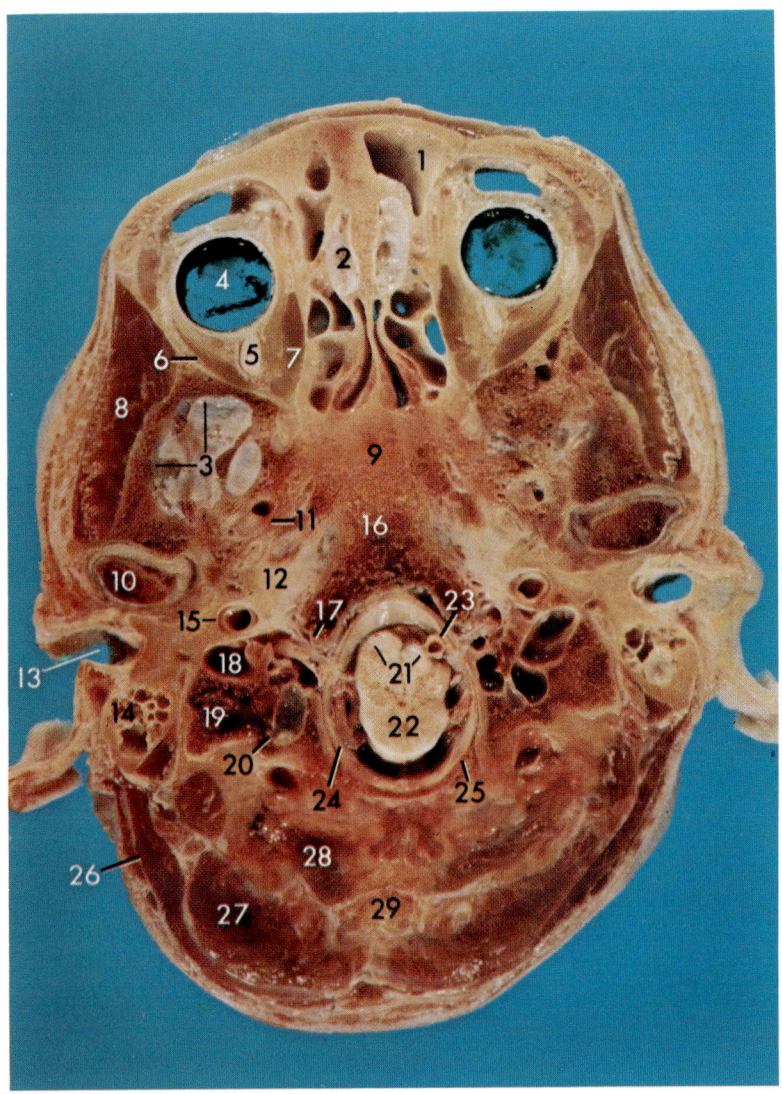

1. Frontal sinus
2. Ethmoid sinus
3. Greater wing of sphenoid
4. Globe
5. Optic nerve (II)
6. Lateral rectus muscle
7. Medial rectus muscle
8. Temporalis muscle
9. Body of sphenoid
10. Mandibular condyle
11. Foramen ovale (mandibular nerve [V₃])
12. Petrous portion of temporal bone
13. External auditory canal
14. Mastoid portion of temporal bone
15. Carotid canal (internal carotid artery)
16. Clivus (basisphenoid and basiocciput)
17. Hypoglossal canal (hypoglossal nerve [XII])
18. Jugular foramen (internal jugular vein)
19. Jugular process of occipital bone
20. Condylar (emissary) vein
21. Pyramids of medulla
22. Medulla oblongata
23. Vertebral artery
24. Posterior inferior cerebellar artery (caudal loop)
25. Dura mater
26. Splenius capitis muscle
27. Semispinalis capitis muscle
28. Rectus capitis posterior muscle
29. Ligamentum nuchae and surrounding fat

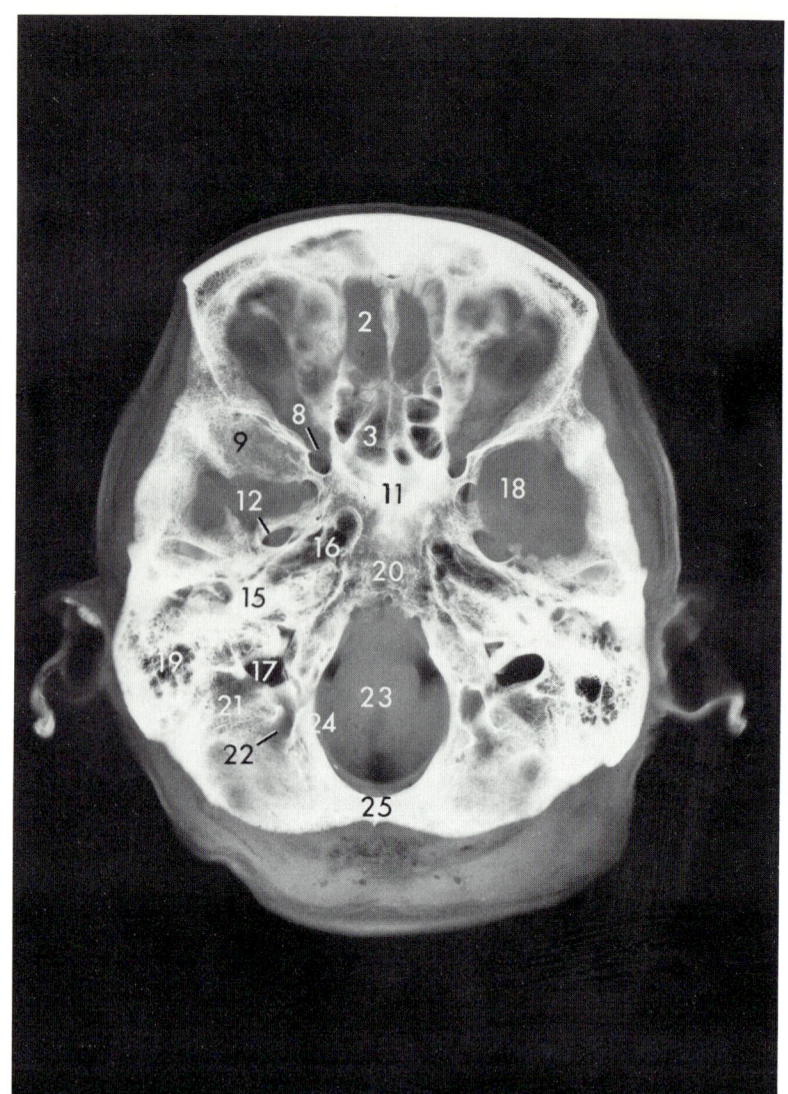
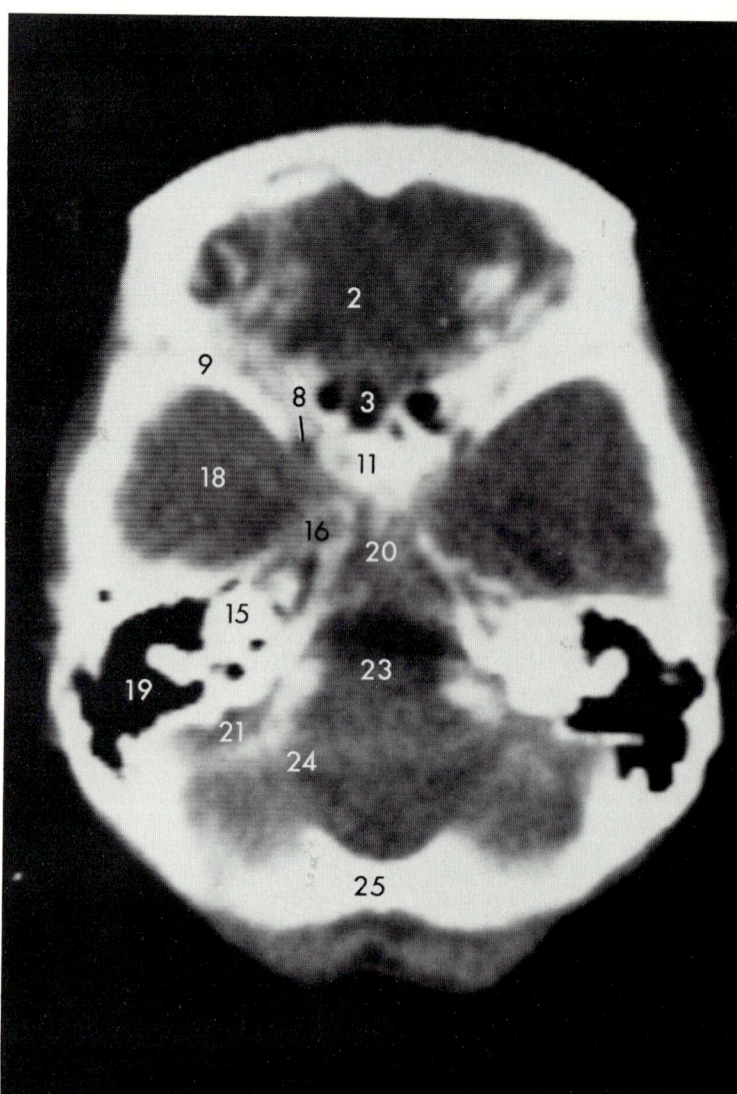
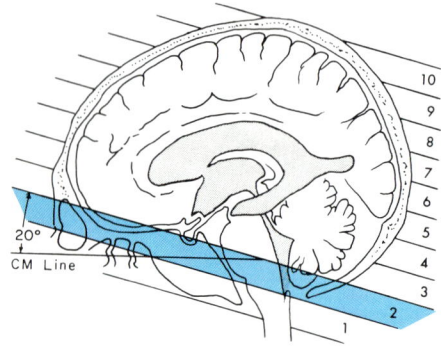

SKULL AND BRAIN

Level 2
(Inferior aspect)

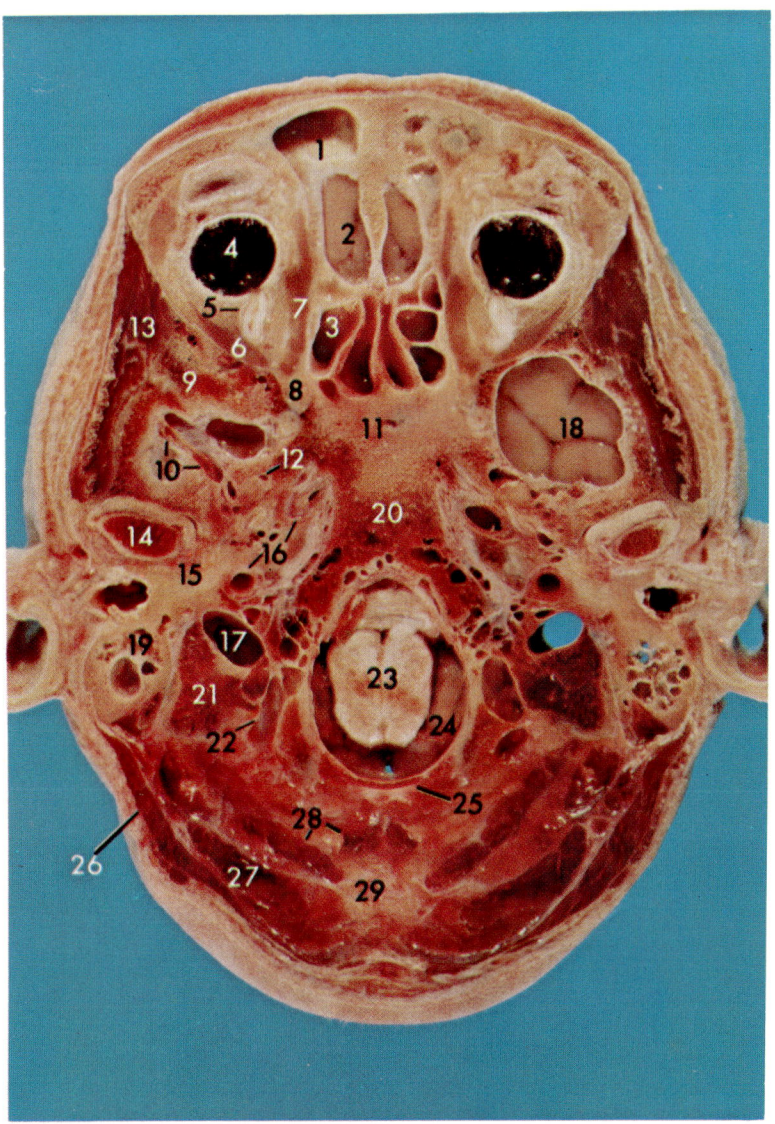

1. Frontal sinus
2. Frontal lobe (gyrus rectus)
3. Sphenoid sinus
4. Globe
5. Optic nerve (II)
6. Lateral rectus muscle
7. Medial rectus muscle
8. Superior orbital fissure
9. Greater wing of sphenoid
10. Middle meningeal artery
11. Body of sphenoid
12. Foramen ovale (mandibular nerve [V₁])
13. Temporalis muscle
14. Mandibular condyle
15. Petrous portion of temporal bone
16. Carotid canal (internal carotid artery)
17. Jugular foramen (internal jugular vein)
18. Temporal lobe
19. Mastoid portion of temporal bone
20. Clivus (basisphenoid)
21. Jugular process of occipital bone
22. Condyloid (emissary) vein
23. Medulla oblongata
24. Cerebellar tonsil
25. Posterior lip of foramen magnum (occipital bone)
26. Splenius capitis muscle
27. Semispinalis capitis muscle
28. Rectus capitis posterior muscle
29. Ligamentum nuchae and surrounding fat

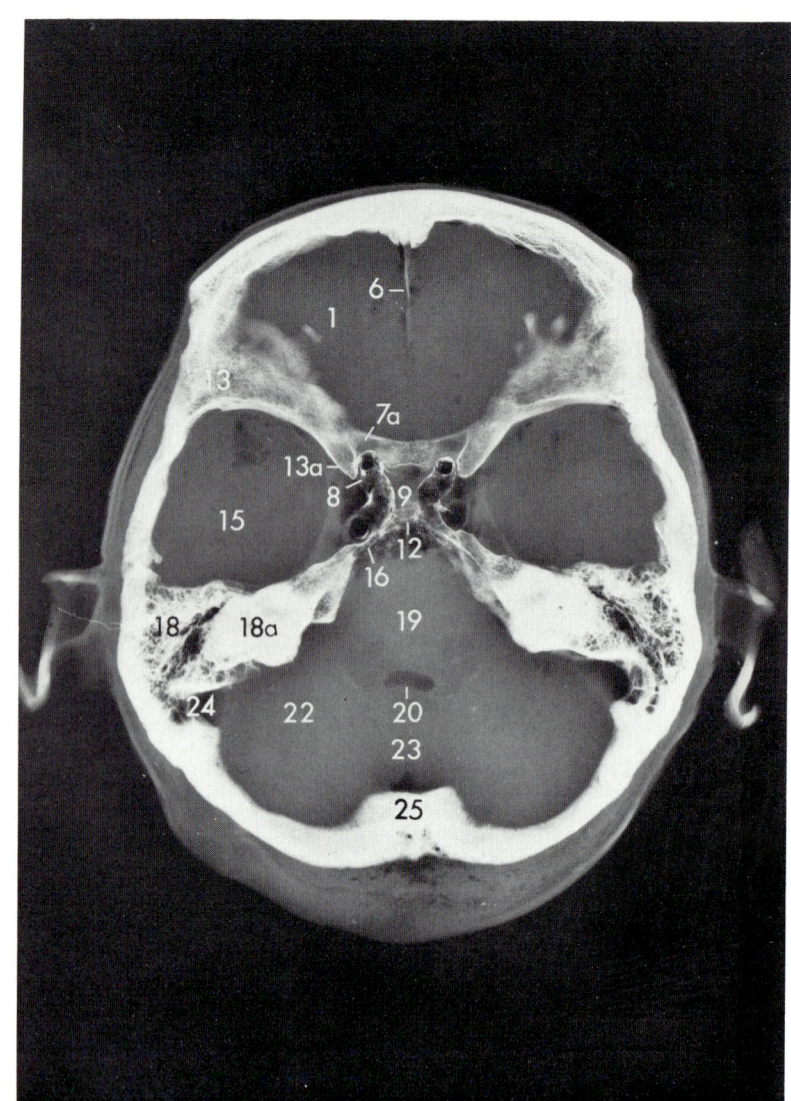
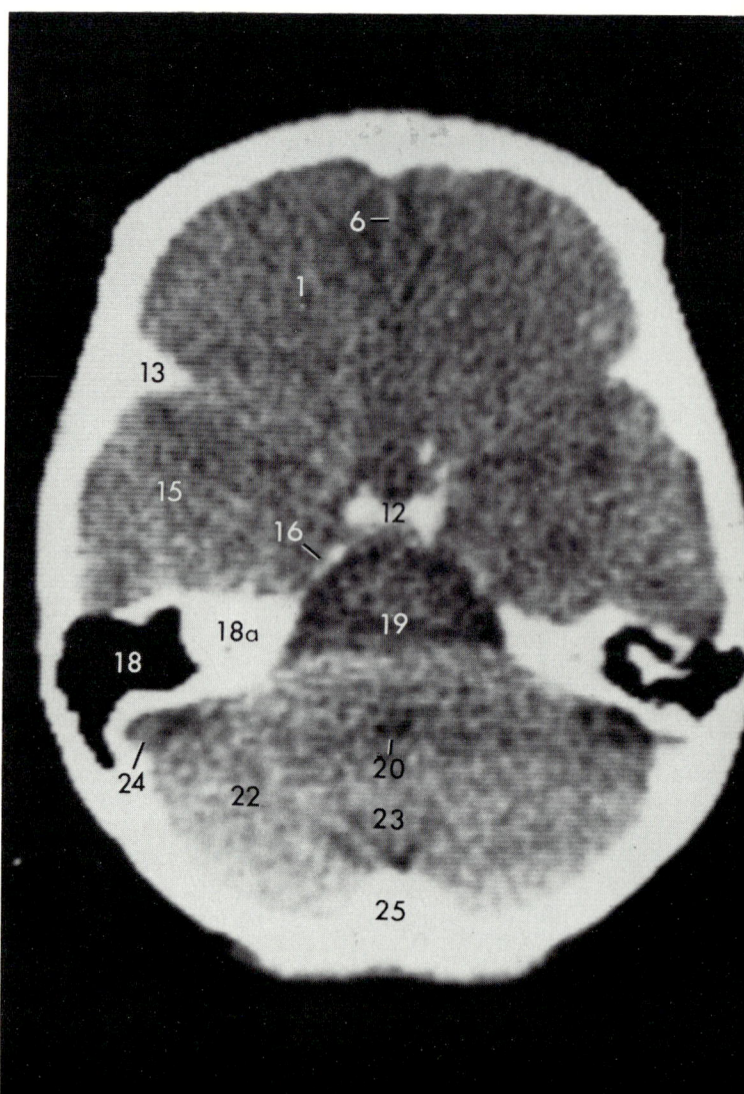
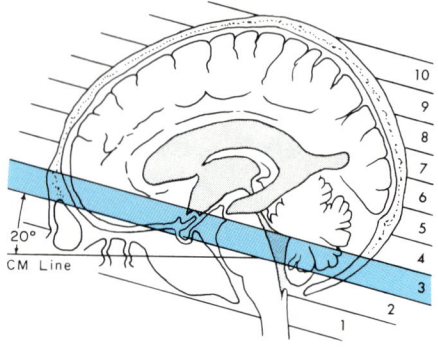

SKULL AND BRAIN

Level 3
(Superior aspect)

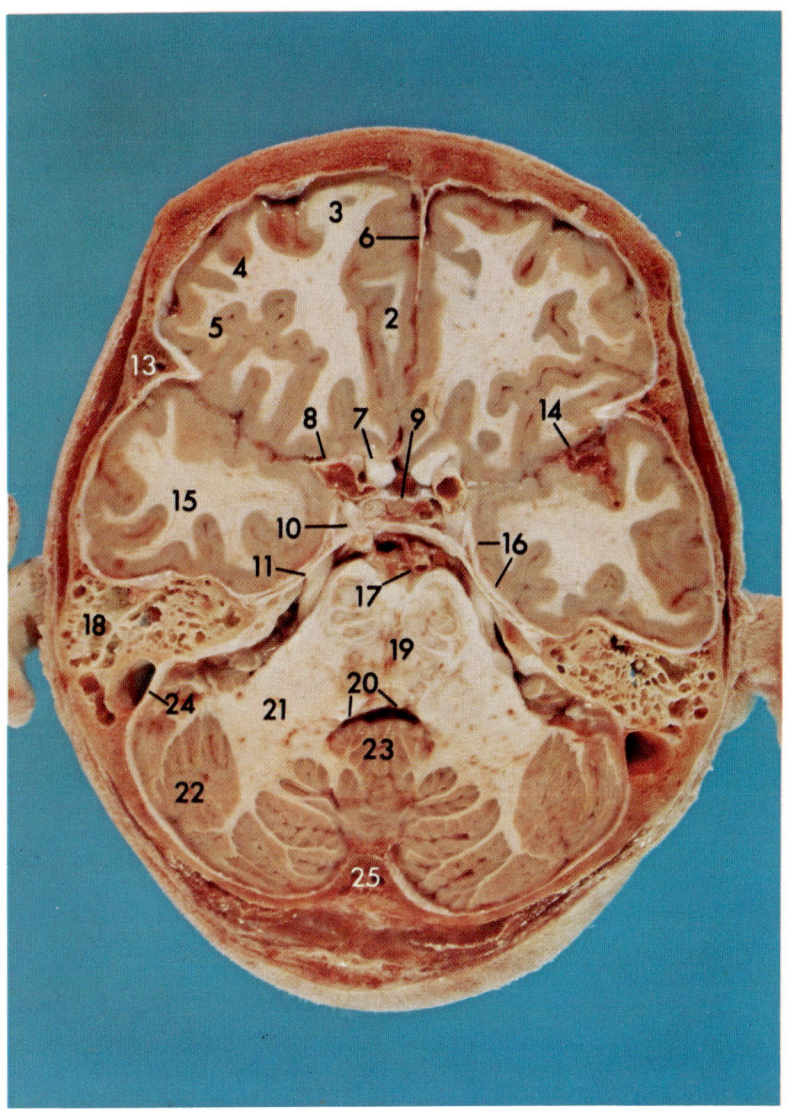

1. Frontal lobe
2. Gyrus rectus
3. Superior frontal gyrus
4. Middle frontal gyrus
5. Inferior frontal gyrus
6. Falx cerebri
7. Optic nerve (II)
7a. Optic canal
8. Internal carotid artery (supraclinoid portion)
9. Infundibulum of pituitary gland
10. Oculomotor nerve (III)
11. Trigeminal nerve (V)
12. Dorsum sellae
13. Greater wing of sphenoid
13a. Anterior clinoid process
14. Middle cerebral artery
15. Temporal lobe
16. Tentorium cerebelli (petroclinoid ligament)
17. Basilar artery
18. Mastoid portion of temporal bone
18a. Petrous portion of temporal bone
19. Pons
20. Fourth ventricle
21. Brachium pontis (middle cerebellar peduncle)
22. Cerebellar hemisphere
23. Cerebellar vermis
24. Sigmoid sinus
25. Internal occipital crest

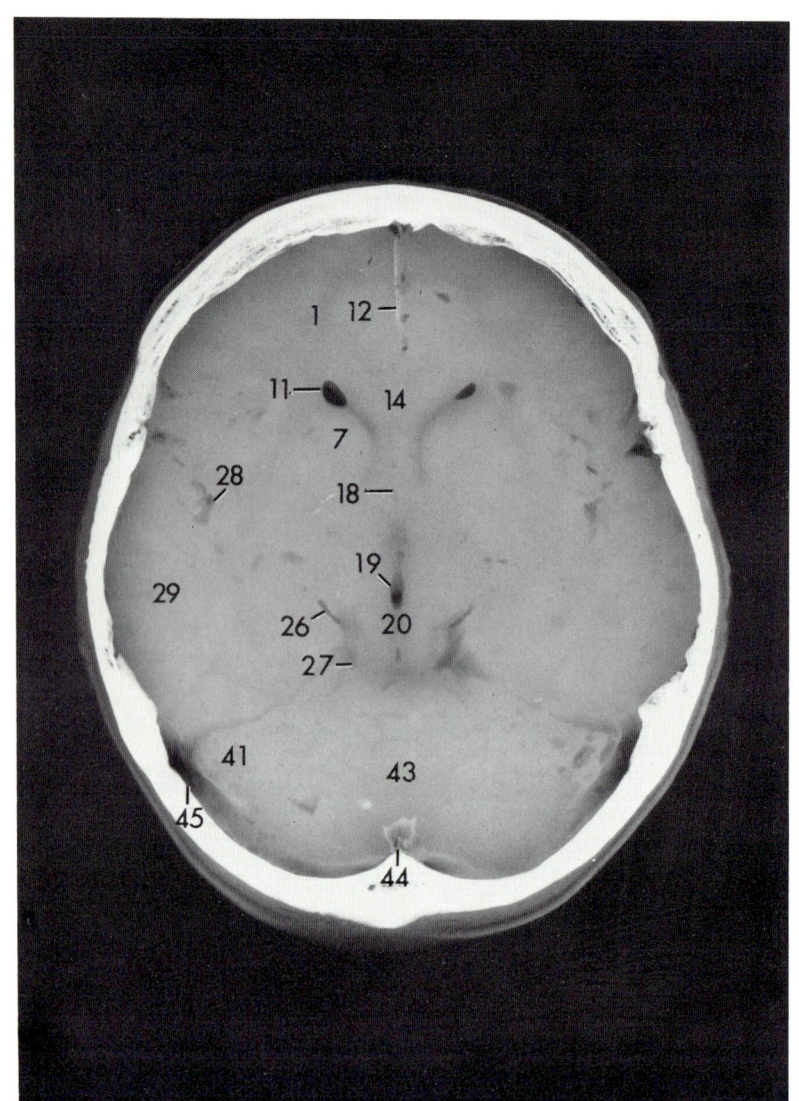
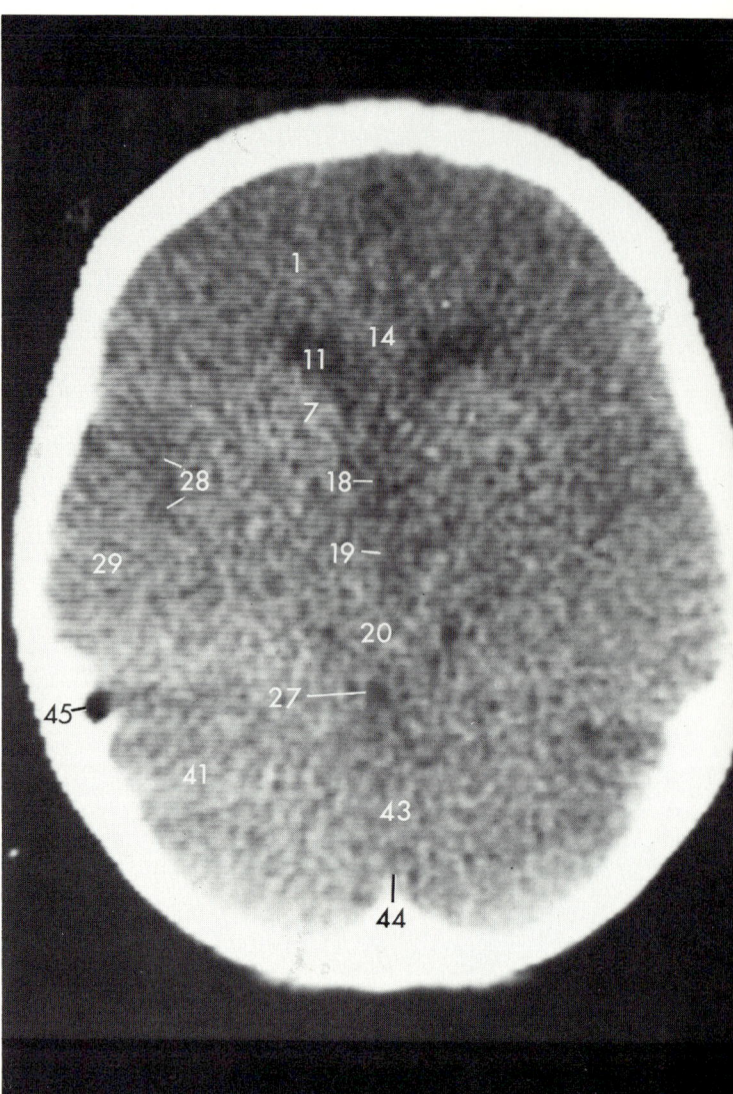
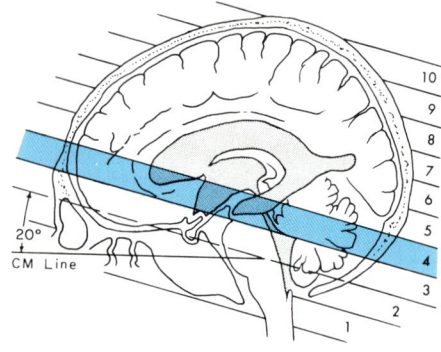

SKULL AND BRAIN

**Level 4
(Inferior aspect)**

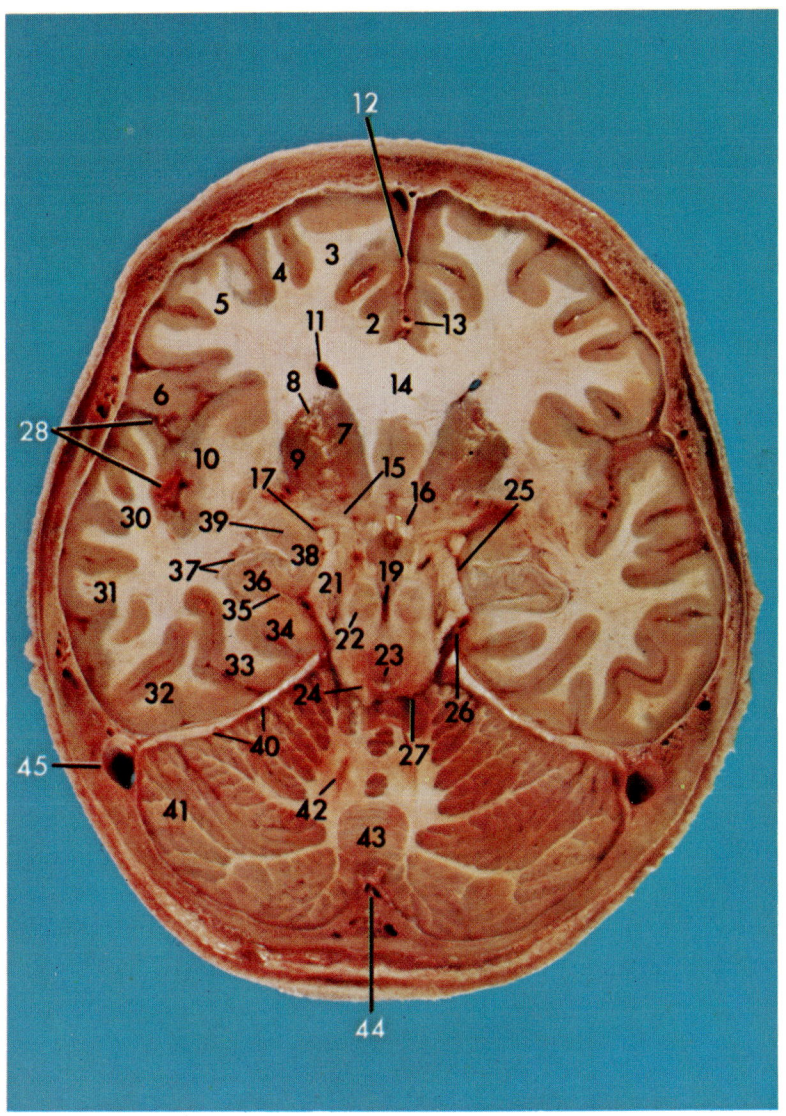

1. Frontal lobe
   2. Cingulate gyrus
   3. Superior frontal gyrus
   4. Middle frontal gyrus
   5. Inferior frontal gyrus
   6. Precentral gyrus
   7. Head of caudate nucleus
   8. Anterior limb of internal capsule
   9. Putamen
   10. Insula
   11. Frontal horn of lateral ventricle
12. Falx cerebri
13. Anterior cerebral artery
14. Genu of corpus callosum
15. Anterior commissure
16. Column of fornix
17. Optic tract
18. Third ventricle
19. Interpeduncular cistern
20. Midbrain
   21. Cerebral peduncle
   22. Red nucleus
   23. Aqueduct of Sylvius
   24. Inferior colliculus
25. Crural cistern
26. Circummesencephalic (ambient) cistern (with posterior cerebral artery)
27. Quadrigeminal cistern
28. Sylvian fissure (with middle cerebral artery branches)
29. Temporal lobe
   30. Superior temporal gyrus
   31. Middle temporal gyrus

Temporal lobe continued
   32. Inferior temporal gyrus
   33. Fusiform gyrus
   34. Parahippocampal gyrus
   35. Choroidal fissure
   36. Hippocampus
   37. Temporal horn of lateral ventricle (anterior tip)
   38. Uncus
   39. Amygdaloid nucleus
40. Tentorium cerebelli
41. Cerebellar hemisphere
42. Dentate nucleus
43. Cerebellar vermis
44. Occipital sinus
45. Sigmoid sinus

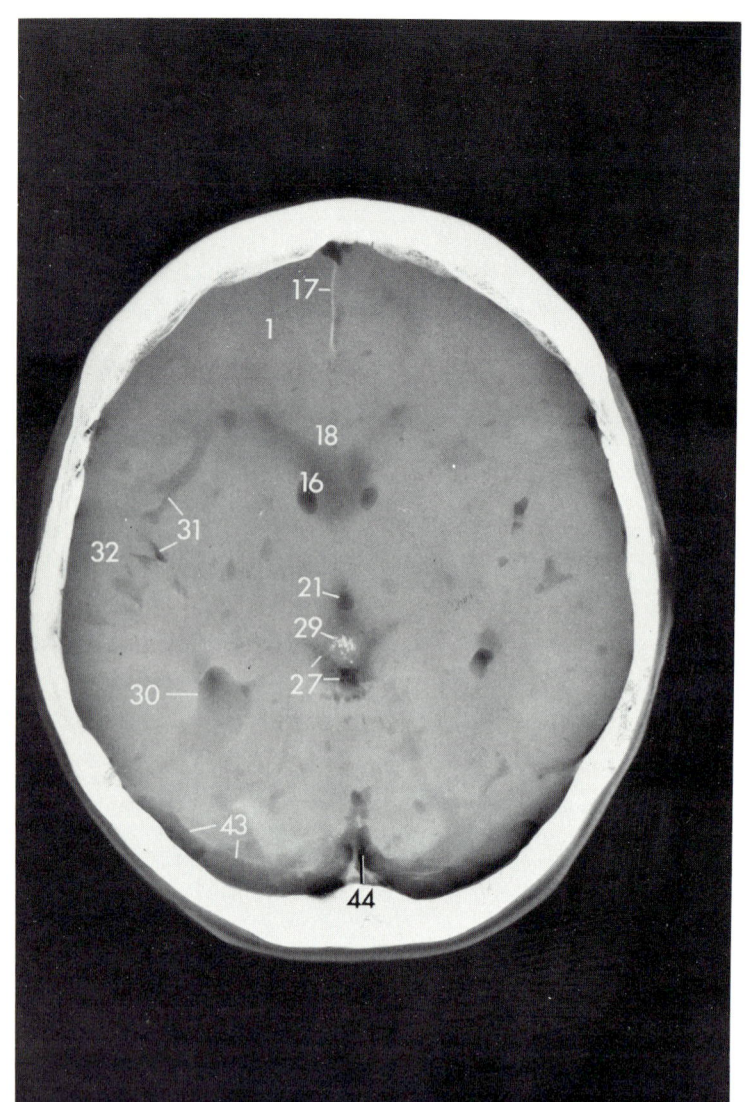
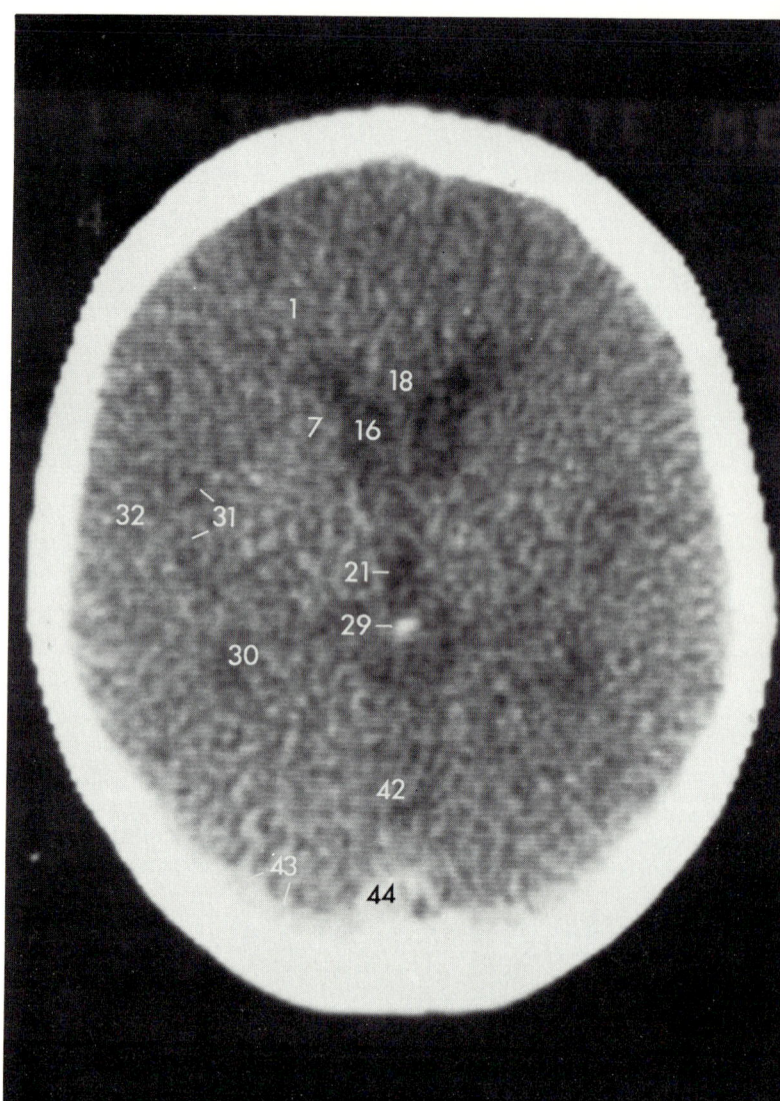
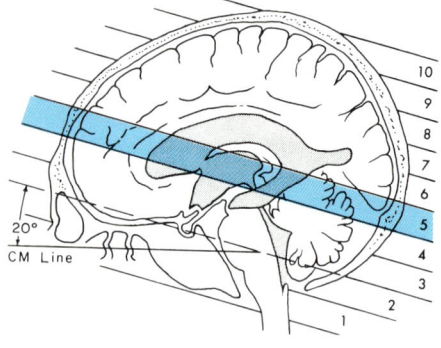

SKULL AND BRAIN

Level 5
(Inferior aspect)

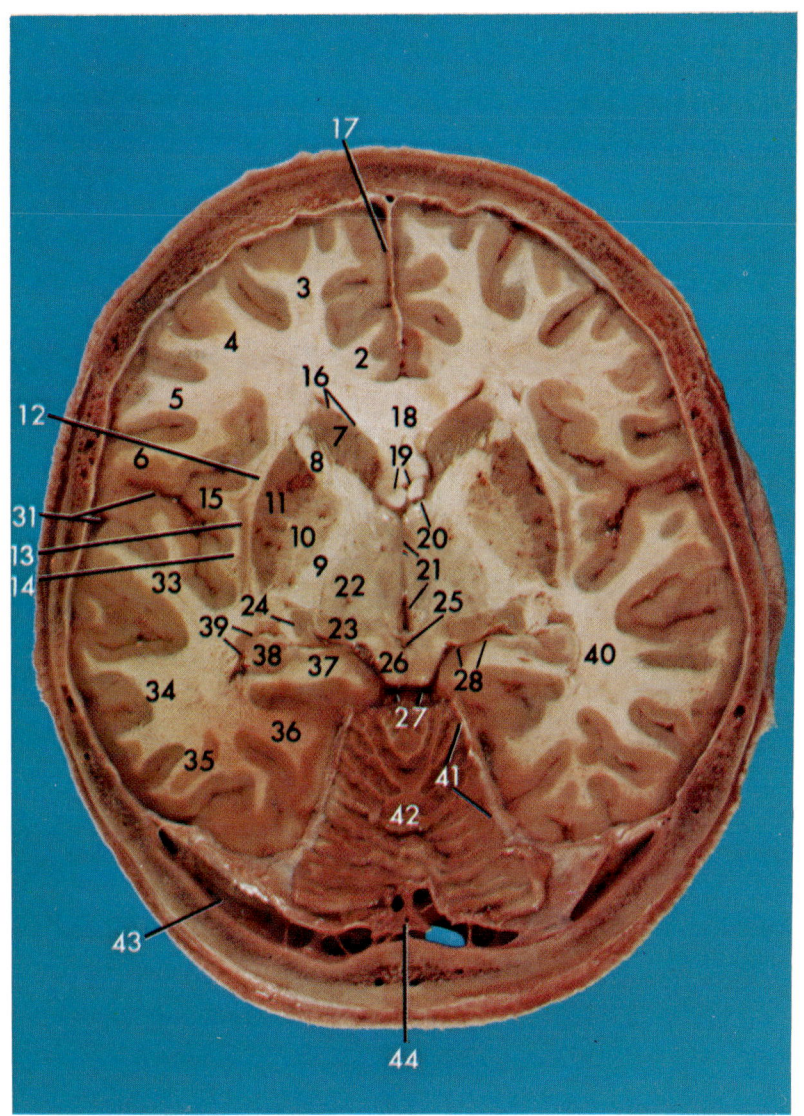

1. Frontal lobe
    2. Cingulate gyrus
    3. Superior frontal gyrus
    4. Middle frontal gyrus
    5. Inferior frontal gyrus
    6. Precentral gyrus
    7. Head of caudate nucleus
    8. Anterior limb of internal capsule
    9. Posterior limb of internal capsule
   10. Globus pallidus
   11. Putamen
   12. External capsule
   13. Claustrum
   14. Extreme capsule
   15. Insula
16. Frontal horn of lateral ventricle
17. Falx cerebri
18. Genu of corpus callosum
19. Columns of fornix
20. Foramen of Monro
21. Third ventricle
22. Thalamus
    23. Pulvinar
24. Lateral geniculate body
25. Aqueduct of Sylvius
26. Superior colliculus
27. Quadrigeminal cistern
28. Retropulvinar cistern (wing of ambient cistern)
29. Pineal gland (calcified)
30. Atrium of lateral ventricle
31. Sylvian fissure
32. Temporal lobe
    33. Superior temporal gyrus
    34. Middle temporal gyrus
    35. Inferior temporal gyrus
    36. Fusiform gyrus
    37. Parahippocampal gyrus
    38. Hippocampus
    39. Temporal horn of lateral ventricle
    40. Optic radiations
41. Tentorium cerebelli
42. Cerebellar vermis
43. Lateral sinus
44. Torcular Herophili

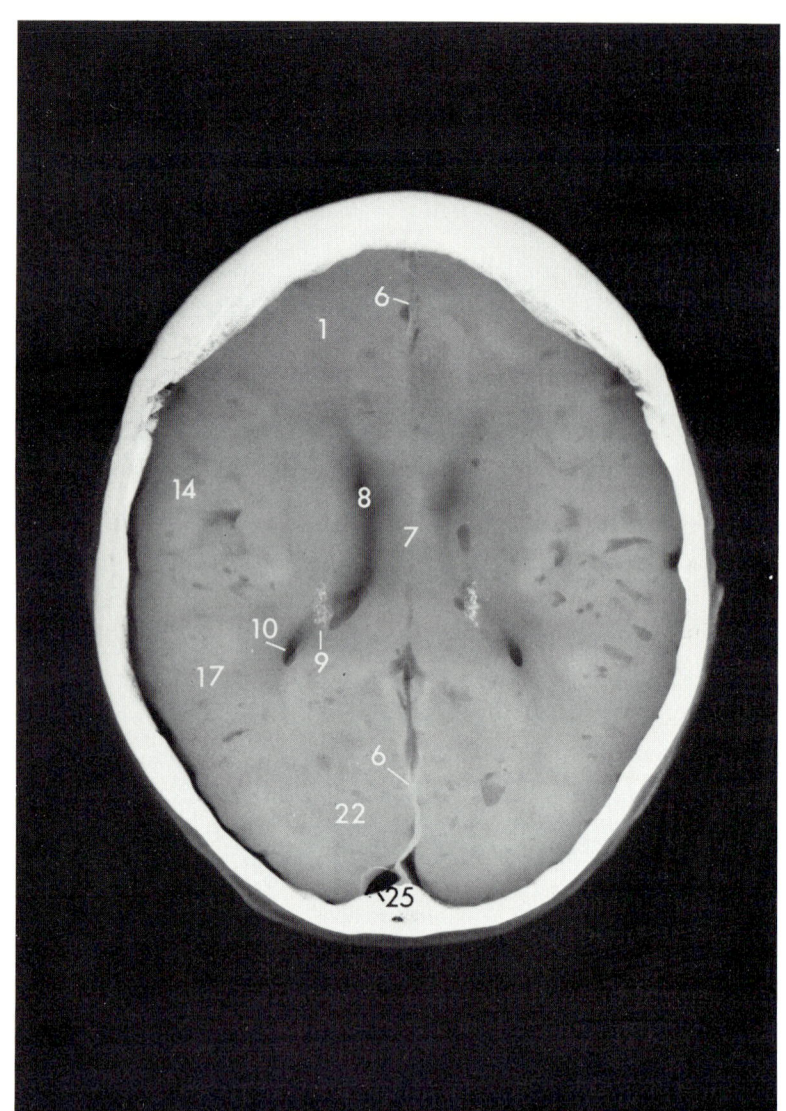
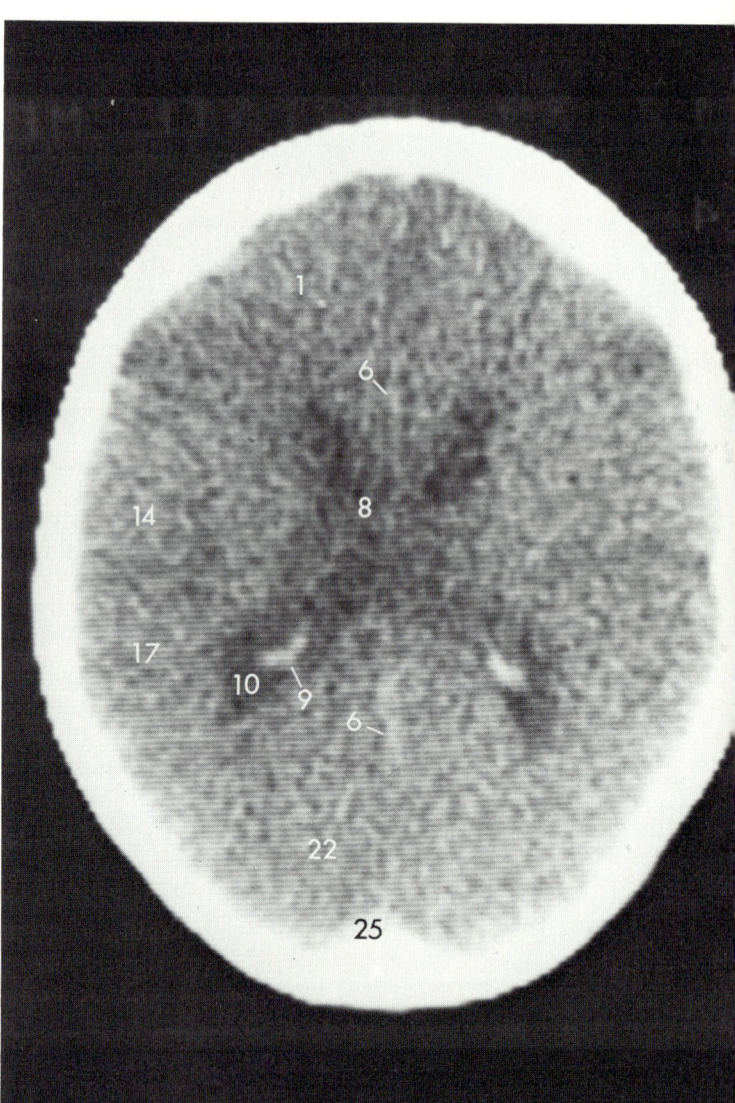
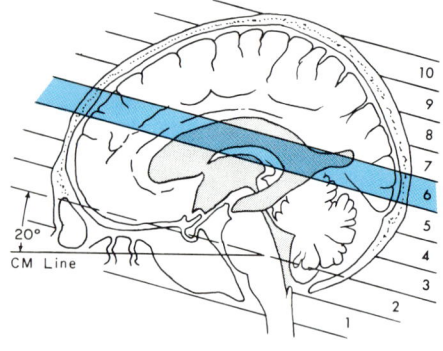

SKULL AND BRAIN

Level 6
(Superior aspect)

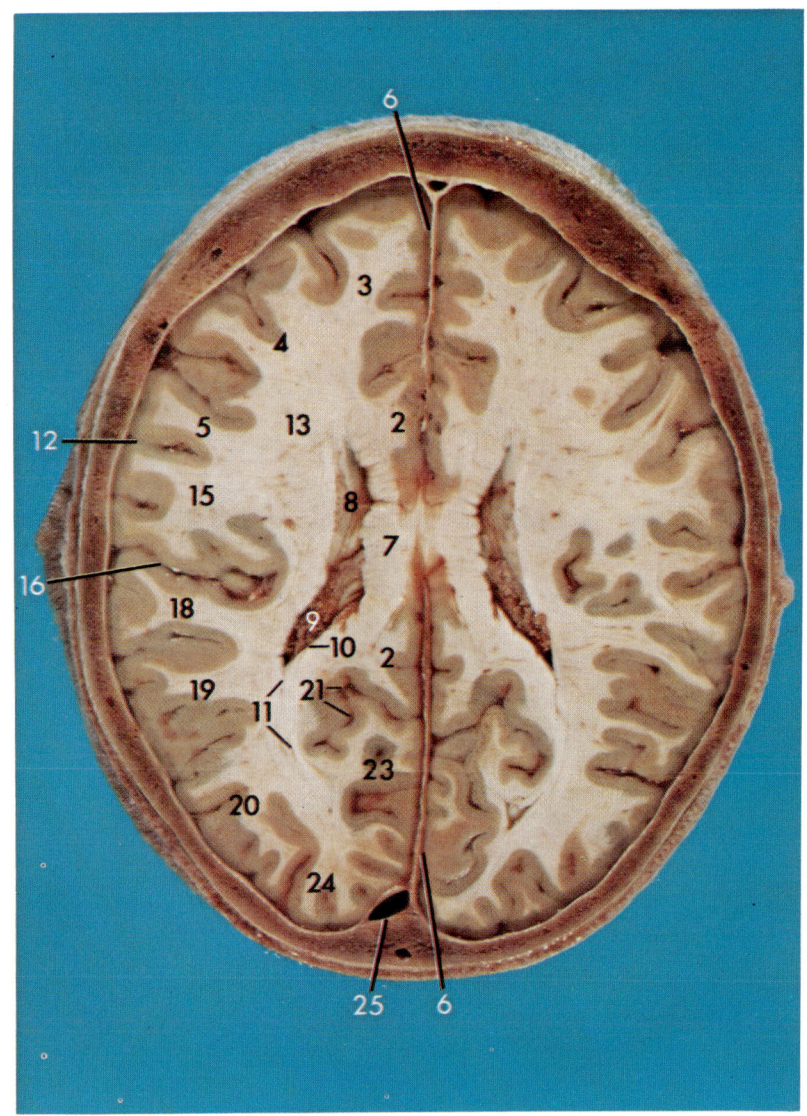

1. Frontal lobe
2. Cingulate gyrus
3. Superior frontal gyrus
4. Middle frontal gyrus
5. Precentral gyrus
6. Falx cerebri
7. Body of corpus callosum
8. Body of lateral ventricle
9. Glomus of choroid plexus of lateral ventricle
10. Atrium of lateral ventricle
11. Occipital horn of lateral ventricle
12. Central (Rolandic) fissure
13. Centrum semiovale
14. Parietal lobe
15. Postcentral gyrus
16. Sylvian fissure
17. Temporal lobe
18. Superior temporal gyrus
19. Middle temporal gyrus

Temporal lobe continued
20. Inferior temporal gyrus
21. Parieto-occipital fissure
22. Occipital lobe
23. Cuneus
24. Lateral occipital gyrus
25. Superior sagittal sinus

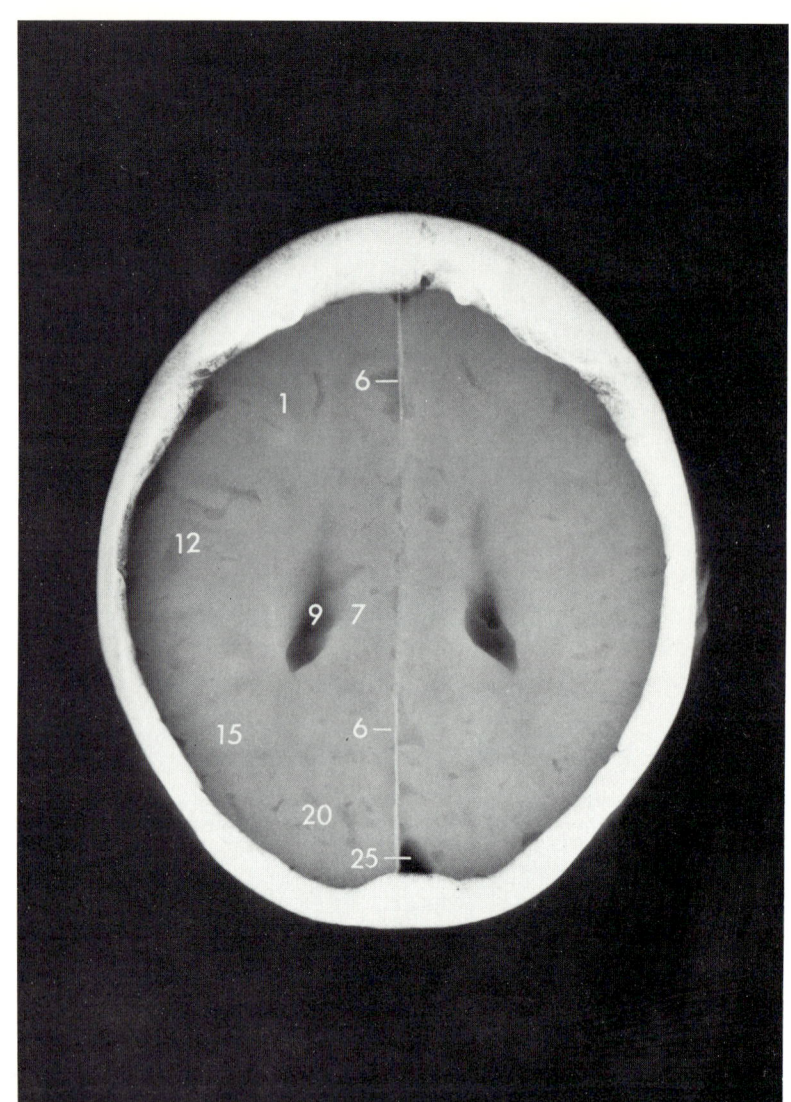
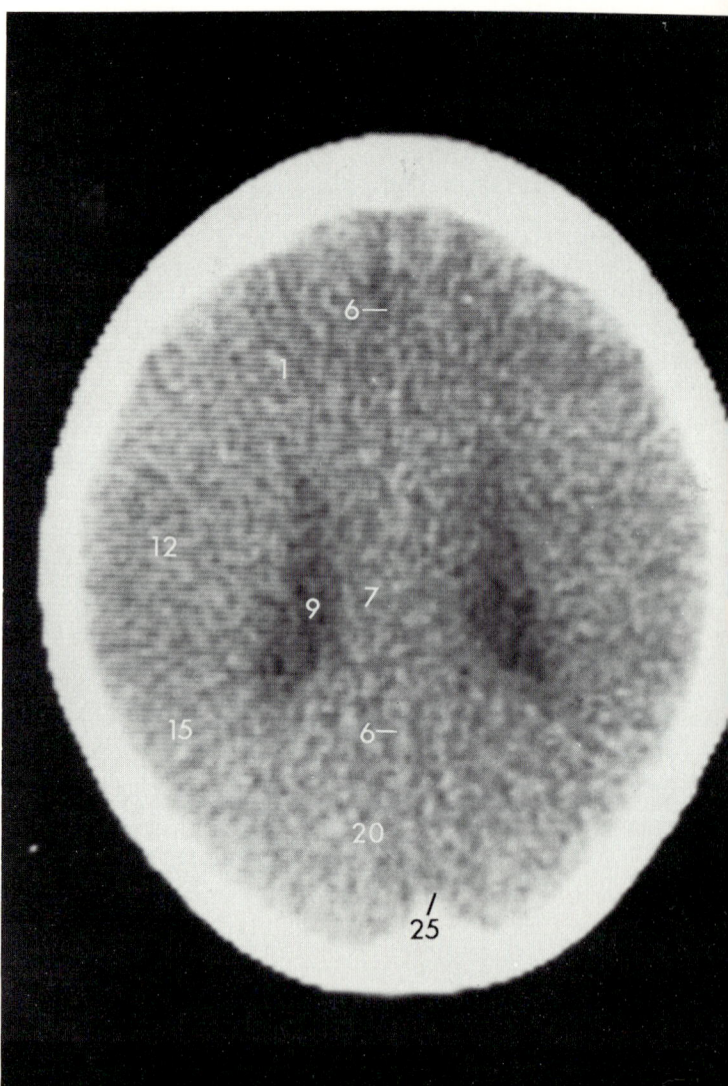
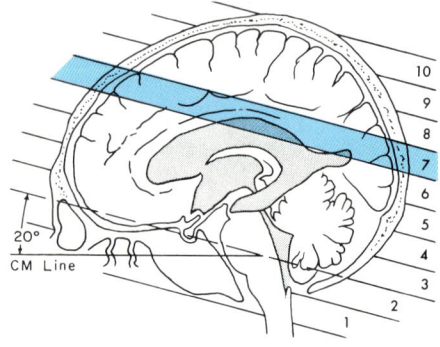

SKULL AND BRAIN

**Level 7
(Inferior aspect)**

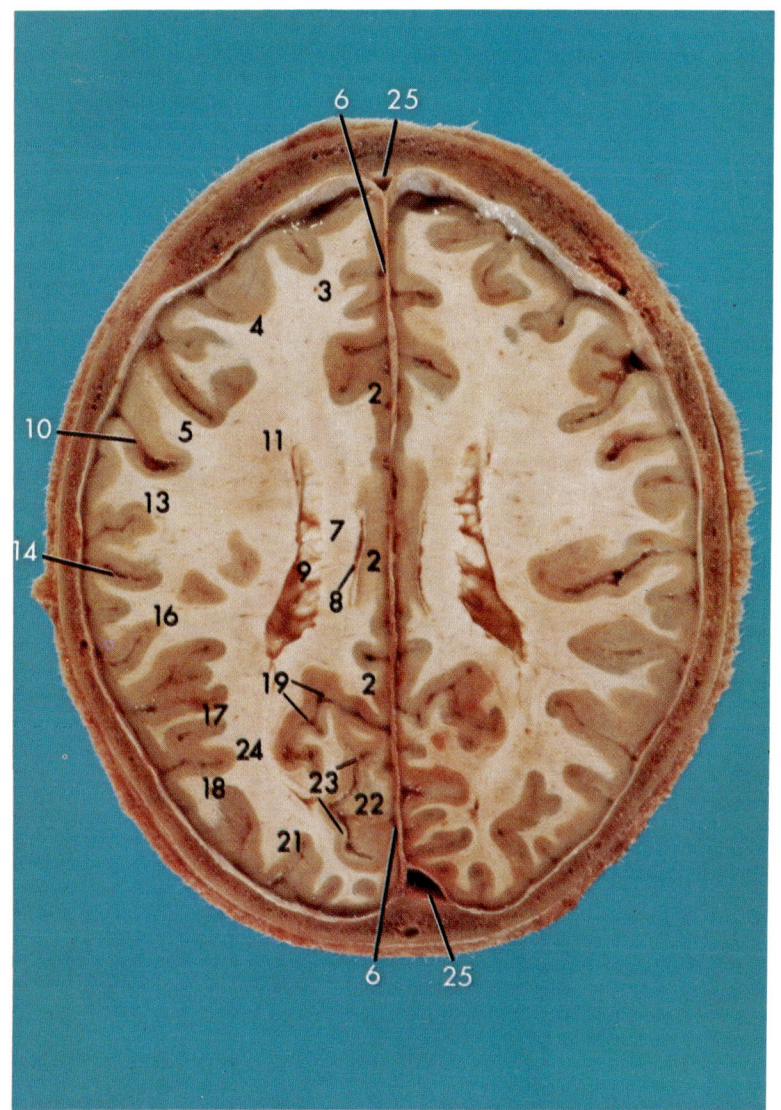

1. Frontal lobe
2. Cingulate gyrus
3. Superior frontal gyrus
4. Middle frontal gyrus
5. Precentral gyrus
6. Falx cerebri
7. Body of corpus callosum
8. Callosal sulcus
9. Body of lateral ventricle
10. Central (Rolandic) fissure
11. Centrum semiovale (corona radiata)
12. Parietal lobe
13. Postcentral gyrus
14. Sylvian fissure
15. Temporal lobe
16. Superior temporal gyrus
17. Middle temporal gyrus
18. Inferior temporal gyrus
19. Parieto-occipital fissure
20. Occipital lobe
21. Lateral occipital gyri
22. Cuneus
23. Calcarine fissure
24. Optic radiations
25. Superior sagittal sinus

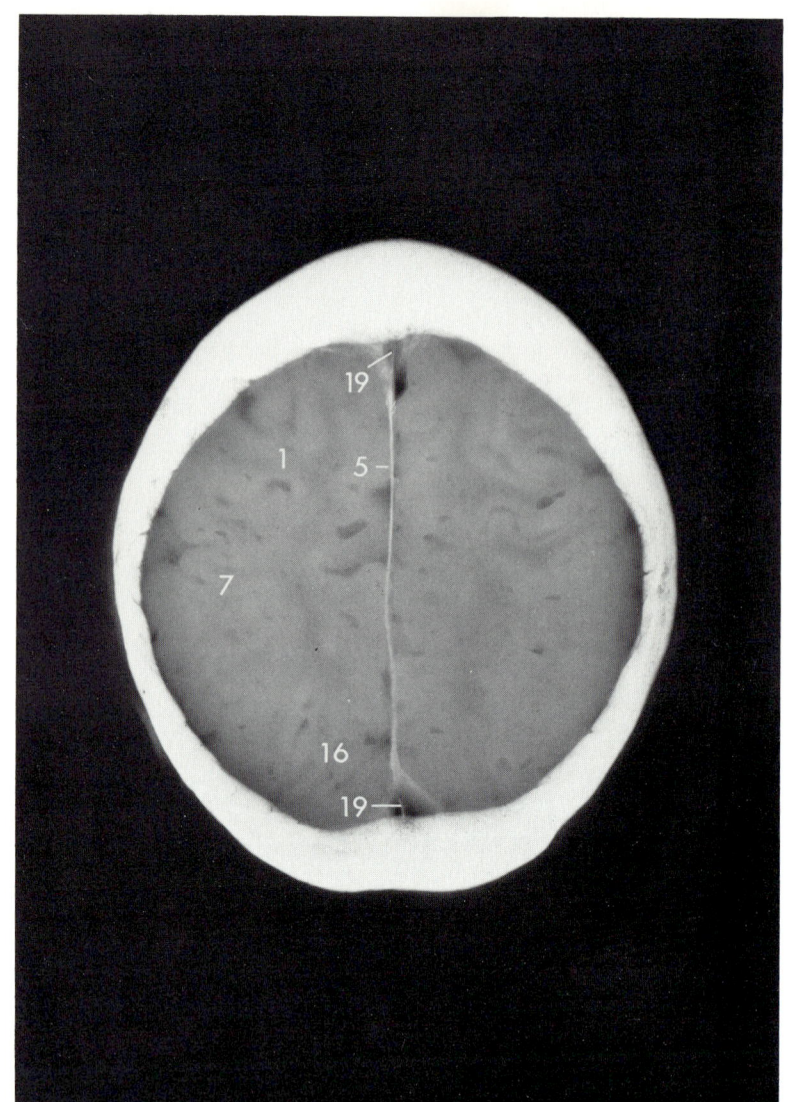
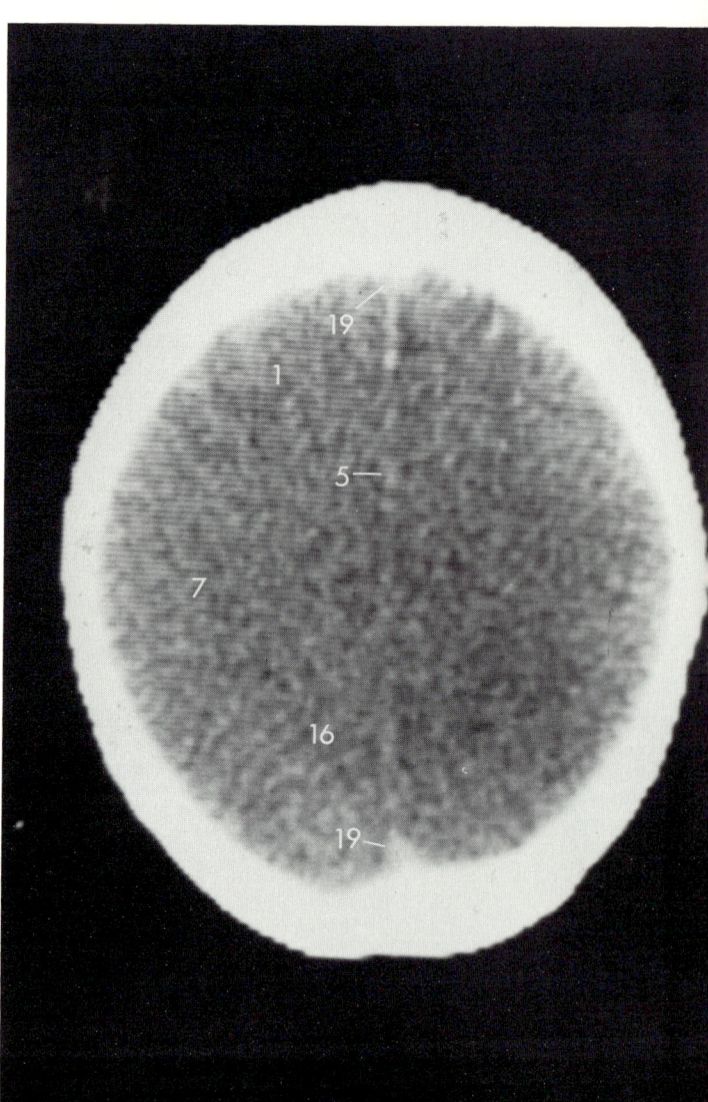
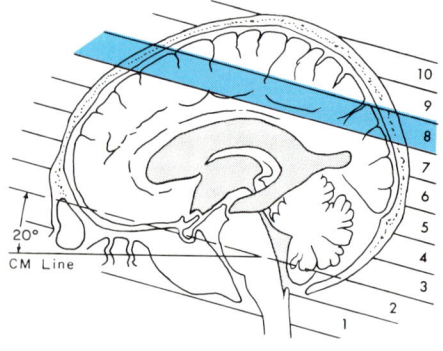

SKULL AND BRAIN

**Level 8
(Inferior aspect)**

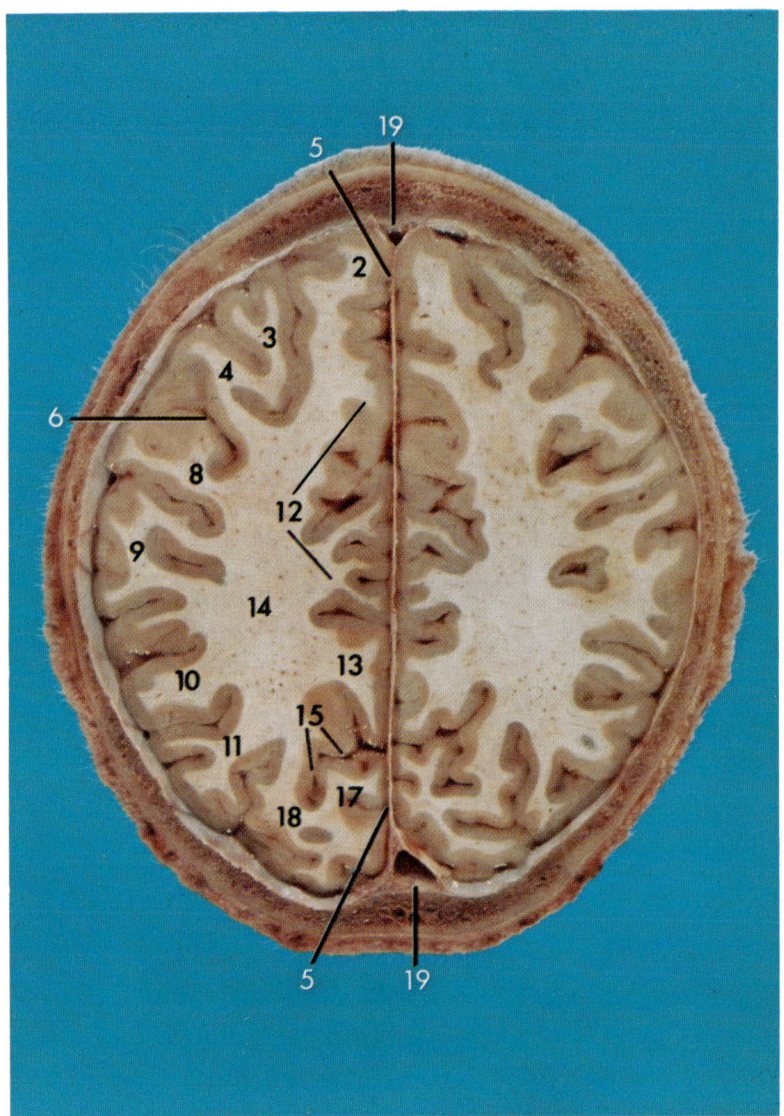

1. Frontal lobe
   2. Superior frontal gyrus
   3. Middle frontal gyrus
   4. Precentral gyrus
5. Falx cerebri
6. Central (Rolandic) fissure
7. Parietal lobe

Parietal lobe continued
   8. Postcentral gyrus
   9. Supramarginal gyrus
   10. Angular gyrus
   11. Inferior parietal lobule
   12. Paracentral lobule
   13. Precuneus

14. Centrum semiovale
15. Parieto-occipital fissure
16. Occipital lobe
   17. Cuneus
   18. Superior occipital gyri
19. Superior sagittal sinus

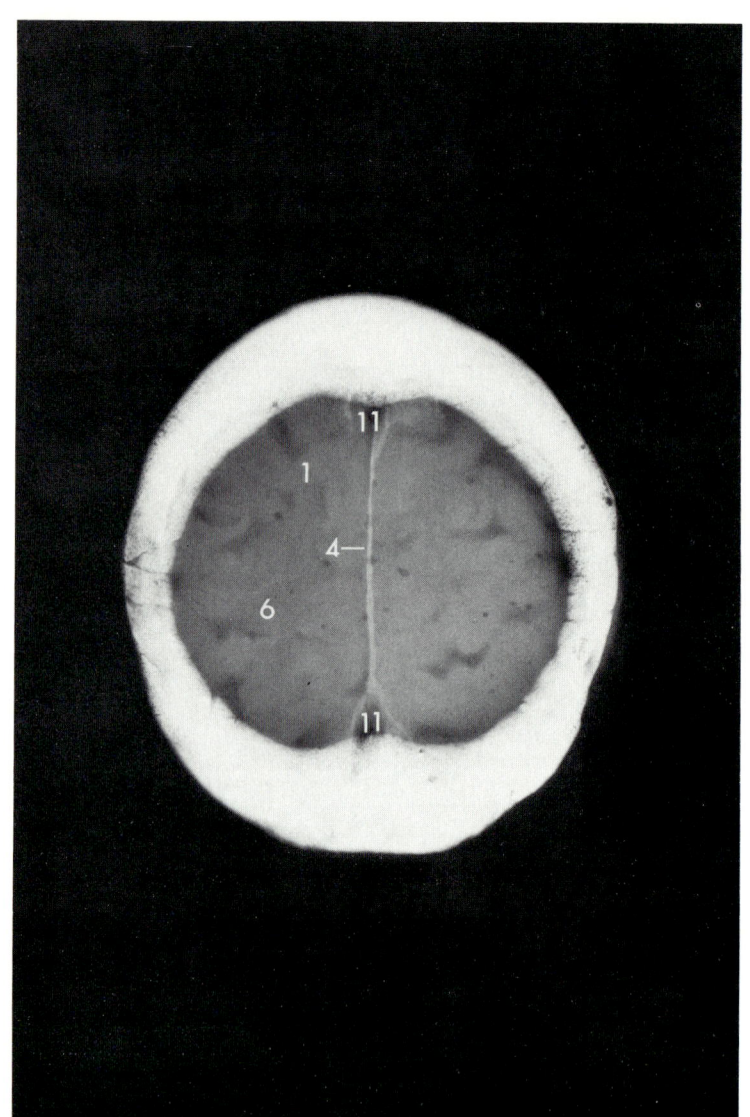
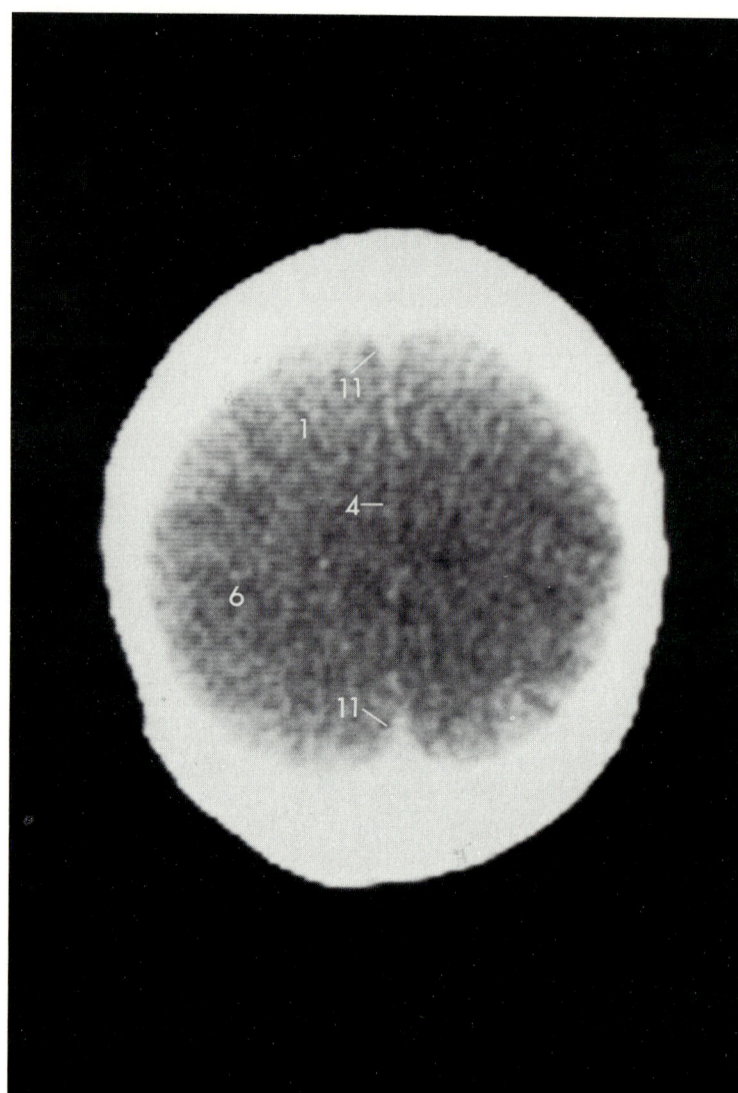
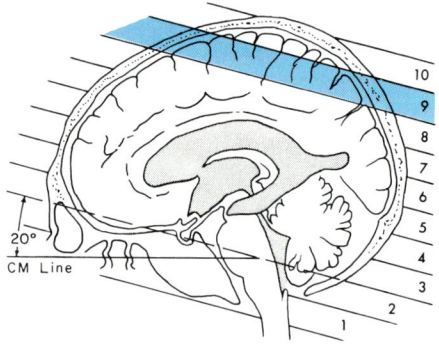

SKULL AND BRAIN

**Level 9
(Inferior aspect)**

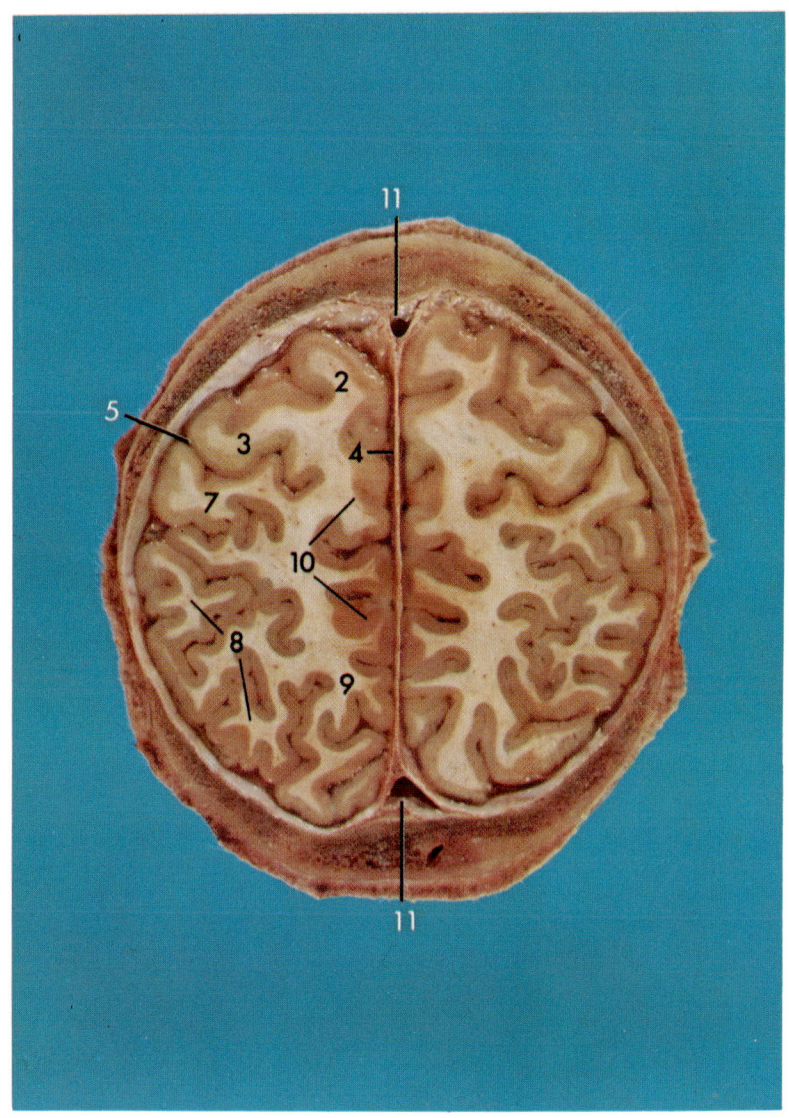

1. Frontal lobe
    2. Superior frontal gyrus
    3. Precentral gyrus
4. Falx cerebri
5. Central (Rolandic) fissure
6. Parietal lobe
    7. Postcentral gyrus
    8. Superior parietal lobule

Parietal lobe continued
    9. Precuneus
    10. Paracentral lobule
11. Superior sagittal sinus

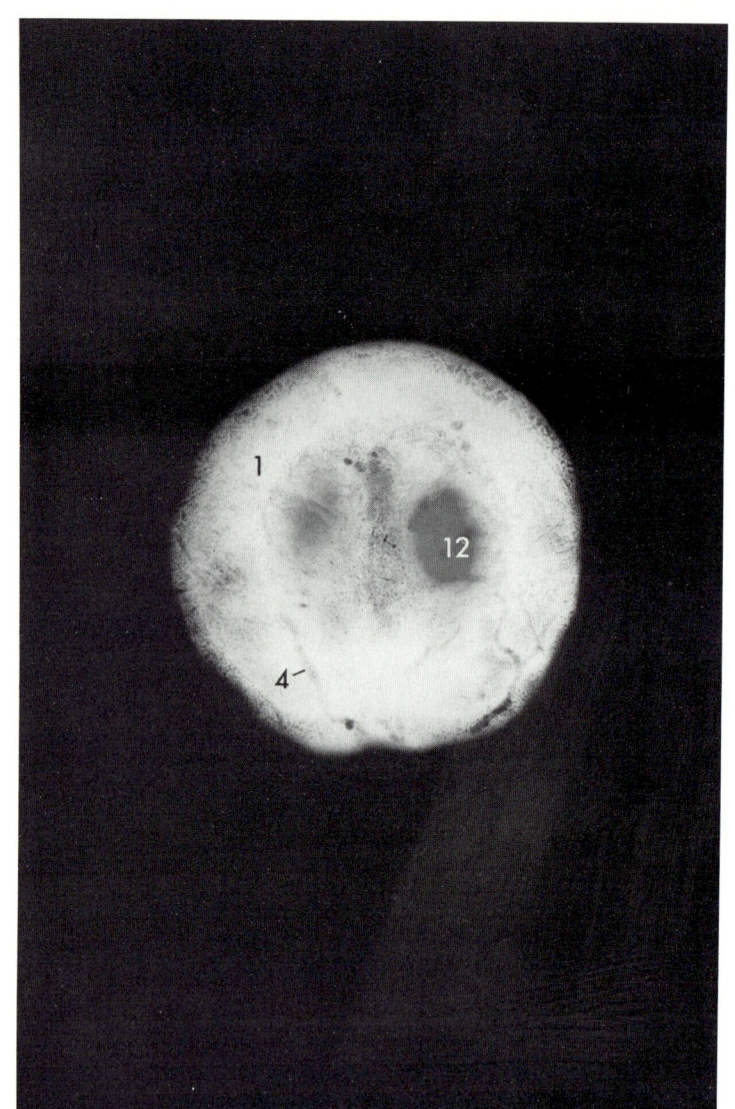
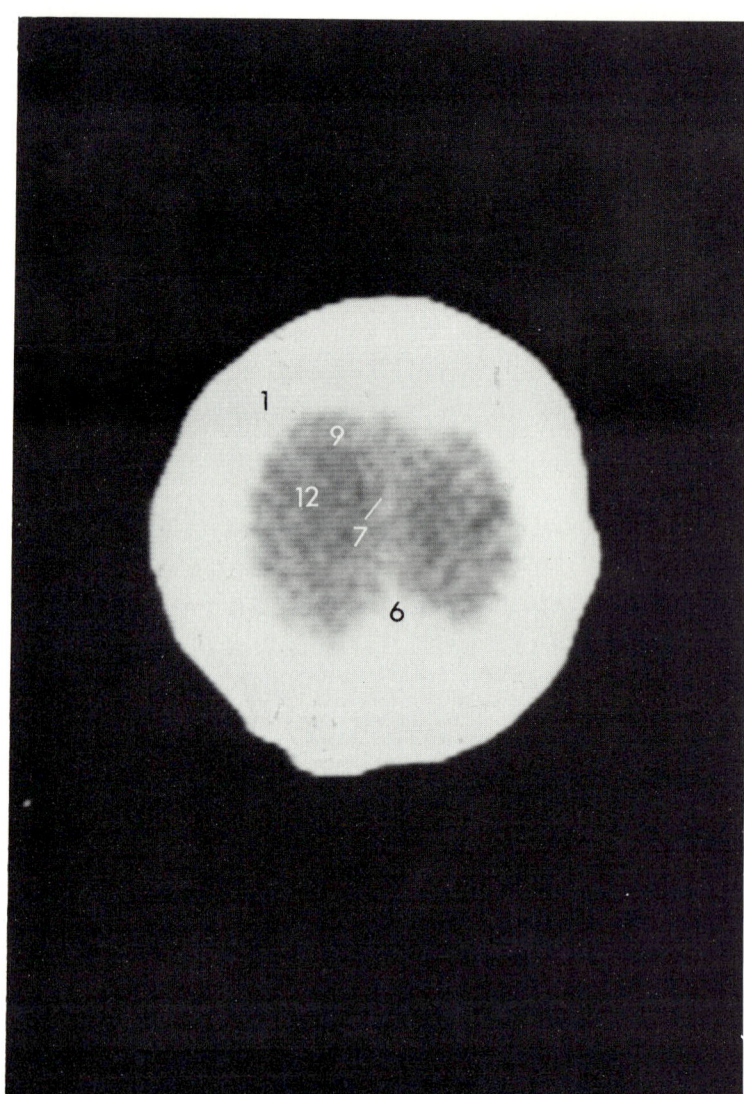
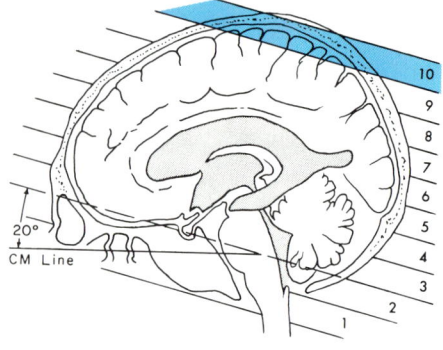

SKULL AND BRAIN

Level 10
(Inferior aspect)

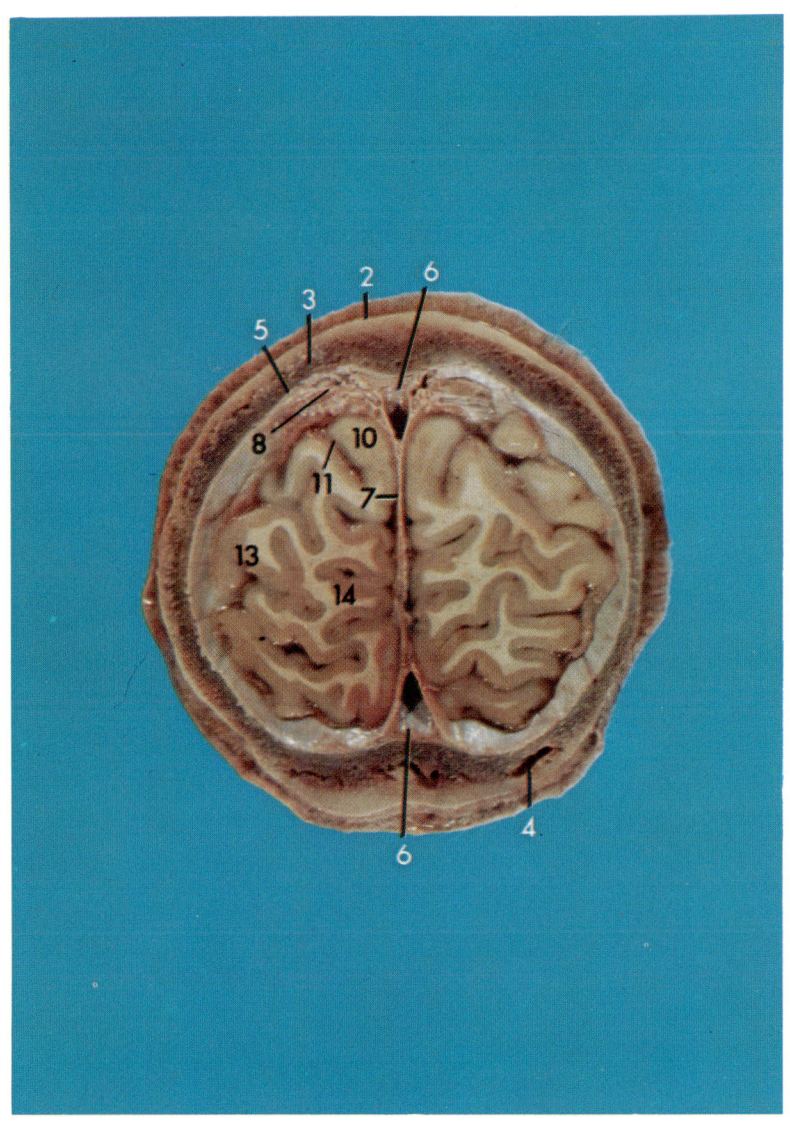

1. Parietal bone
2. Outer table
3. Diploë
4. Diploic vein
5. Inner table
6. Superior sagittal sinus
7. Falx cerebri
8. Arachnoid (Pacchionian) granulation
9. Frontal lobe
10. Precentral gyrus
11. Central (Rolandic) fissure
12. Parietal lobe
13. Superior parietal lobule
14. Paracentral lobule

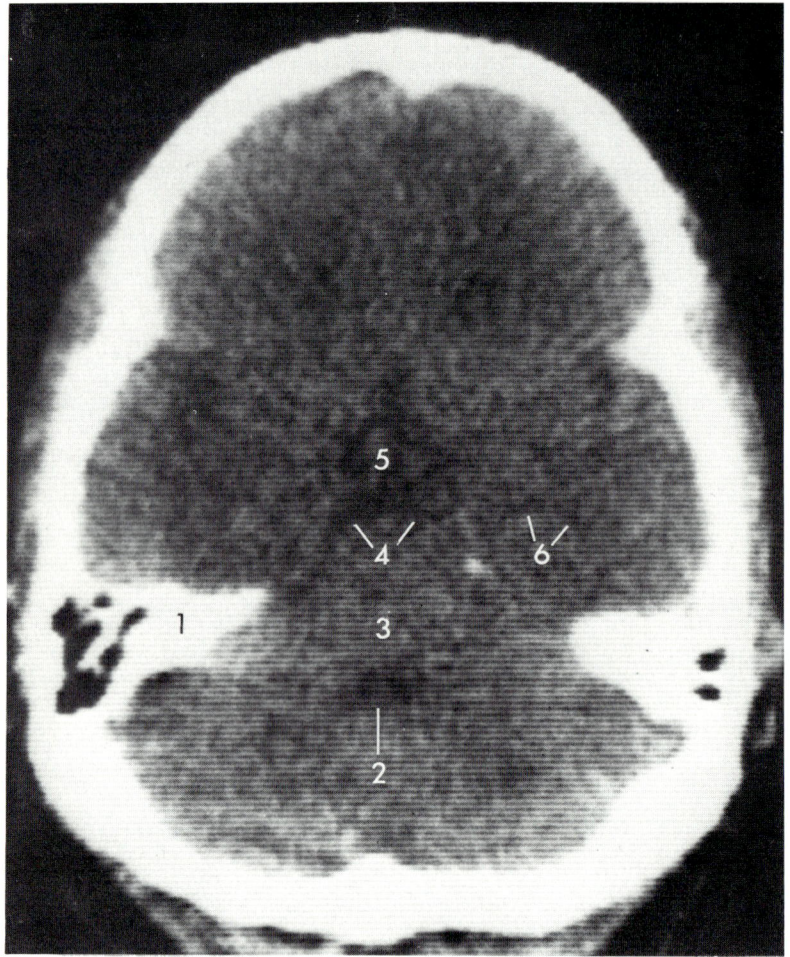 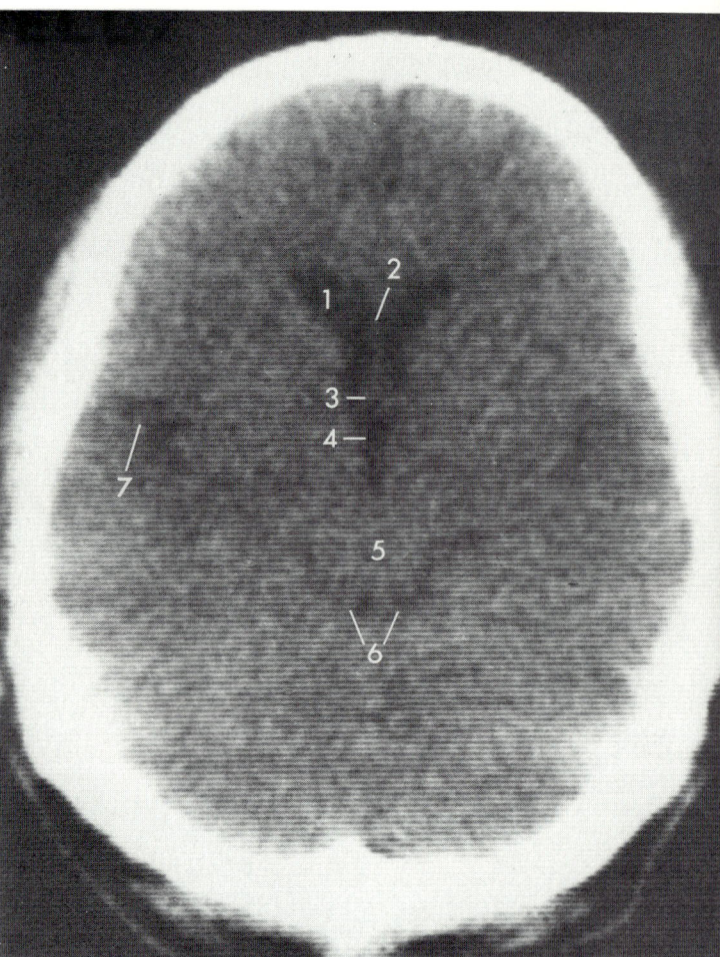

A. Section through fourth ventricle and suprasellar cistern.
  1. Petrous pyramid
  2. Fourth ventricle
  3. Pons
  4. Pontine cistern
  5. Suprasellar cistern
  6. Temporal horn of lateral ventricle

B. Section through frontal horns and third ventricle.
  1. Frontal horn of lateral ventricle
  2. Septum pellucidum
  3. Columns of fornix
  4. Third ventricle
  5. Midbrain
  6. Quadrigeminal cistern
  7. Sylvian fissure

Fig. 1-1. Studies in a 37-year-old female with slightly enlarged ventricles.

SKULL AND BRAIN
Normal *in Vivo* Computed Tomographic Studies

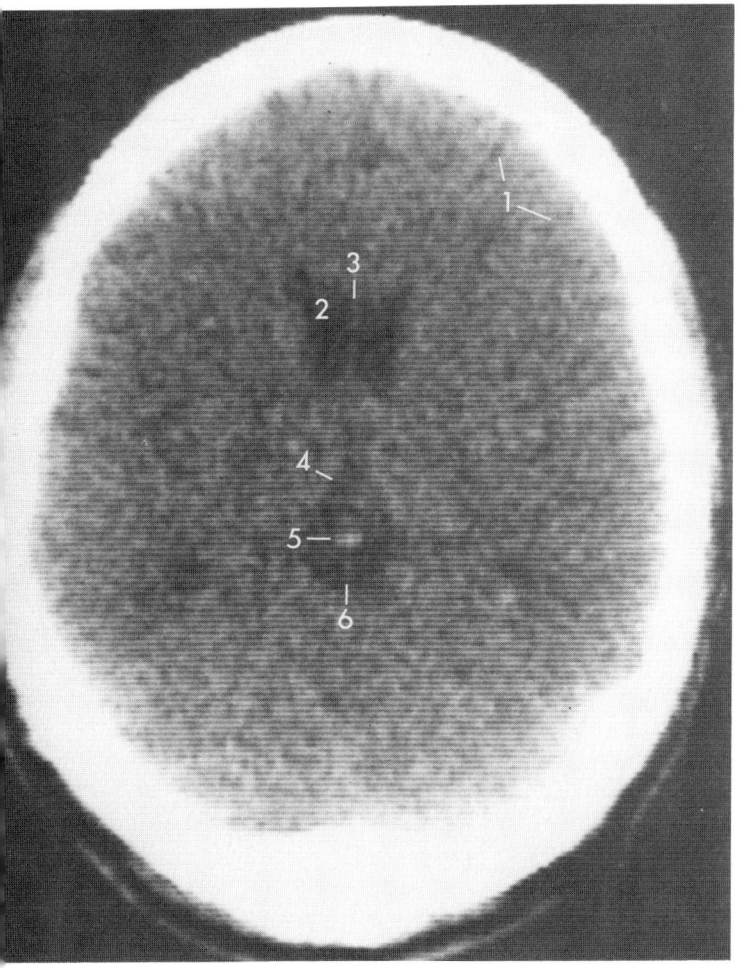
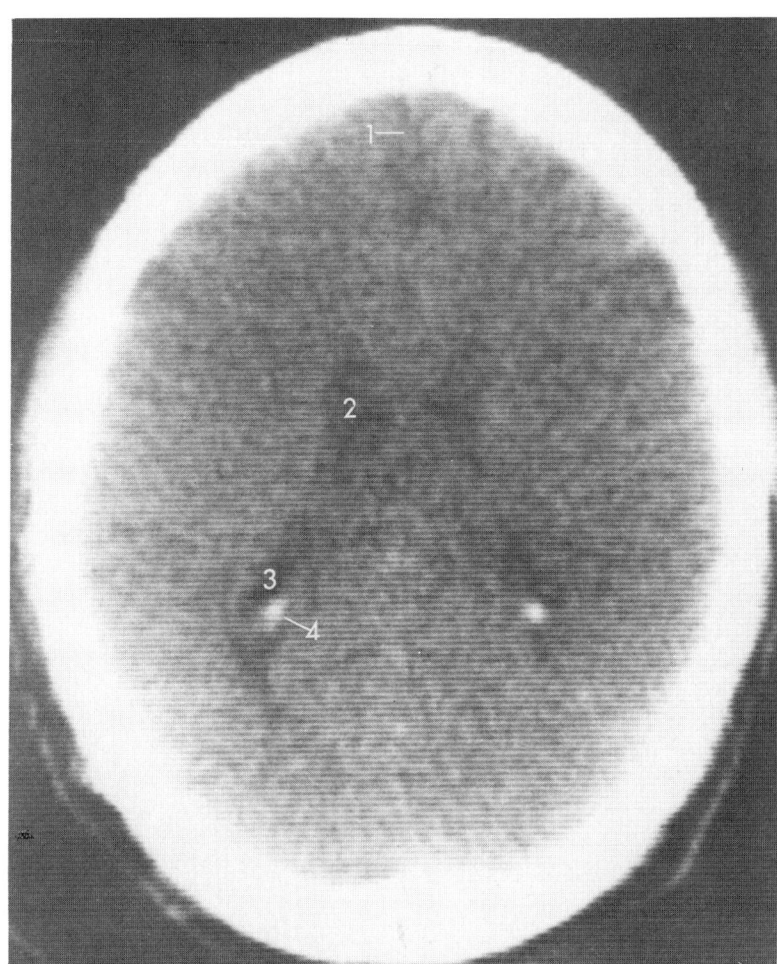

C. Section through cistern of velum interpositum and pineal gland.
 1. Sulci on surface of frontal lobe
 2. Frontal horn of lateral ventricle
 3. Septum pellucidum
 4. Cistern of velum interpositum
 5. Pineal gland (calcified)
 6. Quadrigeminal cistern

D. Section through bodies and atria of lateral ventricles.
 1. Falx cerebri
 2. Body of lateral ventricle
 3. Atrium of lateral ventricle
 4. Choroid plexus glomus

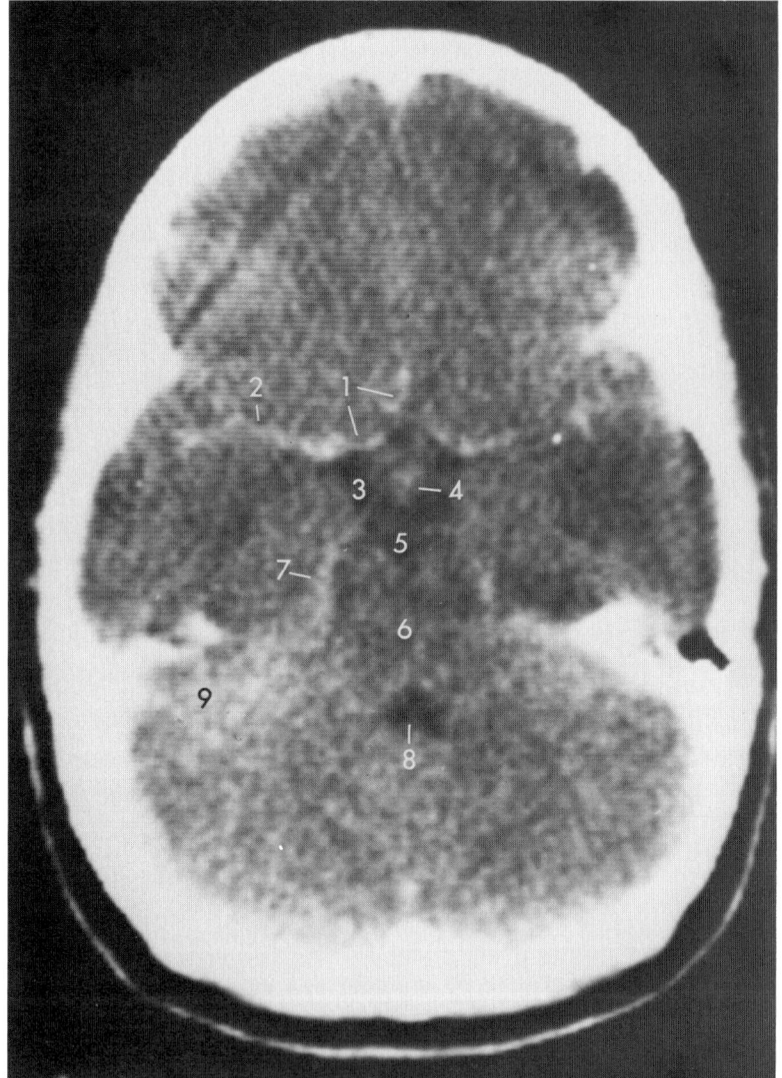 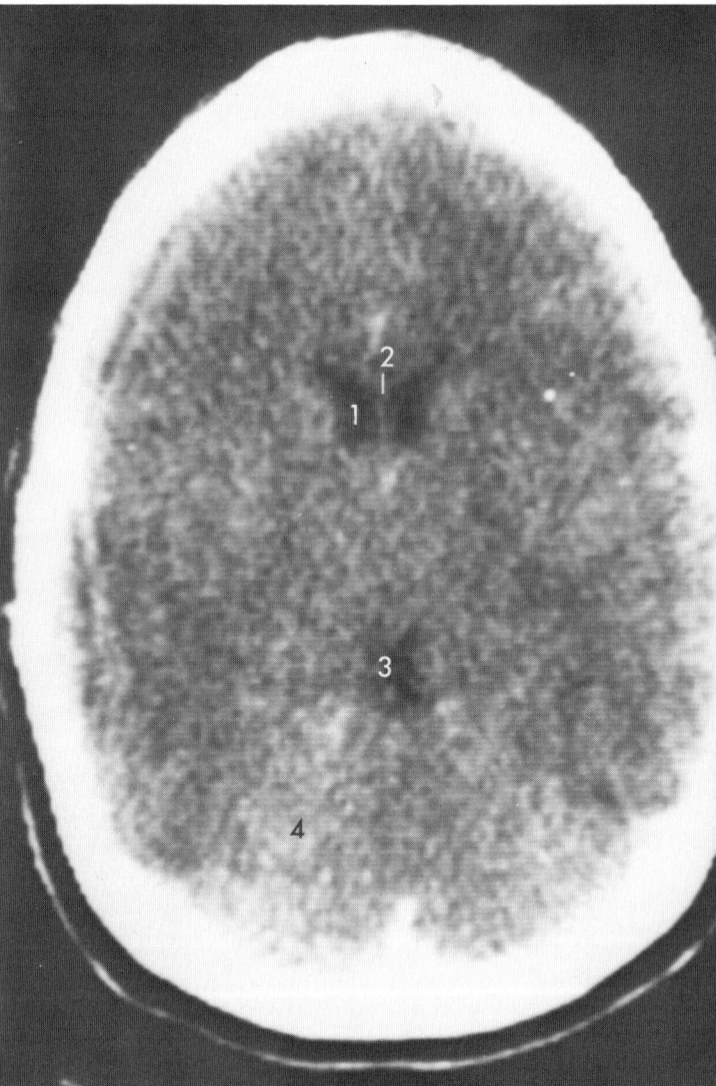

A. Major cerebral arteries at base of brain.
  1. Anterior cerebral artery
  2. Middle cerebral artery
  3. Suprasellar cistern
  4. Infundibulum of pituitary gland
  5. Interpeduncular cistern
  6. Midbrain
  7. Posterior cerebral artery
  8. Fourth ventricle
  9. Tentorium cerebelli

B. Opacification of tentorium.
  1. Frontal horn of lateral ventricle
  2. Septum pellucidum
  3. Quadrigeminal cistern
  4. Tentorium cerebelli

Fig. 1-2. Studies following intravenous bolus injection of contrast medium in a 10-year-old male.

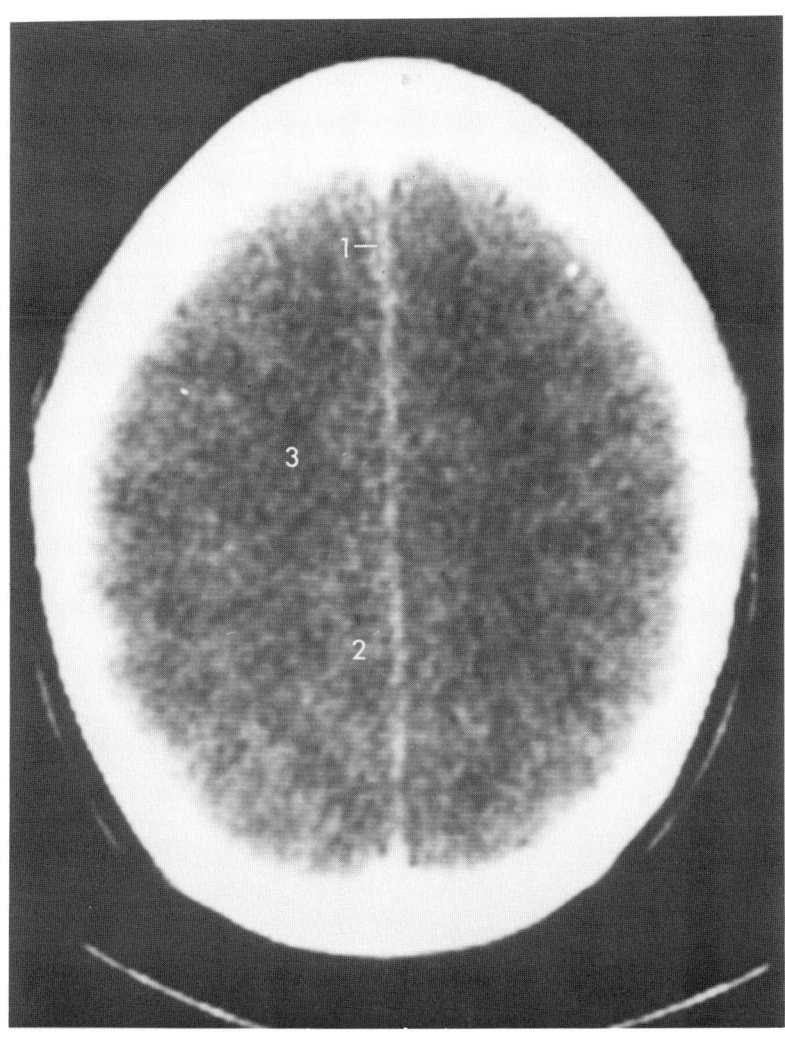

C. Opacification of falx and cerebral cortex.
1. Falx cerebri
2. Cerebral cortex (gray matter)
3. Centrum semiovale (white matter)

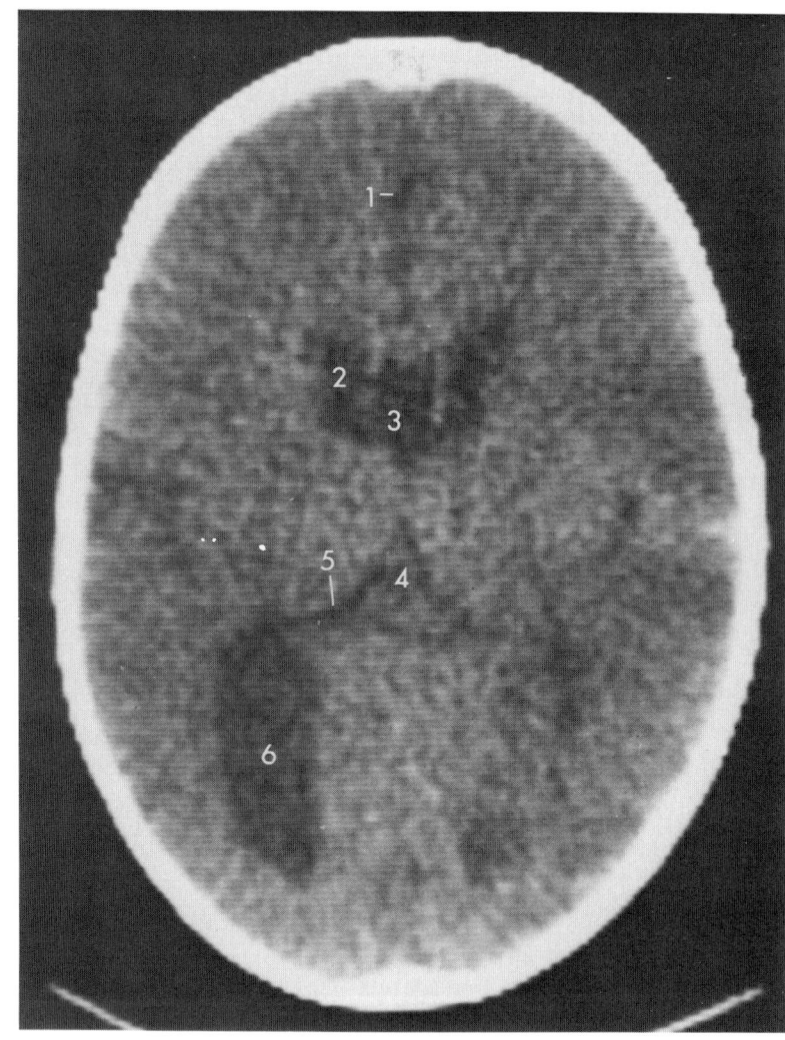

Fig. 1-3. Cavum septum pellucidum in a 1½-year-old male.
1. Interhemispheric fissure
2. Frontal horn of lateral ventricle
3. Cavum septum pellucidum
4. Cistern of velum interpositum
5. Retropulvinar cistern
6. Occipital horn of lateral ventricle

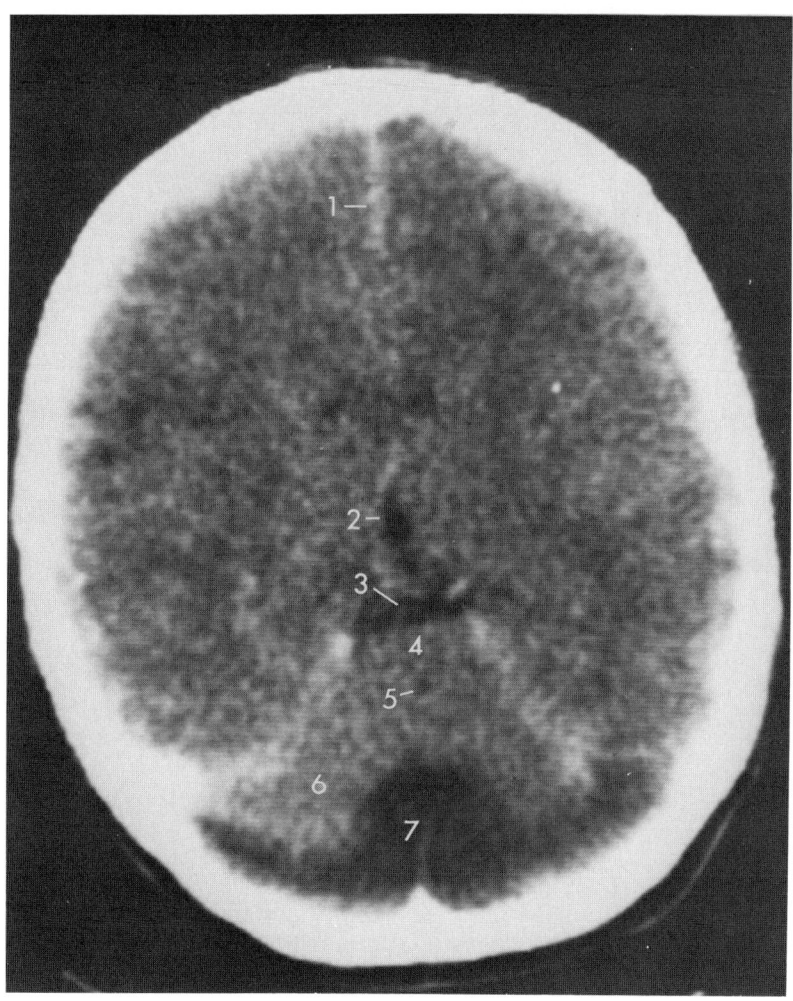

Fig. 1-4. Large cisterna magna in a 12-year-old male: study following intravenous injection of contrast medium.
1. Falx cerebri
2. Third ventricle
3. Pontine cistern
4. Pons
5. Fourth ventricle
6. Cerebellar hemisphere
7. Cisterna magna

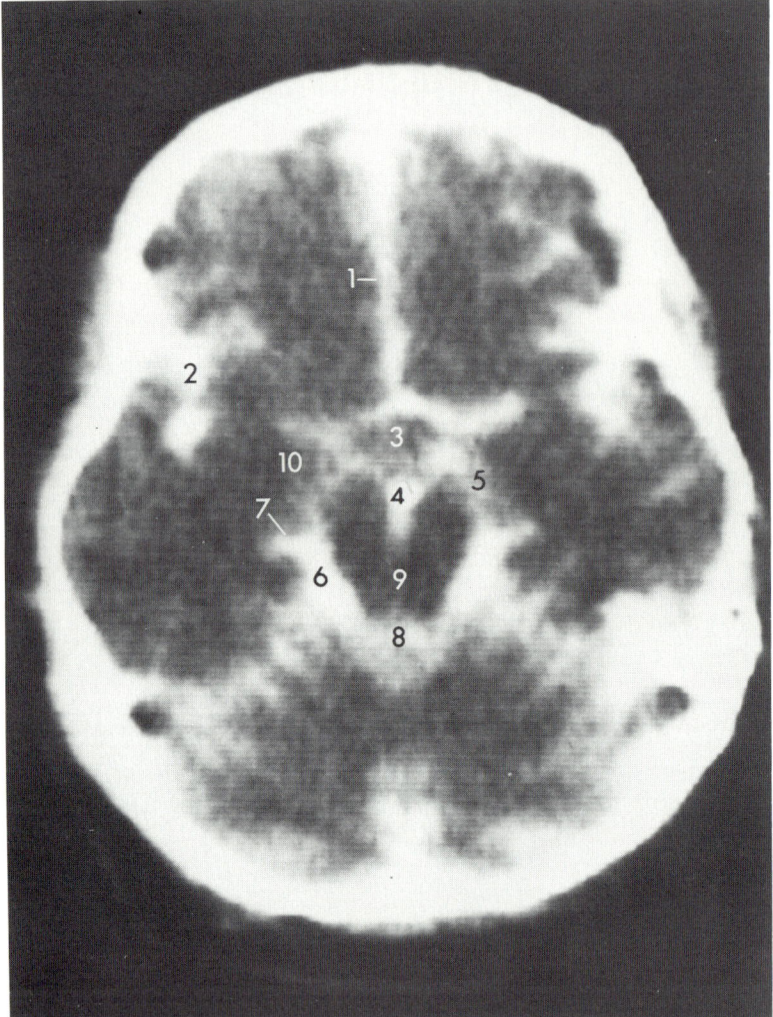
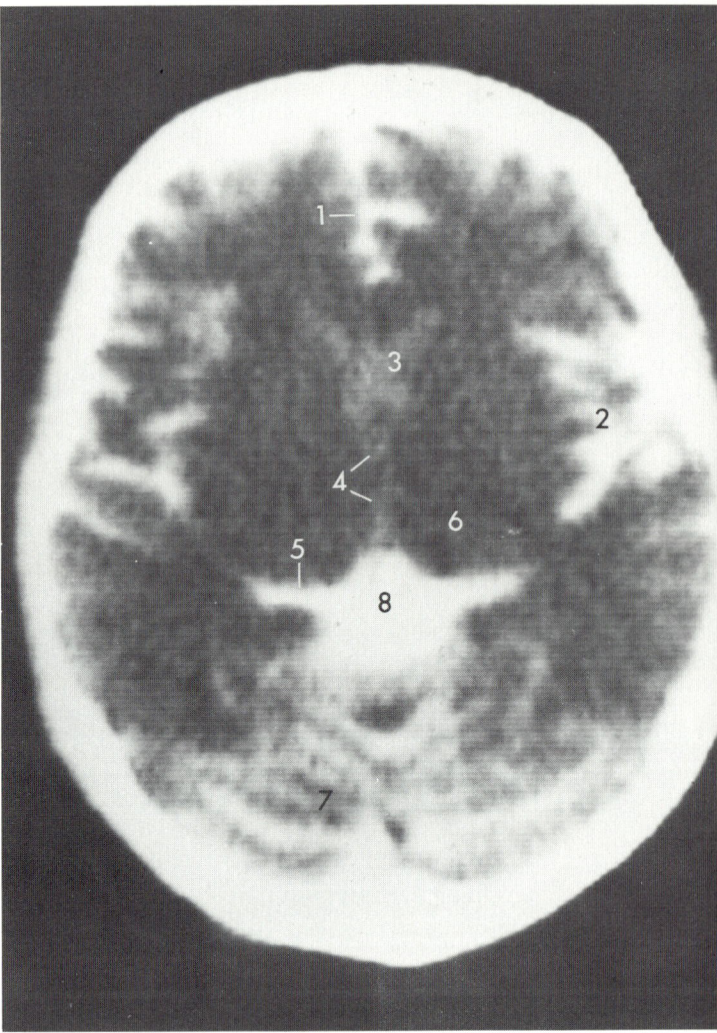

A. Section through midbrain and suprasellar cistern.
  1. Interhemispheric fissure
  2. Sylvian fissure
  3. Optic chiasm (II) and inferior recesses of third ventricle (surrounded by suprasellar cistern)
  4. Interpeduncular cistern
  5. Crural cistern
  6. Circummesencephalic (ambient) cistern
  7. Choroidal fissure
  8. Quadrigeminal cistern
  9. Midbrain
  10. Uncus of temporal lobe

B. Section through quadrigeminal cistern.
  1. Interhemispheric fissure
  2. Sylvian fissure
  3. Frontal horn of lateral ventricle
  4. Third ventricle
  5. Retropulvinar cistern (wing of ambient cistern)
  6. Thalamus
  7. Sulci on superior aspect of cerebellum
  8. Quadrigeminal cistern

Normal *in Vivo* Computed Tomographic Studies: Metrizamide

The computed tomographic images in Figures 1-5, 1-6, and 1-7 demonstrate the normal appearance of the intracranial cisterns and sulci opacified with metrizamide. Those images were obtained between 1½ and 2½ hours after the water-soluble contrast medium had been introduced into the subarachnoid space via lumbar puncture.

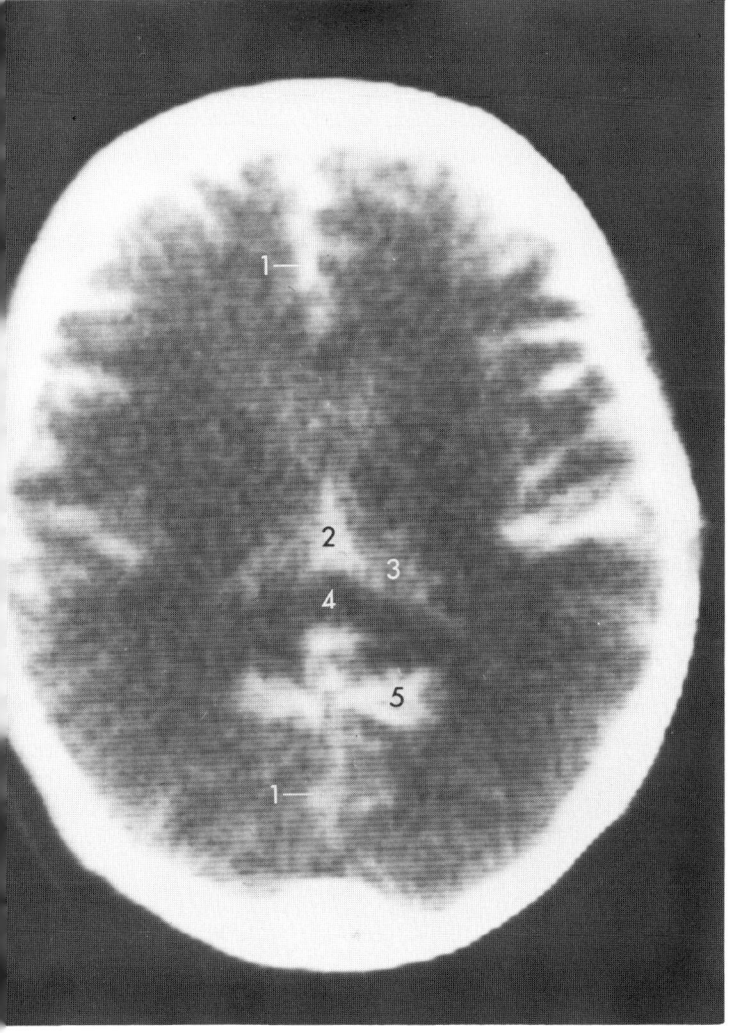
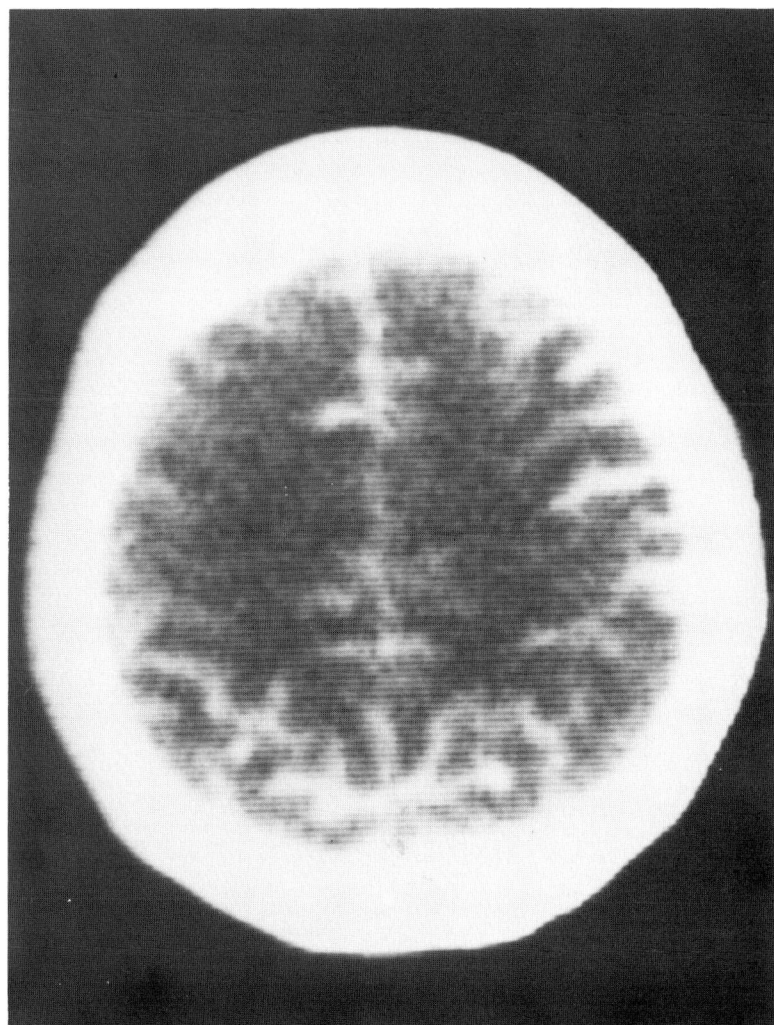

C. Section through splenium of corpus callosum.
  1. Interhemispheric fissure
  2. Cistern of velum interpositum
  3. Posterior portion of body of lateral ventricle
  4. Splenium of corpus callosum
  5. Calcarine fissure

D. Section through cerebral hemispheres near vertex of skull. Note opacification of sulci on medial and lateral aspects of each cerebral hemisphere.

Fig. 1-5. Normal computed tomographic cisternogram, 24-year-old female. Images obtained in standard modified transaxial plane.

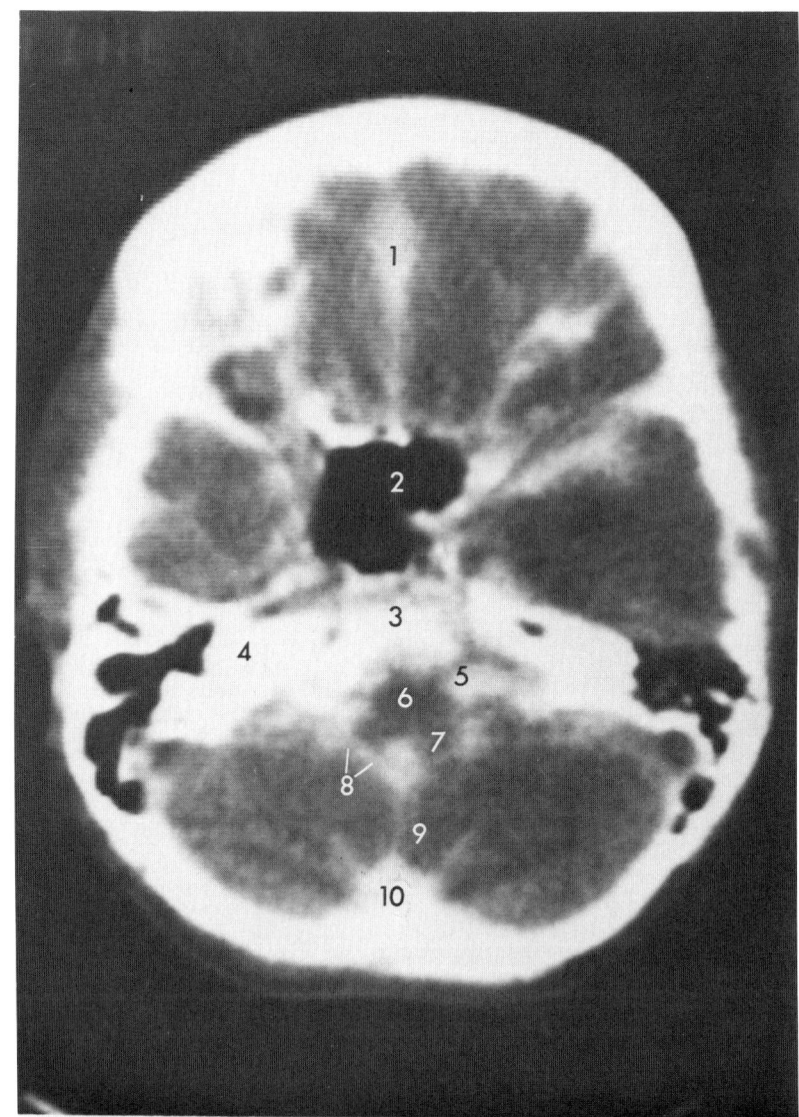

A. Section through sphenoid sinus and inferior portion of brainstem.
  1. Interhemispheric fissure
  2. Sphenoid sinus
  3. Clivus
  4. Petrous portion of temporal bone
  5. Medullary cistern
  6. Medulla oblongata
  7. Restiform body (inferior cerebellar peduncle)
  8. Lateral recess of fourth ventricle
  9. Cerebellar tonsil
  10. Cisterna magna

Fig. 1-6. Normal computed tomographic cisternogram demonstrating anatomy of fourth ventricle, 45-year-old female. Images obtained in standard modified transaxial plane.

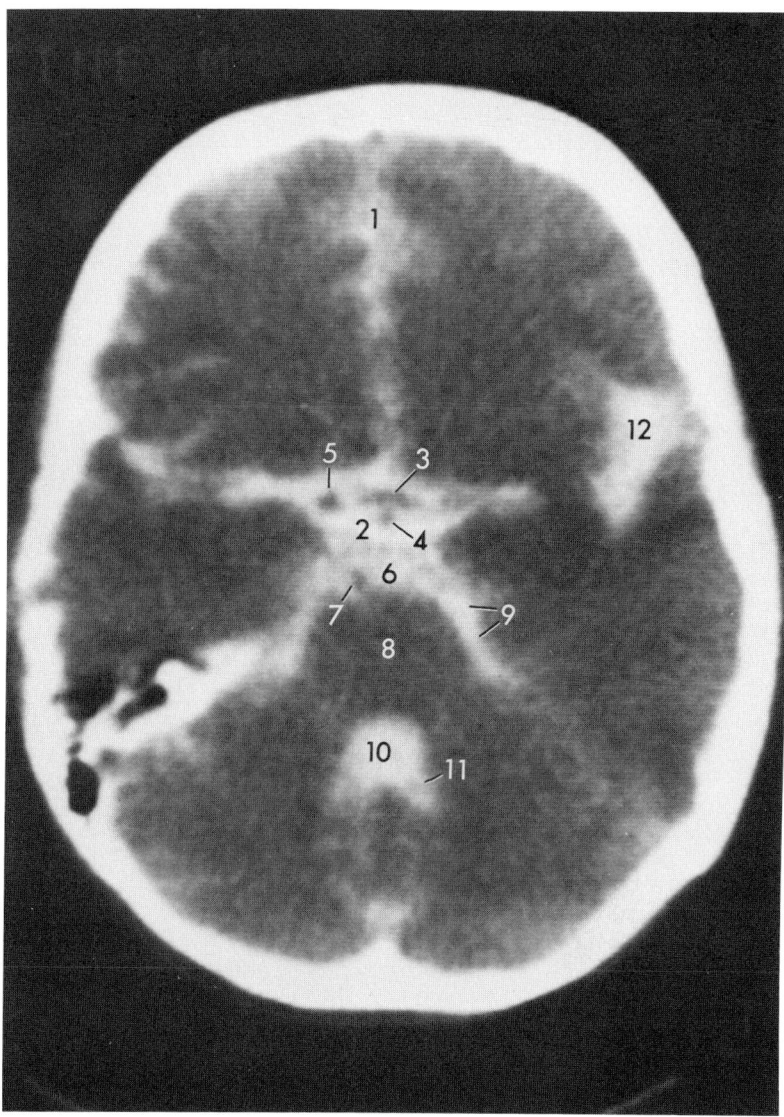

B. Section through suprasellar cistern and fourth ventricle.
1. Interhemispheric fissure
2. Suprasellar cistern
3. Optic chiasm (II)
4. Infundibulum of pituitary gland
5. Internal carotid artery (supraclinoid portion)
6. Pontine cistern
7. Basilar artery
8. Pons
9. Cerebellopontine angle cistern
10. Fourth ventricle
11. Posterior superior recess of fourth ventricle
12. Sylvian fissure

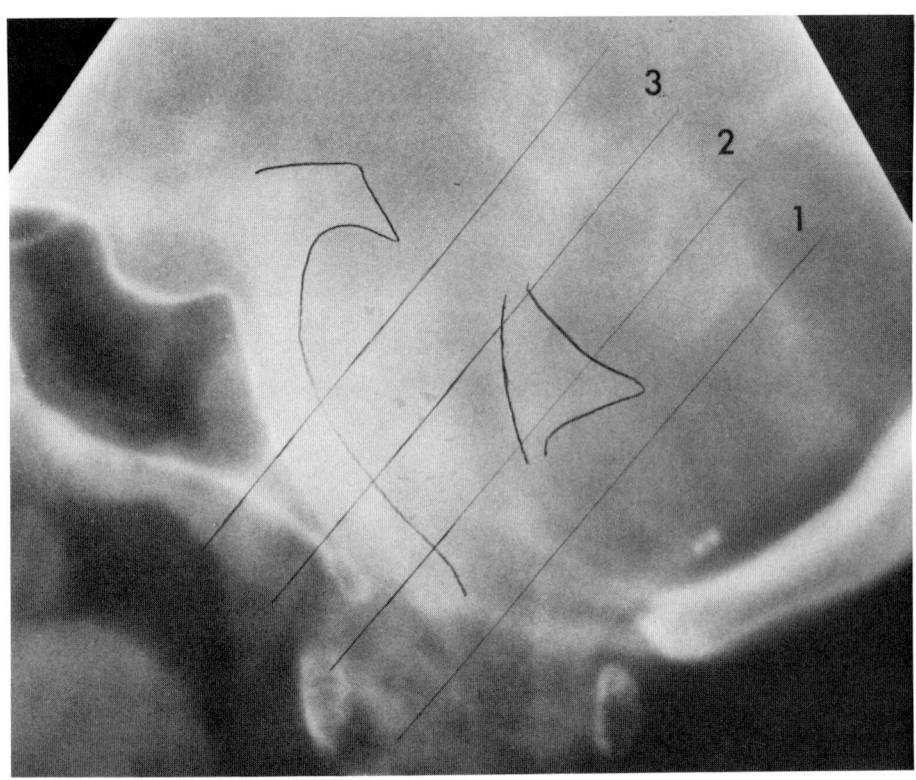

Fig. 1-7. Normal computed tomographic cisternogram, 45-year-old female. Images obtained in a modified coronal plane.

A. Hypocycloidal tomogram in midsagittal plane indicating the levels of the images in the modified coronal plane.

B. Section through Level 1.
1. Superior cerebellar cistern
2. Vallecula of cisterna magna
3. Cerebellar tonsil

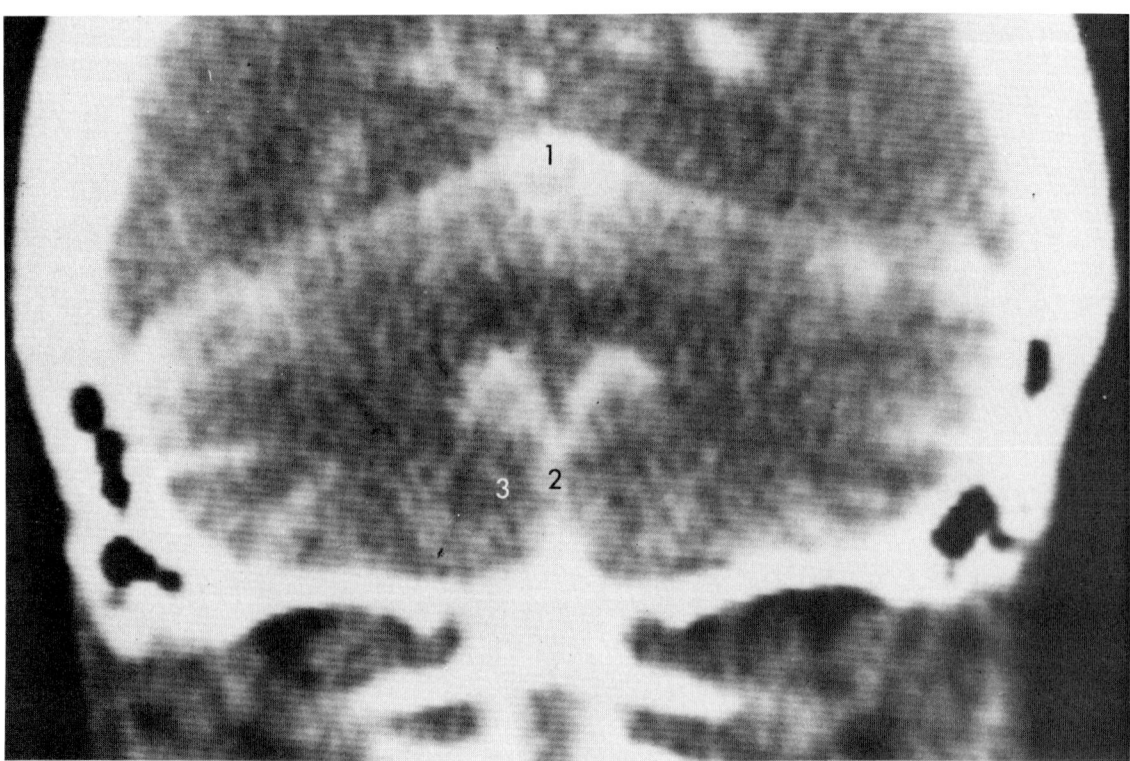

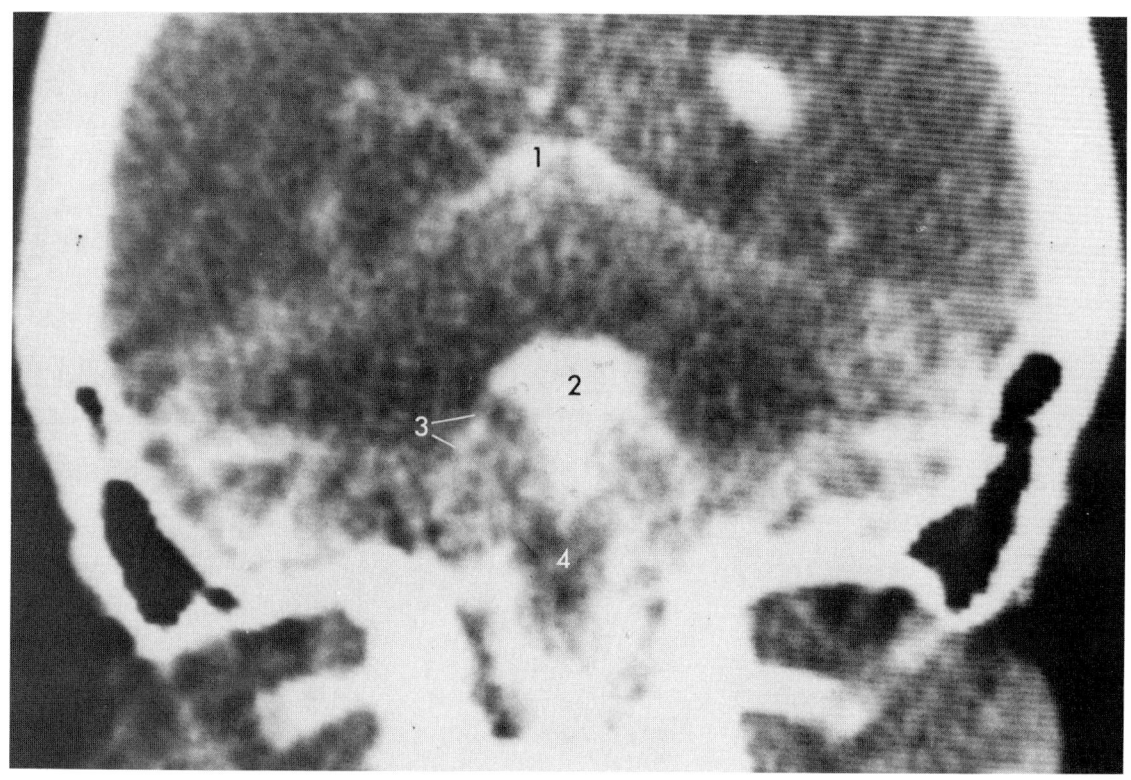

C. Section through Level 2.
1. Superior cerebellar cistern
2. Fourth ventricle
3. Lateral recess of fourth ventricle
4. Medulla oblongata

D. Section through Level 3.
1. Quadrigeminal cistern
2. Inferior colliculi (midbrain)
3. Circummesencephalic (ambient) cistern
4. Pons
5. Cerebellopontine angle cistern
6. Petrous portion of temporal bone

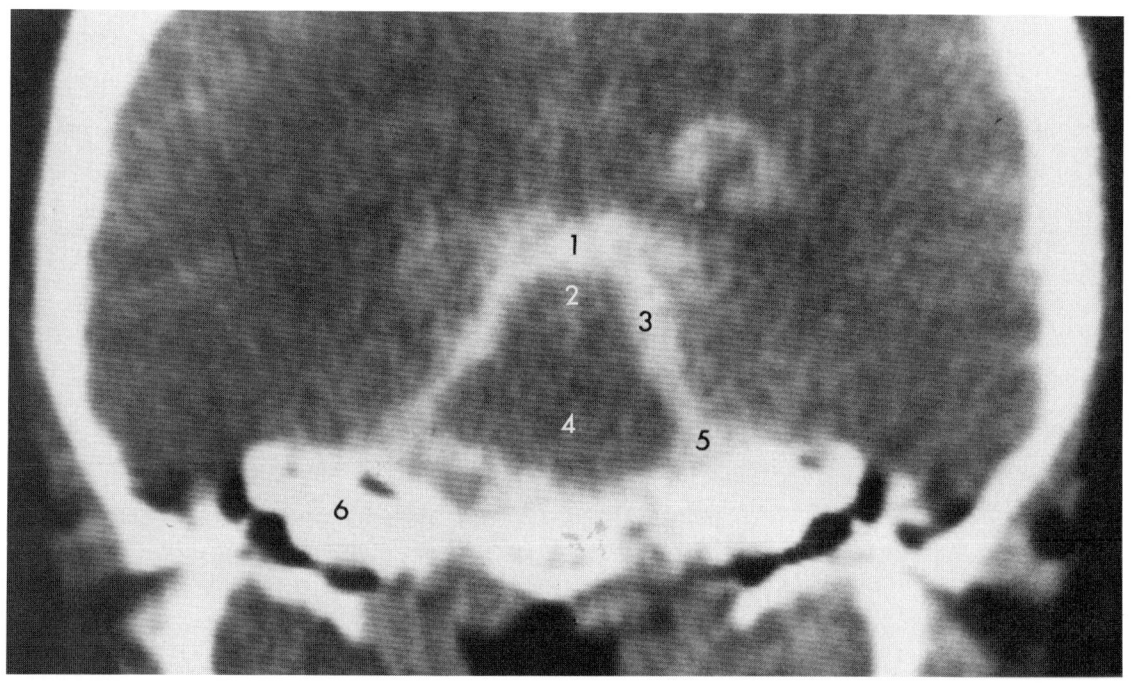

2
Orbit

STEPHEN A. KIEFFER

The plane of section conventionally utilized for computed tomographic examination of the orbit is horizontal (parallel with the orbitomeatal line). However, the long axes of the optic nerve and the extraocular muscles are not horizontal. The optic nerve follows a slight upward course from the posterior surface of the globe to the optic canal, while the extraocular muscles converge from all sides toward the annulus of Zinn immediately anterior to the superior orbital fissure. Thus, in any given horizontal section, portions of these structures will be visualized but not the complete structure.

Because the structures of interest within the orbit are relatively small, the thickness of each section is only 8 mm, as compared with 13 mm in the remainder of this atlas. The considerable amount of fat in the retrobulbar space and surrounding the extraocular muscles permits good radiographic contrast despite the relative thinness of the sections.

All sections are displayed as viewed from below (inferior aspect) with the exception of Level 1, in which anatomy more pertinent to the orbit is seen on the superior aspect, and thus the anatomic illustration for that level is displayed as viewed from above.

Technical factors for the computed tomographic images included a center setting of 0–20 Hounsfield units and a window width of 350–400 Hounsfield units. The diameter of the scanning circle was 29 cm. These correspond closely to the settings used in clinical practice.

A more recent innovation in computed tomographic examination of the orbit is imaging in a modified coronal plane. Apparatus with a sufficiently wide gantry opening will permit the head to be hyperextended and arched backward on the neck so that the plane of section is at an angle of 65–70 degrees with respect to the orbitomeatal plane. An image in this plane of the orbits in a normal patient is displayed in the section Normal *In Vivo* Computed Tomographic Studies at the conclusion of this chapter.

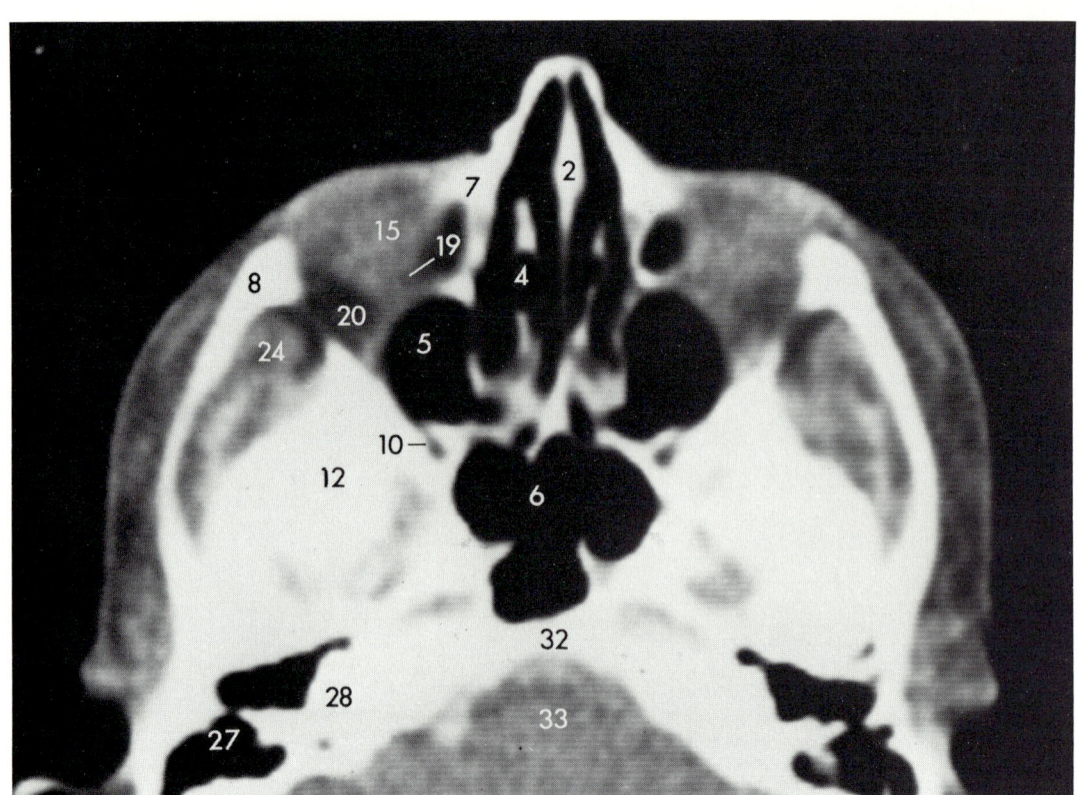

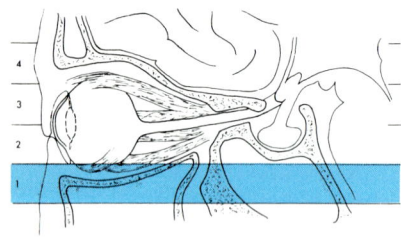

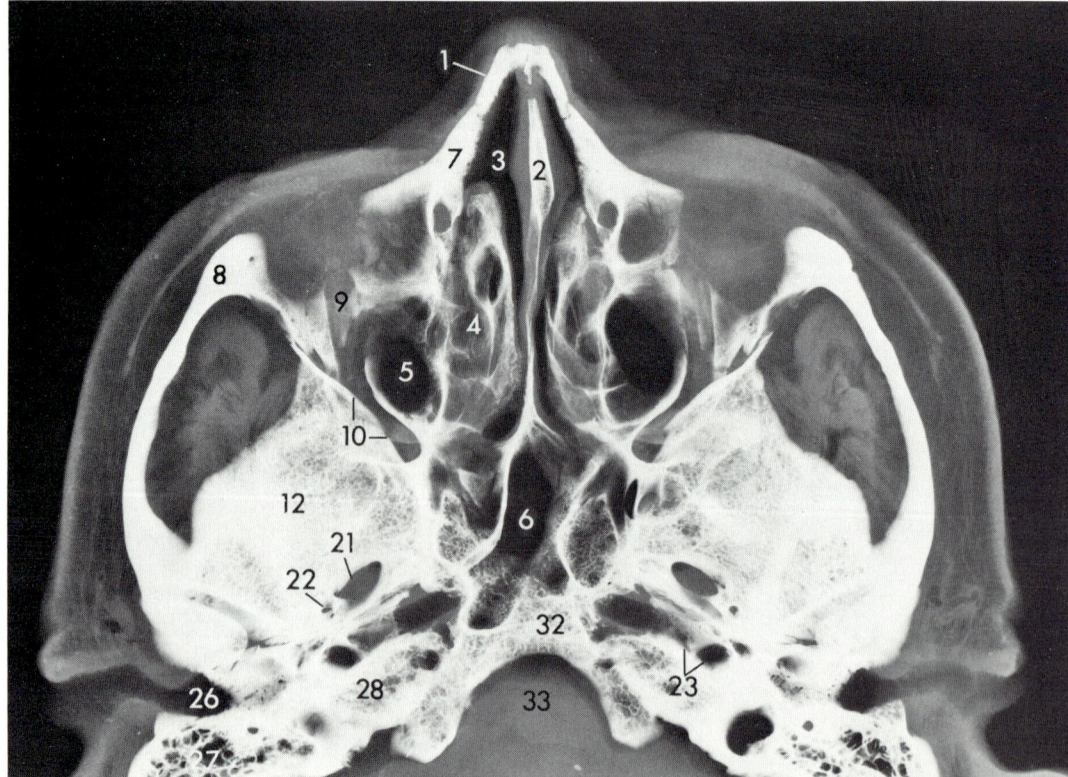

ORBIT

**Level 1
(Superior aspect)**

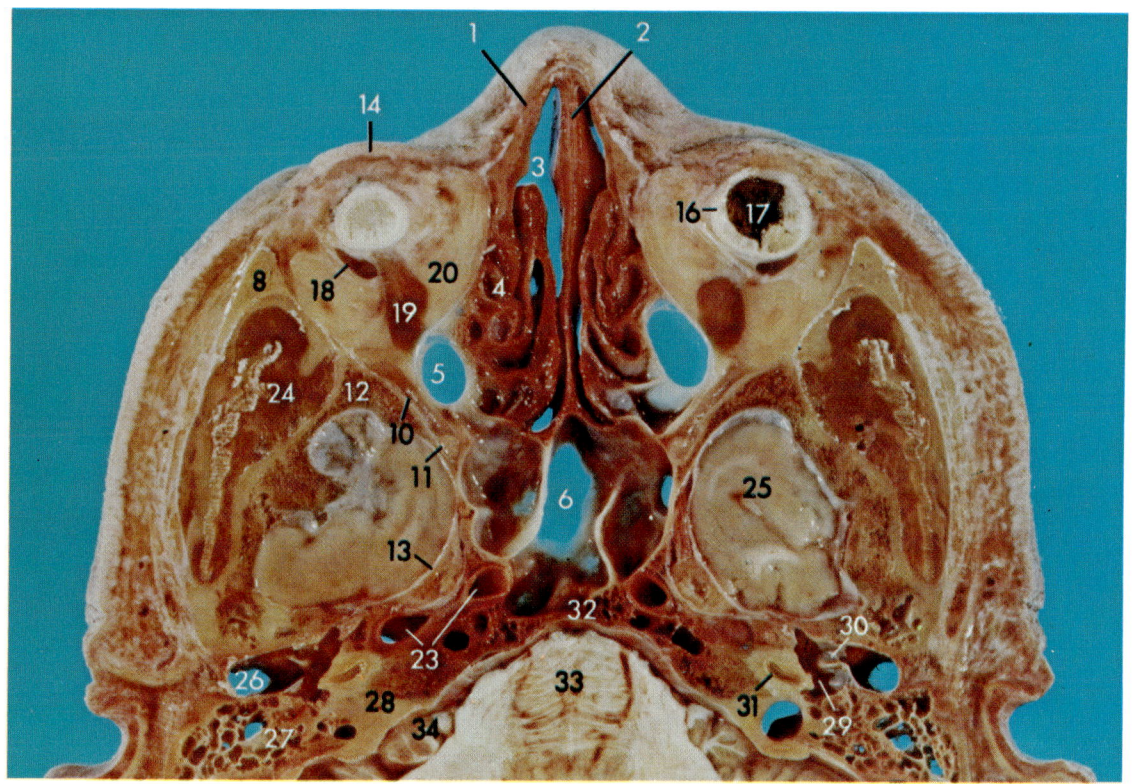

1. Nasal bone
2. Perpendicular plate of ethmoid
3. Nasal fossa
4. Ethmoid sinus
5. Maxillary sinus
6. Sphenoid sinus
7. Maxilla
8. Zygoma
9. Infraorbital canal
10. Inferior orbital fissure
11. Sphenopalatine ganglion
12. Greater wing of sphenoid
13. Meckel's cave (Gasserian ganglion)
14. Lower eyelid
15. Globe
    16. Sclera
    17. Retina
18. Inferior oblique muscle
19. Inferior rectus muscle
20. Orbital fat
21. Foramen ovale
22. Foramen spinosum
23. Carotid canal (internal carotid artery)
24. Temporalis muscle
25. Temporal lobe
26. External auditory canal
27. Mastoid portion of temporal bone
28. Petrous portion of temporal bone
29. Middle ear (tympanic) cavity
30. Tympanic membrane
31. Lateral semicircular canal
32. Clivus (basisphenoid)
33. Pons
34. Flocculus of cerebellum

41

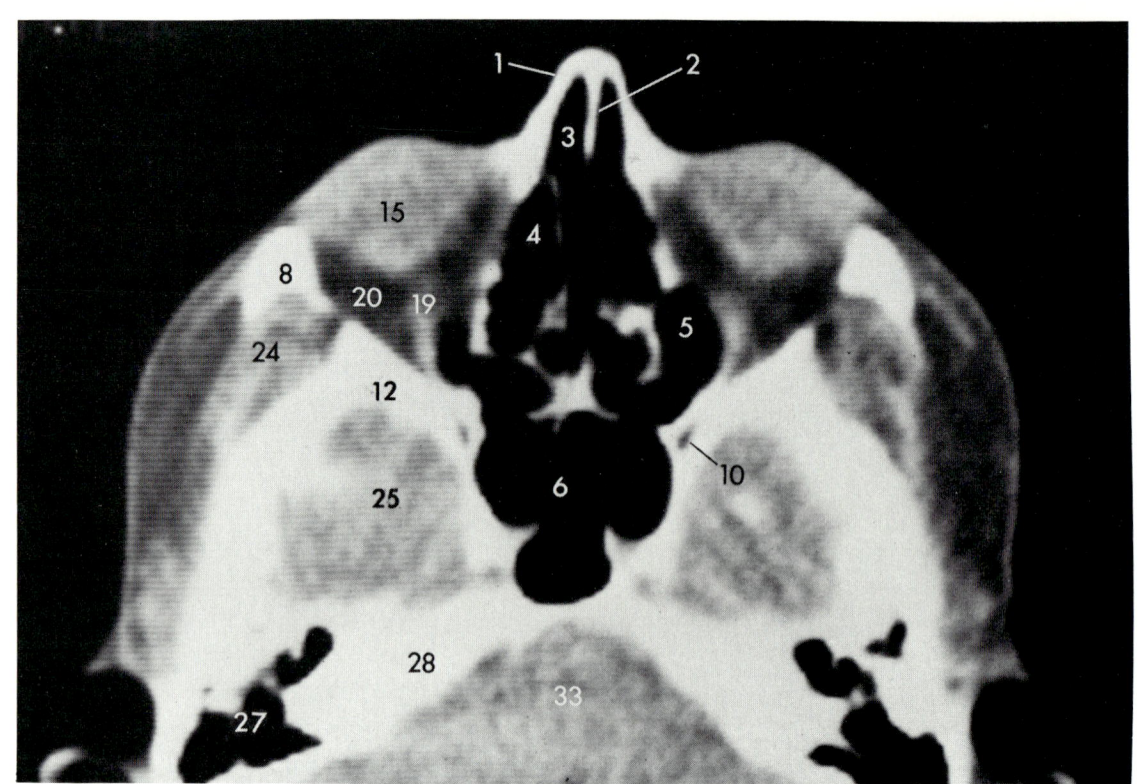

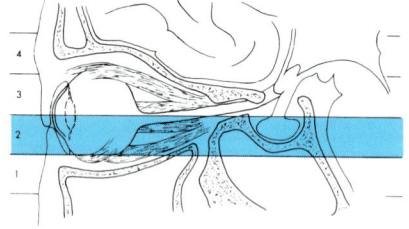

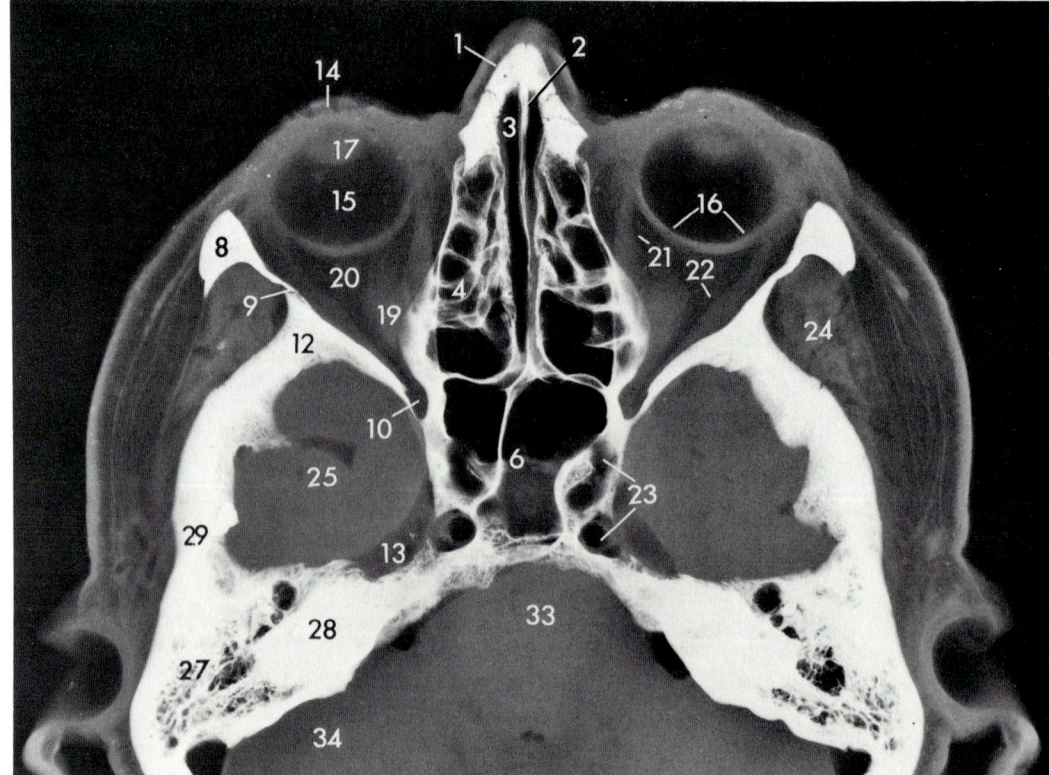

ORBIT

Level 2

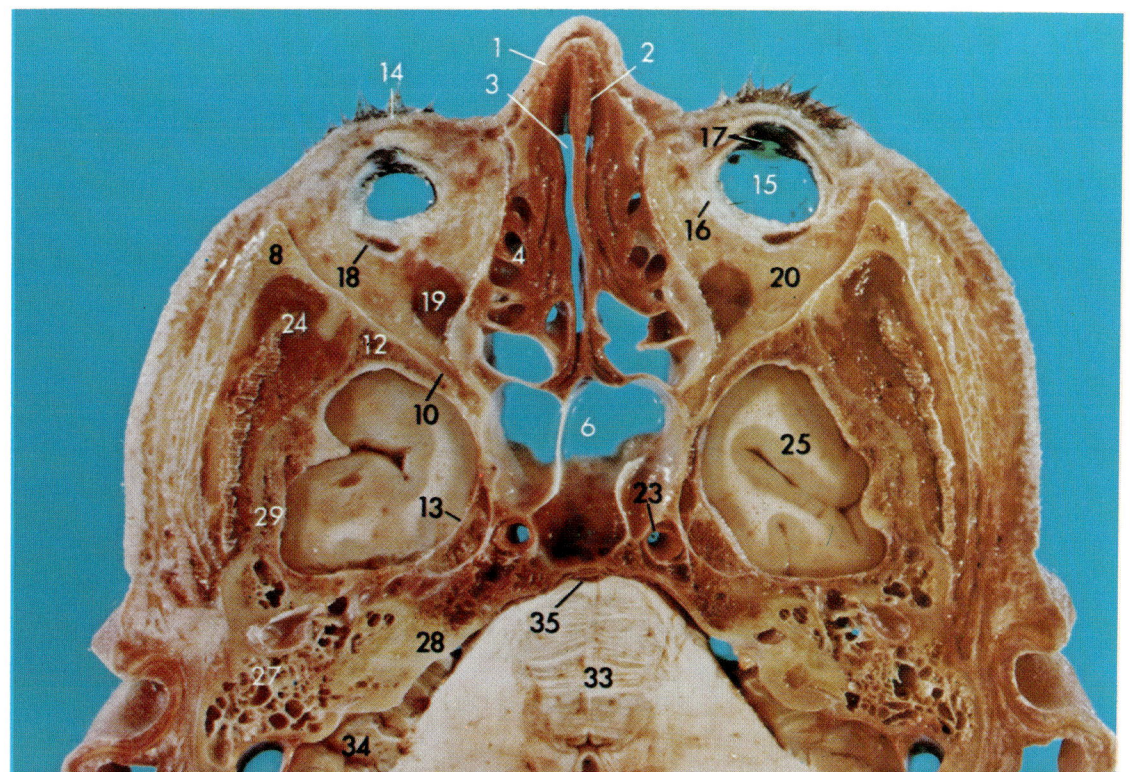

1. Nasal bone
2. Perpendicular plate of ethmoid
3. Nasal fossa
4. Ethmoid sinus
5. Maxillary sinus
6. Sphenoid sinus
8. Zygoma
9. Sphenozygomatic suture
10. Superior orbital fissure
12. Greater wing of sphenoid
13. Meckel's cave (Gasserian ganglion)
14. Upper eyelid
15. Globe (with vitreous humor)
16. Sclera
17. Lens
18. Inferior oblique muscle
19. Inferior rectus muscle
20. Retrobulbar fat
21. Medial rectus muscle
22. Lateral rectus muscle
23. Internal carotid artery (surrounded by cavernous sinus)
24. Temporalis muscle
25. Temporal lobe
27. Mastoid portion of temporal bone
28. Petrous portion of temporal bone
29. Squamous portion of temporal bone
33. Pons
34. Cerebellar hemisphere
35. Basilar artery

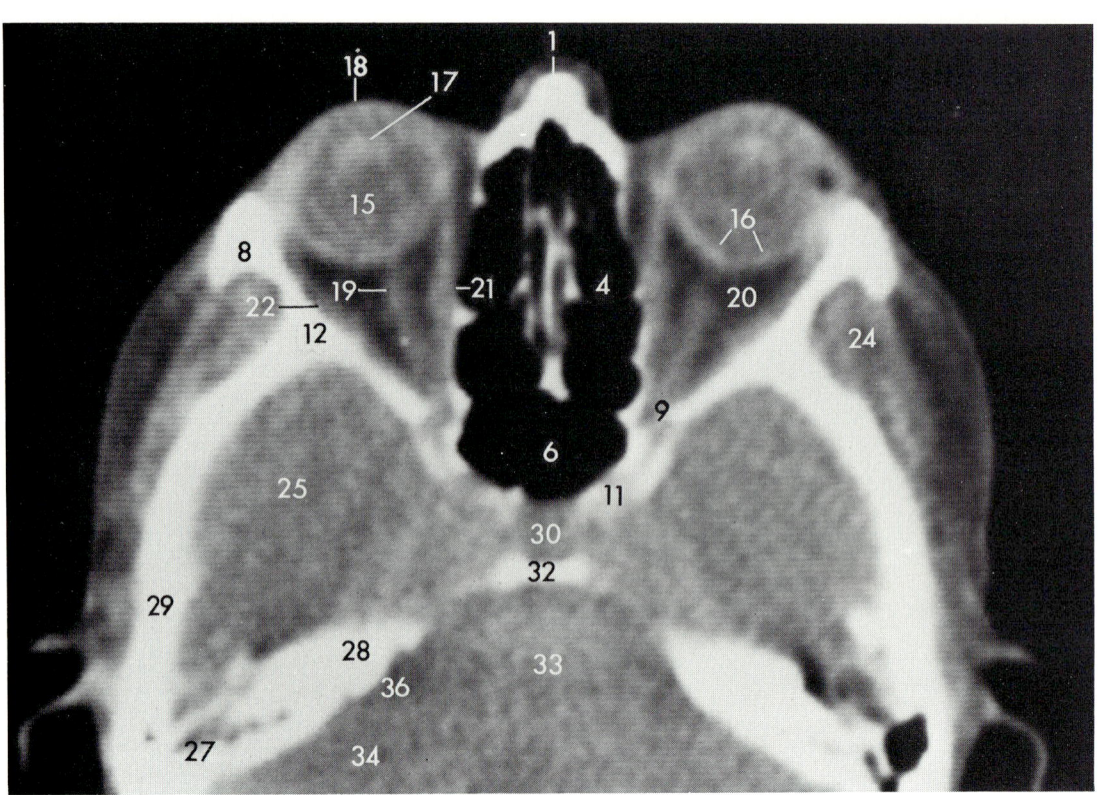

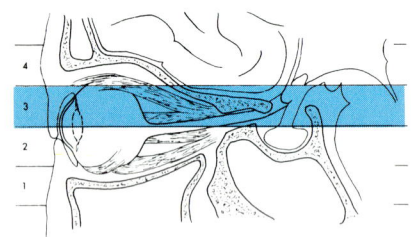

ORBIT

Level 3

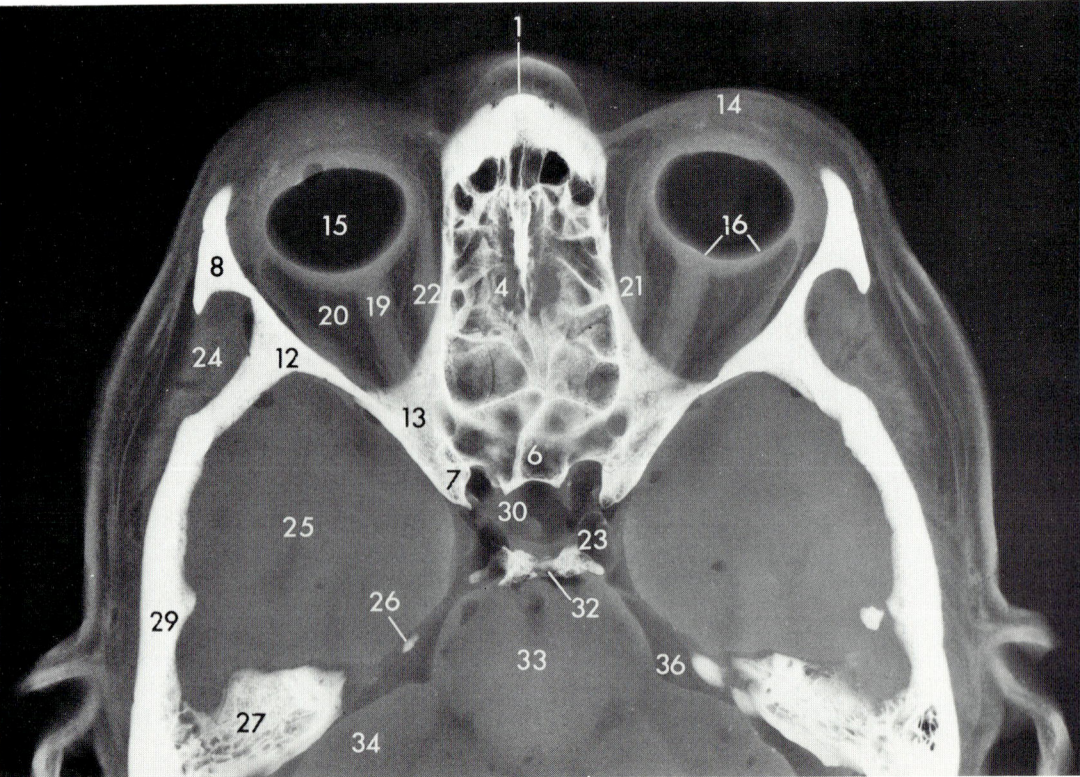

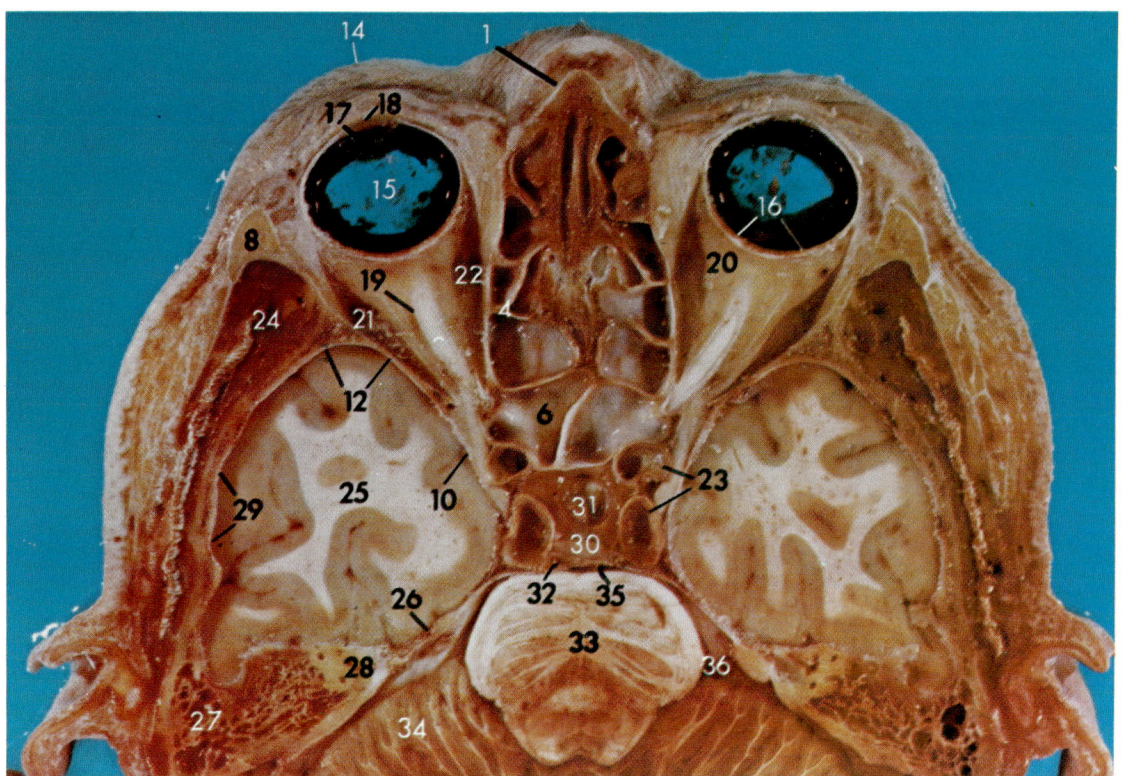

1. Nasal bone
4. Ethmoid sinus
6. Sphenoid sinus
7. Anterior clinoid process
8. Frontal process of zygoma
9. Orbital opening of optic canal
10. Superior orbital fissure (oculomotor nerve [III])
11. Cranial opening of optic canal
12. Greater wing of sphenoid
13. Lesser wing of sphenoid
14. Upper eyelid
15. Globe (with vitreous humor)

Globe (with vitreous humor) continued
    16. Sclera
    17. Lens
    18. Cornea
19. Optic nerve (II)
20. Retrobulbar fat
21. Medial rectus muscle
22. Lateral rectus muscle
23. Internal carotid artery
24. Temporalis muscle
25. Temporal lobe
26. Petroclinoid ligament (dura mater, partially calcified)

27. Mastoid portion of temporal bone
28. Petrous portion of temporal bone
29. Squamous portion of temporal bone
30. Hypophyseal fossa covered by diaphragma sellae
31. Foramen of diaphragma sellae (infundibulum of pituitary gland)
32. Dorsum sellae
33. Pons
34. Cerebellar hemisphere
35. Basilar artery
36. Cerebellopontine angle cistern

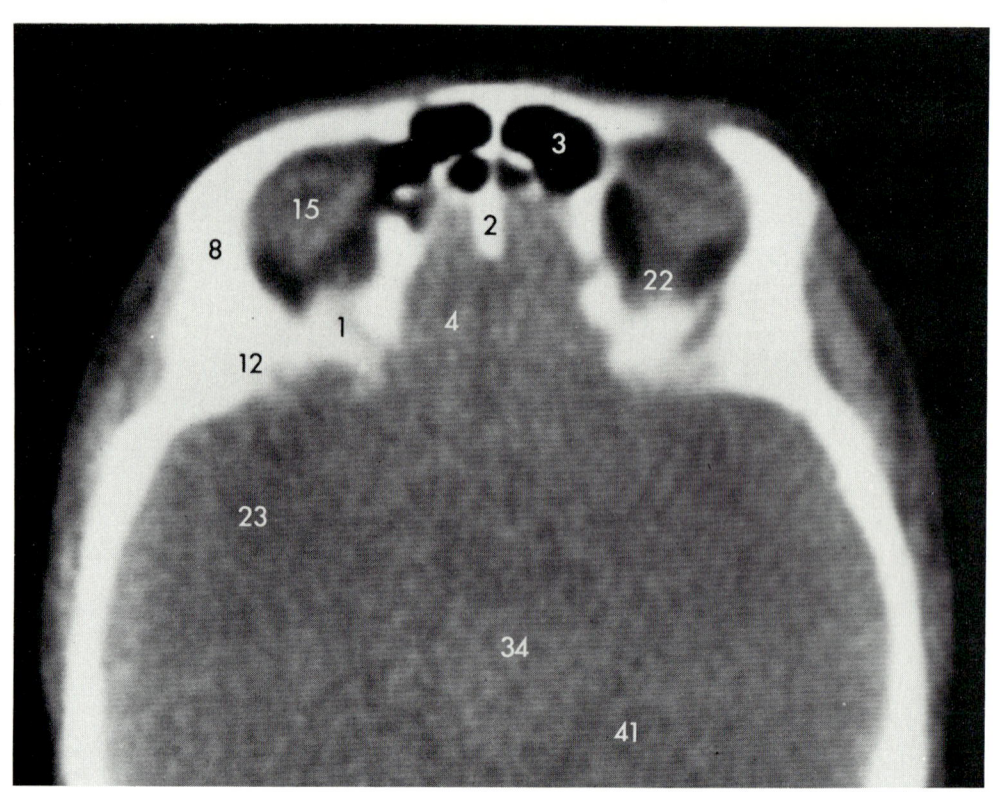
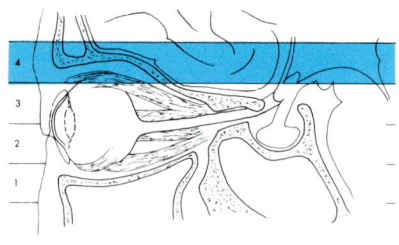
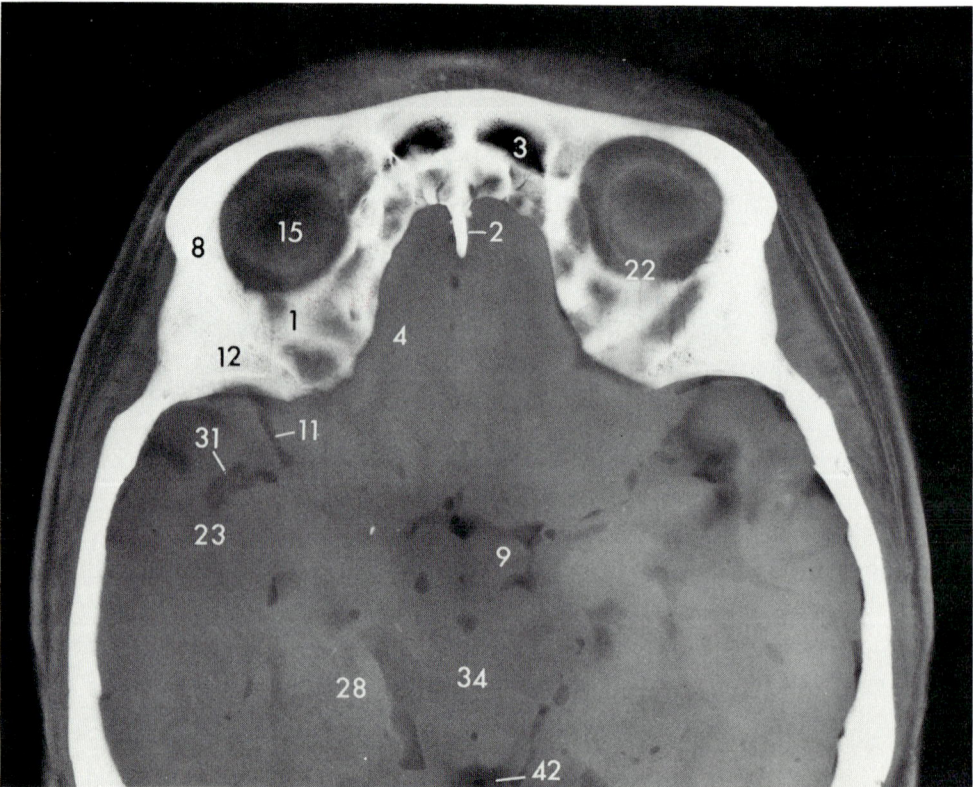

ORBIT

Level 4

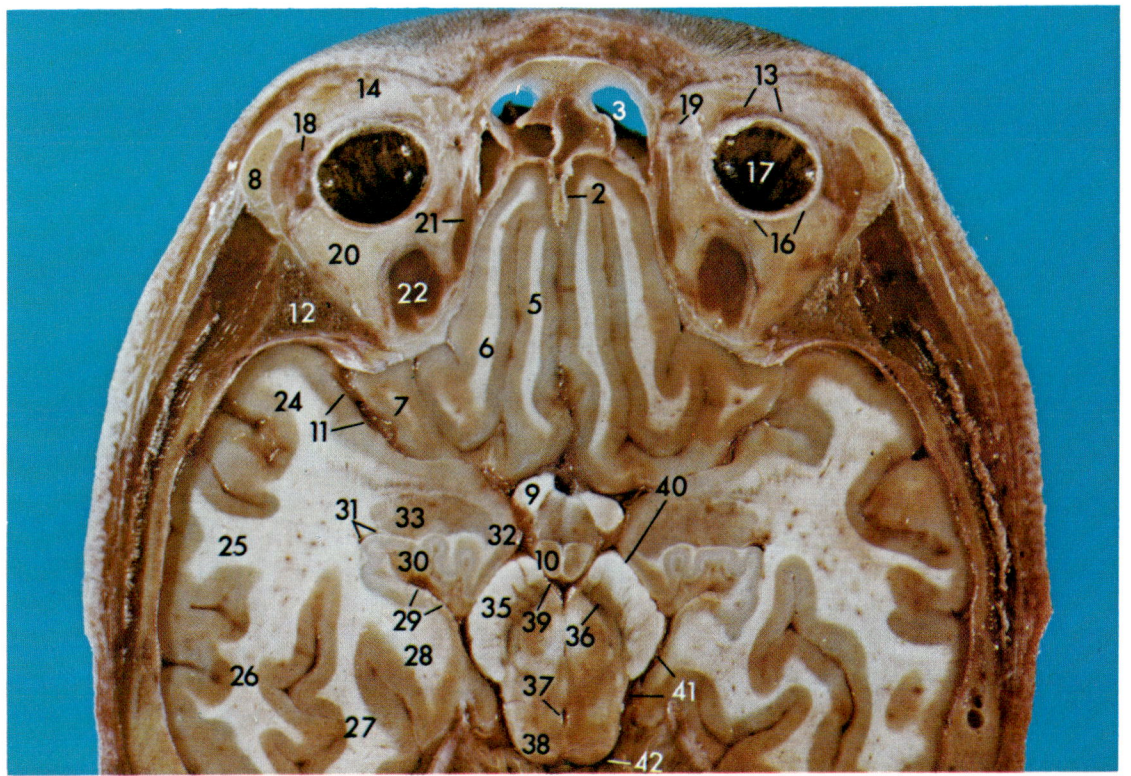

1. Frontal bone (orbital roof)
2. Crista galli
3. Frontal sinus
4. Frontal lobe
    5. Gyrus rectus
    6. Medial orbital gyrus
    7. Posterior orbital gyrus
8. Zygomatic process of frontal bone
9. Optic chiasm
10. Mamillary body
11. Sylvian fissure (with middle cerebral artery branches)
12. Greater wing of sphenoid
13. Orbicularis oculi muscle
14. Upper eyelid
15. Globe

Globe continued
16. Sclera
17. Retina
18. Lacrimal gland
19. Trochlea
20. Orbital fat
21. Superior oblique muscle
22. Superior rectus and levator palpebrae superioris muscles
23. Temporal lobe
    24. Superior temporal gyrus
    25. Middle temporal gyrus
    26. Inferior temporal gyrus
    27. Fusiform gyrus
    28. Parahippocampal gyrus
    29. Choroidal fissure

Temporal lobe continued
    30. Hippocampus
    31. Temporal horn of lateral ventricle (anterior tip)
    32. Uncus
    33. Amygdaloid nucleus
34. Midbrain
    35. Cerebral peduncle
    36. Substantia nigra
    37. Aqueduct of Sylvius
    38. Inferior colliculus
39. Interpeduncular cistern
40. Crural cistern
41. Circummesencephalic (ambient) cistern
42. Quadrigeminal cistern

47

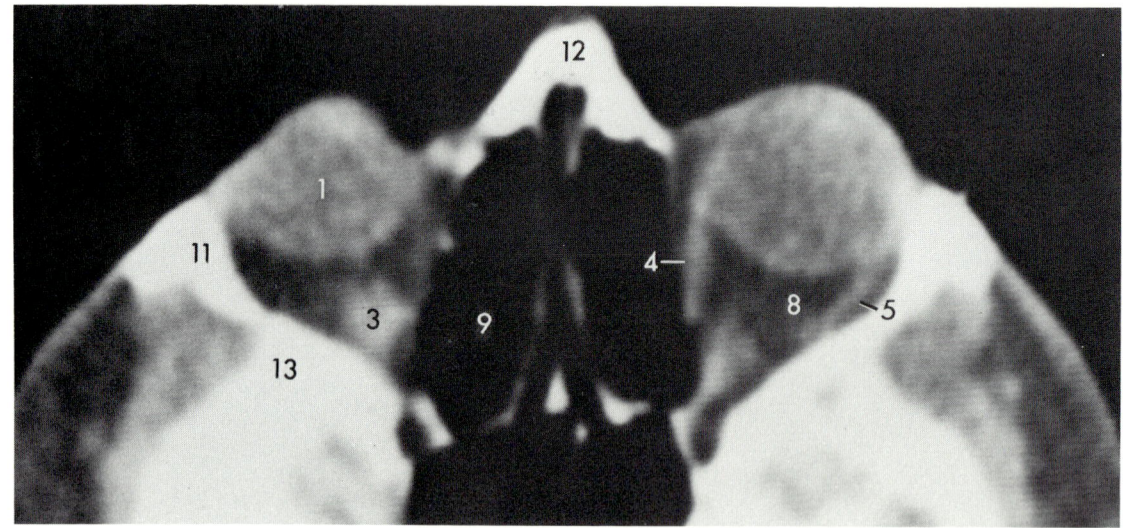

A. Lower level.

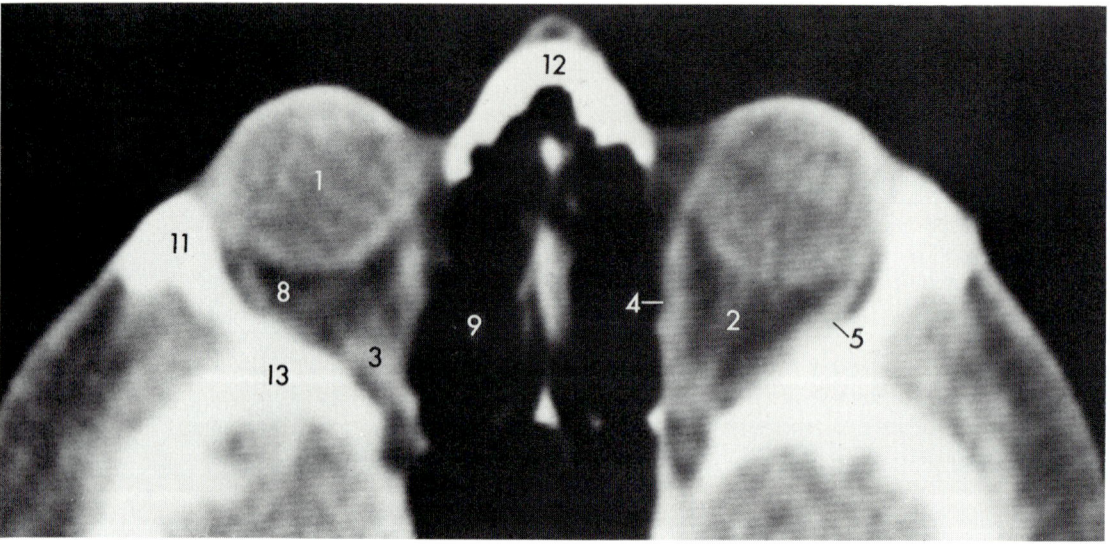

B. Higher level.

Fig. 2-1. Adjacent 8-mm-thick transaxial computed tomographic studies from a normal patient. The patient's head is slightly tilted so that the plane of section is not precisely horizontal; as a result, the structures visualized in the right orbit lie slightly inferior to those in the left orbit.

ORBIT

Normal *in Vivo* Computed Tomographic Studies

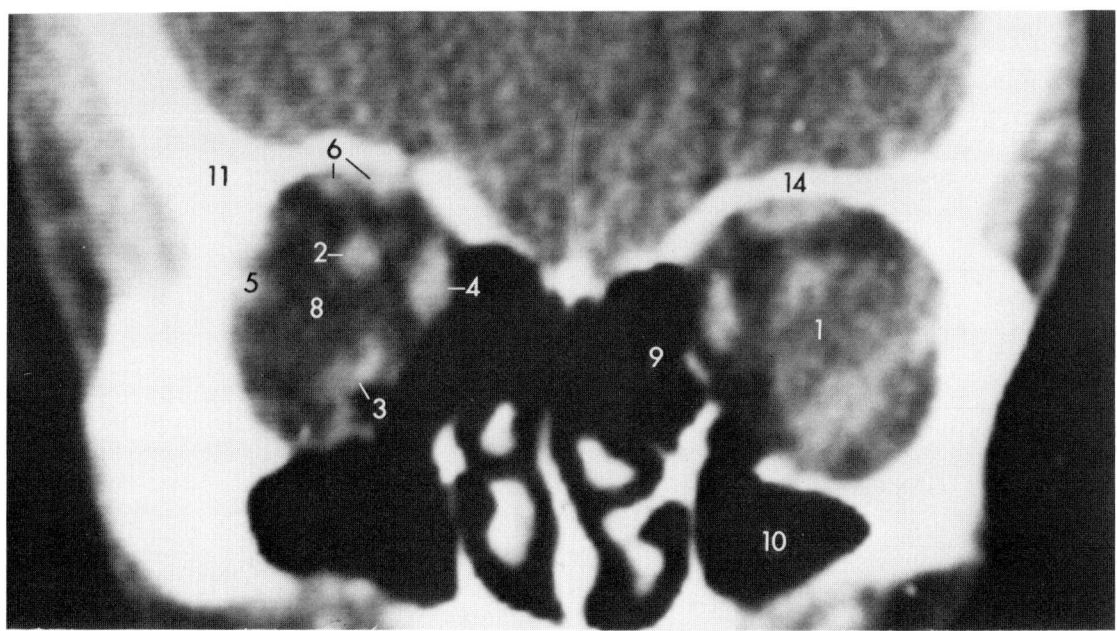

Fig. 2-2. Computed tomographic study in the coronal plane at a level just behind the globes. The patient's head is slightly rotated so that the plane of section passes through the posterior aspect of the left globe but behind the right globe.

1. Globe
2. Optic nerve (II)
3. Inferior rectus muscle
4. Medial rectus muscle
5. Lateral rectus muscle
6. Superior rectus and levator palpebrae superioris muscles
8. Retrobulbar fat
9. Ethmoid sinus
10. Maxillary sinus
11. Zygoma
12. Nasal bone
13. Greater wing of sphenoid
14. Frontal bone (orbital roof)

3
Neck and Face
LEO V. GOULD

This chapter displays the cross-sectional anatomy of the neck and the inferior facial structures. The lowest section (Level 1) is at a level immediately above the uppermost section of Chapter 4, although the illustrations in that chapter are from a different cadaver. Similarly, the higher sections include much of the anatomy of the base of the skull, and the highest section (Level 10) lies immediately below the lowest section of Chapter 2, although the illustrations in that chapter are also from a different cadaver.

The plane of anatomic section was unfortunately not always exactly horizontal so that the soft-tissue structures differ slightly in level from one side of the neck to the other. This is particularly true of the upper levels in this chapter where the obliquity of the plane of section is more apparent. It is a result of distortion of the cadaver while it was being frozen. The positive result of this change is that it provides the opportunity to develop a greater understanding of the differences in transverse surface anatomy at slightly different depths. However, a modest discrepancy is also apparent between the gross anatomic and radiographic images of the cut specimens and the computed tomographic image of the intact cadaver prior to sectioning. Nevertheless, the correspondence between the various images at any given level is sufficiently close to provide a clear roentgen–anatomic correlation.

The reader will note that many of the major blood vessels displayed on the computed tomographic images in this chapter appear lucent (black) and that the posterior cranial fossa is empty. The skullcap of this cadaver was opened, and the brain was transected at the cervicomedullary junction and removed from the cranial cavity, thus allowing air to enter some of the vessels prior to computed tomography. This also explains the artifact which is evident beneath the base of the skull on the right side of the computed tomographic image of Level 8.

The window and center settings selected for the computed tomographic images of the neck are most appropriate for the demonstration of soft-tissue anatomy. These generally fall in the range of 150–200 Hounsfield units for the window width, with a center of 50–80 Hounsfield units. The more inferior levels include a greater thickness of both soft tissues and bone and required a wider window. A more detailed evaluation of the bony anatomy of the cervical spine on computed tomography (utilizing a higher center and a wider window) may be found in Chapter 4. Center settings for the upper sections including the base of the skull are in the range of 80–100 Hounsfield units, with a window width of 300–400 Hounsfield units. The diameter of the scanning circle was 45 cm for Level 1 and 29 cm for Levels 2–10.

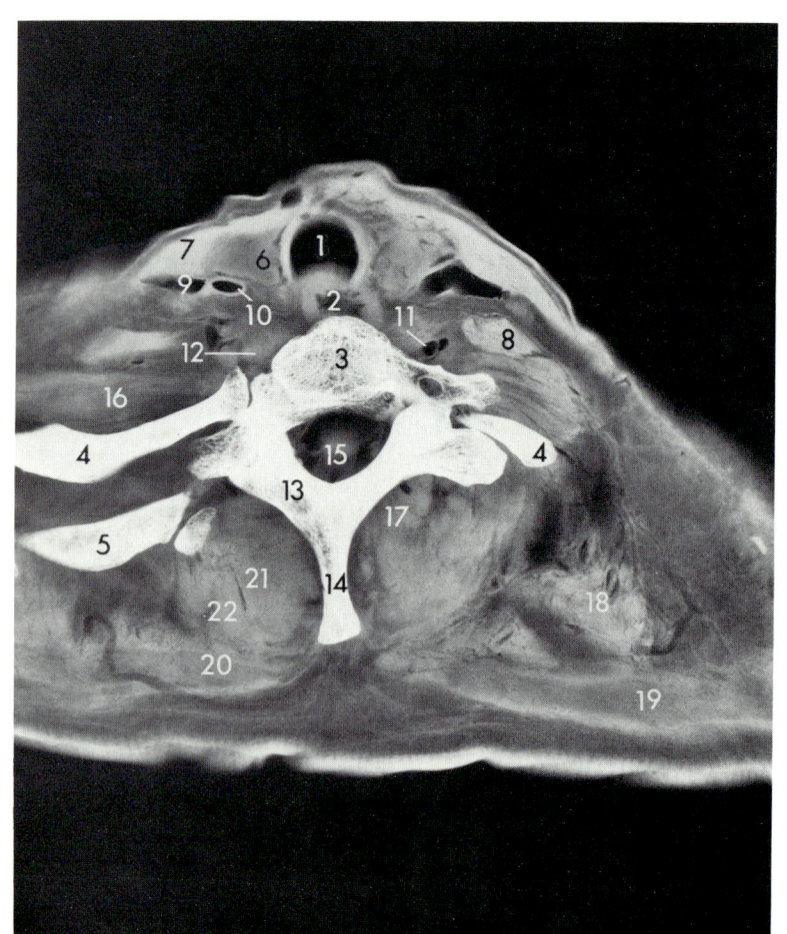
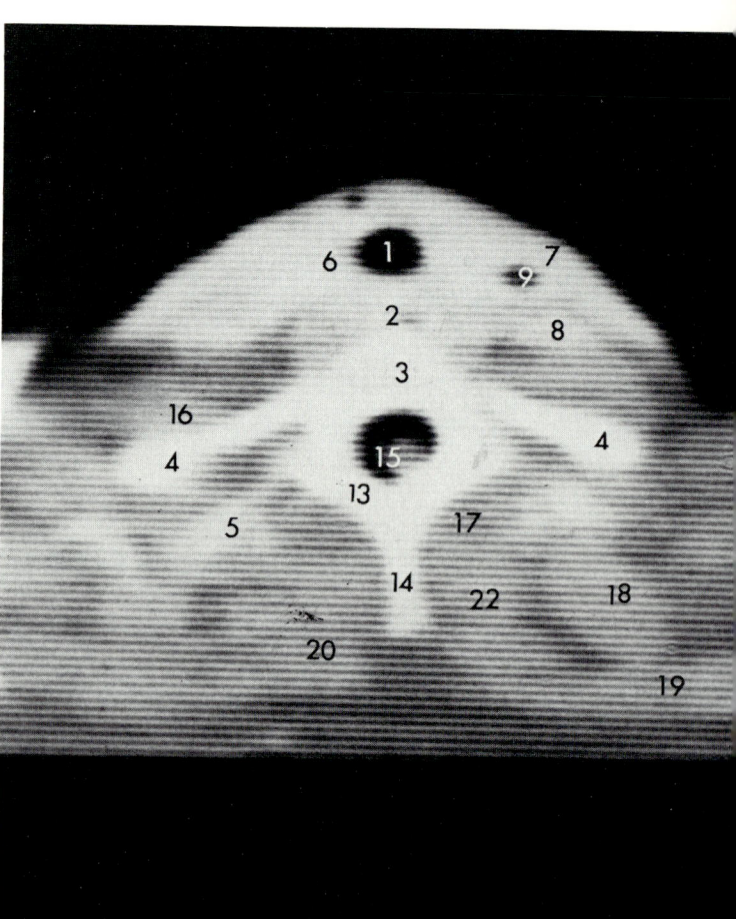
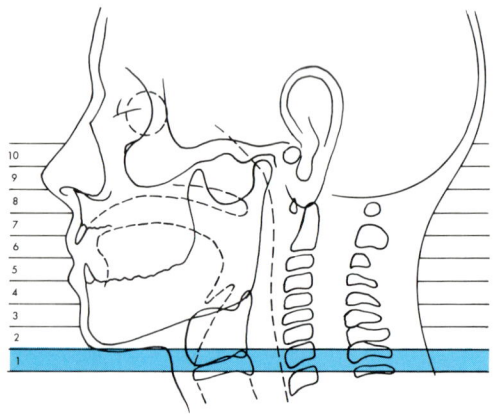

NECK AND FACE

Level 1

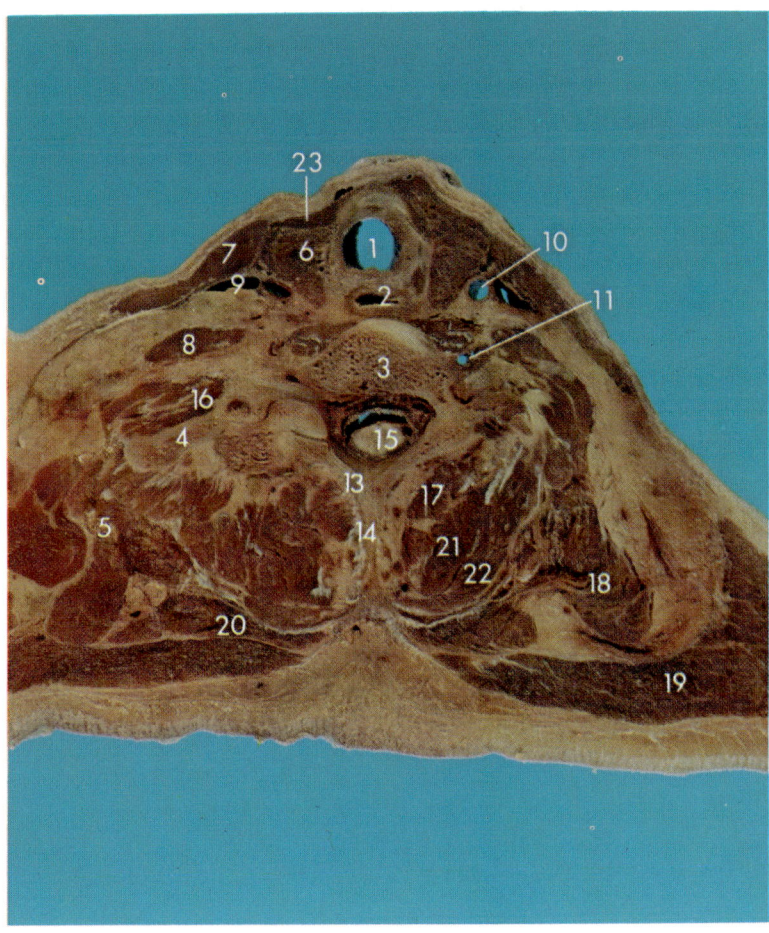

1. Trachea
2. Esophagus
3. Body of first thoracic vertebra
4. First rib
5. Second rib
6. Lateral lobe of thyroid gland
7. Sternocleidomastoid muscle
8. Scalenus anterior muscle
9. Internal jugular vein
10. Common carotid artery
11. Vertebral artery
12. Longus colli muscle
13. Lamina of first thoracic vertebra
14. Spinous process of first thoracic vertebra
15. Spinal cord
16. Scalenus medius and scalenus posterior muscles
17. Multifidus muscle
18. Levator scapulae muscle
19. Trapezius muscle
20. Rhomboideus minor muscle
21. Semispinalis cervicis and semispinalis capitis muscles
22. Splenius cervicis and splenius capitis muscles
23. Sternohyoid and sternothyroid muscles

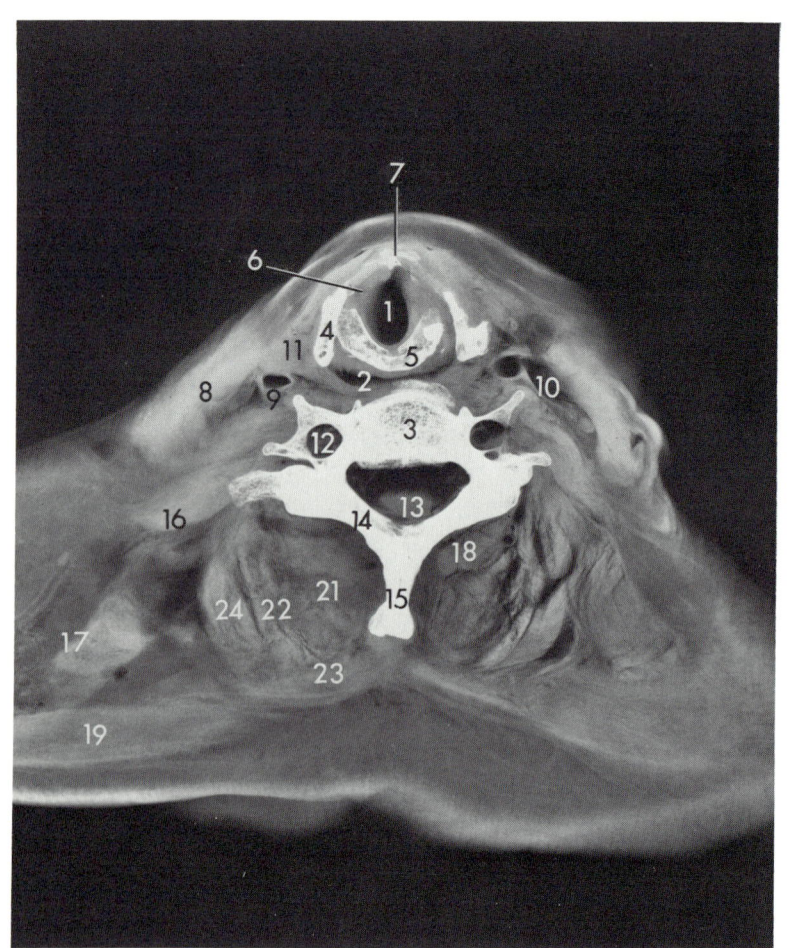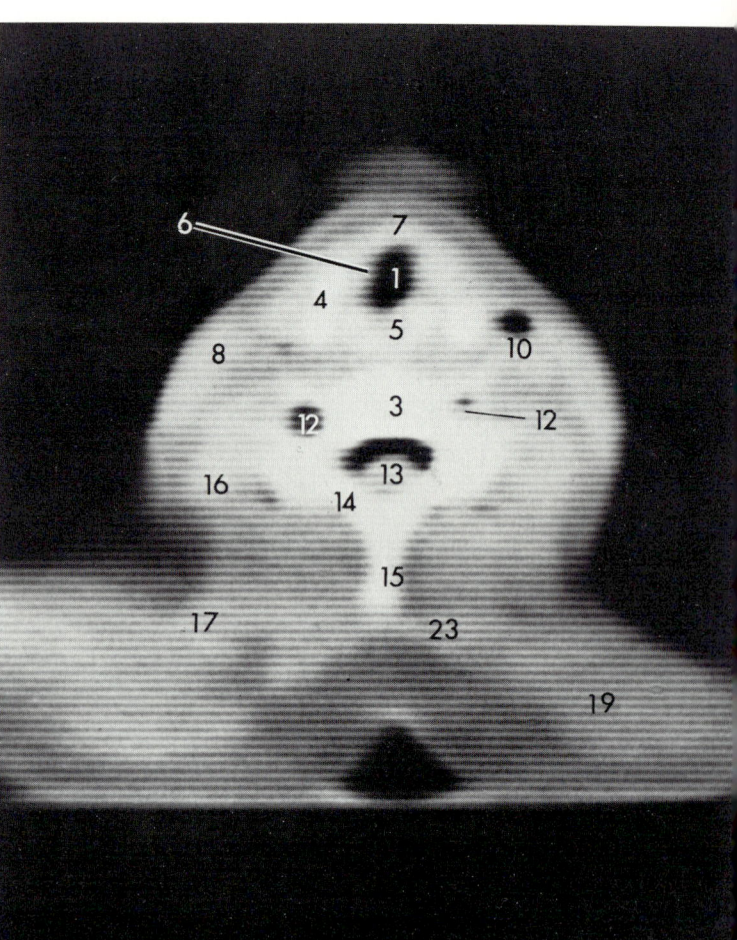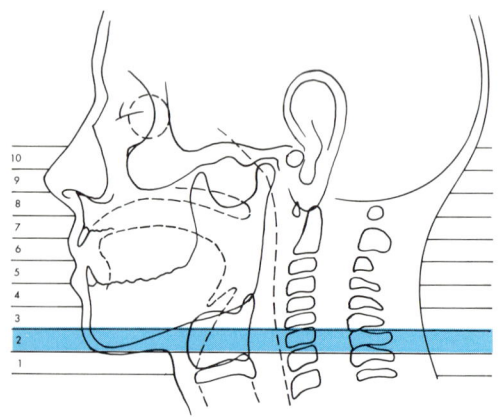

NECK AND FACE

Level 2

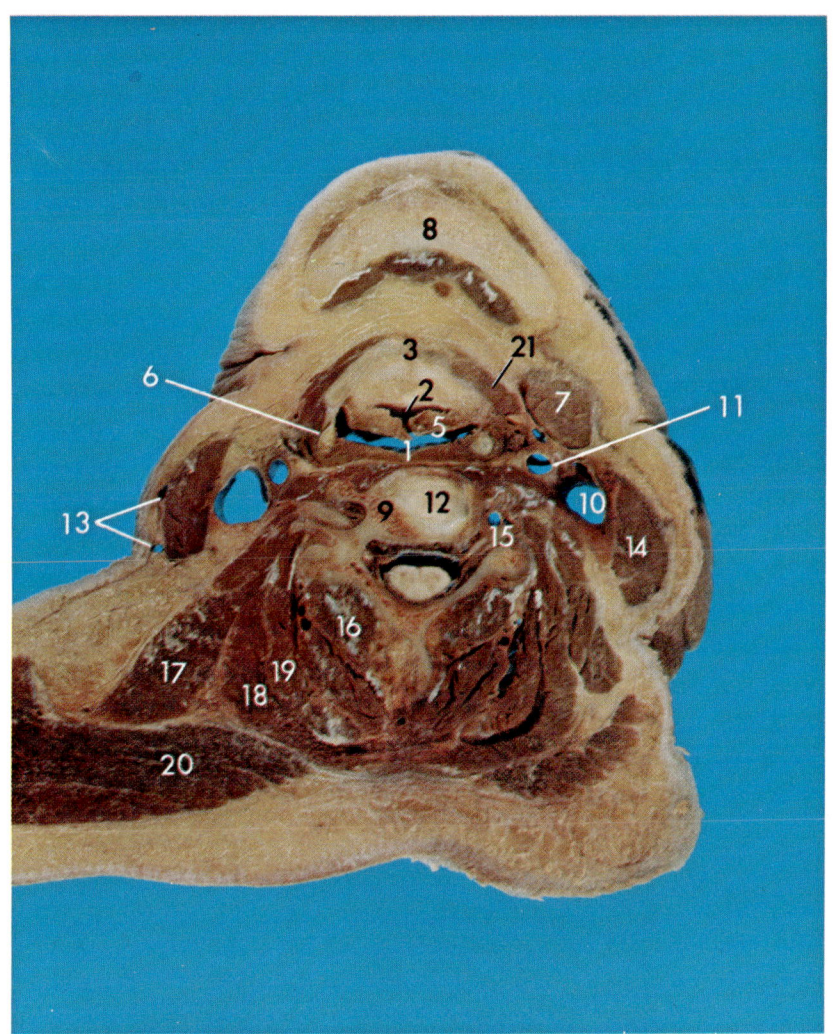

1. Hypopharynx
2. Vallecula of larynx
3. Body of hyoid bone
4. Greater cornu of hyoid bone
5. Aryepiglottic fold
6. Superior cornu of thyroid cartilage
7. Submaxillary gland
8. Mandible
9. Body of fifth cervical vertebra
10. Internal jugular vein
11. Common carotid artery
12. C5-6 intervertebral disc
13. External jugular vein branches
14. Sternocleidomastoid muscle
15. Vertebral artery (in foramen transversarium)
16. Multifidus muscle
17. Levator scapulae muscle
18. Splenius capitis muscle
19. Semispinalis capitis muscle
20. Trapezius muscle
21. Sternohyoid and omohyoid muscles
22. Base of epiglottic cartilage

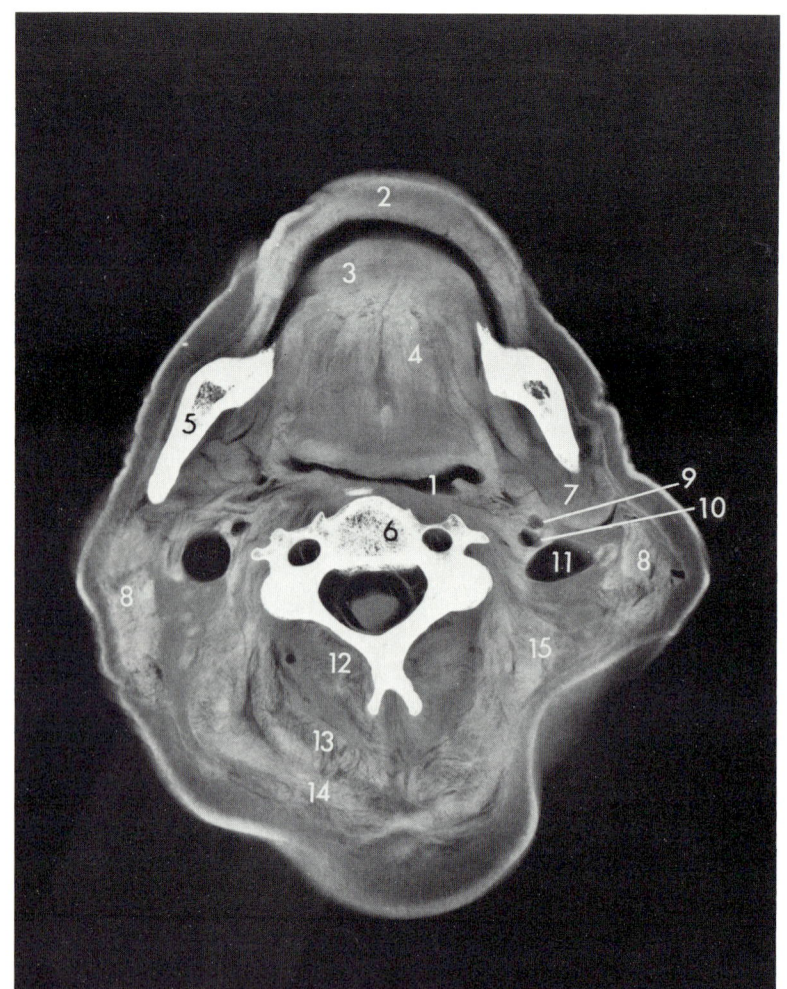
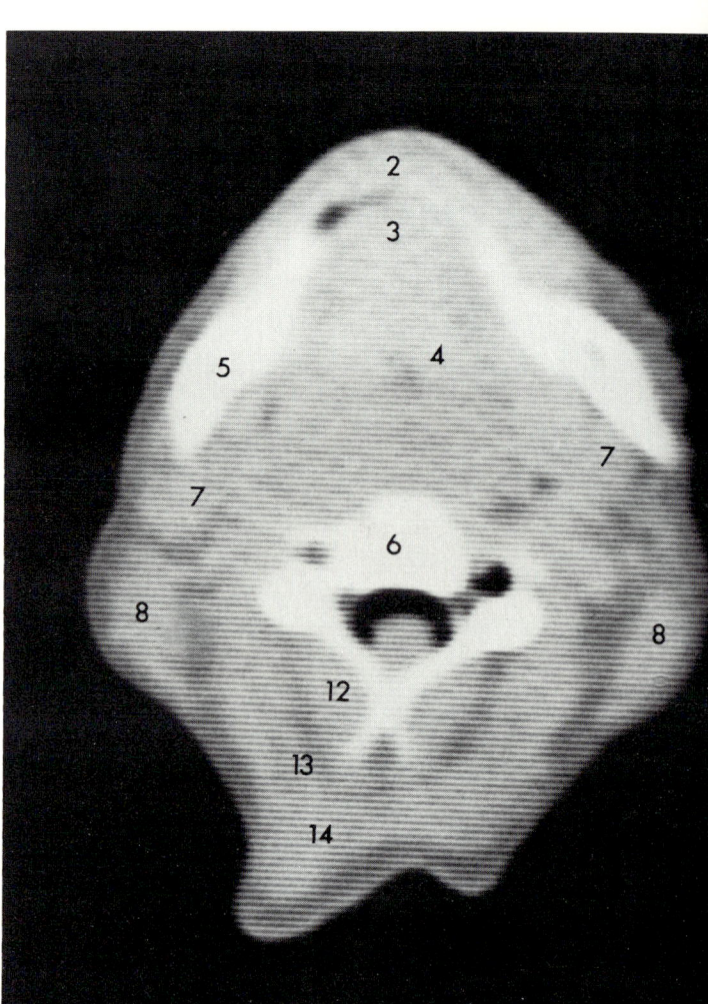
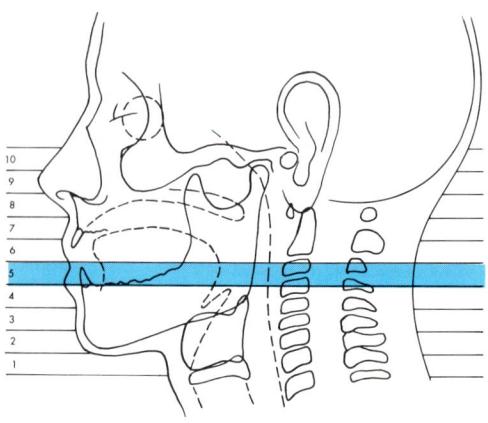

NECK AND FACE

Level 5

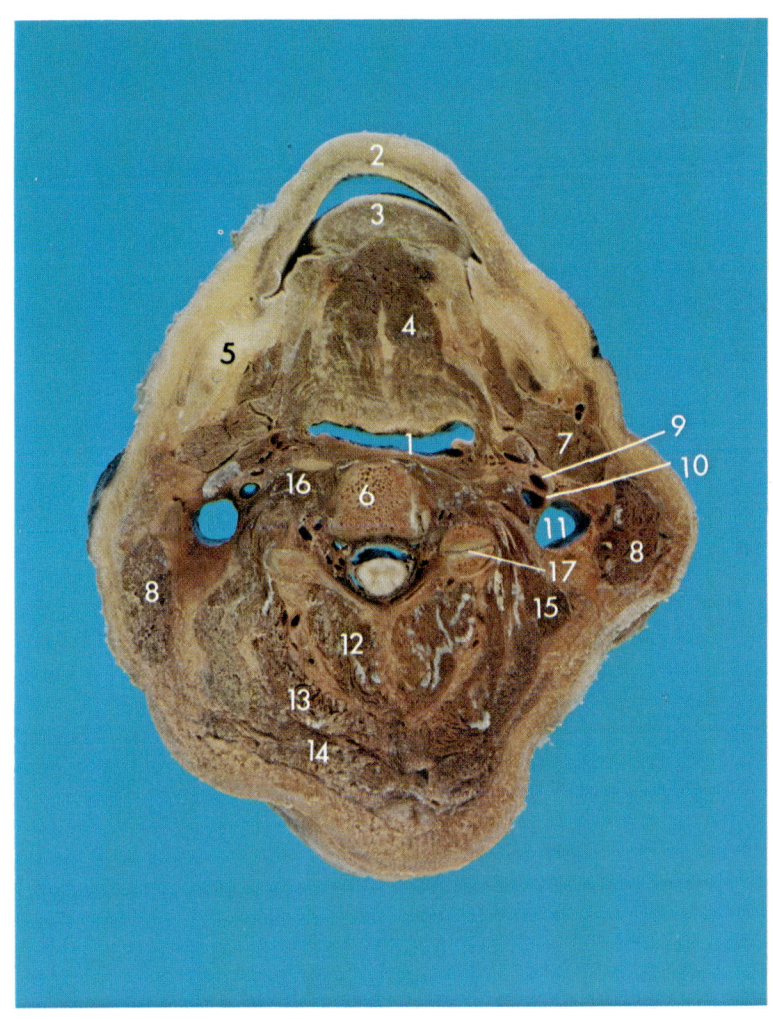

1. Oropharynx
2. Lower lip
3. Tongue
4. Genioglossus muscle
5. Mandible
6. Body of fourth cervical vertebra
7. Submaxillary gland
8. Sternocleidomastoid muscle
9. External carotid artery
10. Internal carotid artery
11. Internal jugular vein
12. Multifidus and semispinalis cervicis muscles
13. Semispinalis capitis muscle
14. Splenius capitis muscle
15. Levator scapulae muscle
16. Longus colli muscle
17. C4–5 apophyseal joint

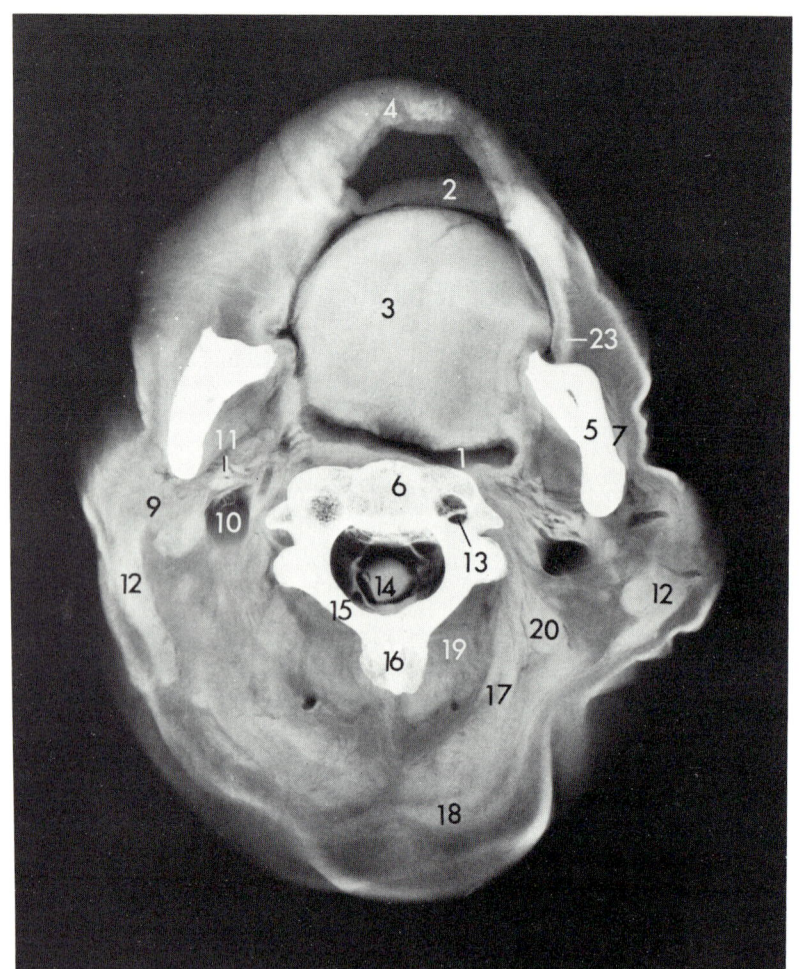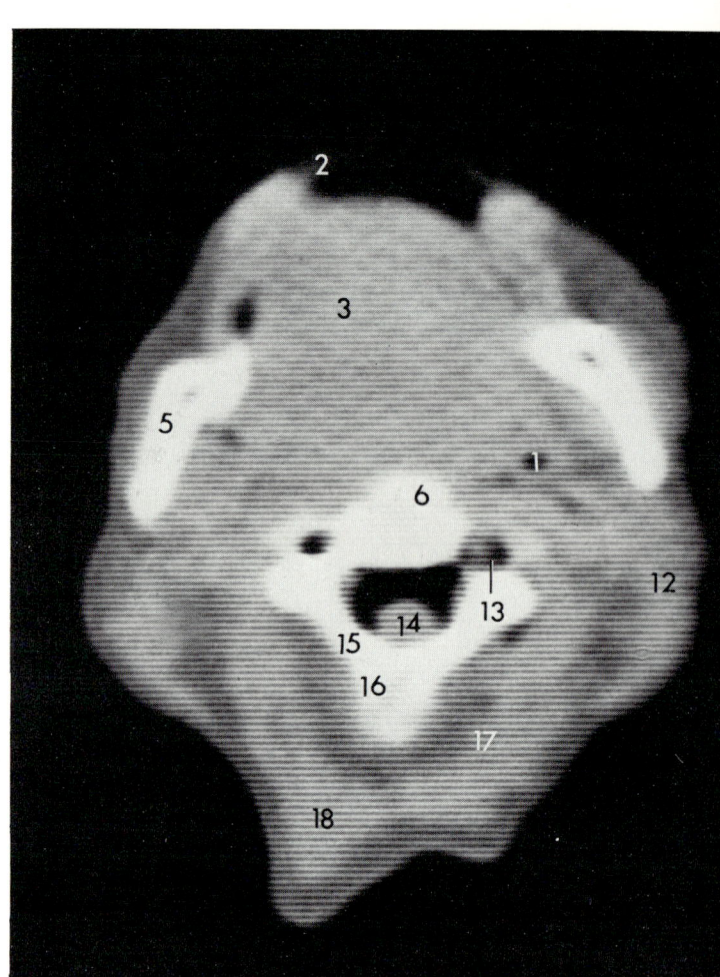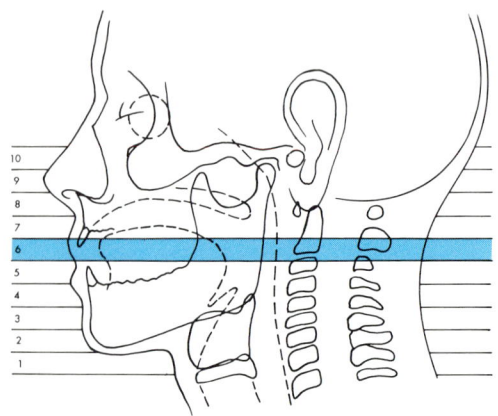

NECK AND FACE

Level 6

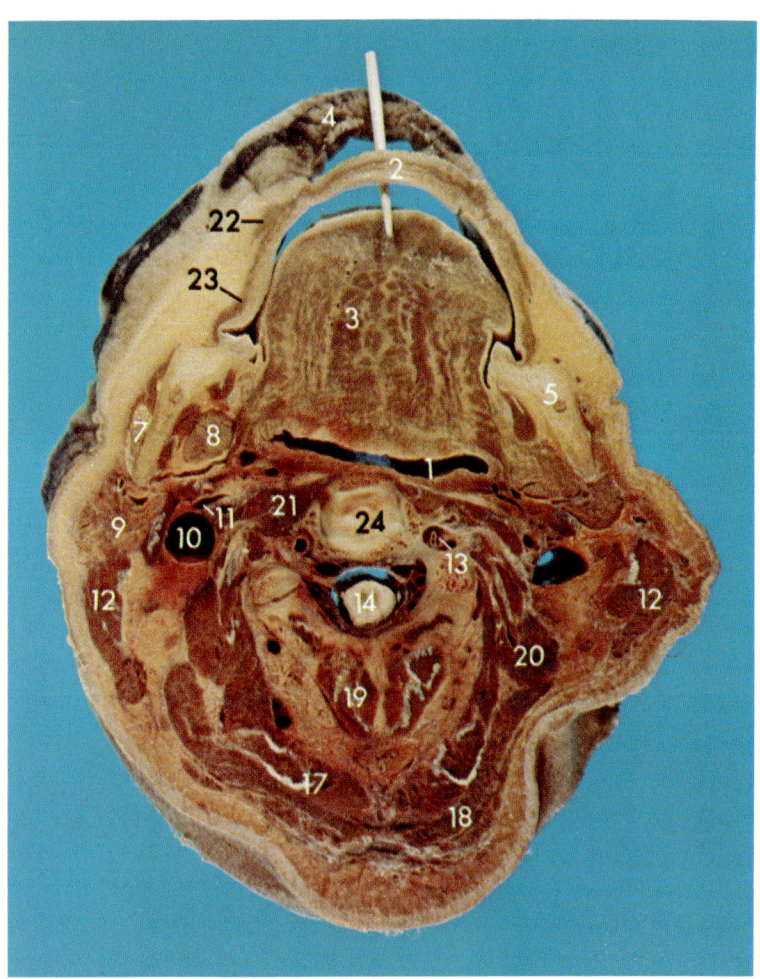

1. Oropharynx
2. Lower lip
3. Tongue
4. Upper lip
5. Ramus of mandible
6. Body of second cervical vertebra
7. Masseter muscle and tendon
8. Submaxillary gland
9. Parotid gland
10. Internal jugular vein
11. Internal carotid artery
12. Sternocleidomastoid muscle
13. Vertebral artery (in foramen transversarium)
14. Spinal cord
15. Lamina of second cervical vertebra
16. Spinous process of second cervical vertebra
17. Semispinalis capitis muscle
18. Splenius capitis muscle
19. Semispinalis cervicis muscle
20. Longissimus capitis muscle
21. Longus colli muscle
22. Orbicularis oris muscle
23. Buccinator muscle
24. C2–3 intervertebral disc

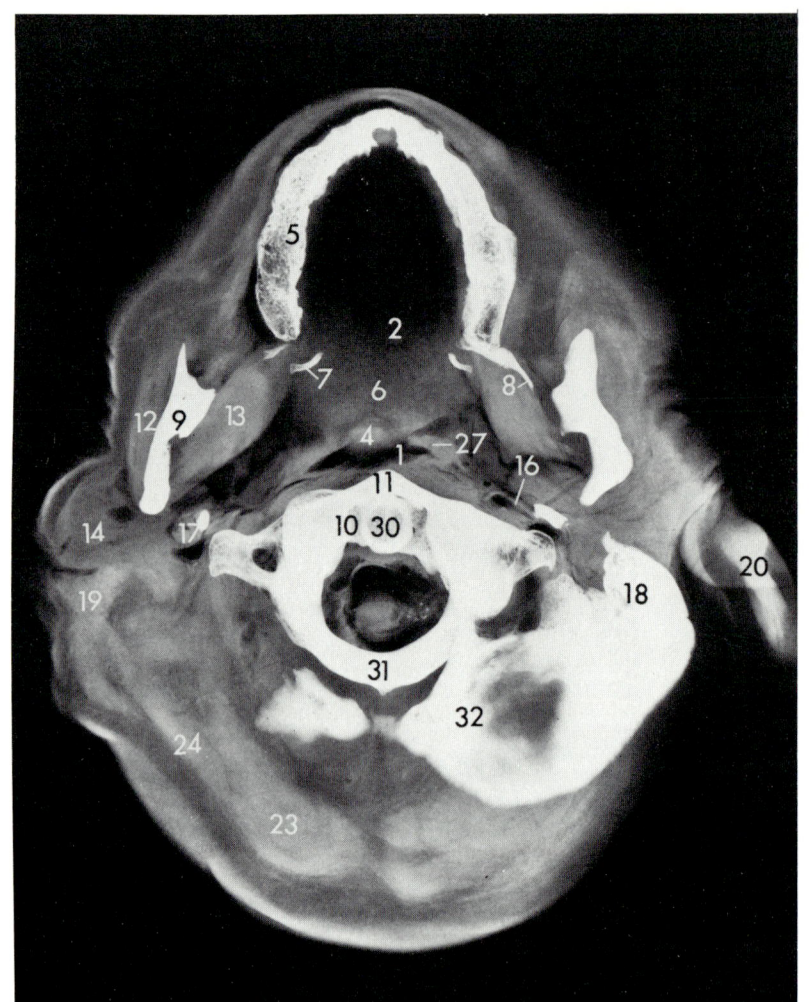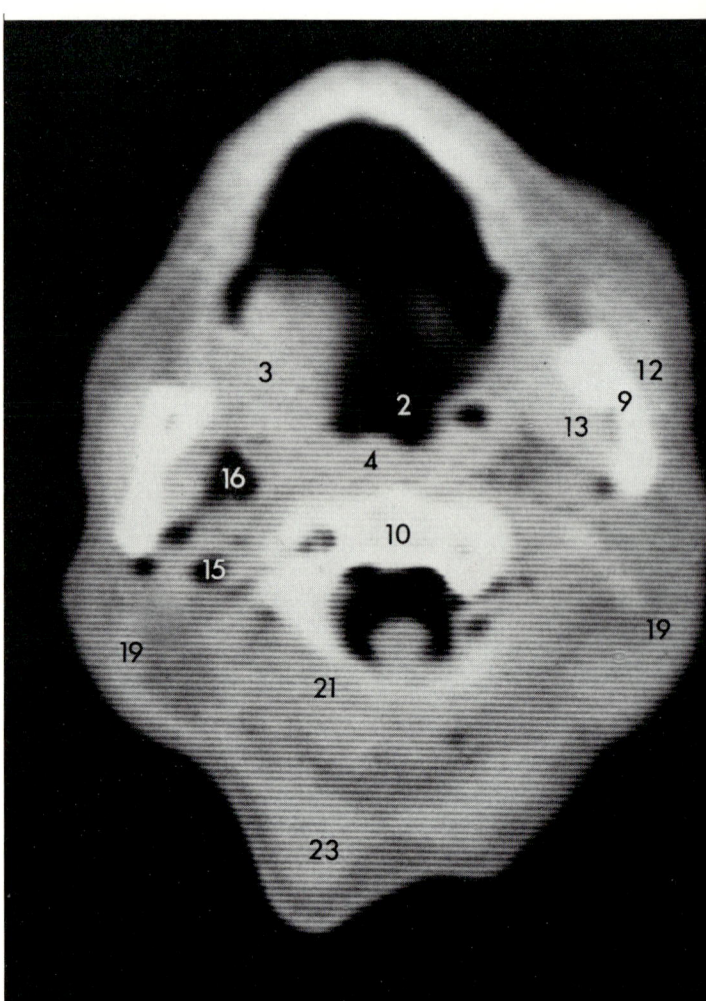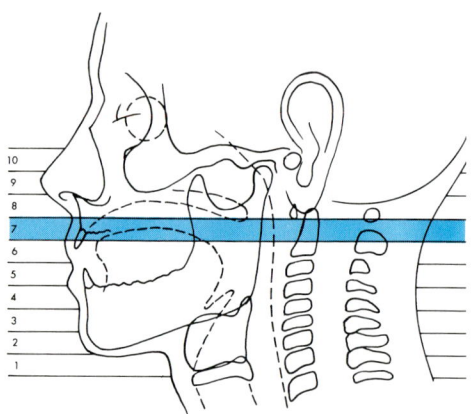

NECK AND FACE

Level 7

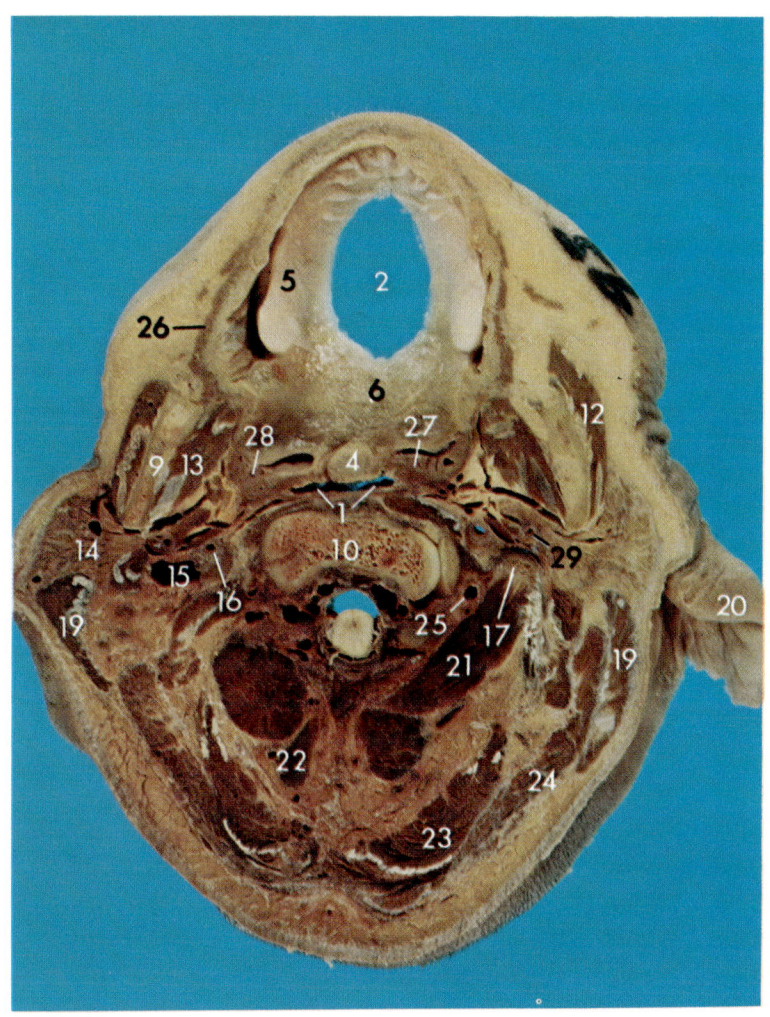

1. Oropharynx
2. Oral cavity
3. Tongue
4. Uvula
5. Superior alveolar ridge of maxilla
6. Soft palate
7. Pterygoid hamulus
8. Lateral pterygoid plate
9. Ramus of mandible
10. Body of second cervical vertebra
11. Anterior arch of first cervical vertebra
12. Masseter muscle and tendon
13. Internal pterygoid muscle
14. Parotid gland
15. Internal jugular vein
16. Internal carotid artery
17. Styloid process of temporal bone
18. Mastoid portion of temporal bone
19. Sternocleidomastoid muscle
20. Pinna
21. Obliquus capitis inferior muscle
22. Rectus capitis posterior muscle
23. Semispinalis capitis muscle
24. Splenius capitis muscle
25. Vertebral artery
26. Buccinator muscle
27. Pharyngopalatine muscle and arch (posterior faucial pillar)
28. Palatine tonsil
29. External carotid artery
30. Odontoid process of second cervical vertebra
31. Posterior arch of first cervical vertebra
32. Occipital bone

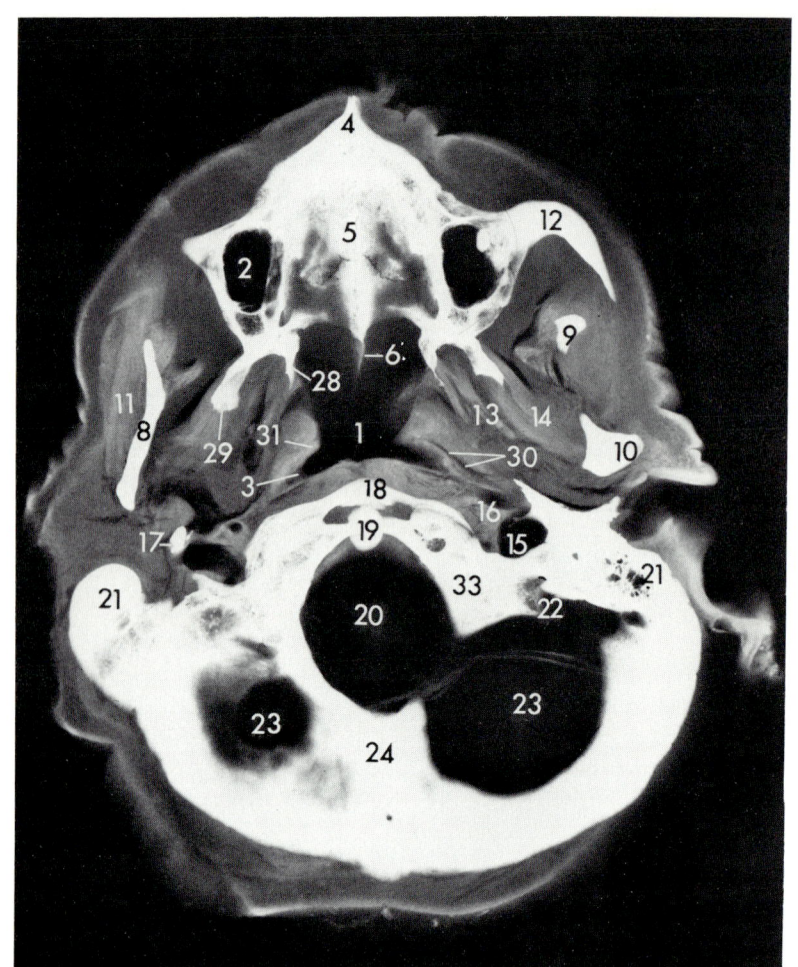
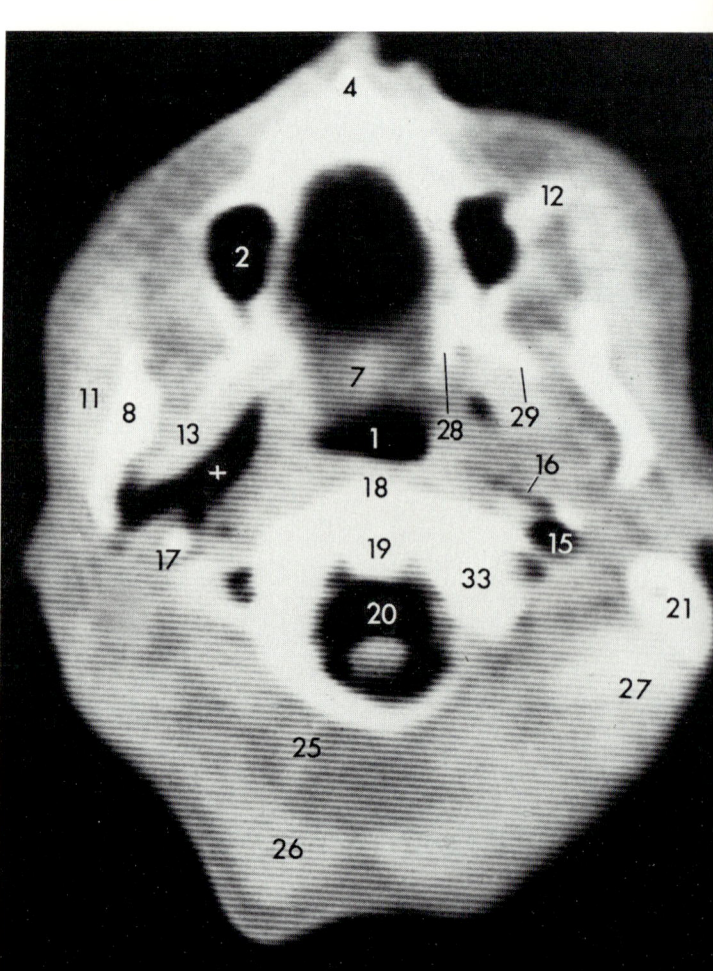
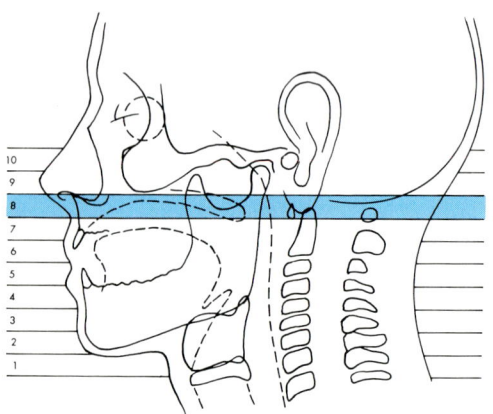

NECK AND FACE

Level 8

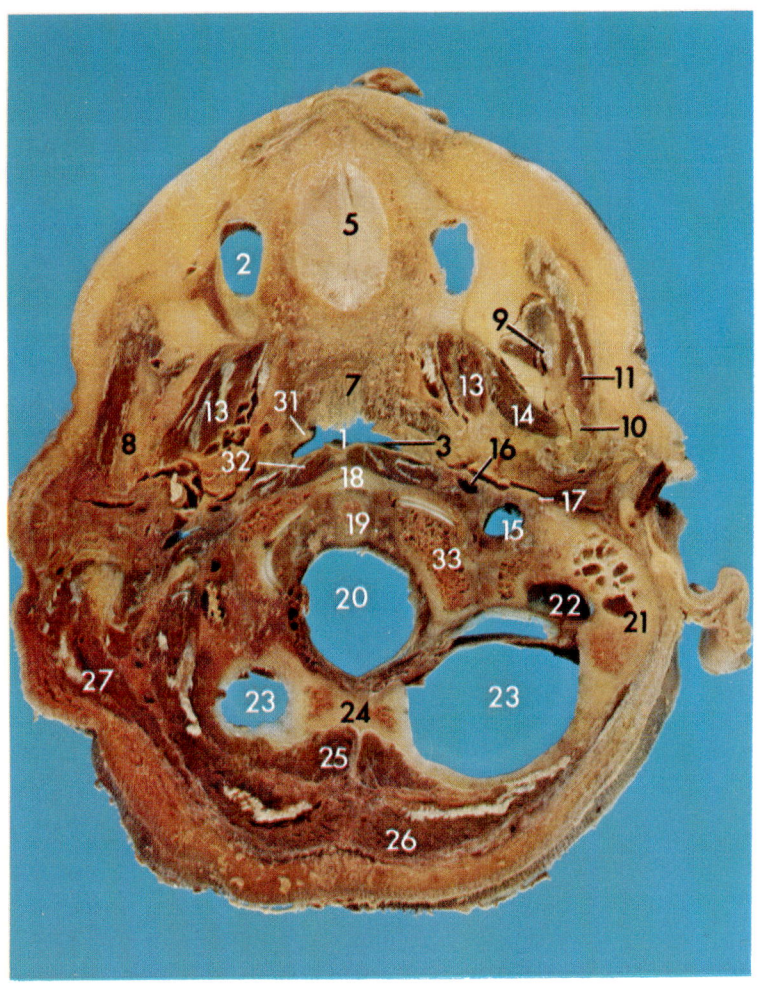

1. Nasopharynx
2. Maxillary sinus
3. Pharyngeal recess (fossa of Rosenmüller)
4. Anterior nasal spine of maxilla
5. Palatine process of maxilla (hard palate)
6. Vomer (bony nasal septum)
7. Soft palate
8. Ramus of mandible
9. Coronoid process of mandible
10. Condyle of mandible
11. Masseter muscle and tendon
12. Zygoma
13. Internal pterygoid muscle
14. External pterygoid muscle
15. Internal jugular vein
16. Internal carotid artery
17. Styloid process of temporal bone
18. Anterior arch of first cervical vertebra
19. Odontoid process of second cervical vertebra
20. Foramen magnum
21. Mastoid portion of temporal bone
22. Sigmoid sinus
23. Posterior cranial fossa
24. Occipital bone
25. Rectus capitis posterior muscle
26. Semispinalis capitis muscle
27. Sternocleidomastoid muscle
28. Medial pterygoid plate
29. Lateral pterygoid plate
30. Auditory (Eustachian) tube
31. Torus tubarius
32. Longus capitis muscle
33. Occipital condyle
+ Artifact

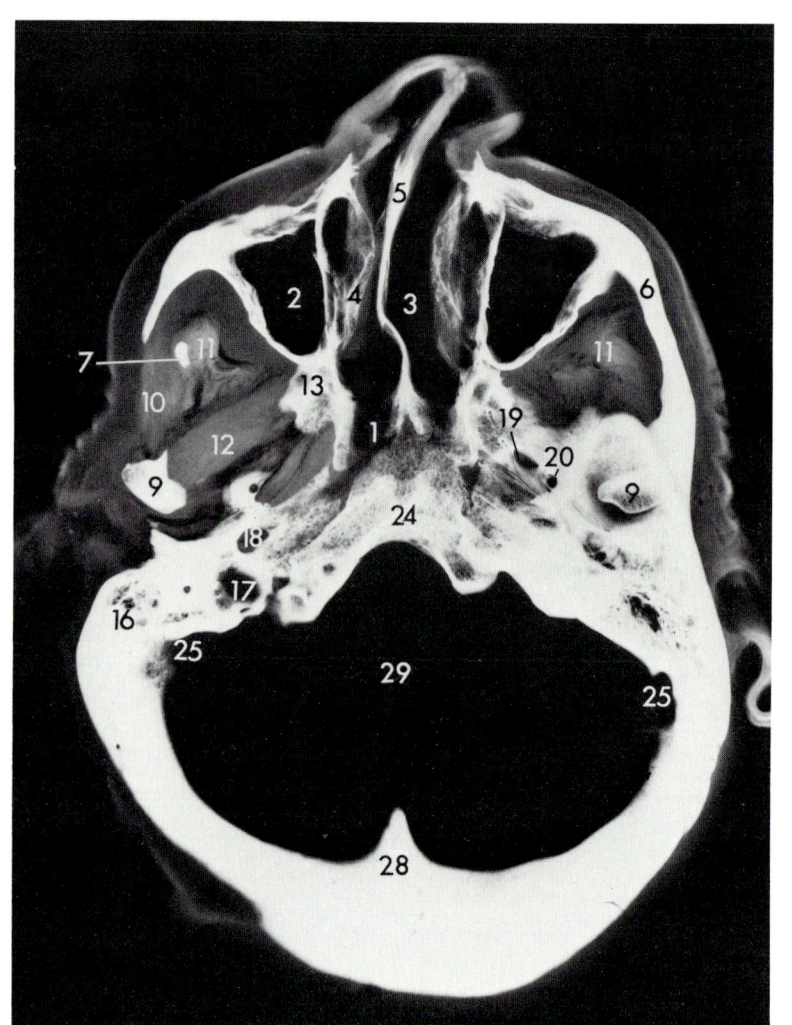
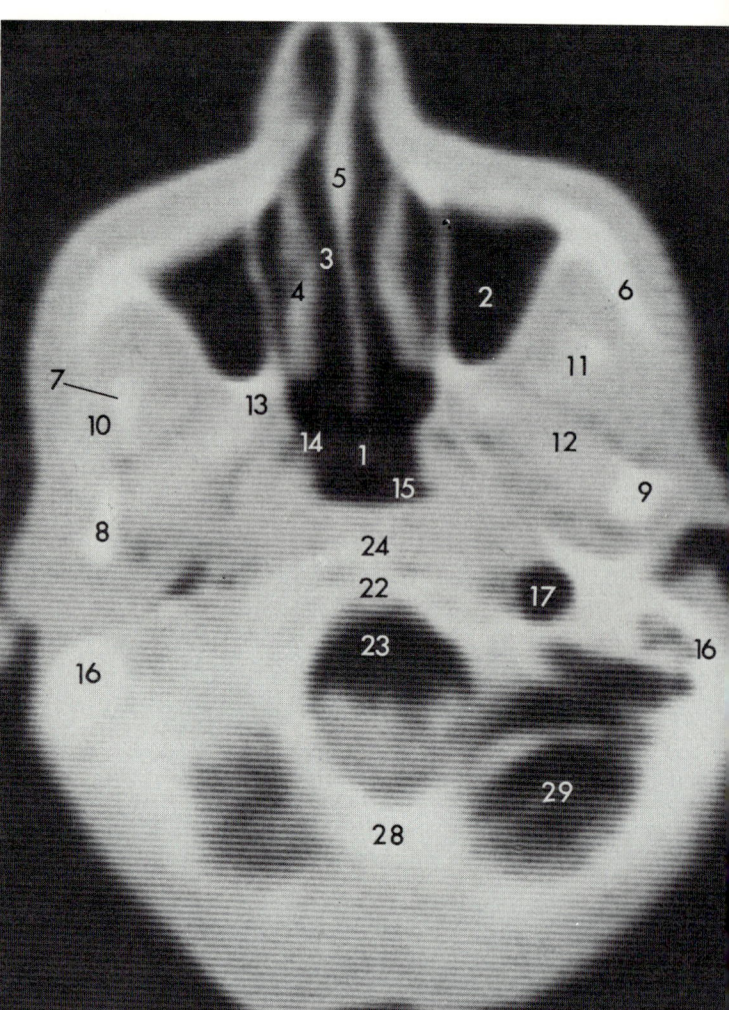
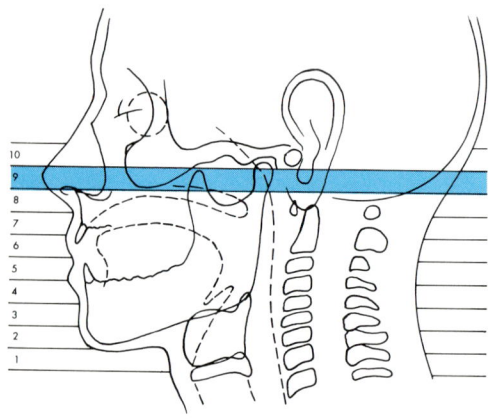

NECK AND FACE

LEVEL 9

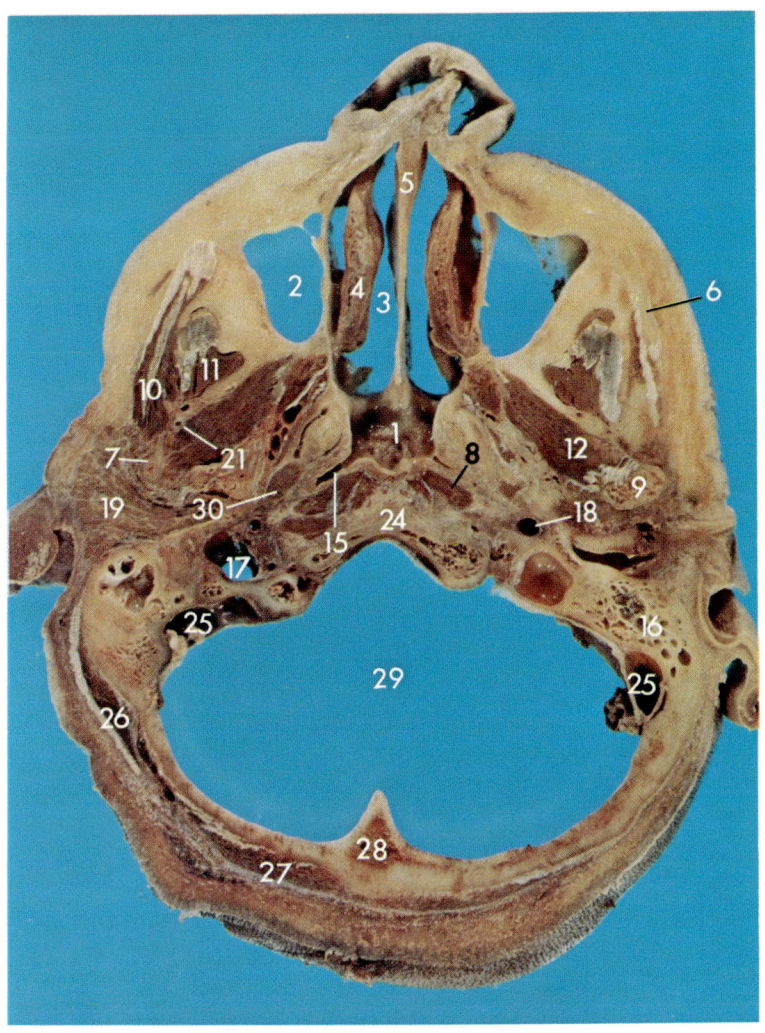

1. Nasopharynx
2. Maxillary sinus
3. Nasal fossa
4. Inferior nasal concha
5. Vomer (bony nasal septum)
6. Zygoma
7. Coronoid process of mandible
8. Longus capitis muscle
9. Condyle of mandible
10. Masseter muscle and tendon
11. Temporalis muscle and tendon
12. External pterygoid muscle
13. Pterygoid process of sphenoid bone
14. Auditory (Eustachian) tube orifice
15. Pharyngeal recess (fossa of Rosenmüller)
16. Mastoid portion of temporal bone
17. Jugular foramen
18. Carotid canal (internal carotid artery)
19. Foramen ovale
20. Foramen spinosum
21. Internal maxillary artery
22. Anterior arch of first cervical vertebra
23. Foramen magnum
24. Clivus (basisphenoid)
25. Transverse sinus
26. Sternocleidomastoid muscle
27. Semispinalis capitis muscle
28. Internal occipital crest
29. Posterior cranial fossa
30. Levator veli palatini muscle

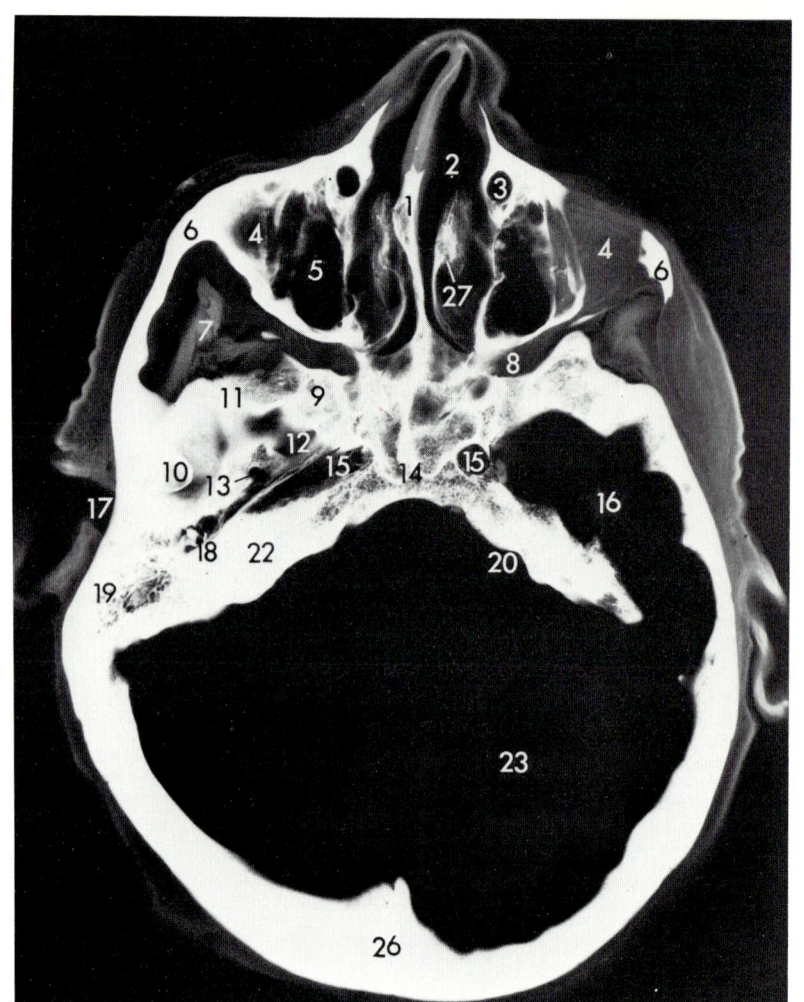
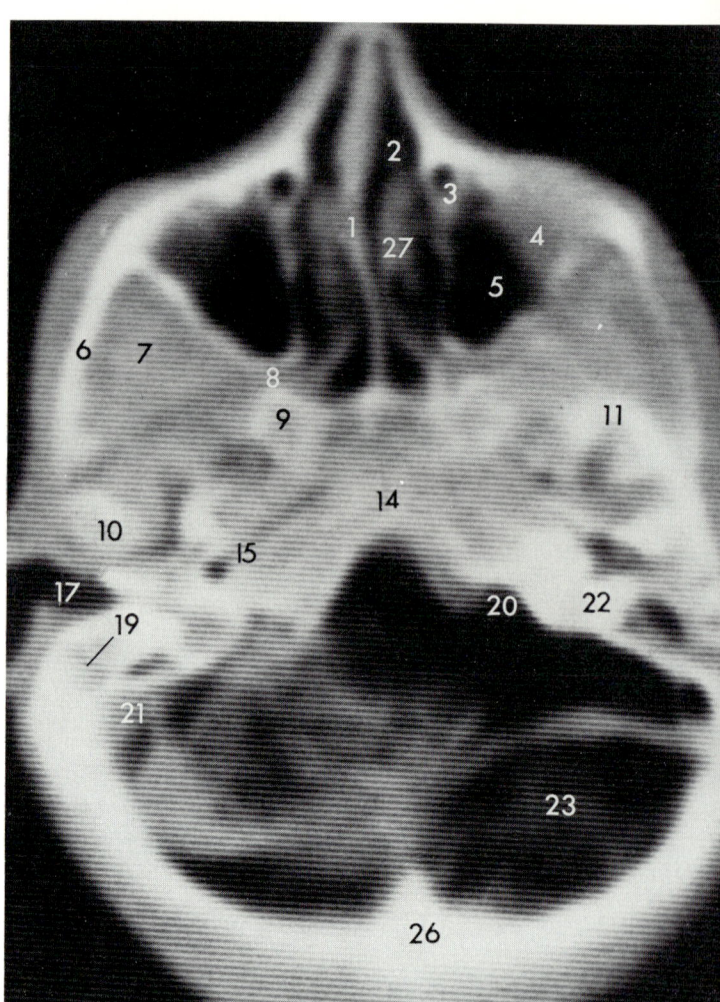
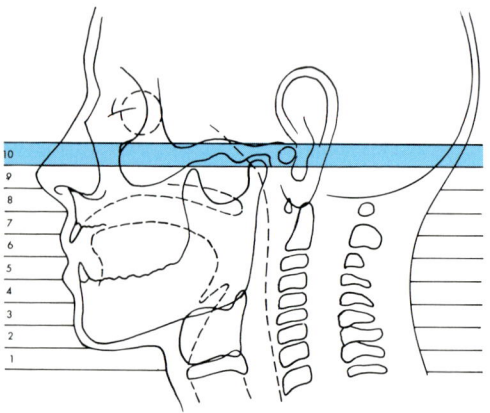

NECK AND FACE

Level 10

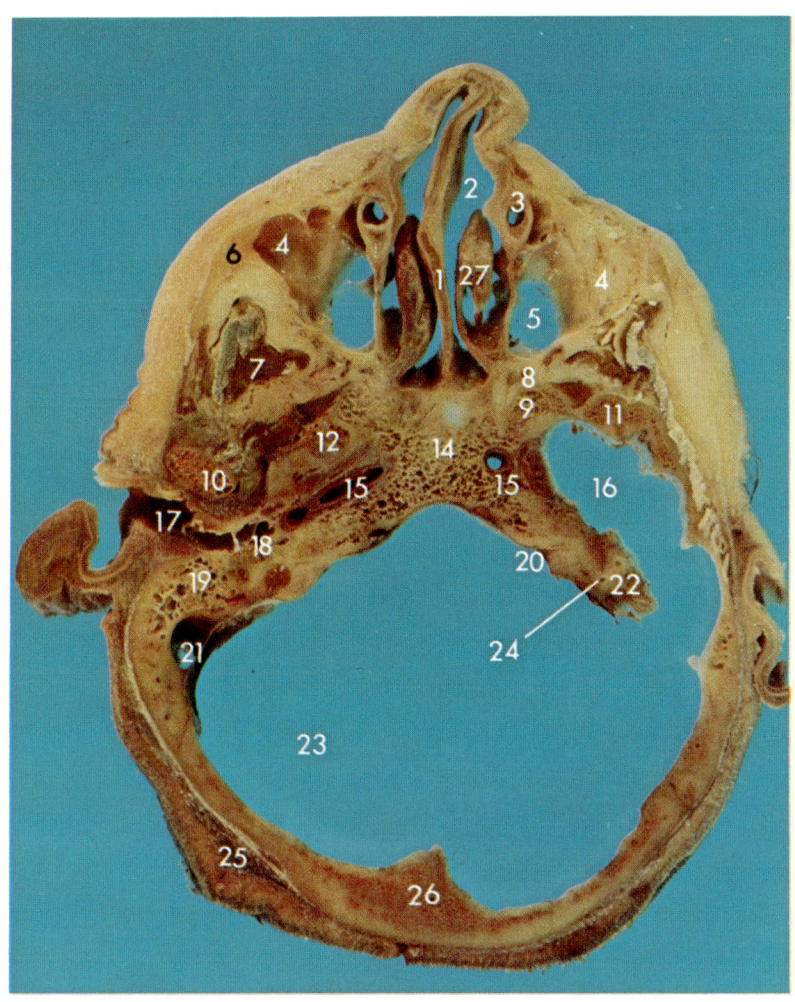

1. Vomer (bony nasal septum)
2. Nasal fossa
3. Nasolacrimal canal
4. Floor of orbit (orbital fat)
5. Maxillary sinus
6. Zygoma
7. Temporalis muscle and tendon
8. Pterygopalatine fossa
9. Pterygoid process of sphenoid
10. Condyle of mandible
11. Greater wing of sphenoid
12. Foramen ovale
13. Foramen spinosum
14. Body of sphenoid
15. Carotid canal (internal carotid artery)
16. Middle cranial fossa
17. External auditory canal
18. Tympanic (middle ear) cavity
19. Mastoid portion of temporal bone
20. Internal auditory meatus
21. Transverse sinus
22. Petrous portion of temporal bone
23. Posterior cranial fossa
24. Superior semicircular canal
25. Occipitalis muscle
26. Internal occipital crest
27. Middle nasal concha

4
Spine

EUGENE F. BINET

The complexity of the vertebral column, the contents of the spinal canal, and the paravertebral soft tissues require the inclusion of a separate chapter on the spine in this atlas. Representative cross sections from the midportions of the lumbar, thoracic, and cervical spine have been supplemented by sections through the lumbosacral and thoracolumbar junctions and three sections of the upper cervical spine.

Because of the curvatures of the normal spine, portions of two adjacent vertebrae are included within a single section at several levels. This is most notable in the lumbosacral region (Level 2), where the horizontal plane of section passes obliquely through the anteroinferior portion of the body of L_5, the midportion of the L_5–S_1 intervertebral disc, and the posterosuperior portion of the body of S_1. At other levels, portions of the posterior neural arches of two adjacent vertebrae together with the intervening apophyseal joints are included in the same section.

The anatomic sections in this chapter were selected from three different cadavers. In Levels 1–8, the cadavers were partially fixed in formalin prior to freezing and sectioning. In Levels 9 and 10, the cadaver was frozen and sectioned without prior fixation; the lack of chemical fixation explains the fleshy tones of the tissues in the anatomic illustrations of these levels.

As elsewhere in this volume, most sections are displayed as viewed from below (inferior aspect). Exceptions to this rule are Levels 1, 2, 3, and 7, in which the pertinent anatomy on the gross specimen is best seen on the superior aspect, and thus the anatomic illustrations for these levels are displayed as viewed from above.

Technical factors for the computed tomographic images included a center of 150–200 Hounsfield units and a window width of 450–550 Hounsfield units. These settings correspond closely to those used in clinical practice for discerning bony detail. However, because of the relatively wide window, differentiation of soft-tissue structures is somewhat diminished. The diameter of the scanning circle for the computed tomographic images of the sacral, lumbar, and thoracic spine was 45 cm and for the images of the cervical spine 29 cm.

The availability of metrizamide (Amipaque), a water-soluble contrast medium for myelography, has made possible the identification of the spinal cord within the opacified spinal subarachnoid space on computed tomography. A series of representative transaxial images from living patients has therefore been included at the conclusion of this chapter.

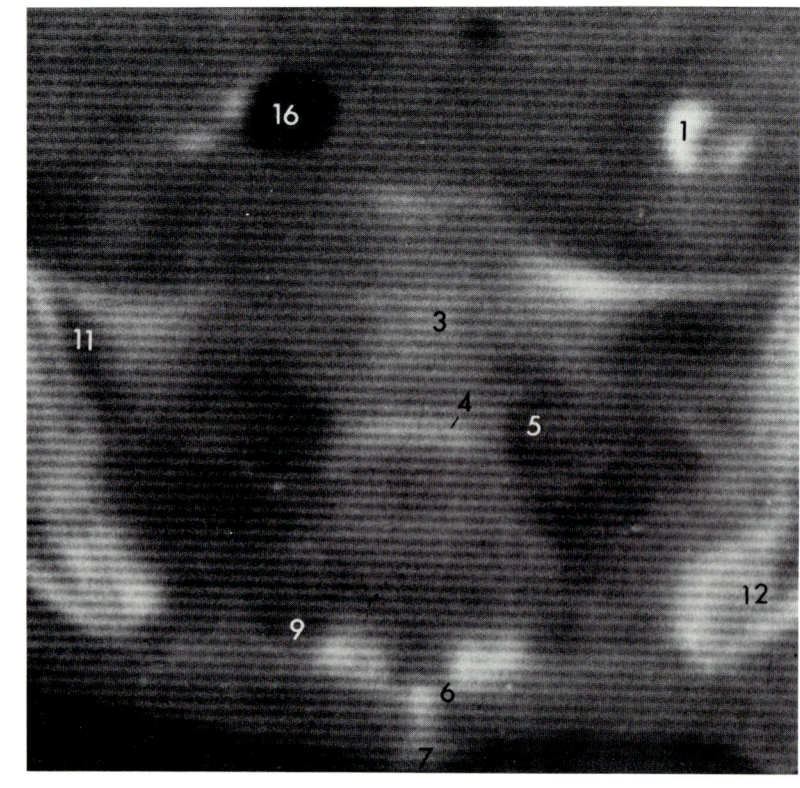

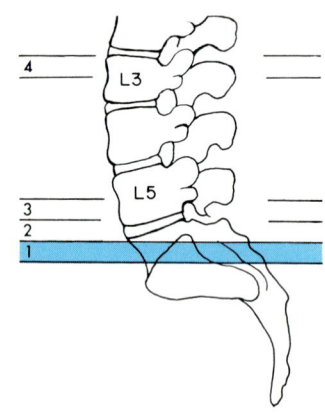

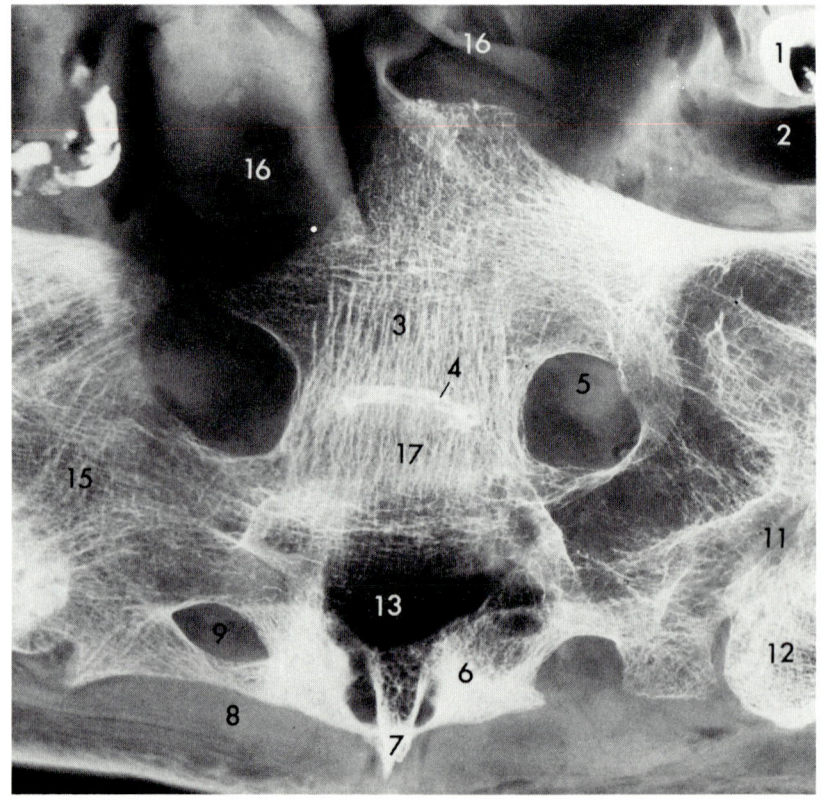

SPINE

**Level 1
(Superior aspect)**

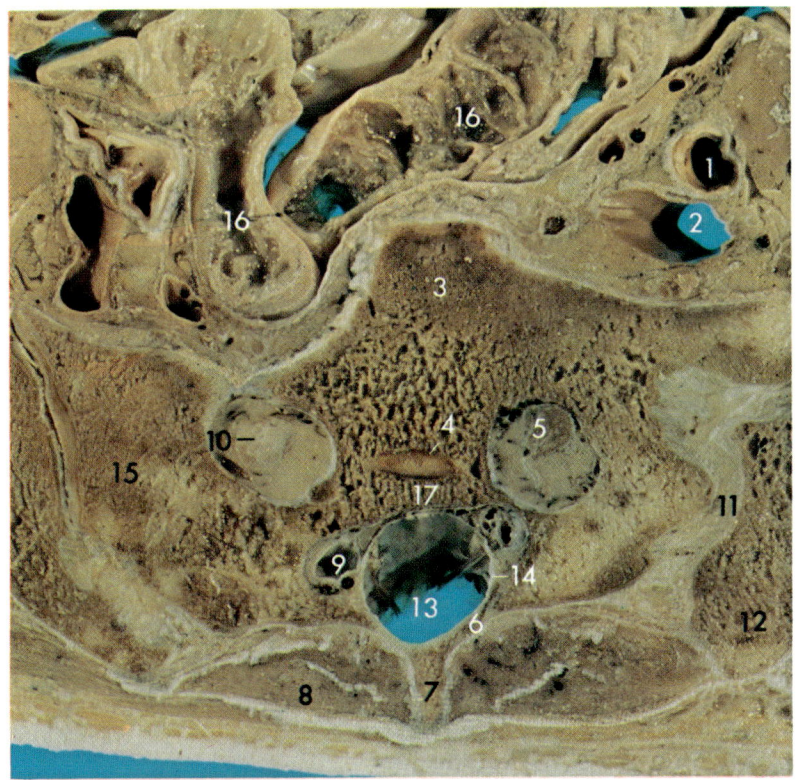

1. External iliac artery
2. External iliac vein
3. Body of first sacral vertebra
4. S1–2 intervertebral disc
5. Anterior sacral foramen
6. Lamina of second sacral vertebra
7. Spinous process of second sacral vertebra
8. Multifidus muscle
9. Posterior sacral foramen
10. First sacral nerve
11. Sacroiliac joint
12. Wing of ilium
13. Spinal canal
14. Spinal dura mater
15. Wing of sacrum
16. Small bowel
17. Body of second sacral vertebra

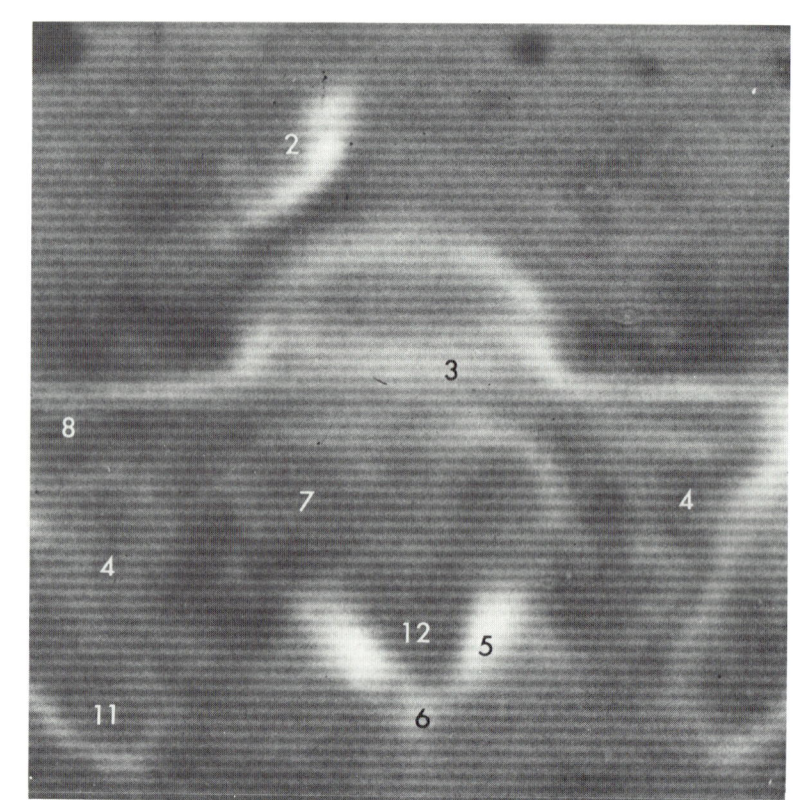

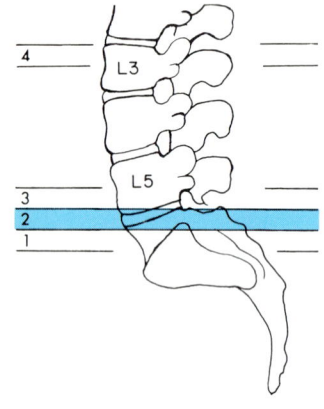

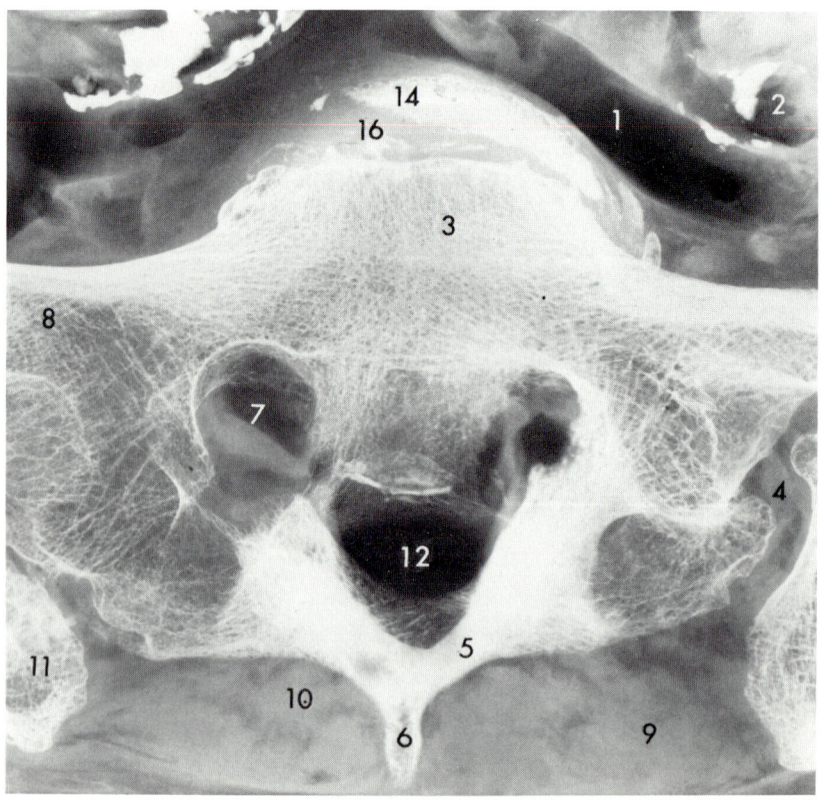

SPINE

**Level 2
(Superior aspect)**

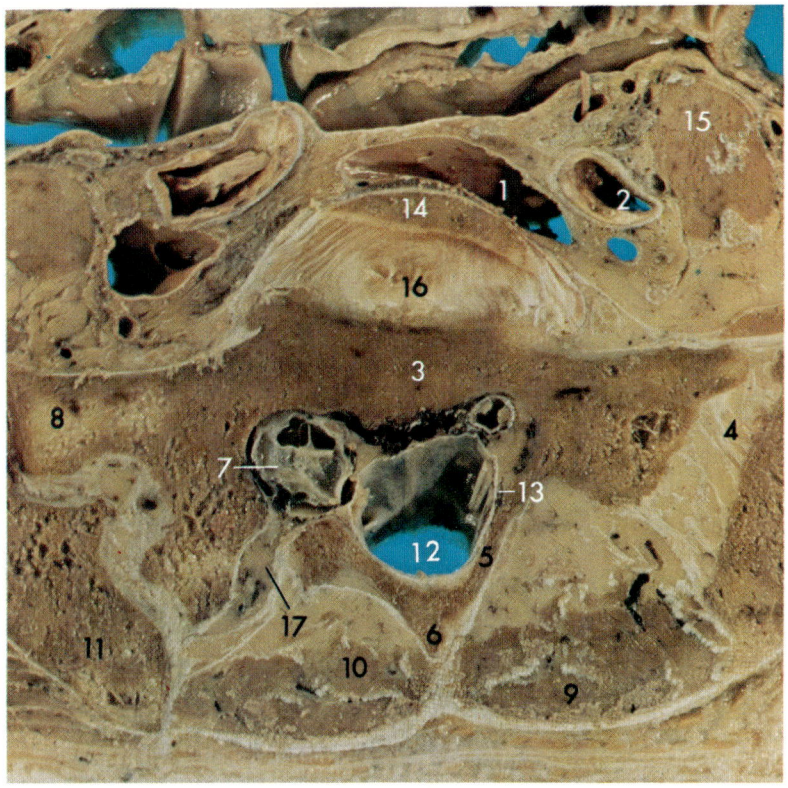

1. Common iliac vein
2. Common iliac artery
3. Body of first sacral vertebra
4. Sacroiliac joint
5. Lamina of first sacral vertebra
6. Spinous process of first sacral vertebra
7. Anterior sacral foramen
8. Wing of sacrum
9. Erector spinae muscle
10. Multifidus muscle
11. Wing of Ilium
12. Spinal canal
13. Spinal dura mater
14. Body of fifth lumbar vertebra
15. Psoas muscle
16. L5–S1 intervertebral disc
17. Posterior sacral foramen

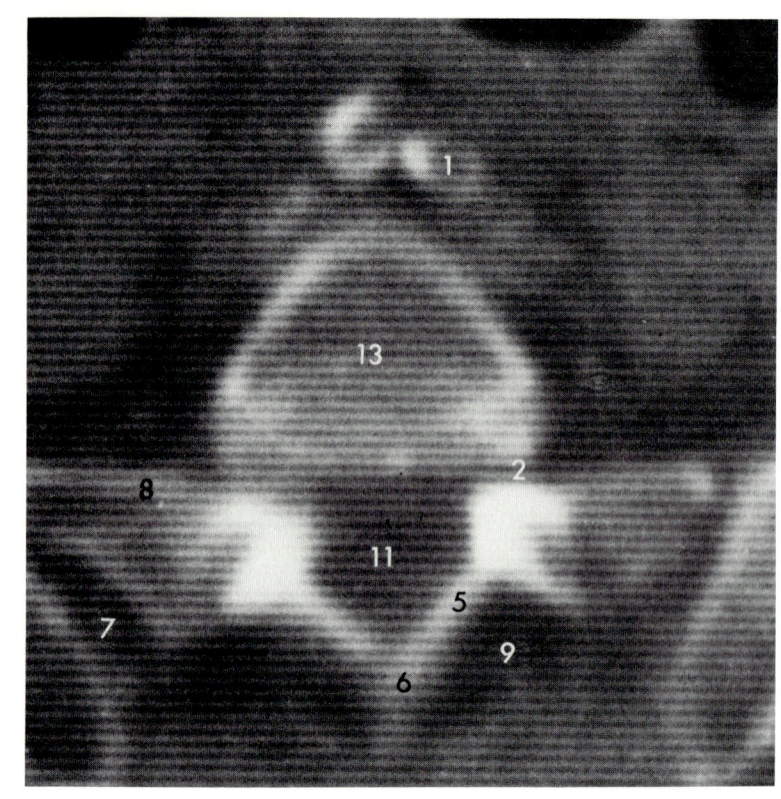

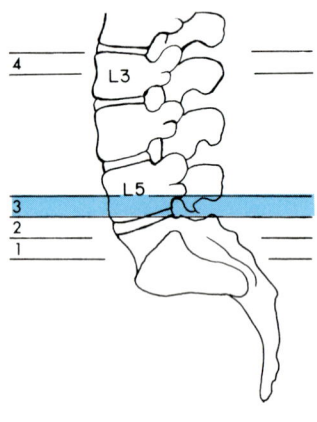

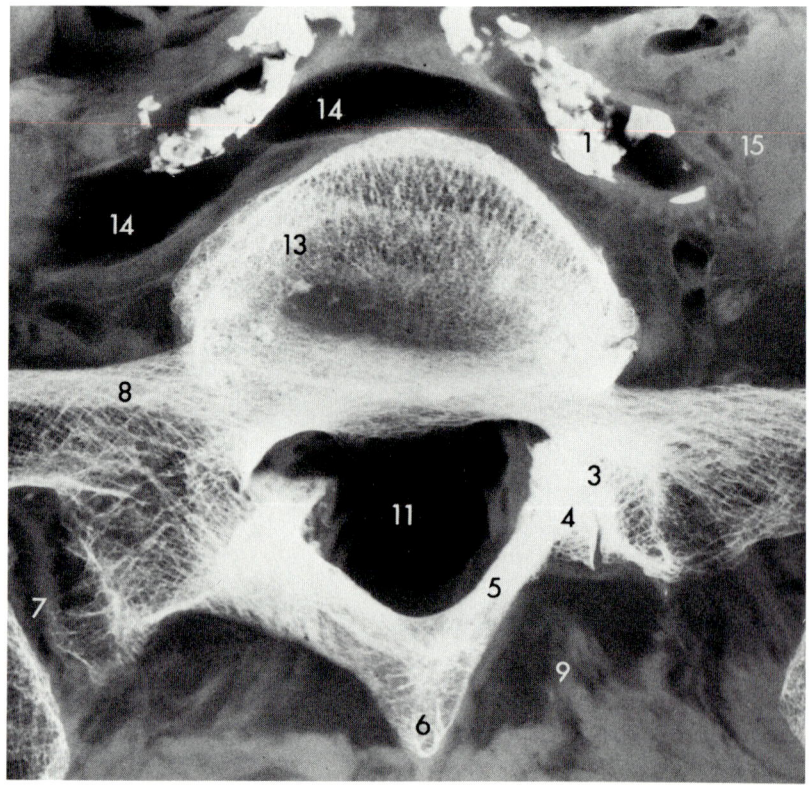

SPINE

**Level 3
(Superior aspect)**

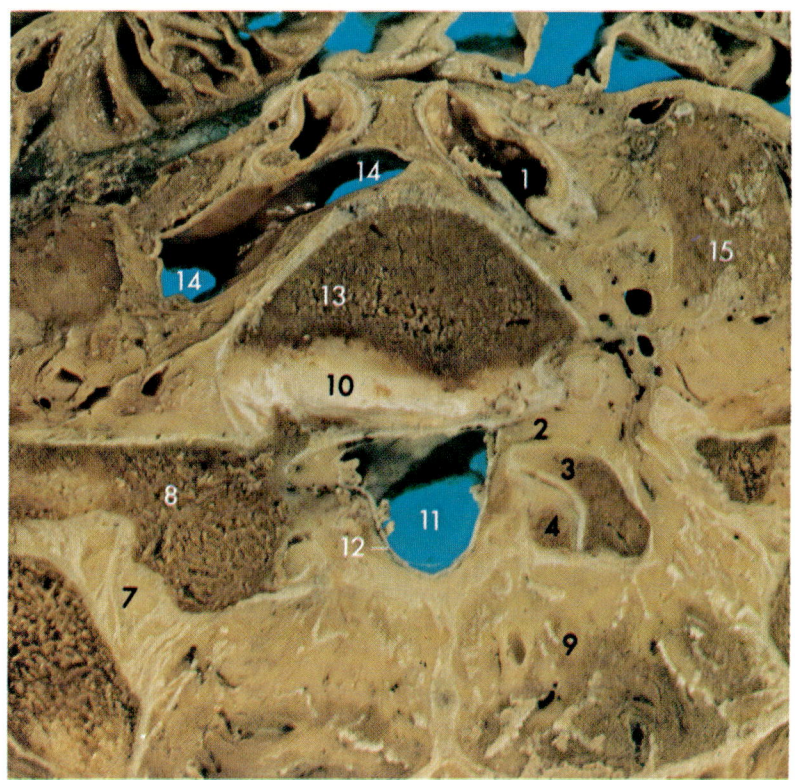

1. Common iliac artery
2. L5–S1 intervertebral foramen
3. Superior articular facet of first sacral vertebra
4. Inferior articular facet of fifth lumbar vertebra
5. Lamina of fifth lumbar vertebra
6. Spinous process of fifth lumbar vertebra
7. Sacroiliac joint
8. Wing of sacrum
9. Multifidus muscle
10. L5–S1 intervertebral disc
11. Spinal canal
12. Spinal dura mater
13. Body of fifth lumbar vertebra
14. Common iliac vein
15. Psoas muscle

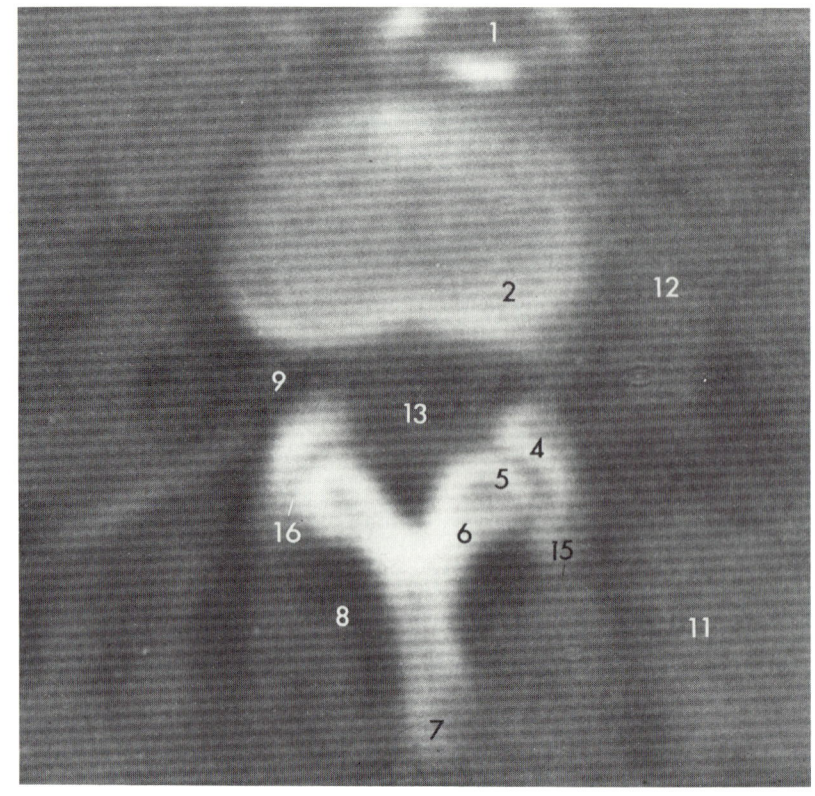
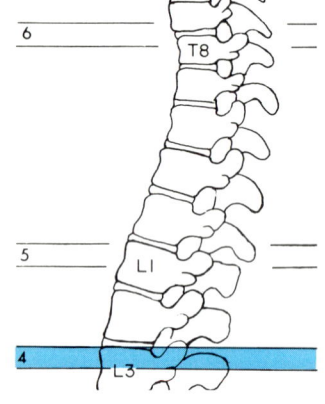
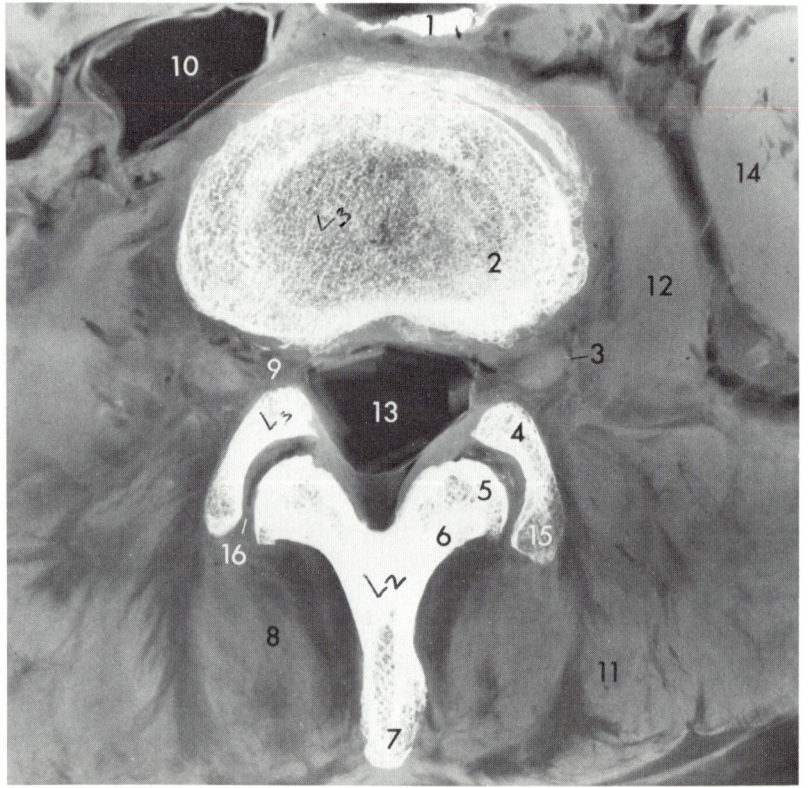

SPINE

Level 4

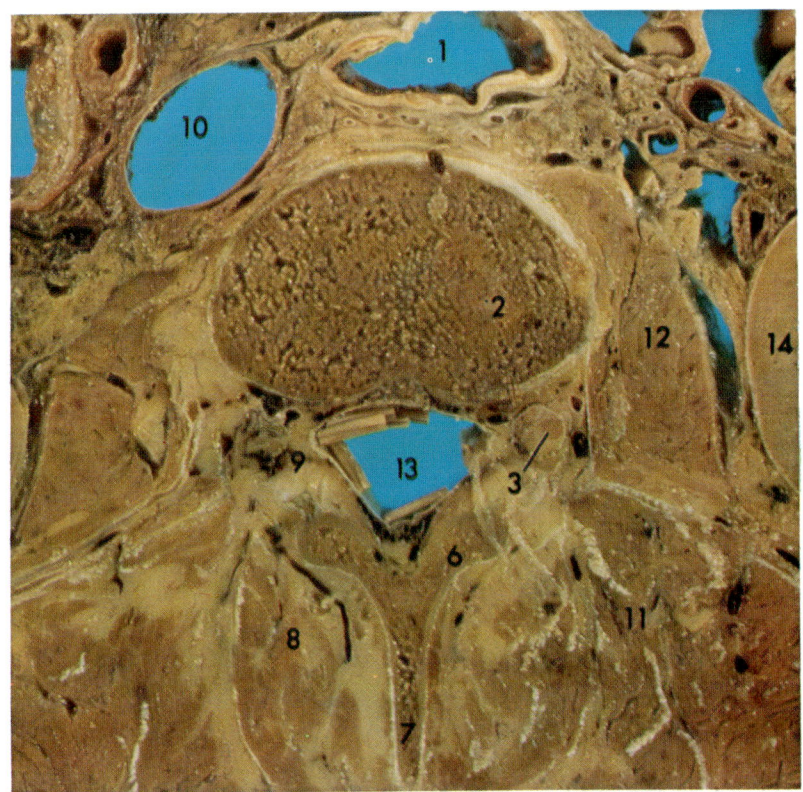

1. Abdominal aorta
2. Body of third lumbar vertebra
3. Second lumbar nerve
4. Superior articular facet of third lumbar vertebra
5. Inferior articular facet of second lumbar vertebra
6. Lamina of second lumbar vertebra
7. Spinous process of second lumbar vertebra
8. Multifidus muscle
9. L2-3 intervertebral foramen
10. Inferior vena cava
11. Erector spinae muscle
12. Psoas muscle
13. Spinal canal
14. Left kidney
15. Mamillary process
16. L2-3 apophyseal joint

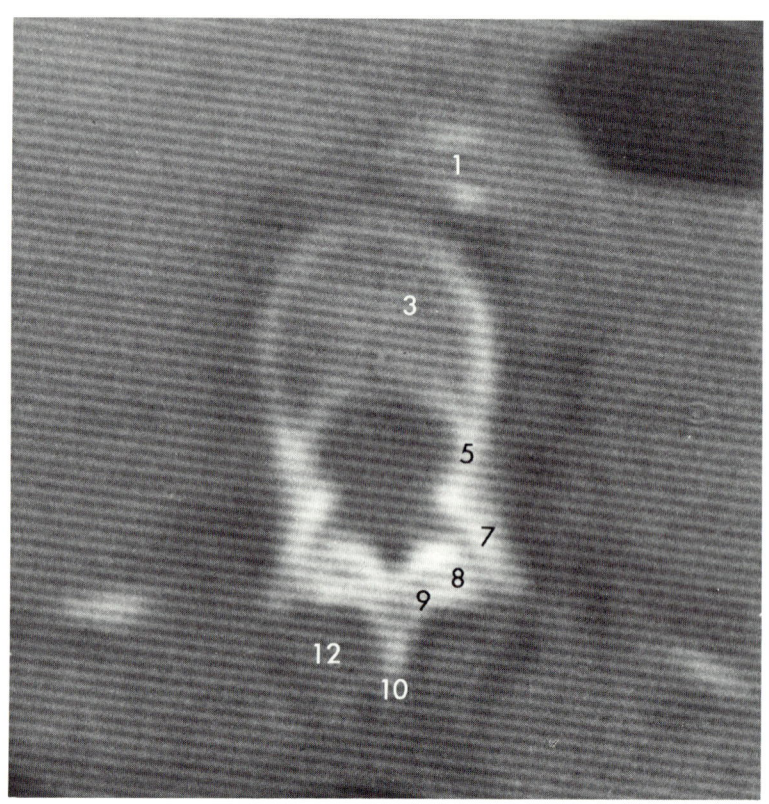

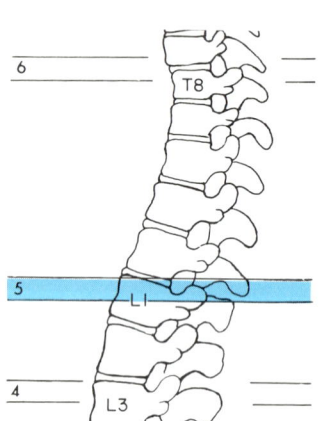

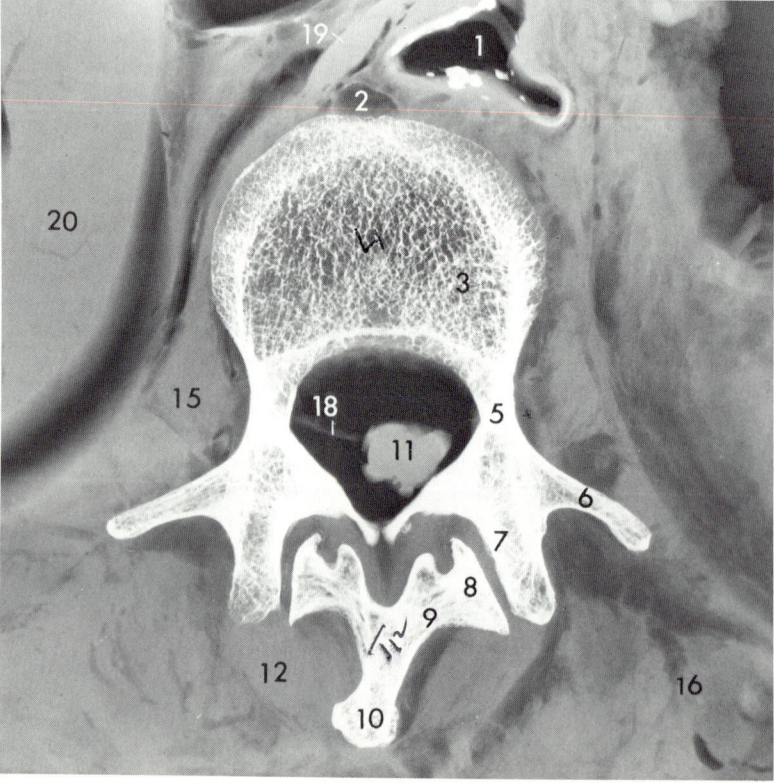

SPINE

Level 5

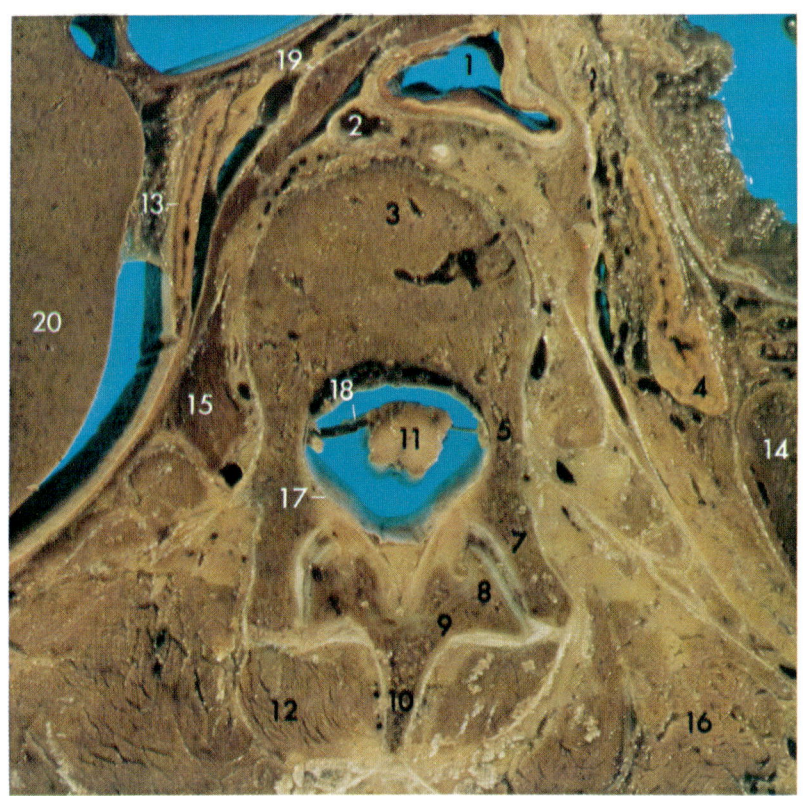

1. Abdominal aorta
2. Azygos vein
3. Body of first lumbar vertebra
4. Left adrenal gland
5. Pedicle of first lumbar vertebra
6. Transverse process of first lumbar vertebra
7. Superior articular facet of first lumbar vertebra
8. Inferior articular facet of twelfth thoracic vertebra
9. Lamina of twelfth thoracic vertebra
10. Spinous process of twelfth thoracic vertebra
11. Conus medullaris of spinal cord
12. Multifidus muscle
13. Right adrenal gland
14. Left kidney
15. Psoas muscle
16. Erector spinae muscle
17. Spinal dura mater
18. Dentate ligament
19. Right crus of diaphragm
20. Liver

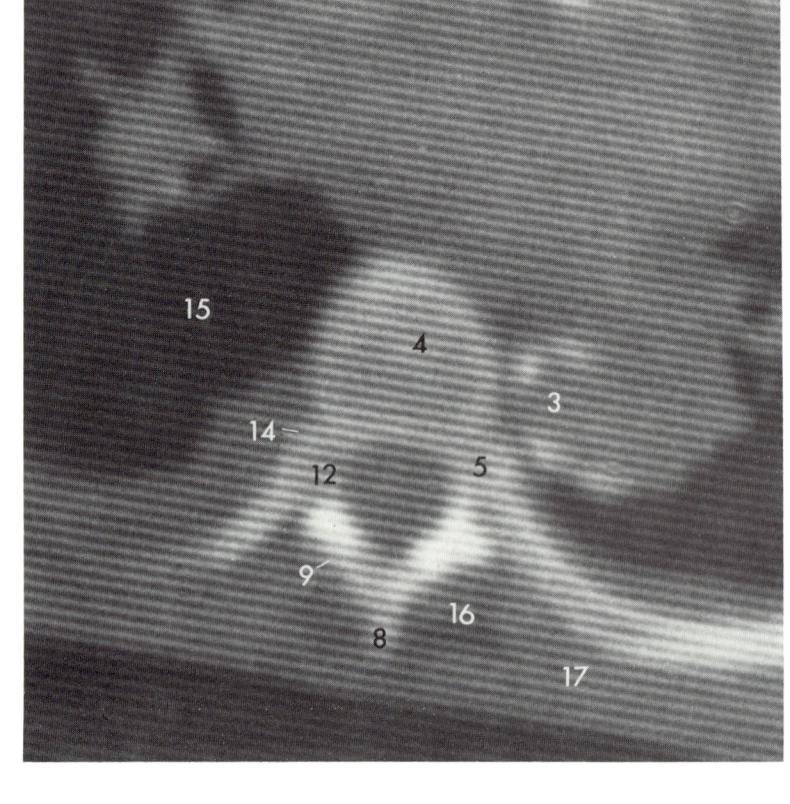

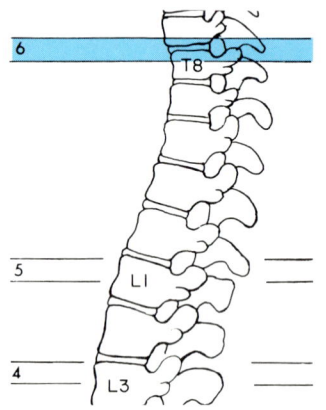

SPINE

Level 6

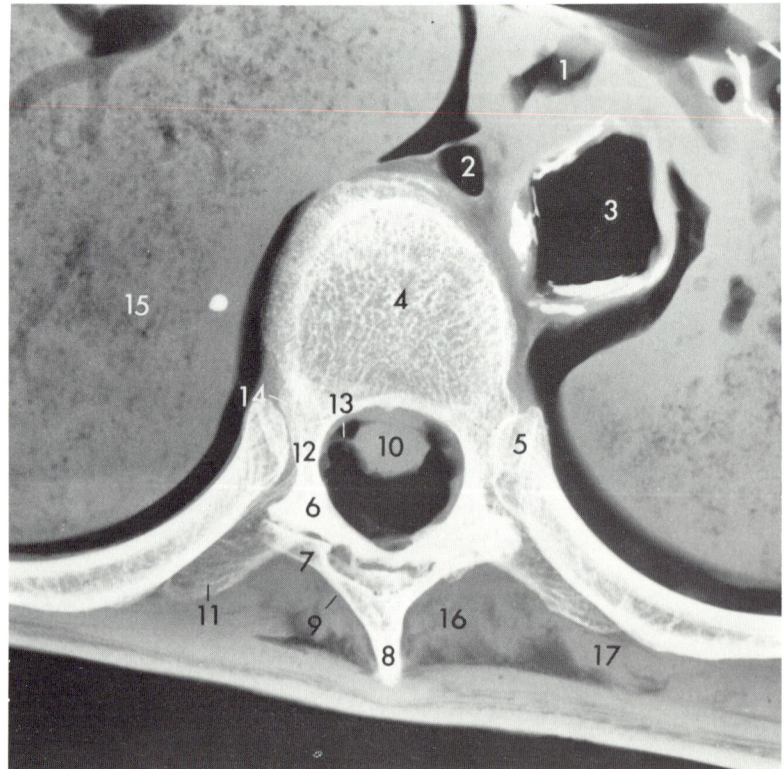

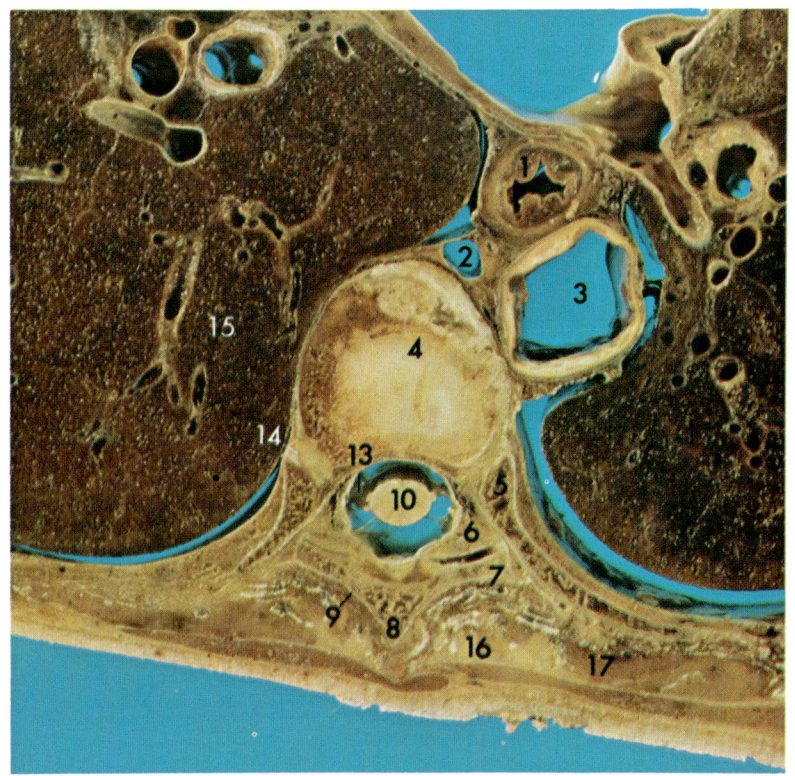

1. Esophagus
2. Azygos vein
3. Thoracic aorta
4. T7–8 intervertebral disc
5. Eighth rib
6. Superior articular process of eighth thoracic vertebra
7. Inferior articular process of seventh thoracic vertebra
8. Spinous process of seventh thoracic vertebra
9. Lamina of seventh thoracic vertebra
10. Spinal cord
11. Transverse process of seventh thoracic vertebra
12. Pedicle of eighth thoracic vertebra
13. Dentate ligament
14. Demifacet for head of eighth rib
15. Right lung
16. Multifidus muscle
17. Erector spinae muscle

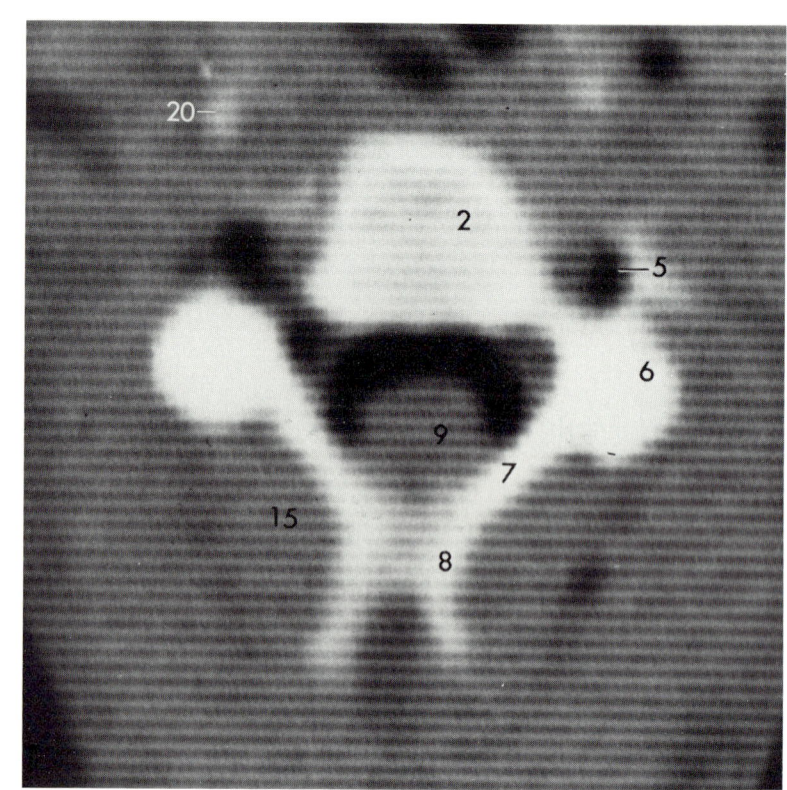

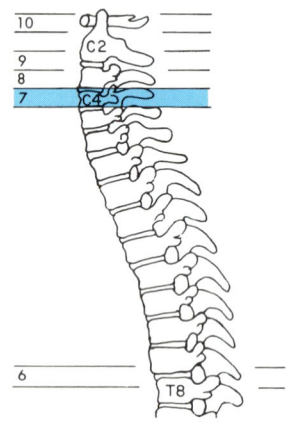

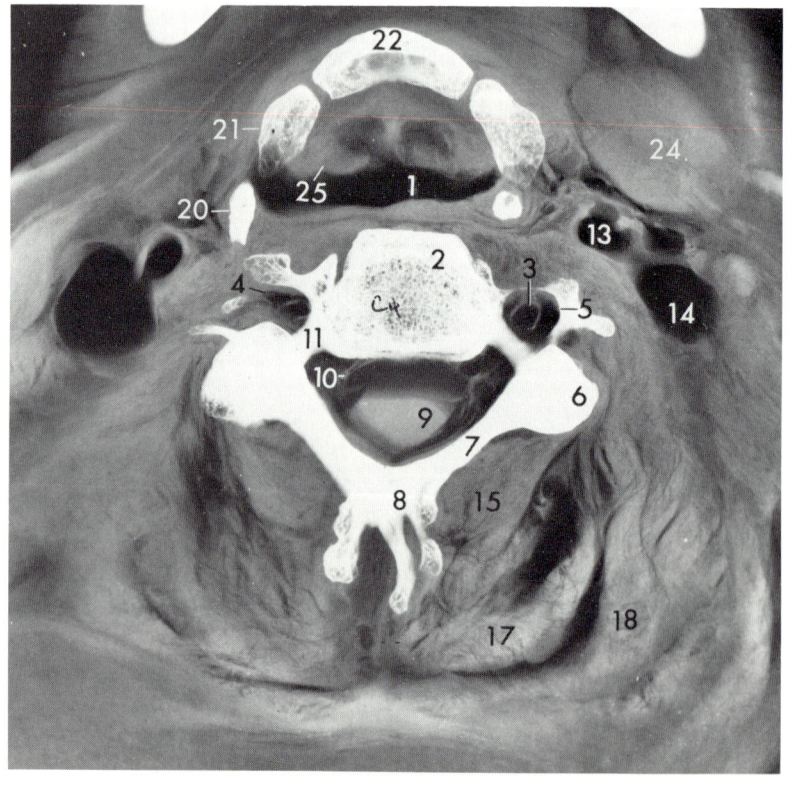

SPINE

**Level 7
(Superior aspect)**

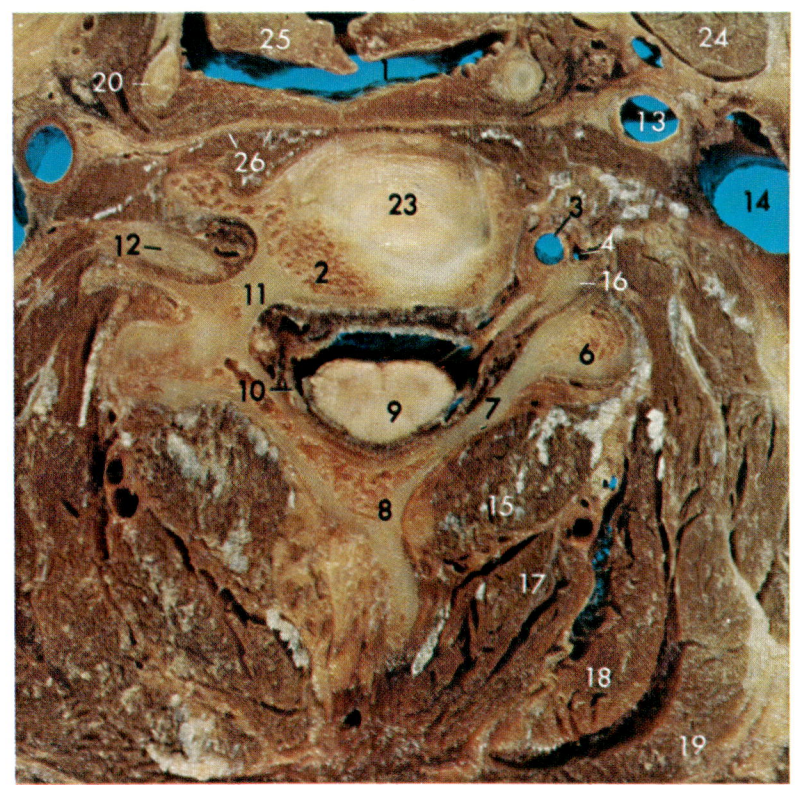

1. Hypopharynx
2. Body of fourth cervical vertebra
3. Vertebral artery
4. Vertebral vein
5. Foramen transversarium
6. Lateral mass of fourth cervical vertebra
7. Lamina of fourth cervical vertebra
8. Spinous process of fourth cervical vertebra
9. Spinal cord
10. Spinal dura mater
11. Pedicle of fourth cervical vertebra
12. Fourth cervical nerve
13. Internal carotid artery
14. Internal jugular vein
15. Multifidus muscle
16. Dorsal root ganglion of fourth cervical nerve
17. Semispinalis cervicis muscle
18. Semispinalis capitis muscle
19. Splenius capitis muscle
20. Superior cornu of thyroid cartilage
21. Greater cornu of hyoid bone
22. Body of hyoid bone
23. C3-4 intervertebral disc
24. Submaxillary gland
25. Aryepiglottic folds
26. Prevertebral fascia

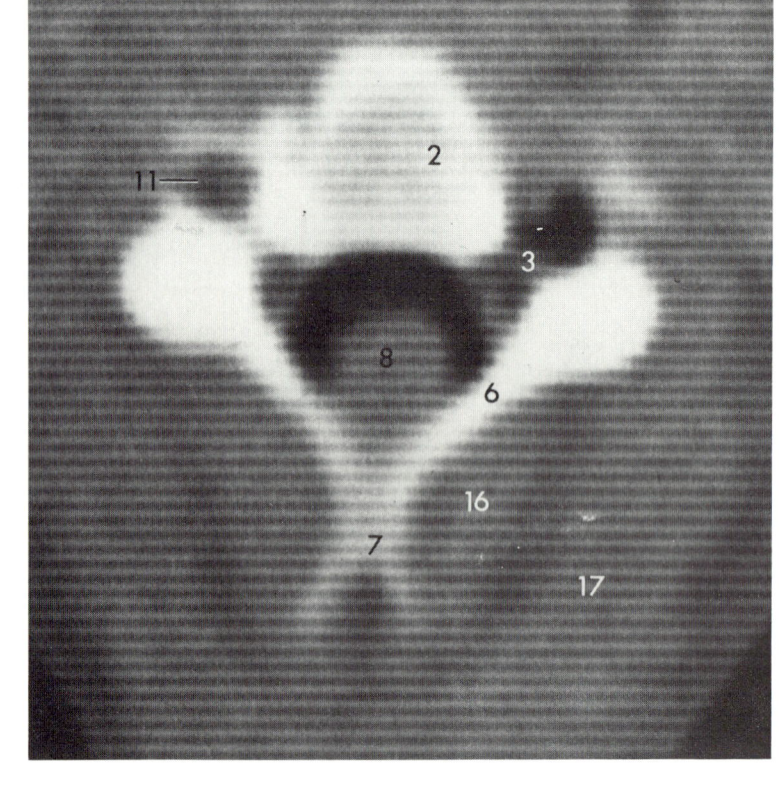

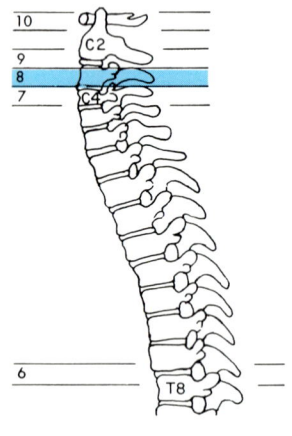

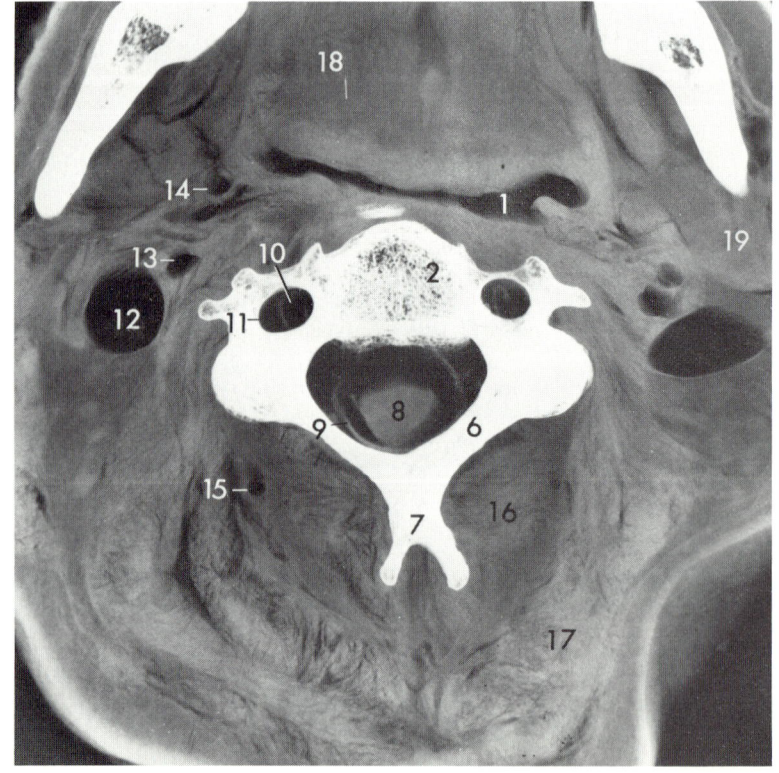

SPINE

Level 8

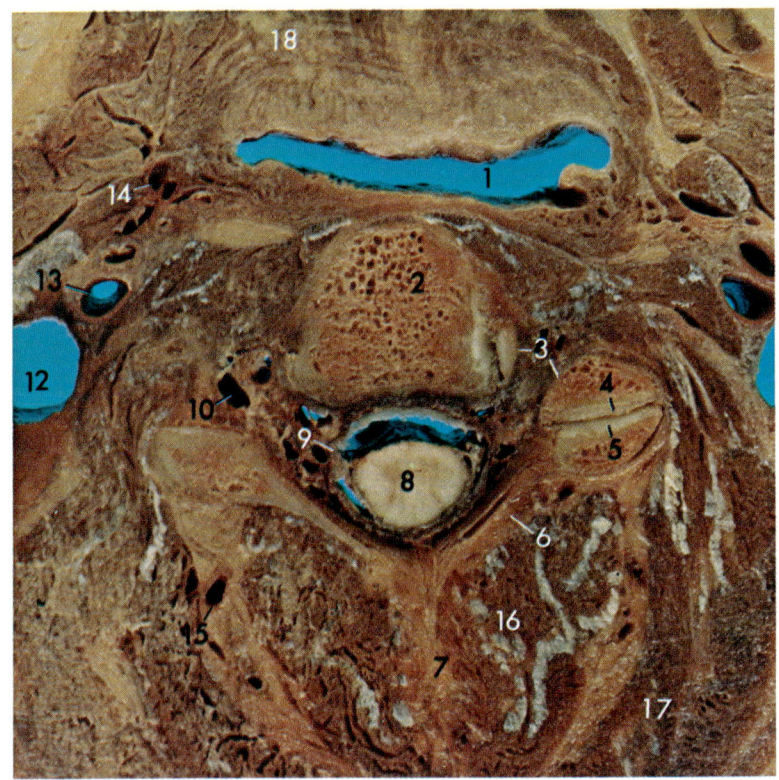

1. Oropharynx
2. Body of third cervical vertebra
3. C3–4 intervertebral foramen
4. Superior articular facet of fourth cervical vertebra
5. Inferior articular facet of third cervical vertebra
6. Lamina of third cervical vertebra
7. Spinous process of third cervical vertebra
8. Cervical spinal cord
9. Spinal dura mater
10. Vertebral artery
11. Foramen transversarium
12. Internal jugular vein
13. Internal carotid artery
14. External carotid artery
15. Deep cervical artery
16. Multifidus muscle
17. Semispinalis cervicis muscle
18. Tongue
19. Submaxillary gland

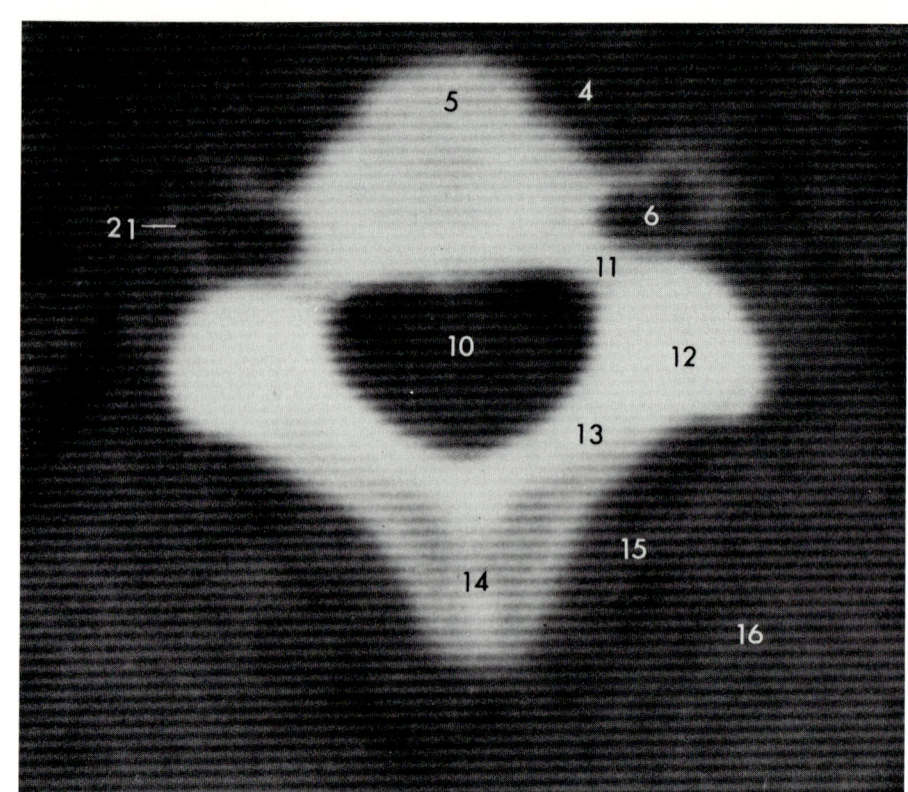

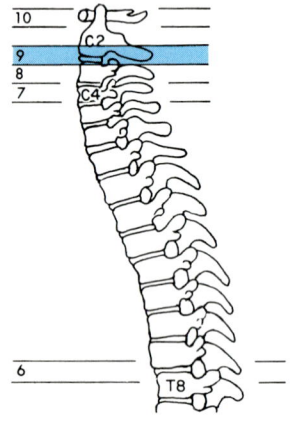

SPINE

Level 9

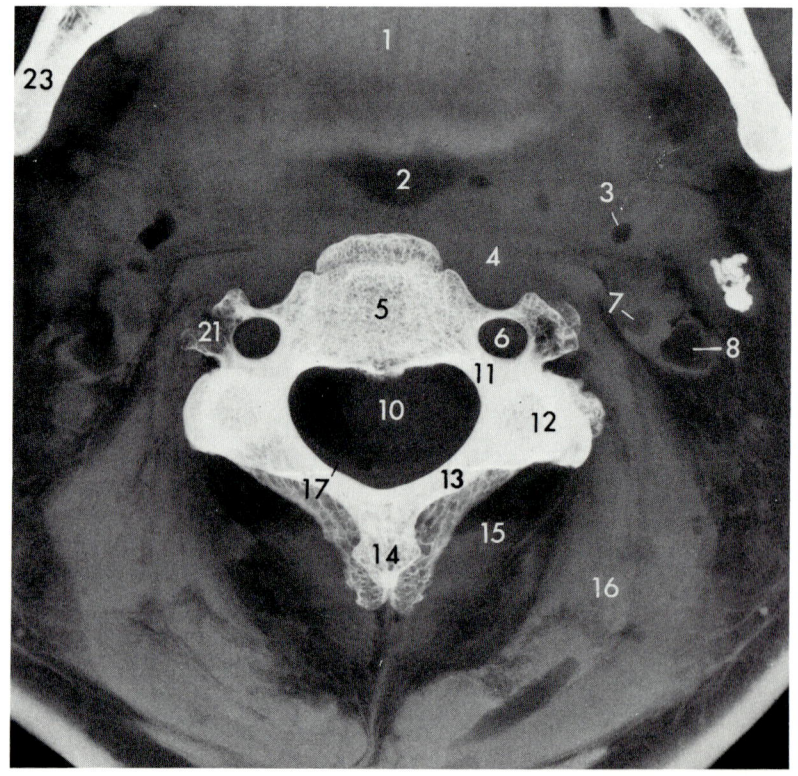

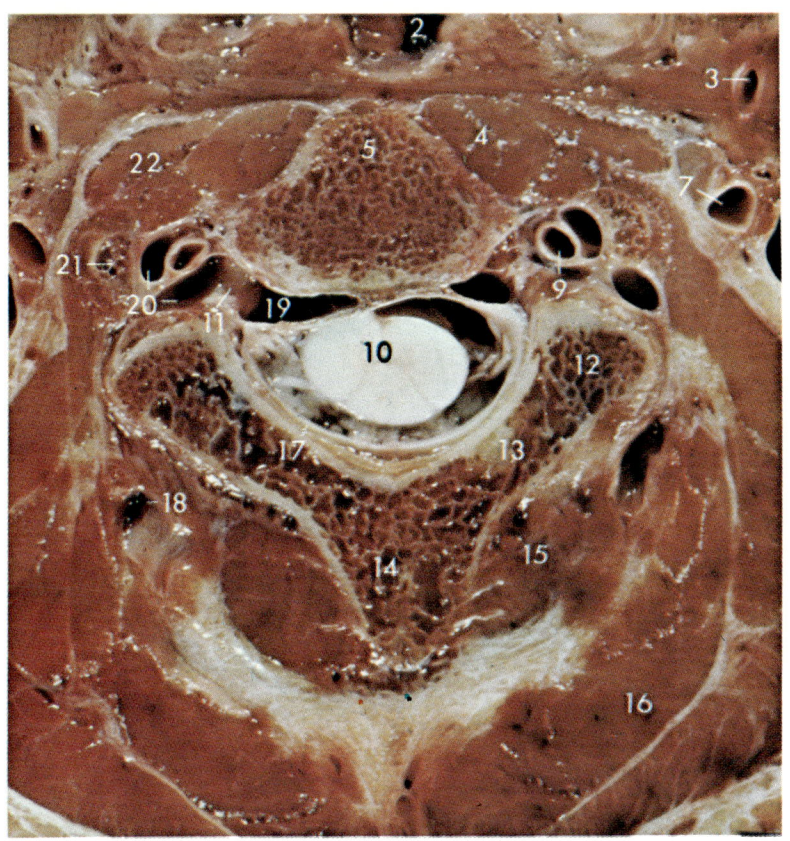

1. Tongue
2. Oropharynx
3. External carotid artery
4. Longus colli muscle
5. Body of third cervical vertebra
6. Foramen transversarium
7. Internal carotid artery
8. Internal jugular vein
9. Vertebral artery
10. Spinal cord
11. Pedicle of third cervical vertebra
12. Lateral mass of third cervical vertebra
13. Lamina of third cervical vertebra
14. Spinous process of third cervical vertebra
15. Rectus capitis posterior muscle
16. Semispinalis capitis muscle
17. Spinal dura mater
18. Deep cervical artery
19. Epidural venous plexus
20. Vertebral veins
21. Transverse process of third cervical vertebra
22. Longus capitis muscle
23. Mandible

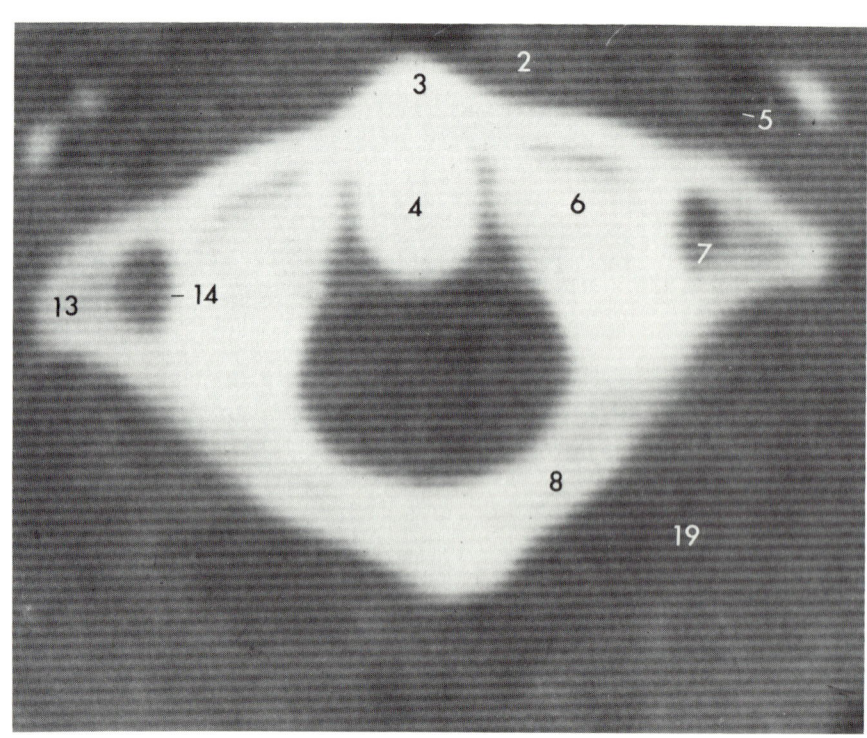

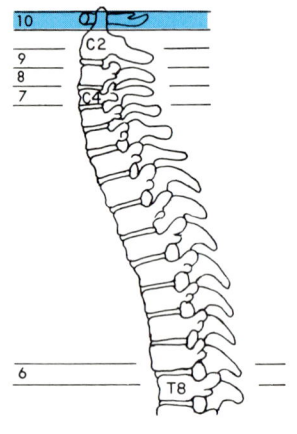

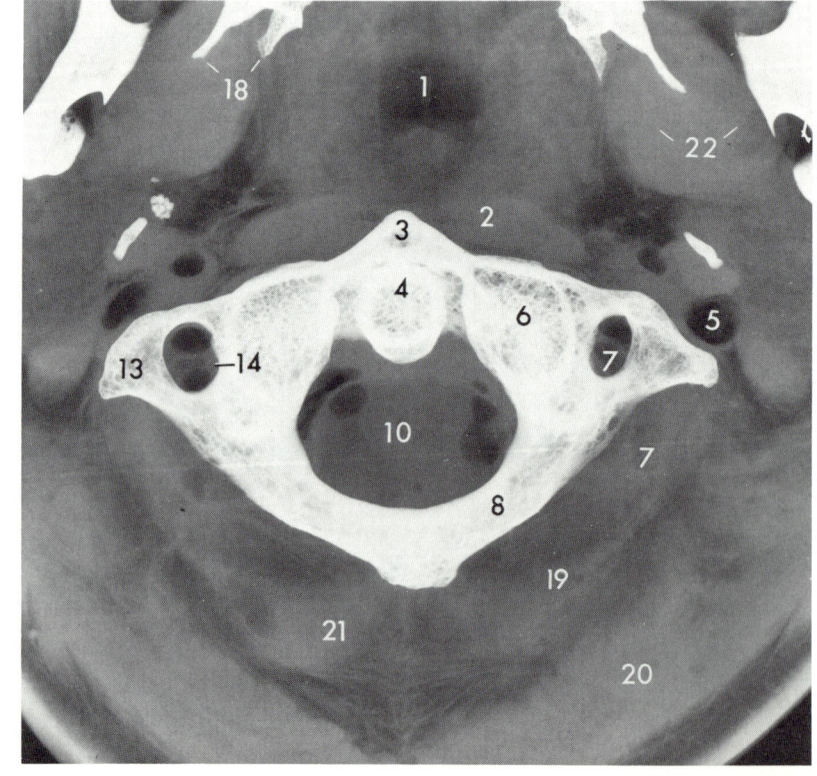

SPINE

Level 10

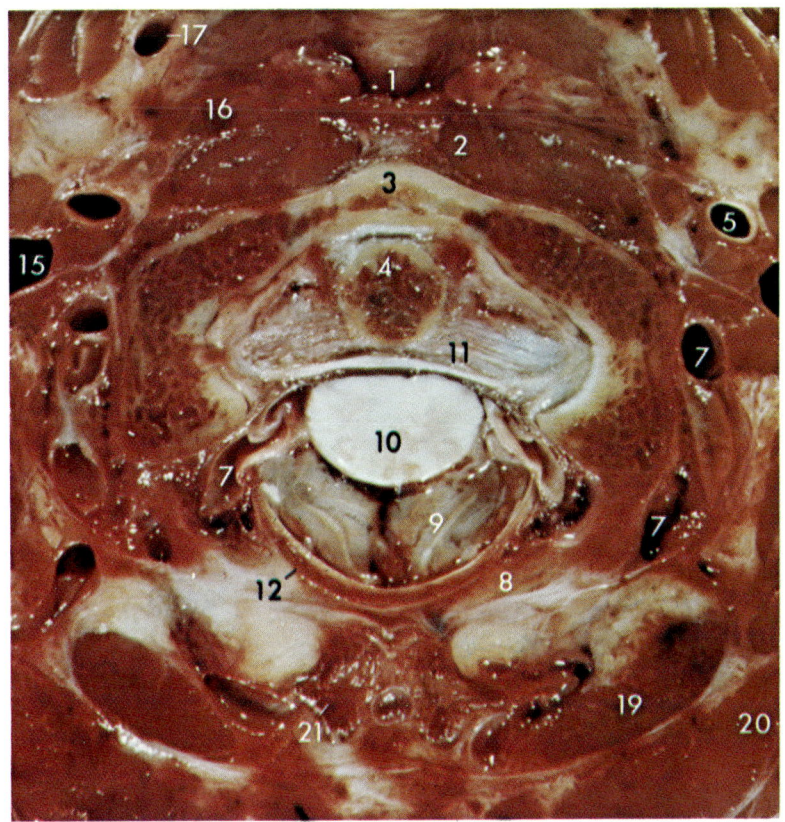

1. Nasopharynx
2. Longus colli muscle
3. Anterior arch of first cervical vertebra
4. Odontoid process of second cervical vertebra
5. Internal carotid artery
6. Superior articular facet of first cervical vertebra
7. Vertebral artery
8. Posterior arch of first cervical vertebra
9. Cerebellar tonsil
10. Cervical spinal cord
11. Transverse odontoid ligament
12. Spinal dura mater
13. Transverse process of first cervical vertebra
14. Foramen transversarium
15. Internal jugular vein
16. Longus capitis muscle
17. External carotid artery
18. Medial and lateral pterygoid plates
19. Semispinalis capitis muscle
20. Splenius capitis muscle
21. Rectus capitis posterior muscle
22. Internal and external pterygoid muscles

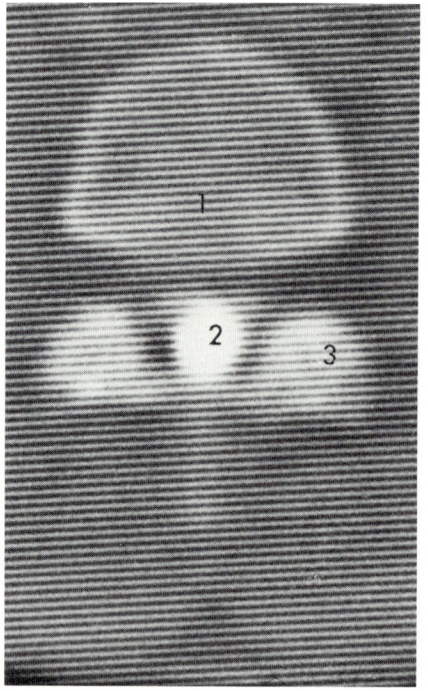

Fig. 4-1. Level of fourth lumbar vertebra.

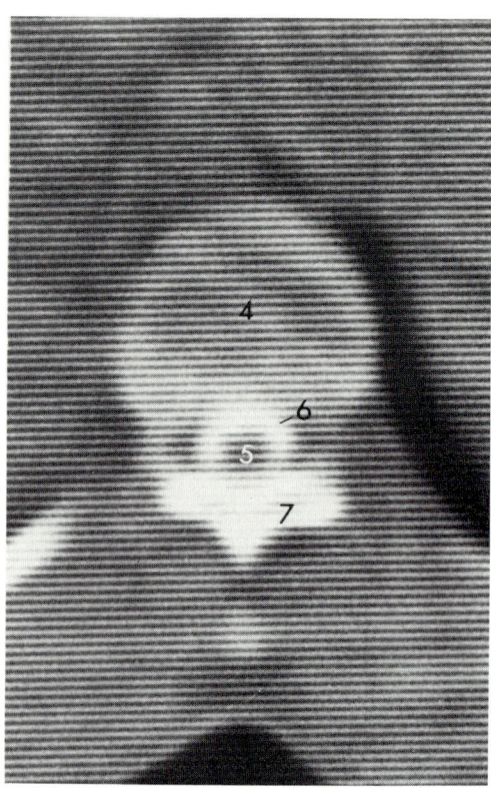

Fig. 4-2. Level of twelfth lumbar vertebra.

SPINE

Normal *in Vivo* Computed Tomographic Studies: Metrizamide

These six CT images are taken from a normal metrizamide myelogram. They demonstrate the spinal subarachnoid space filled with water-soluble contrast medium which outlines the cervical and thoracic spinal cord.

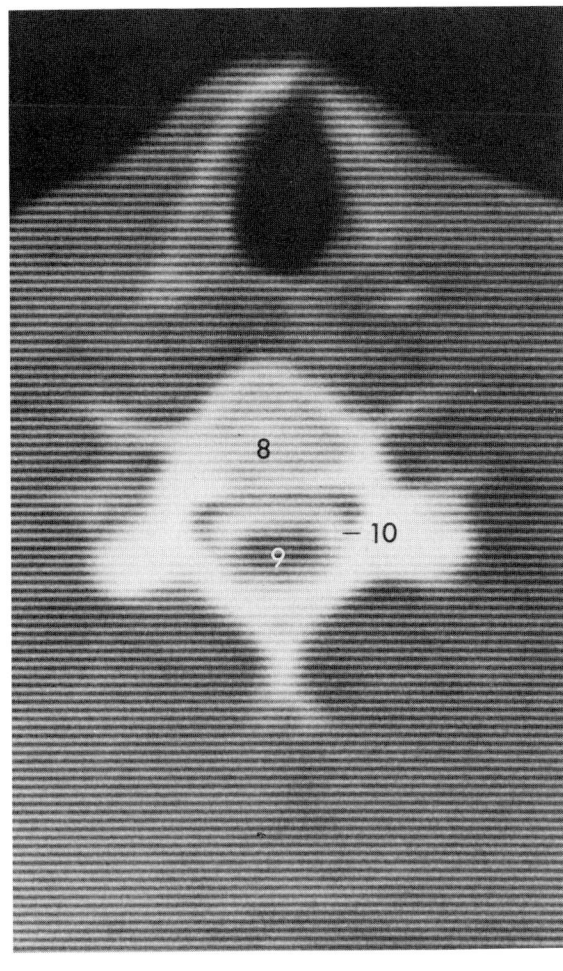

Fig. 4-3. Level of sixth cervical vertebra.

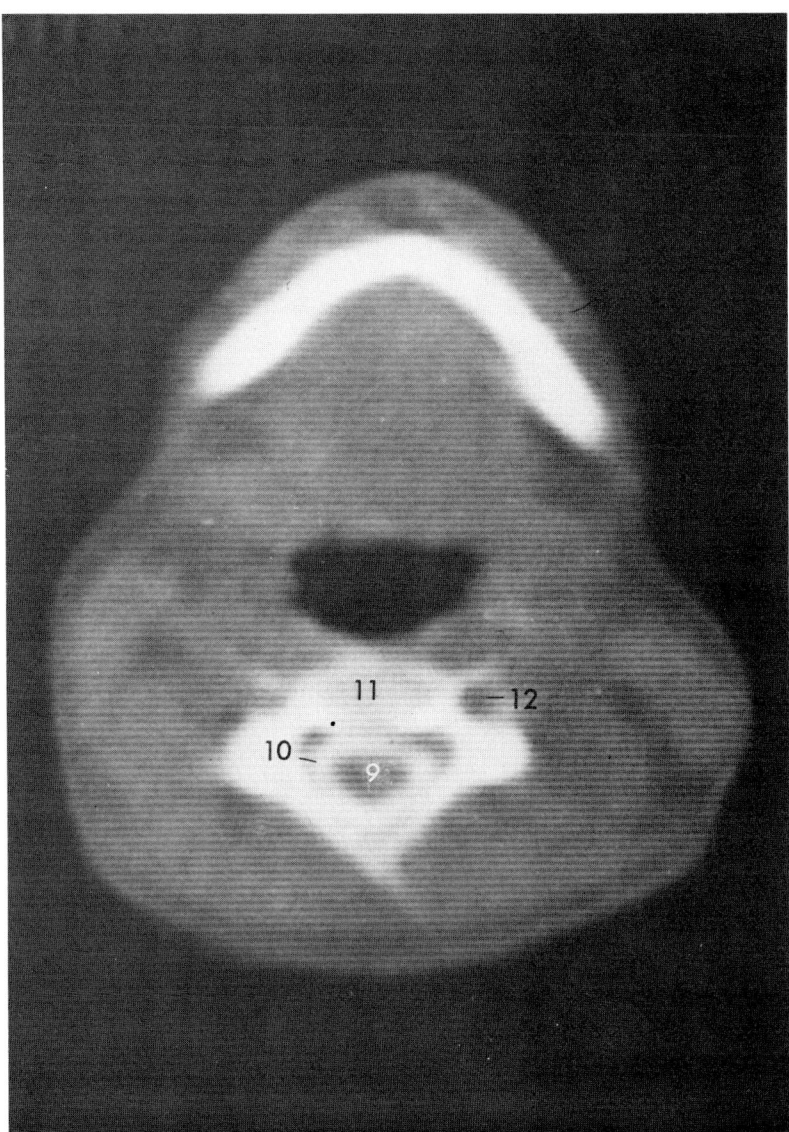

Fig. 4-4. Level of third cervical vertebra.

1. Body of fourth lumbar vertebra
2. Lumbar subarachnoid space
3. Articular facet, L3-4
4. Body of twelfth thoracic vertebra
5. Thoracic spinal cord
6. Thoracic subarachnoid space
7. Lamina of twelfth thoracic vertebra
8. Body of sixth cervical vertebra
9. Cervical spinal cord
10. Cervical subarachnoid space
11. Body of third cervical vertebra
12. Foramen transversarium

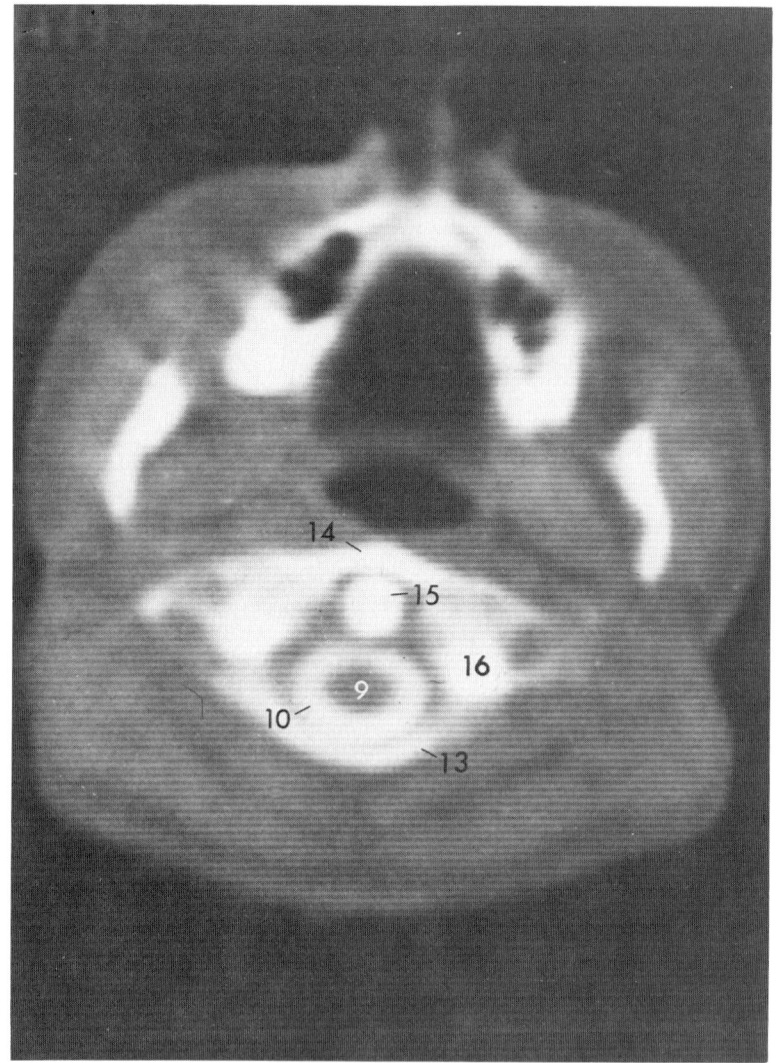
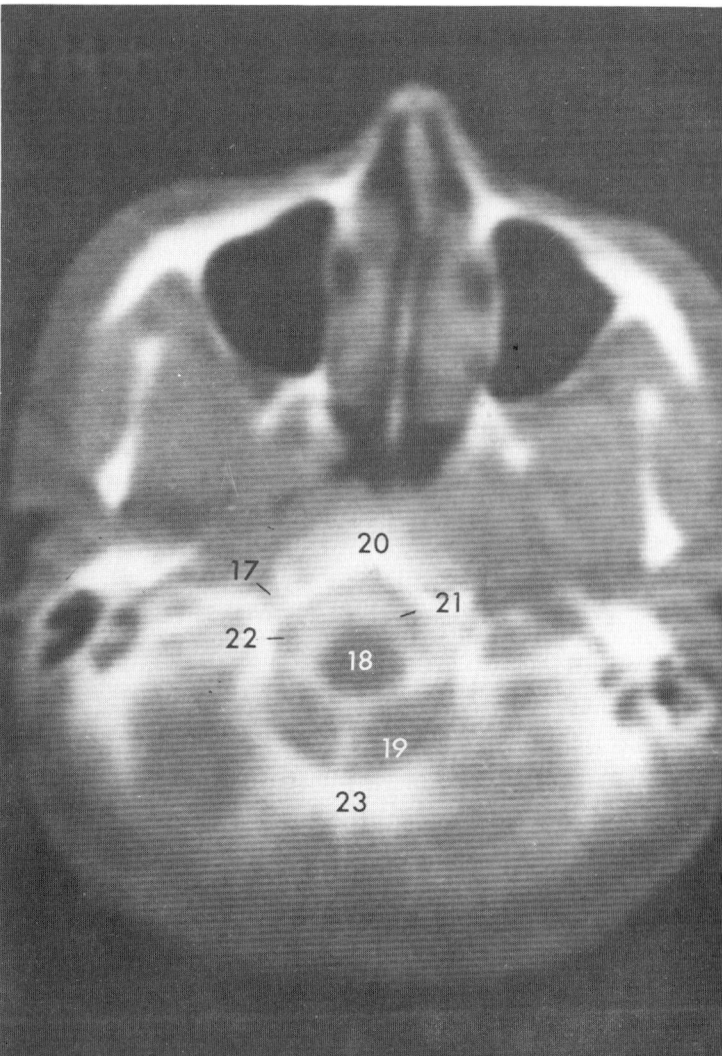

Fig. 4-5. Level of first cervical vertebra.

Fig. 4-6. Level of foramen magnum.

9. Cervical spinal cord
10. Cervical subarachnoid space
13. Posterior arch of first cervical vertebra
14. Anterior arch of first cervical vertebra
15. Odontoid process of second cervical vertebra
16. Inferior articular facet of first cervical vertebra
17. Hypoglossal canal
18. Medulla oblongata
19. Cerebellar tonsil
20. Anterior margin of foramen magnum
21. Medullary cistern
22. Vertebral artery
23. Posterior margin of foramen magnum

5
Chest

ANTHONY V. PROTO

RICHARD L. GOLDWIN

E. ROBERT HEITZMAN

In this chapter, the anatomy of the thorax is displayed in 17 levels extending from diaphragm to pulmonary apex. The sections have been numbered from the diaphragm cephalad. The structures of the shoulder girdle are covered more completely in Chapter 7, The Extremities; those of the thoracic spine and its contents in Chapter 4, The Spine.

In this chapter, two computed tomographic (CT) images are shown for each level. These have been made with a scanning circle diameter of 45 cm and with different center and window settings so that mediastinal and parenchymal lung detail can be demonstrated optimally. In general, to identify mediastinal structures, a relatively narrow window setting is used with a center of about 50–150 Hounsfield units, while examination of the pulmonary parenchyma and vasculature requires a much wider window with center settings of about −200 to −500 Hounsfield units. Occasionally, a wider window is advantageous for the study of mediastinal structures because it accentuates the shape of their interfaces with lung; the images made with a wide window are included in this section for this reason. Although such wide window images usually display details of the pulmonary parenchyma, bronchi, and vessels well *in vivo*, these structures could not be demonstrated satisfactorily in our cadaver material because of the presence of pneumonia and pulmonary edema.

In several sections, some areas or interfaces are identified by terms which are common radiologic parlance. These terms and their definitions are

Anterior junction line The contact of the two lungs across the visceral and parietal pleura anterior to the great vessels and, sometimes, the heart.

Aortic–pulmonic window A space marginated superiorly by the aortic arch and inferiorly by the left pulmonary artery. Lymph nodes at the medial aspect of the window can be considered in the group of left tracheobronchial nodes. Nodes at the lateral aspect of the window have been termed ductus nodes.

Azygoesophageal recess A real or potential mediastinal recess allowing intrusion of the right lower lobe into the mediastinum in relationship to the azygos vein posteriorly and the esophagus anteriorly or medially; the space of Holzknecht.

Cardiophrenic angle An area formed by the junction of the heart and diaphragm.

Interlobar pulmonary artery That portion of either pulmonary artery lying in the major fissure distal to the origin of the artery to the upper lobe.

Parietal trigone An area formed by the contact of the visceral and parietal pleurae of the azygos fissure with the posterior chest wall.

Right paratracheal stripe An interface produced by the contact of the right upper lobe with the right lateral wall of the trachea.

Certain facts concerning the display of thoracic anatomy should be emphasized. The computed tomograms show a ring shadow within the trachea which represents an endotracheal tube used to keep the lungs inflated; this was removed before body sectioning was performed. On some sections, a black line is evident on the skin of the chest wall; this line served as a guide to improve our correlation of levels. The shoulders were disarticulated after the computed tomographic scans were made but before the cadaver was frozen and sectioned. This explains why the humeral heads are present on the computed tomographic images only.

The anatomy in the color photographs of the gross sections may differ slightly from either the x-ray of the section or the computed tomographic image of the same level. This is in part due to the fact that the gross section and the tomographic image are not exactly comparable at all levels. In addition, the photograph demonstrates just the surface anatomy of the slice, while the computed tomogram and the x-ray show anatomic details of its full thickness.

On the computed tomographic images, the superior vena cava seems denser than the other vessels; in fact, during sectioning we found the clotted blood in the vena cava to differ in consistency from clots elsewhere in the heart and vessels. The presence of clotting in dependent portions of the great vessels and cardiac chambers also explains the greater density of these areas on the computed tomograms. In the cadaver used for the correlative study of the thorax, there is a right pleural effusion, best seen on the images made with wide window settings. Some pulmonary edema and patches of bronchopneumonia also were present, accounting for the unsharpness of some of the vessels. These pneumonic areas could be identified on the gross sections.

These scans, of course, do not show the physiologic motion seen in a living patient. At the end of this chapter are several scans carried out *in vivo* which demonstrate that most of the structures of the thorax are well identified even in the presence of respiratory and cardiac motion; examples of some normal variants are also presented. The following table indicates the frequency of identification of many major anatomic structures compiled from 100 random computed tomograms.

TABLE 5-1. Frequency of Identification of Some Anatomic Structures On Computed Tomograms of the Thorax

Structure	Percent identified	No. of observations*
Anterior junction line	49	78
Aorta		
origin	82	87
ascending	68	84
Azygoesophageal recess	77	83
Azygos arch	89	72
Brachiocephalic (innominate) veins	77	66
Bronchus, right main (posterior wall)	100	83
Crura of diaphragm	87	46
Esophagus (with air)	64	76
Left subclavian artery	88	68
Preaortic lung	55	80
Pulmonary artery		
origin	71	87
left (intrapericardial)	7	81
right (intrapericardial)	21	80
Pulmonary veins (entering left atrium)	100	89
Superior vena cava	100	84
Trachea		
retrotracheal lung	52	69
right paratracheal stripe	80	71

*Disease sometimes precluded evaluation of an anatomic structure; hence, the variation in number of observations.

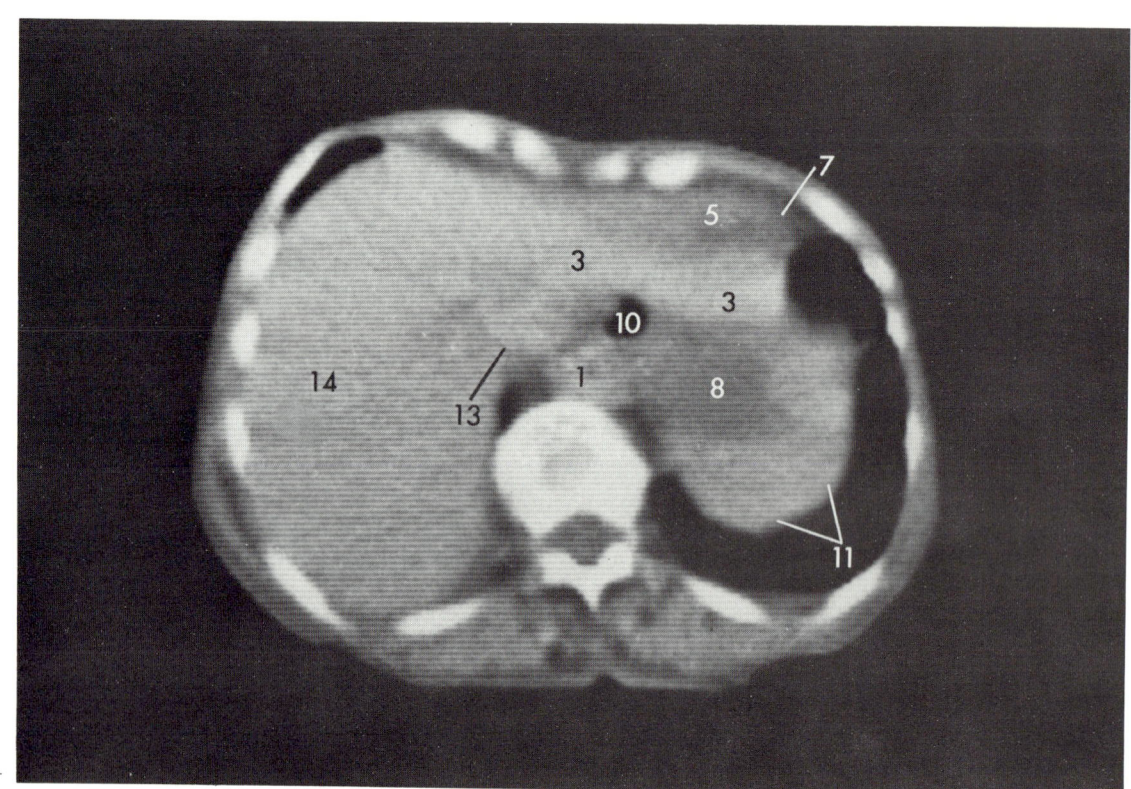

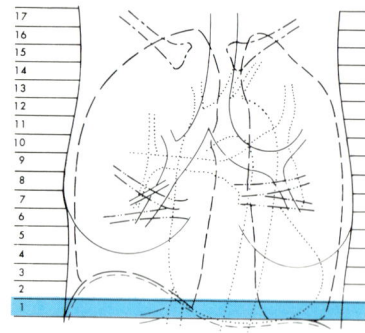

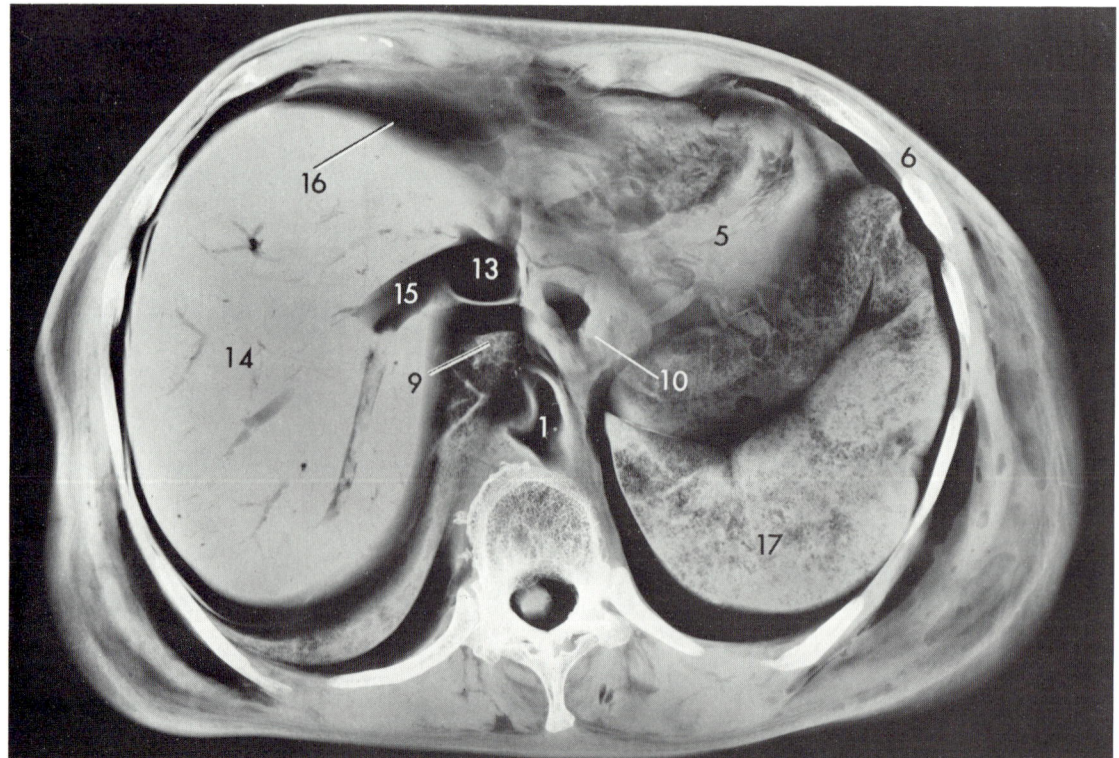

CHEST

Level 1

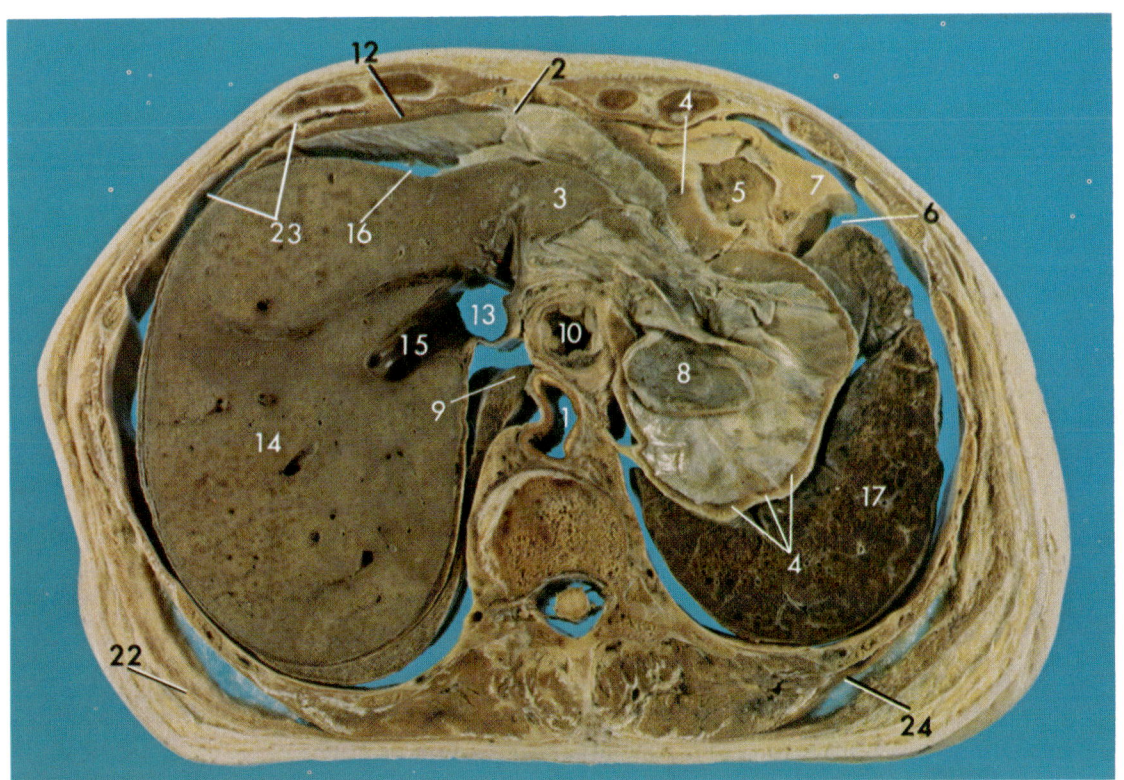

1. Descending thoracic aorta
2. Falciform ligament
3. Left lobe of liver
4. Left hemidiaphragm
5. Cardiac apex
6. Left cardiophrenic angle
7. Left epipericardial fat pad
8. Fundus of stomach
9. Right lower lobe of lung (retrocaval)
10. Esophagus (with gas on CT images) at esophageal hiatus
11. Spleen
12. Right hemidiaphragm
13. Inferior vena cava
14. Right lobe of liver
15. Hepatic vein entering inferior vena cava
16. Peritoneal cavity
17. Left lower lobe of lung
22. Latissimus dorsi muscle
23. Pleural space
24. Serratus posterior inferior muscle

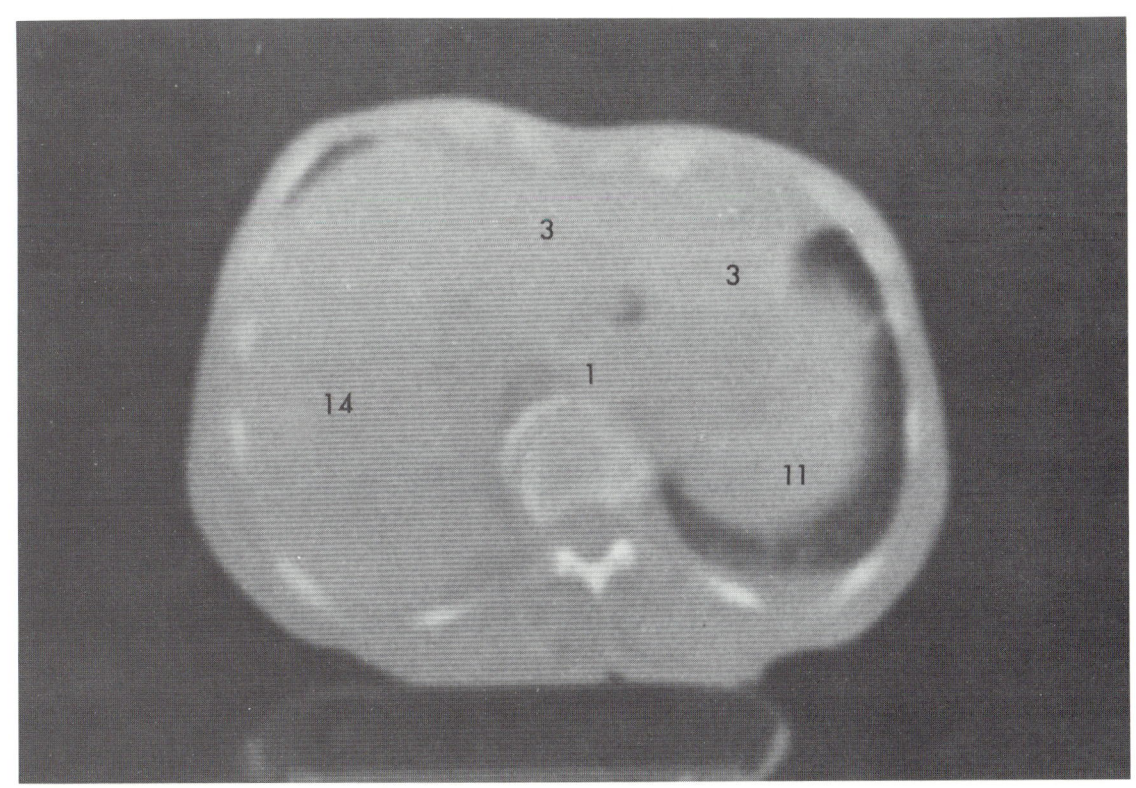

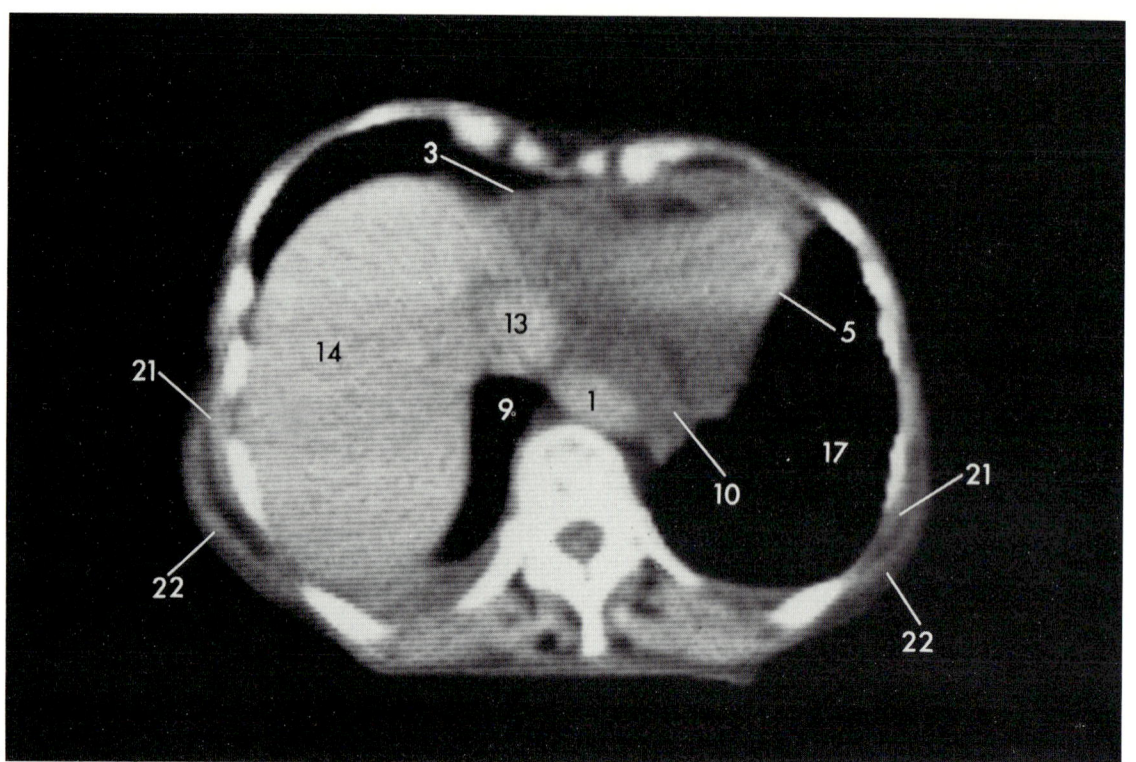

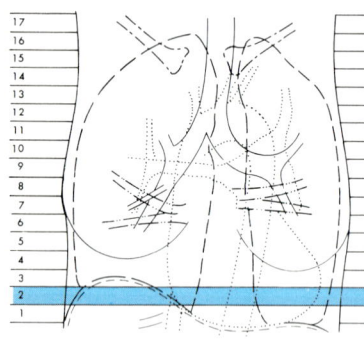

CHEST

Level 2

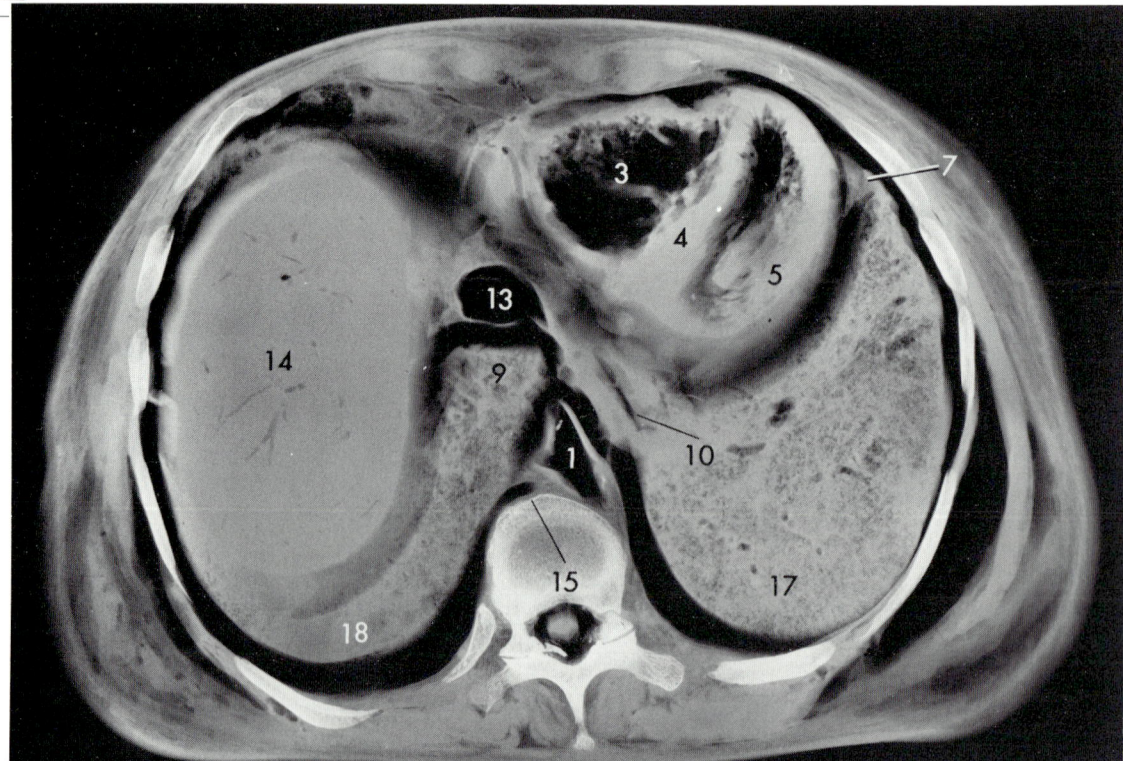

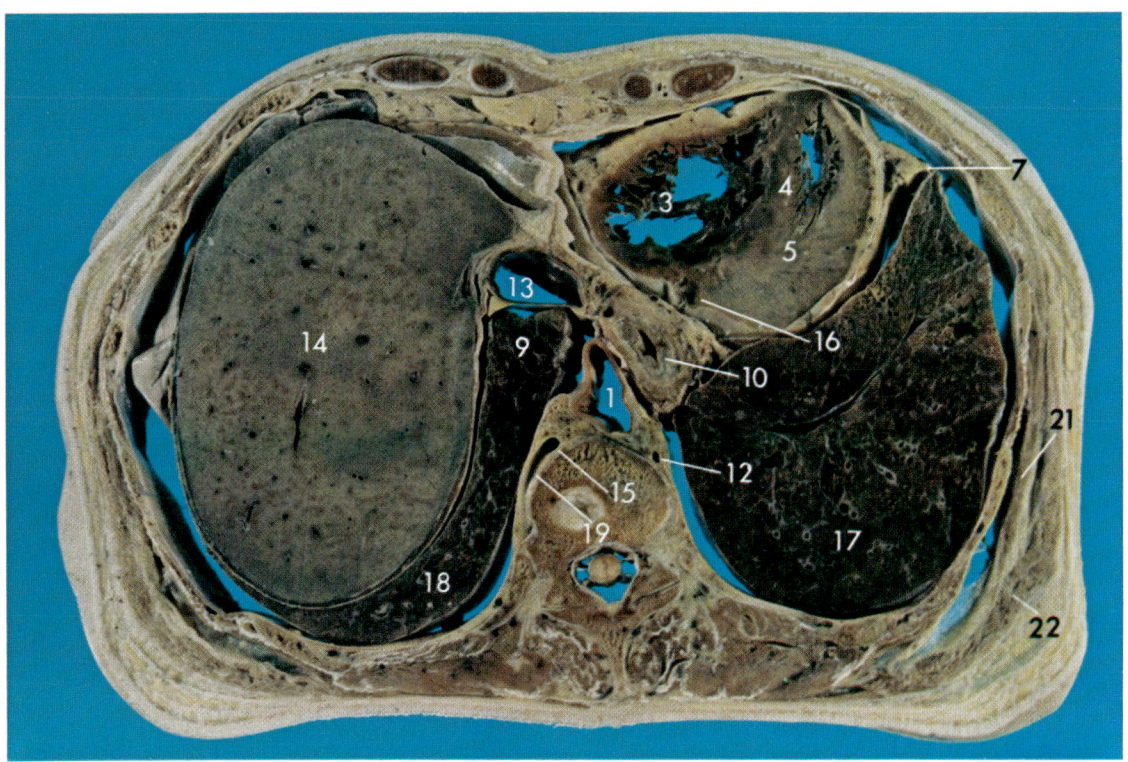

1. Descending thoracic aorta
3. Right ventricle
4. Interventricular septum
5. Left ventricle
7. Left epipericardial fat pad
8. Dome of left hemidiaphragm
9. Right lower lobe of lung (retrocaval)
10. Esophagus
12. Hemiazygos vein
13. Inferior vena cava
14. Right lobe of liver
15. Azygos vein
16. Right posterior descending coronary artery and middle cardiac vein
17. Left lower lobe of lung
18. Right lower lobe of lung
19. Intercostal vein entering azygos vein
21. Serratus anterior muscle
22. Latissimus dorsi muscle

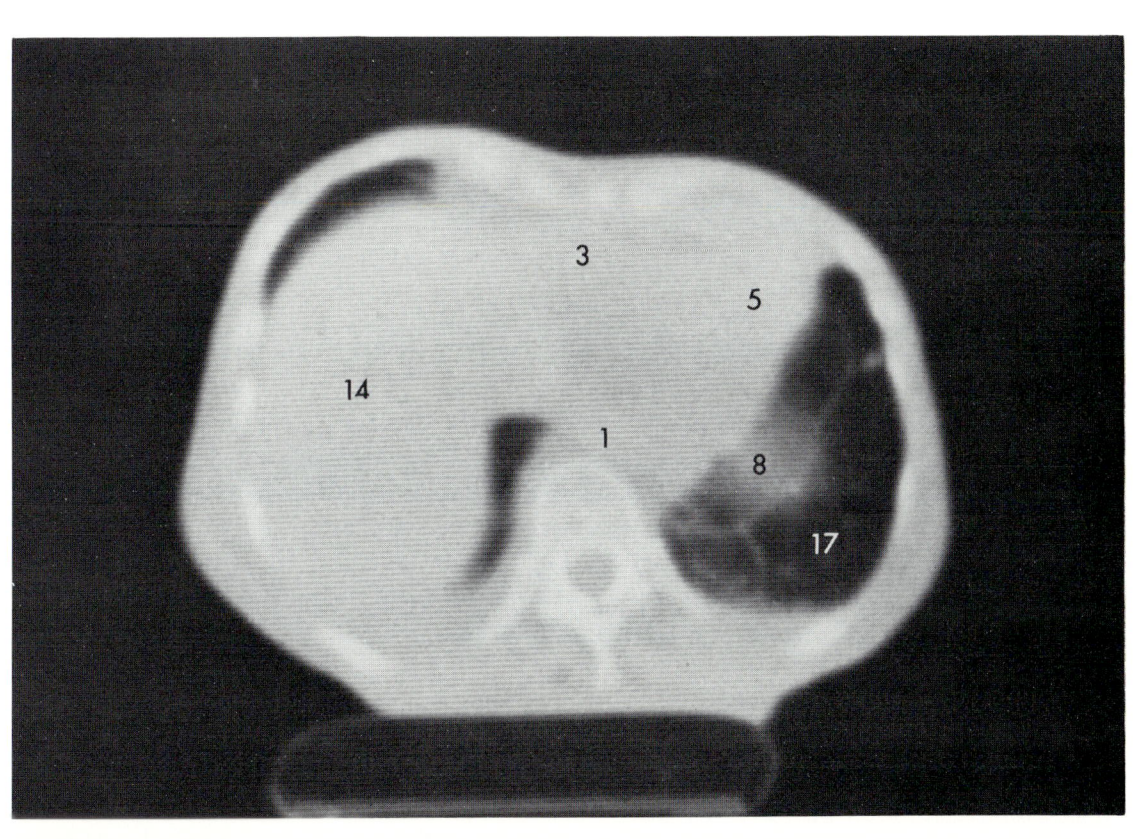

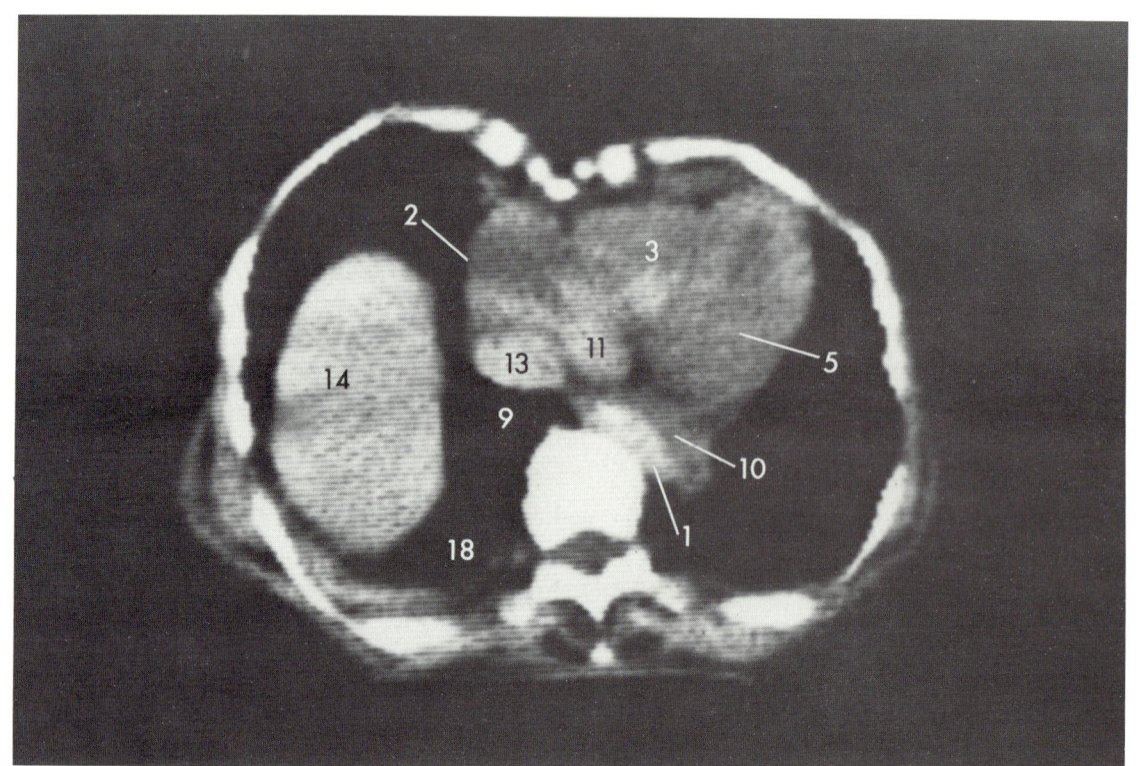

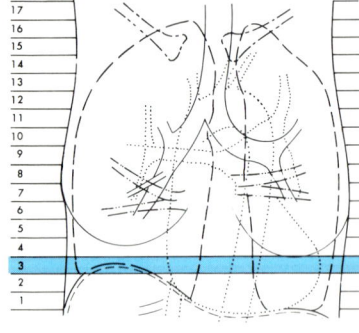

CHEST

Level 3

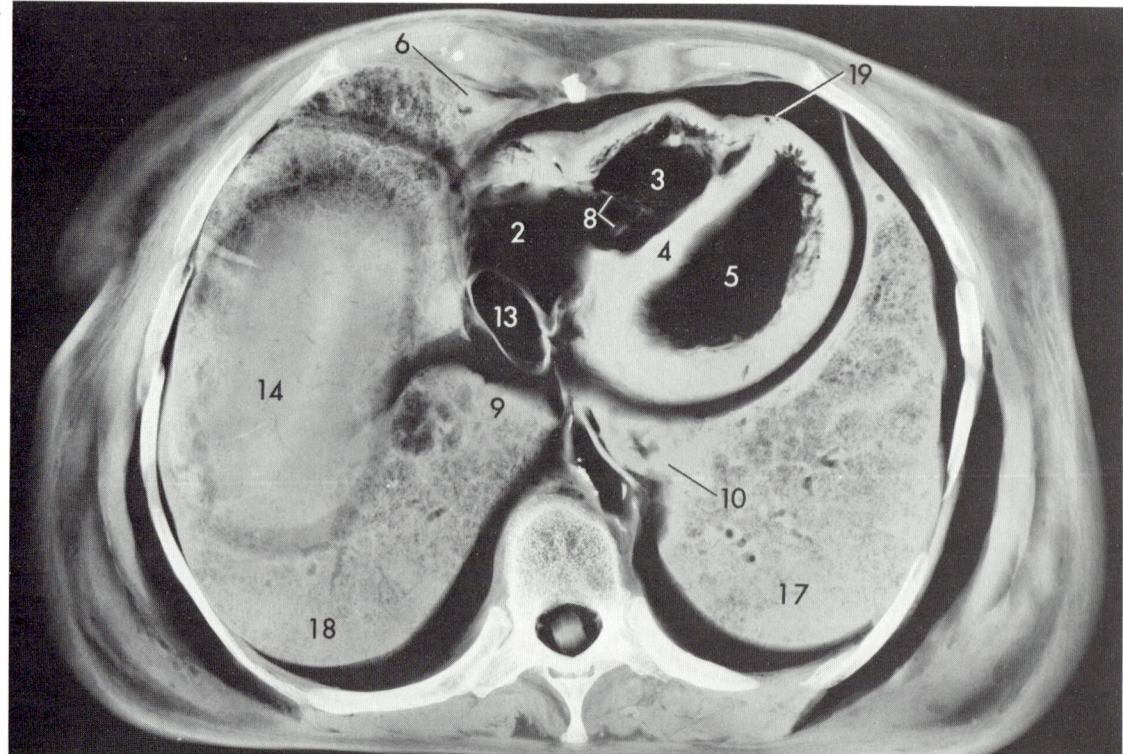

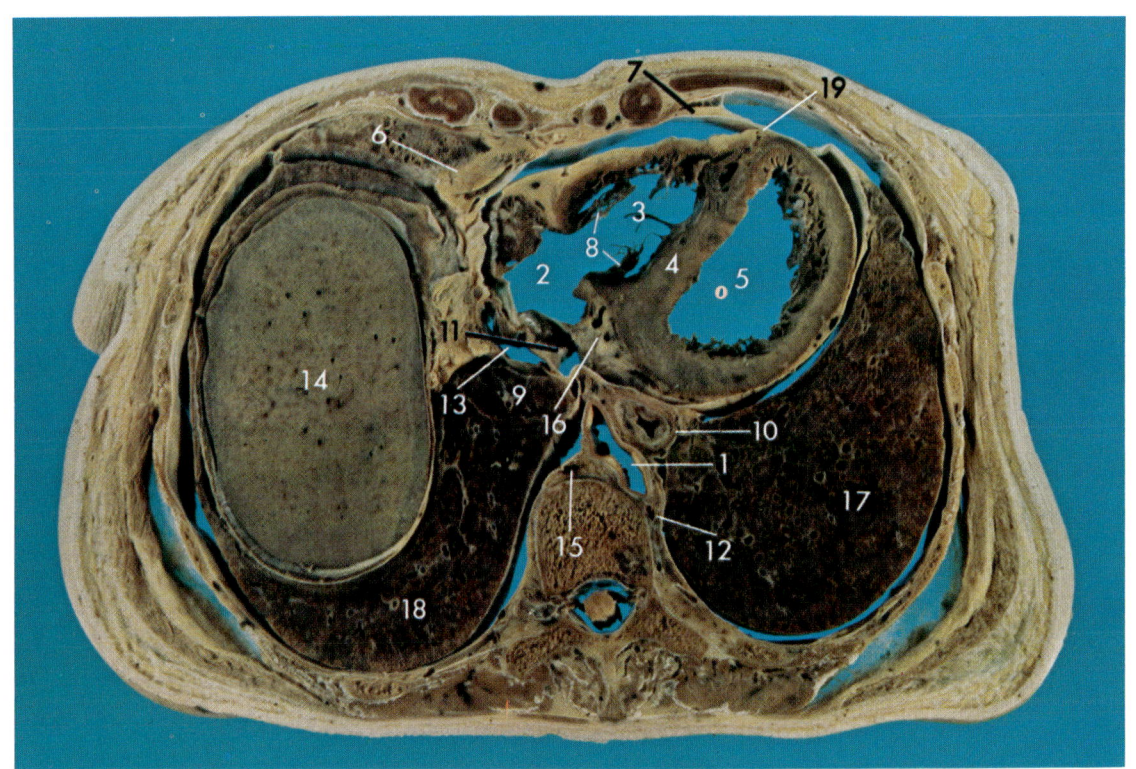

1. Descending thoracic aorta
2. Right atrium
3. Right ventricle
4. Interventricular septum
5. Left ventricle
6. Right epipericardial fat pad
7. Pericardium
8. Tricuspid valve
9. Right lower lobe of lung (retrocaval)
10. Esophagus
11. Coronary sinus
12. Hemiazygos vein
13. Inferior vena cava
14. Right lobe of liver
15. Azygos vein
16. Right posterior descending coronary artery and middle cardiac vein
17. Left lower lobe of lung
18. Right lower lobe of lung
19. Left anterior descending coronary artery and great cardiac vein

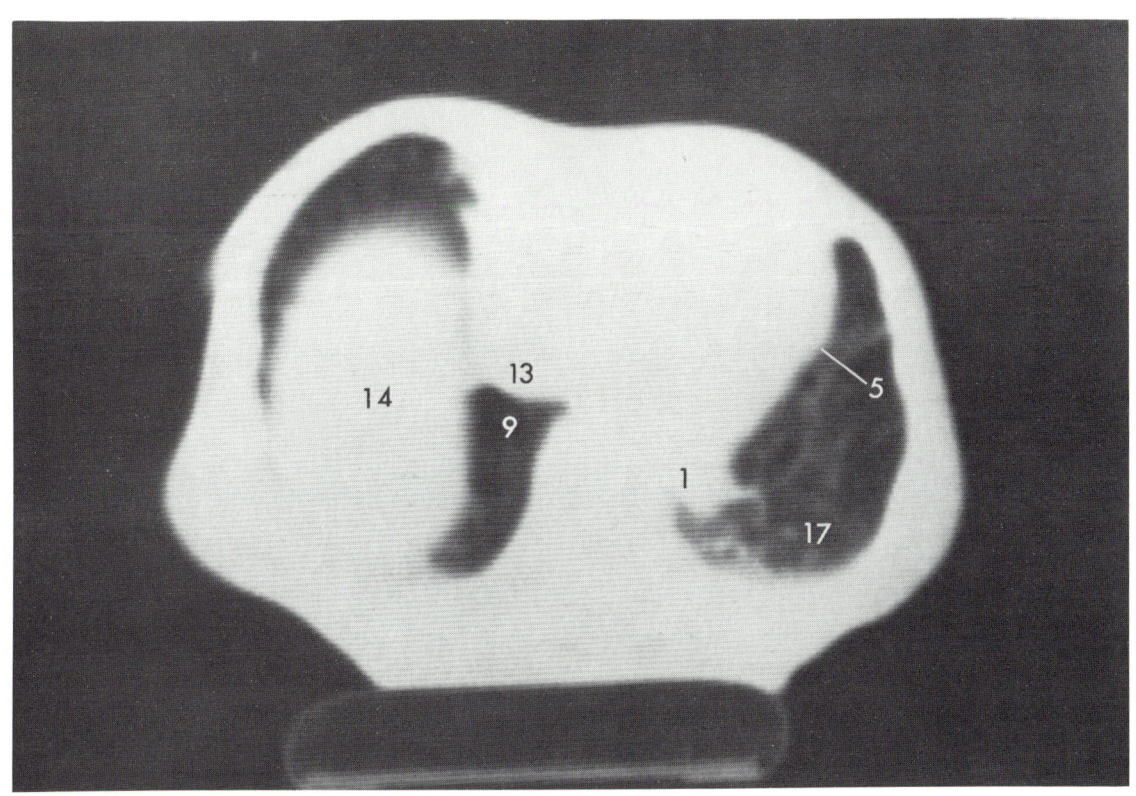

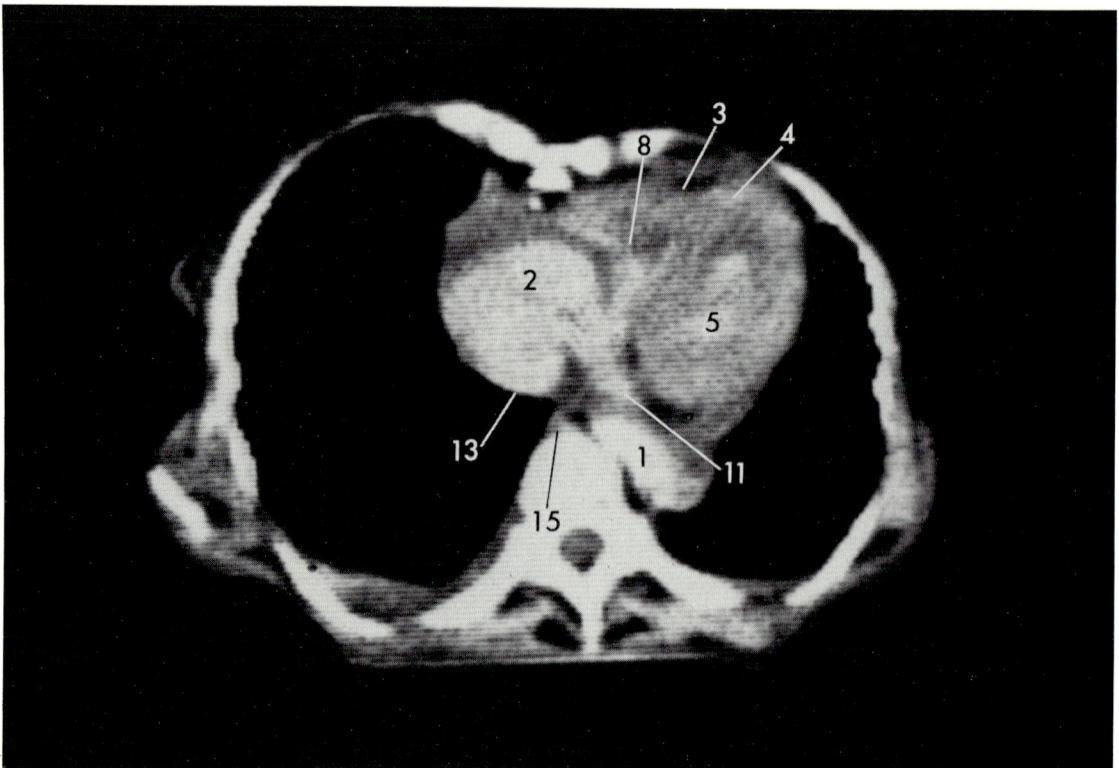

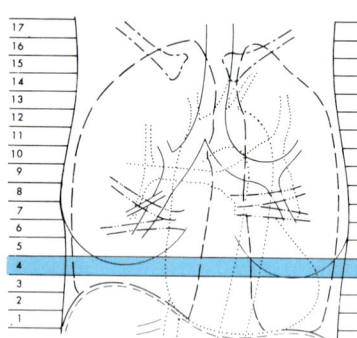

1. Descending thoracic aorta
2. Right atrium
3. Right ventricle
4. Interventricular septum
5. Left ventricle

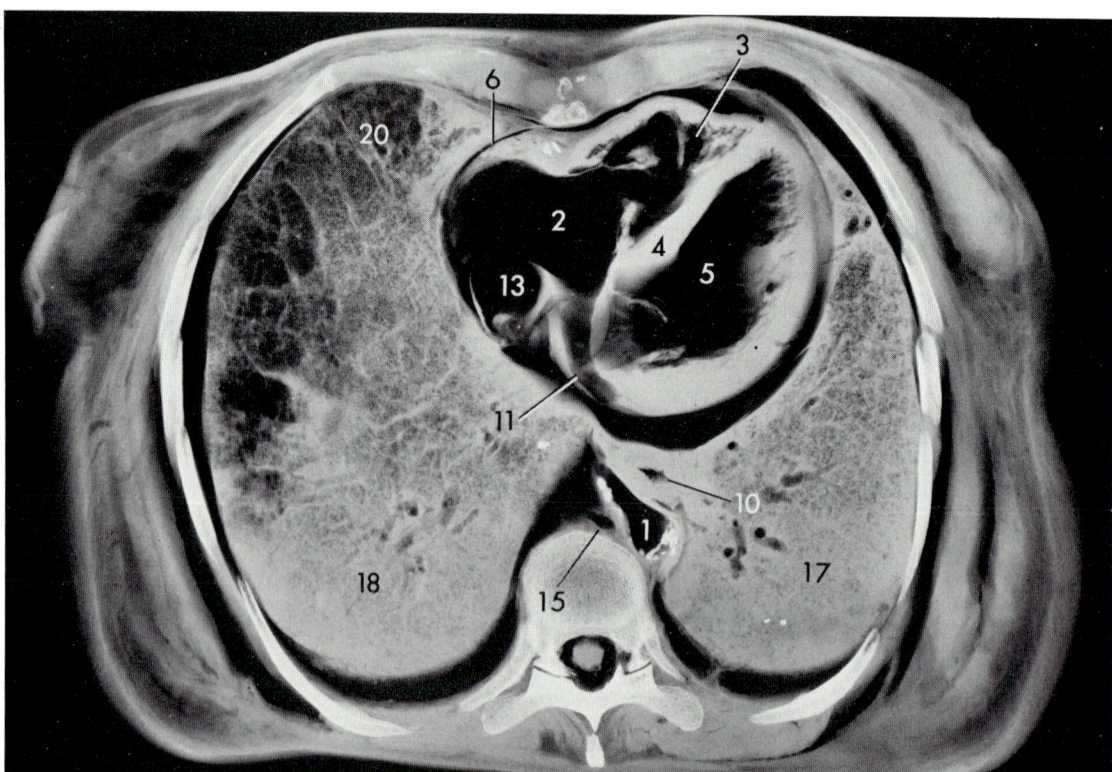

CHEST

Level 4

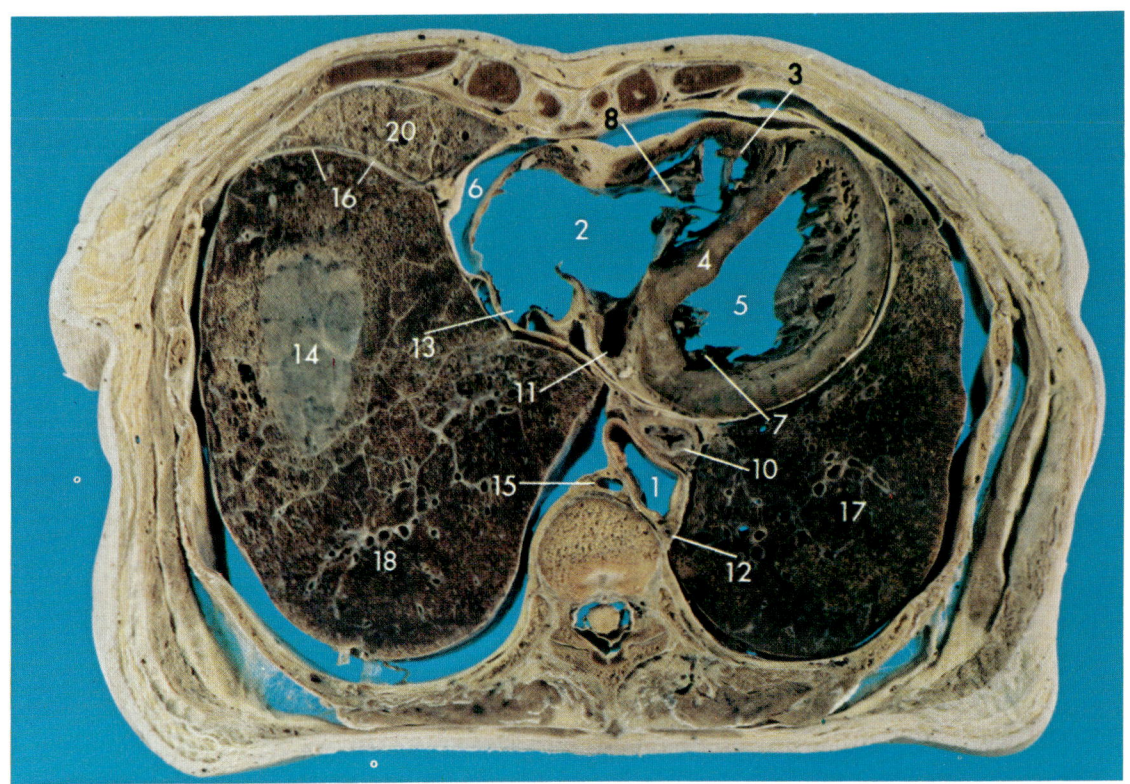

6. Pericardial cavity
7. Mitral valve
8. Tricuspid valve
10. Esophagus
11. Coronary sinus
12. Accessory hemiazygos vein
13. Inferior vena cava entering right atrium
14. Dome of right hemidiaphragm
15. Azygos vein
16. Right major fissure
17. Left lower lobe of lung
18. Right lower lobe of lung
20. Right middle lobe of lung

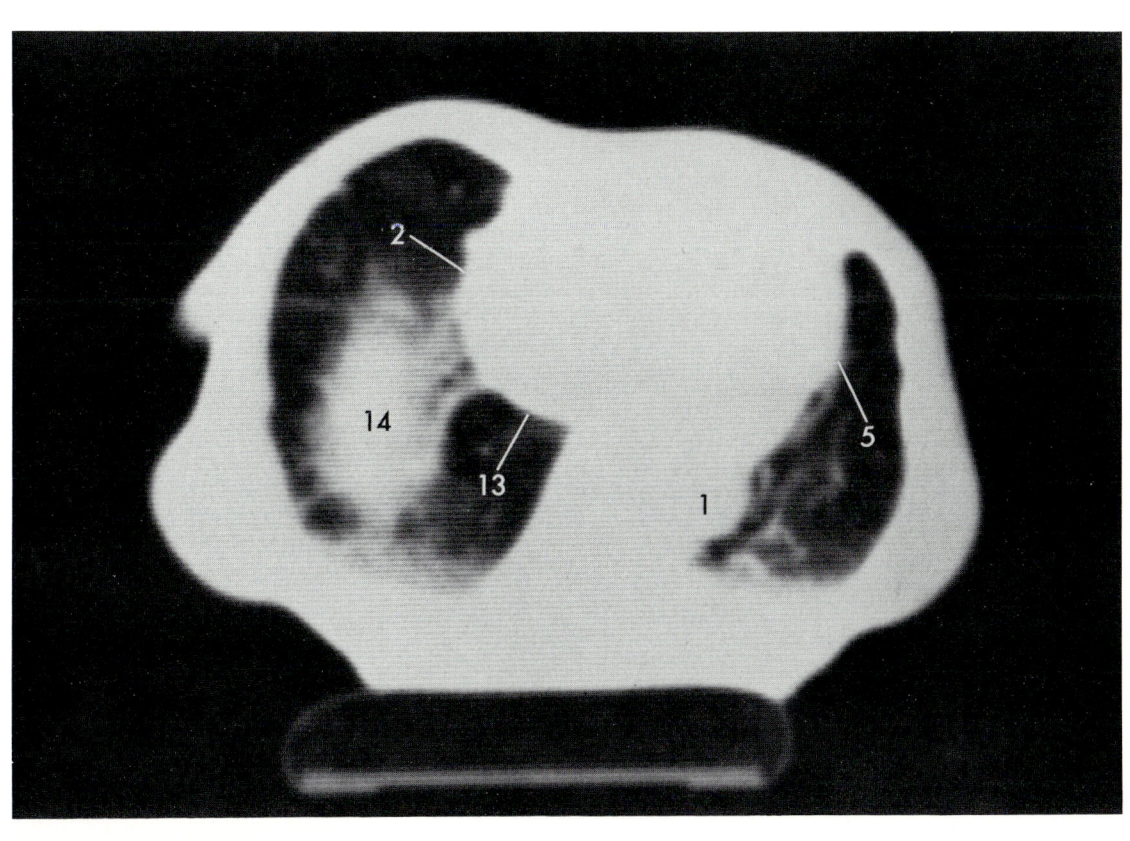

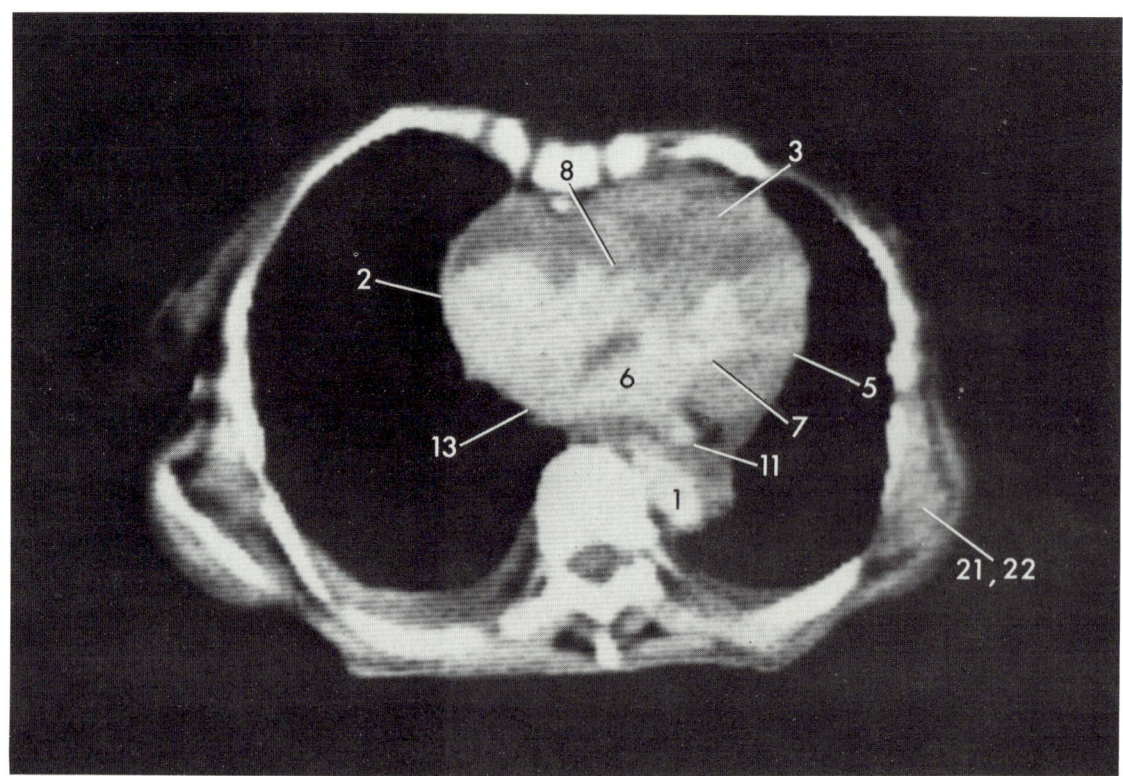

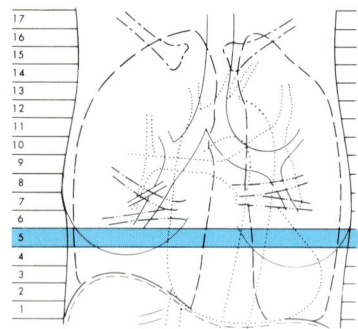

1. Descending thoracic aorta
2. Right atrium
3. Right ventricle
4. Interventricular septum
5. Left ventricle
6. Left atrium

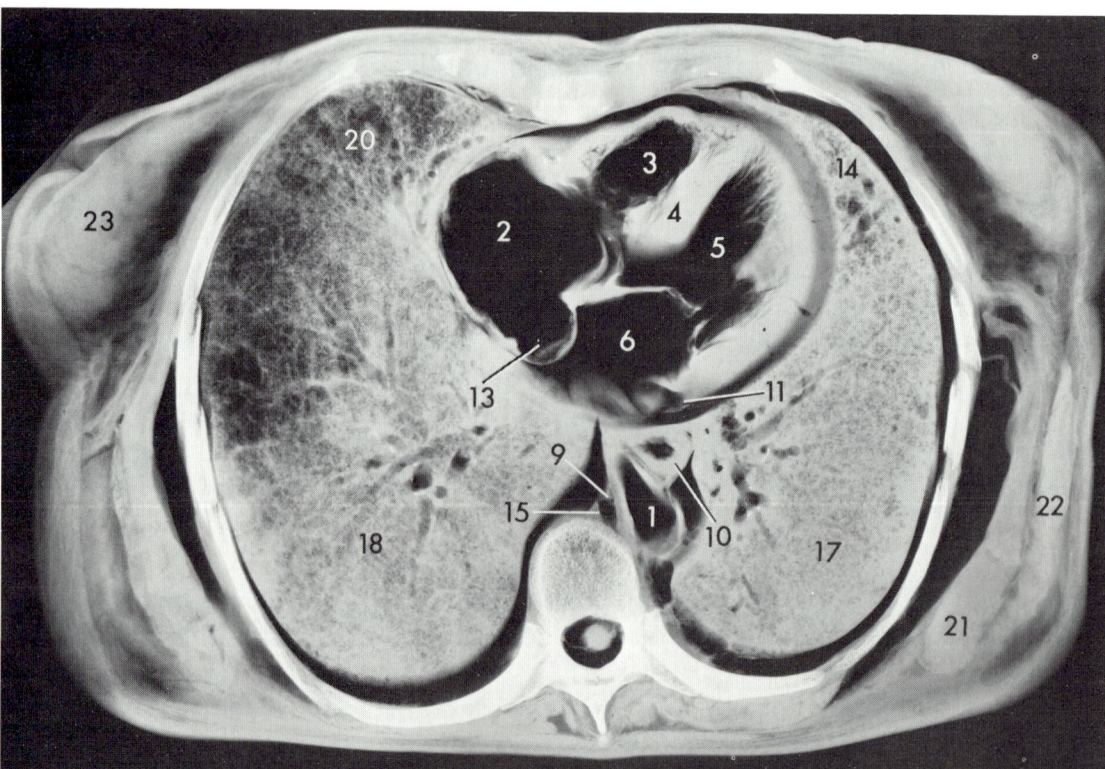

CHEST

Level 5

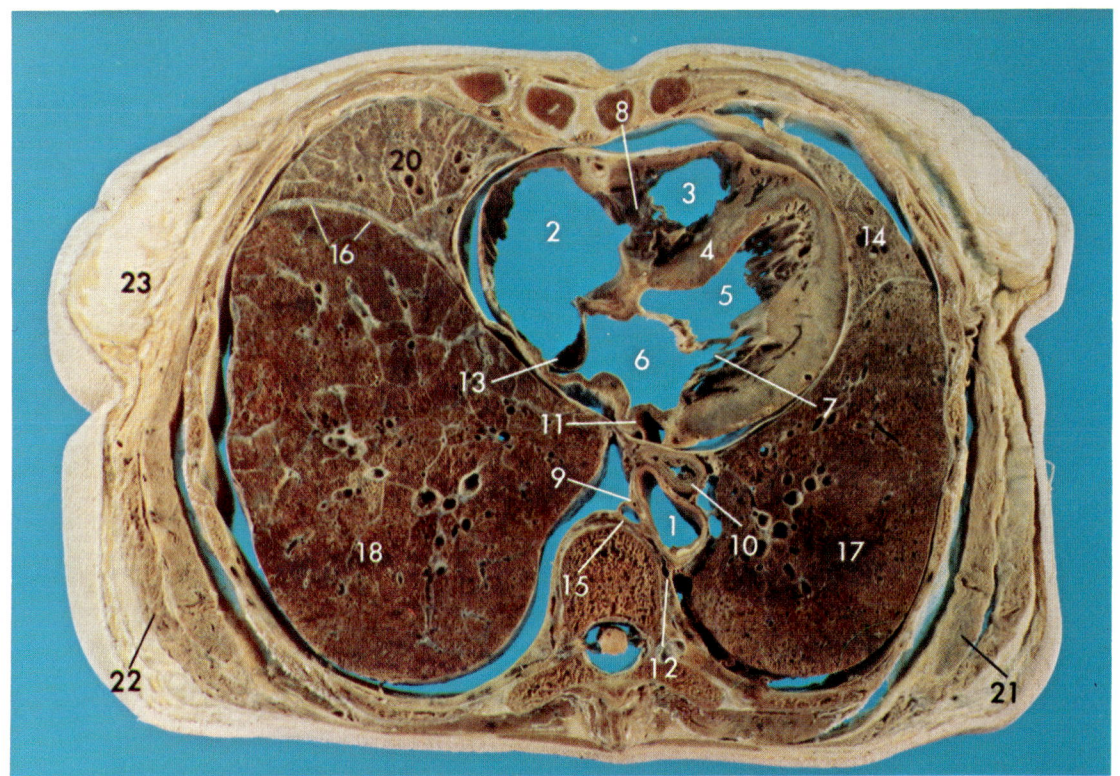

7. Mitral valve
8. Tricuspid valve
9. Thoracic duct
10. Esophagus
11. Coronary sinus
12. Accessory hemiazygos vein
13. Inferior vena cava entering right atrium
14. Lingula of left lung
15. Azygos vein
16. Right major fissure
17. Left lower lobe of lung
18. Right lower lobe of lung
20. Right middle lobe of lung
21. Serratus anterior muscle
22. Latissimus dorsi muscle
23. Breast

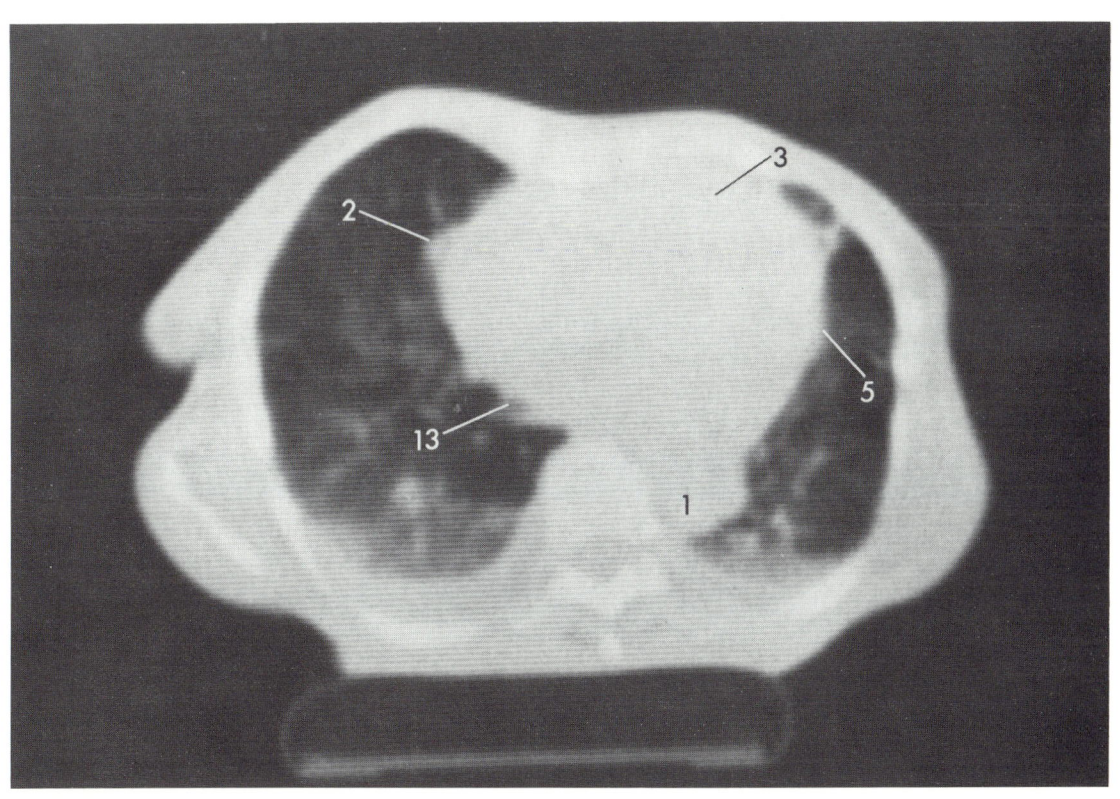

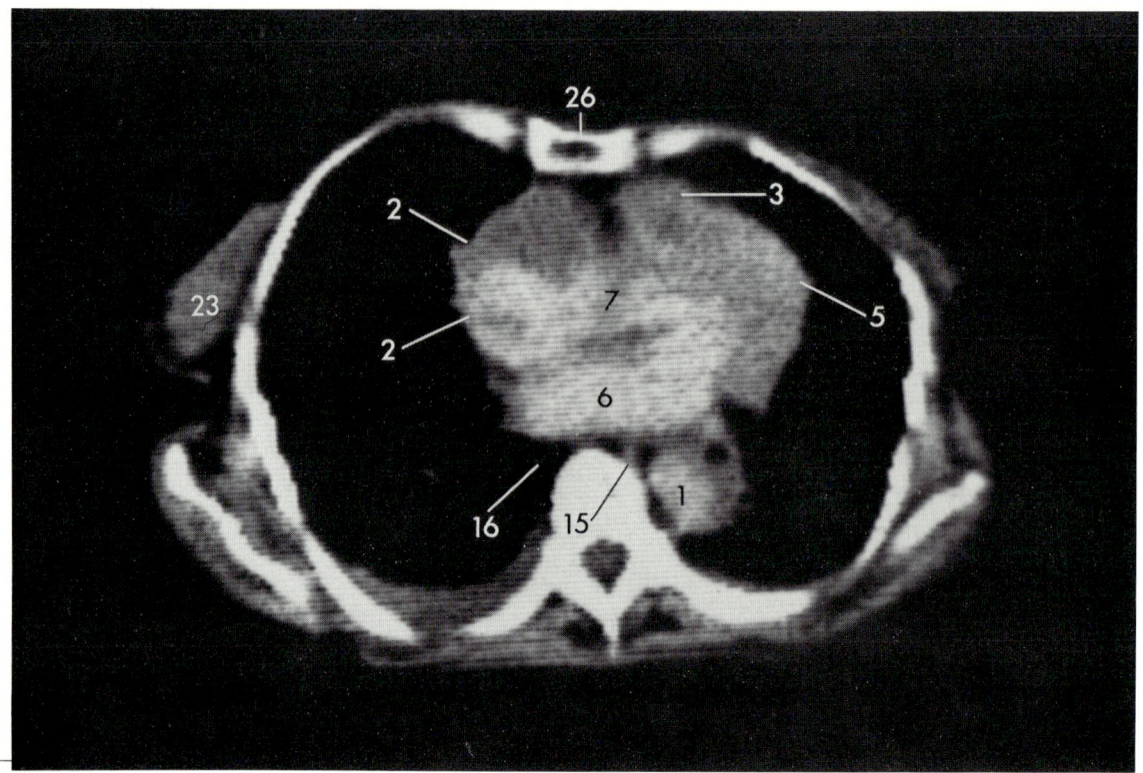

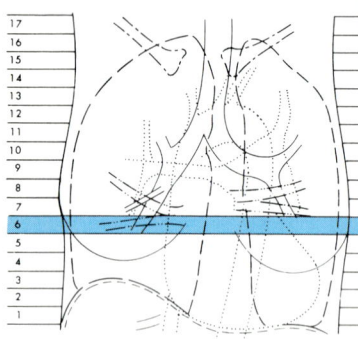

1. Descending thoracic aorta
2. Right atrium
3. Right ventricle
4. Interventricular septum
5. Left ventricular wall
6. Left atrium
7. Aortic valve

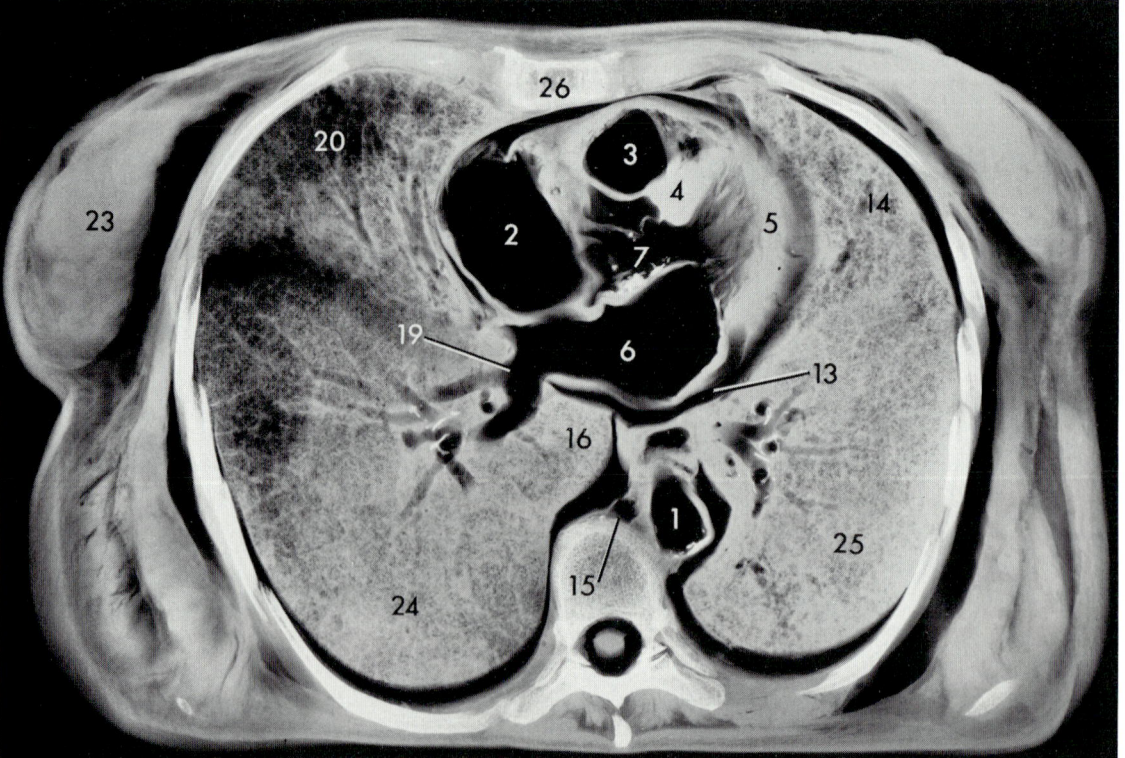

CHEST

Level 6

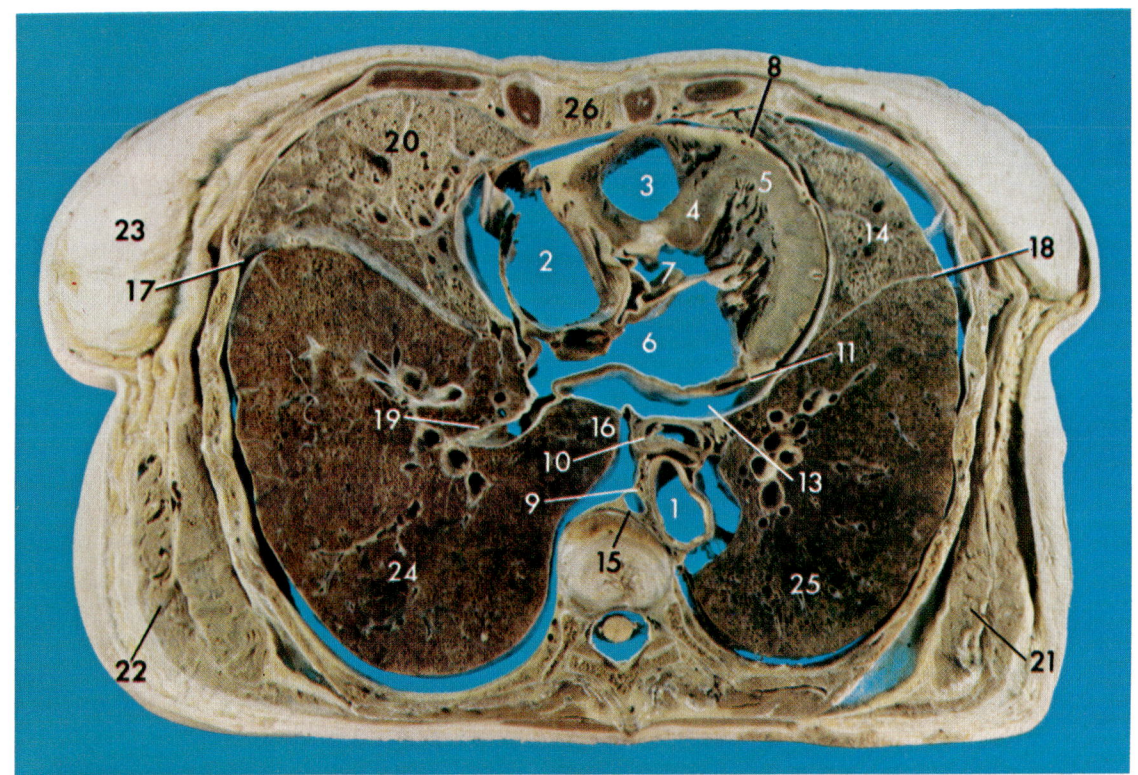

8. Left anterior descending coronary artery and great cardiac vein
9. Thoracic duct
10. Esophagus
11. Coronary sinus
13. Oblique pericardial sinus
14. Lingula of left lung
15. Azygos vein
16. Right lower lobe of lung in azygoesophageal recess
17. Right major fissure
18. Left major fissure
19. Right inferior pulmonary vein
20. Right middle lobe of lung
21. Serratus anterior muscle
22. Latissimus dorsi muscle
23. Breast
24. Right lower lobe of lung
25. Left lower lobe of lung
26. Sternum

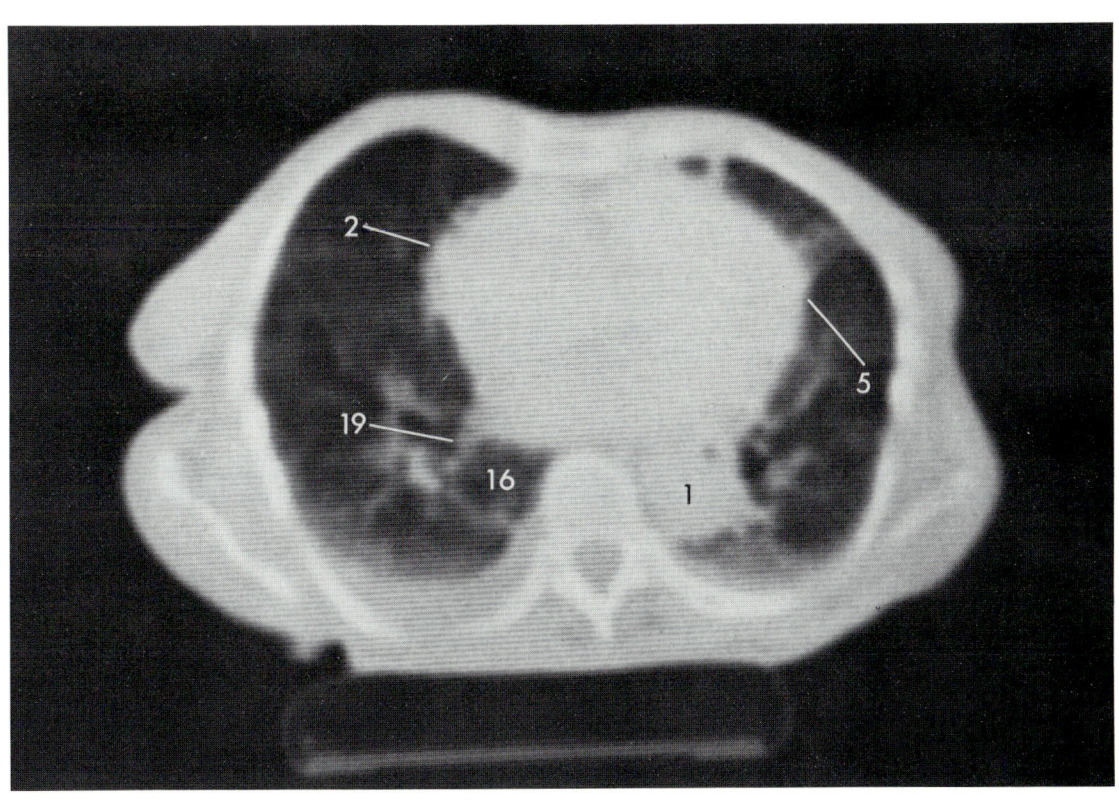

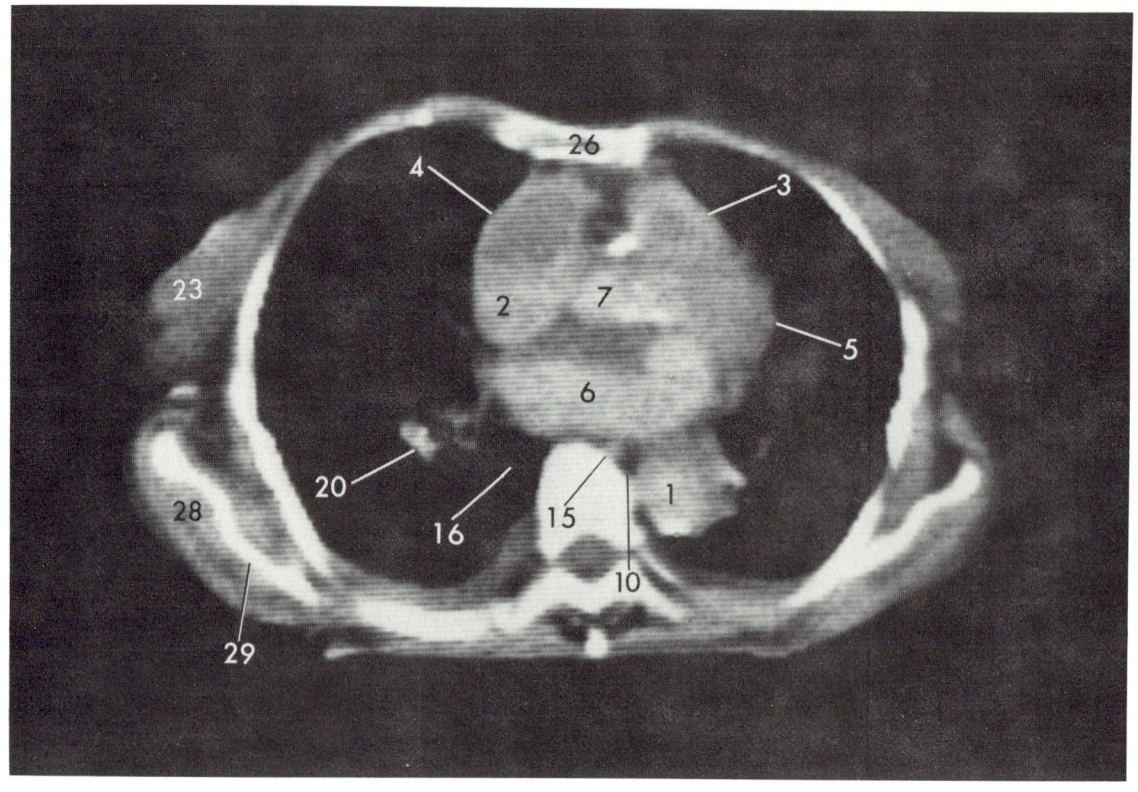

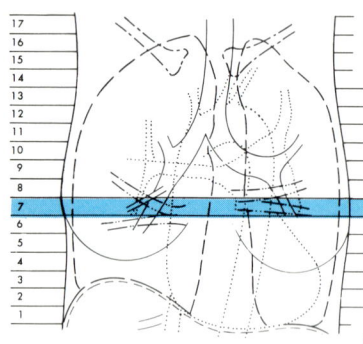

1. Descending thoracic aorta
2. Superior vena cava
3. Right ventricle (outflow tract)
4. Right atrial appendage (with clot)
5. Left ventricular wall
6. Left atrium
7. Aortic valve
8. Segmental bronchi, left lower lobe
9. Thoracic duct
10. Esophagus (with gas on CT images)
11. Coronary sinus
13. Left lower lobe of lung (preaortic)

CHEST

Level 7

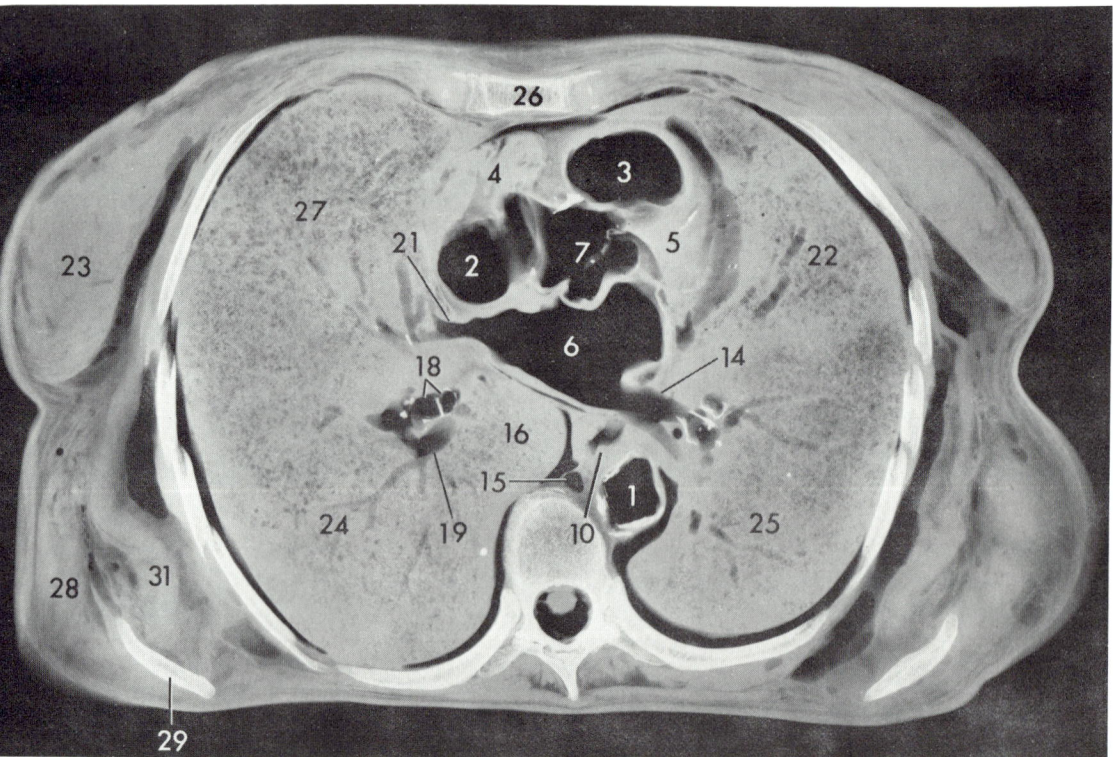

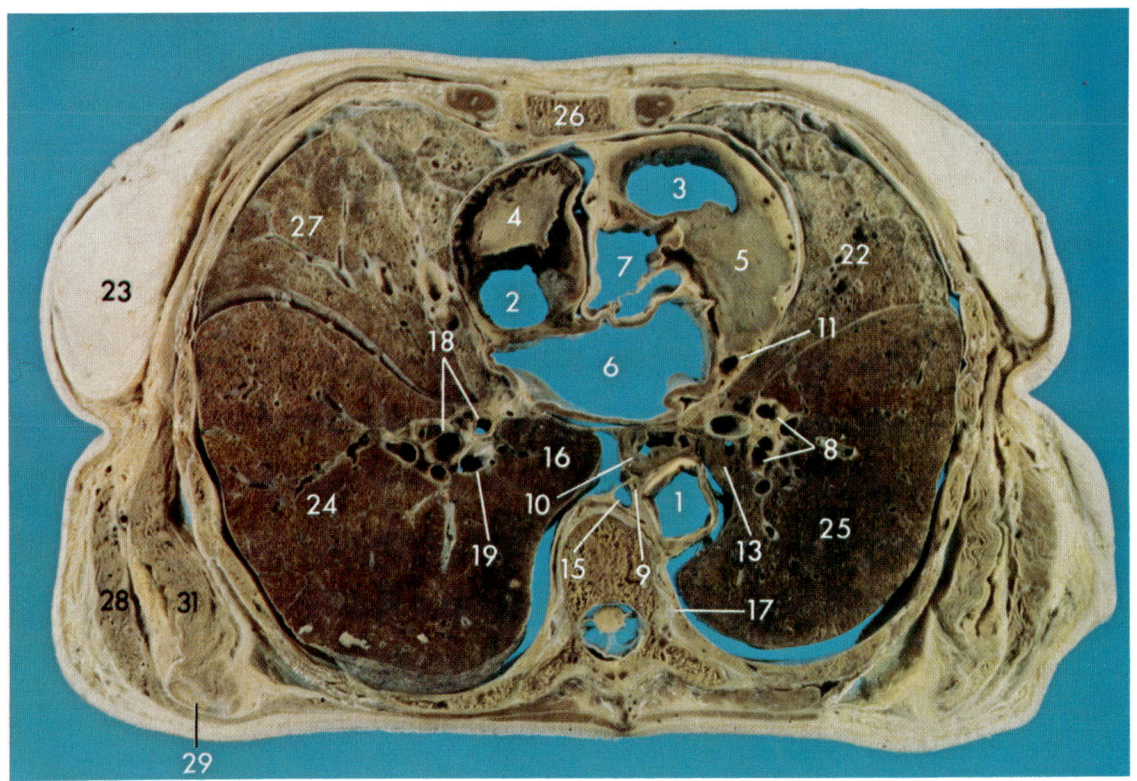

14. Left inferior pulmonary vein
15. Azygos vein
16. Right lower lobe in azygoesophageal recess
17. Left paraspinal area
18. Segmental bronchi, right lower lobe
19. Right inferior pulmonary vein
20. Right lower lobe pulmonary artery
21. Right superior pulmonary vein
22. Lingula of left lung
23. Breast
24. Right lower lobe of lung
25. Left lower lobe of lung
26. Sternum
27. Right middle lobe of lung
28. Latissimus dorsi muscle
29. Scapula
31. Serratus anterior muscle

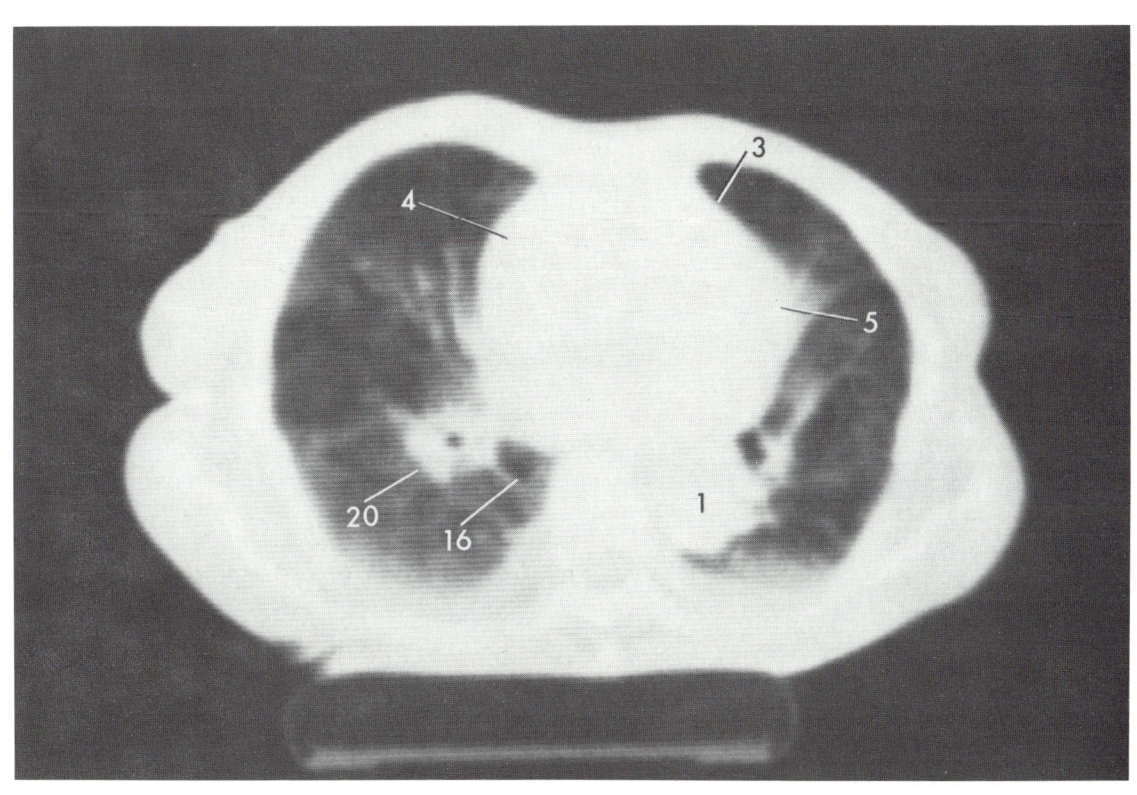

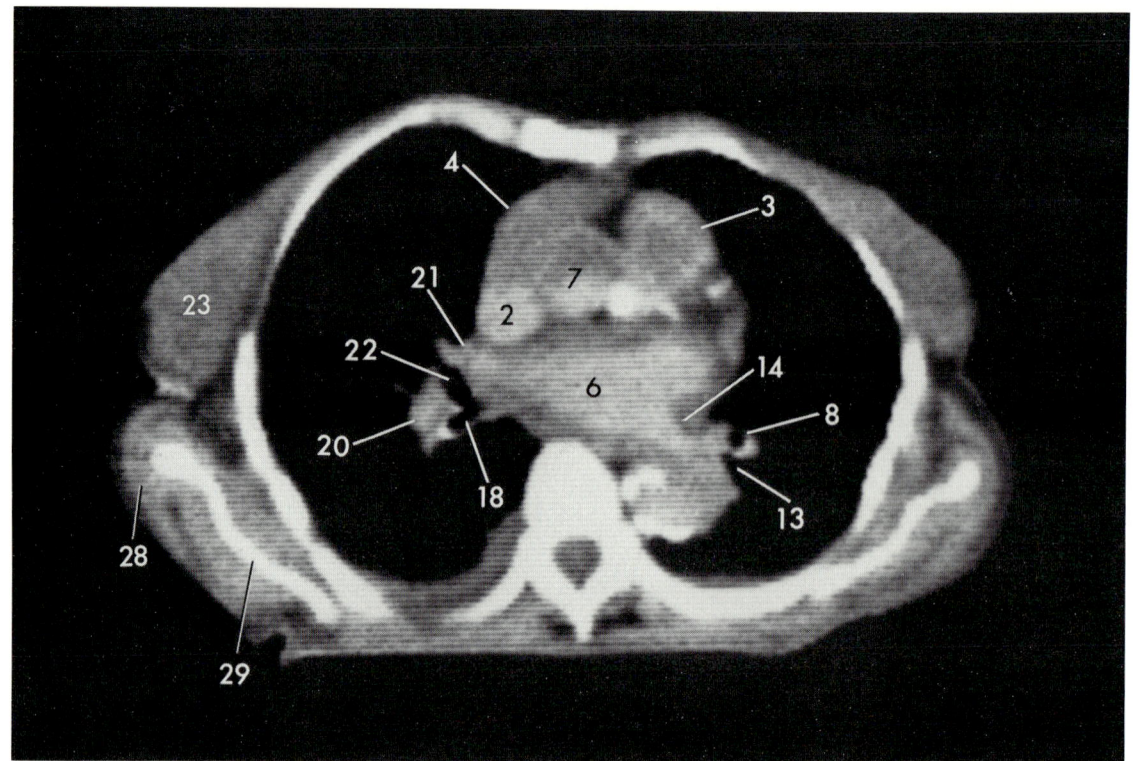

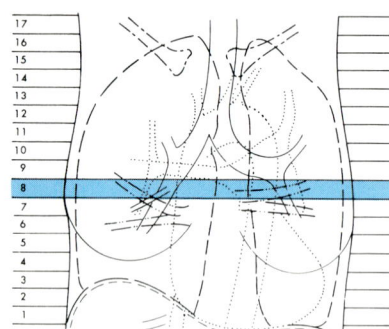

1. Descending thoracic aorta
2. Superior vena cava
3. Pulmonary valve
4. Right atrial appendage
5. Lingula of left lung
6. Left atrium
7. Ascending thoracic aorta
8. Left lower lobe bronchus
9. Thoracic duct

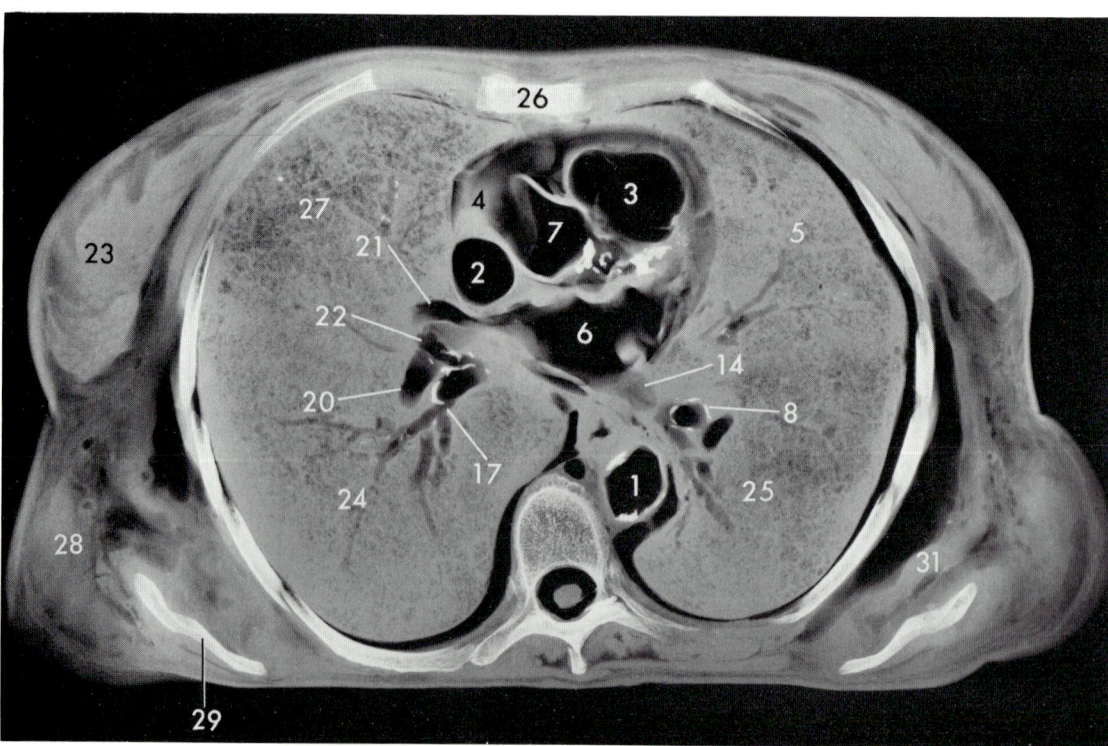

CHEST

Level 8

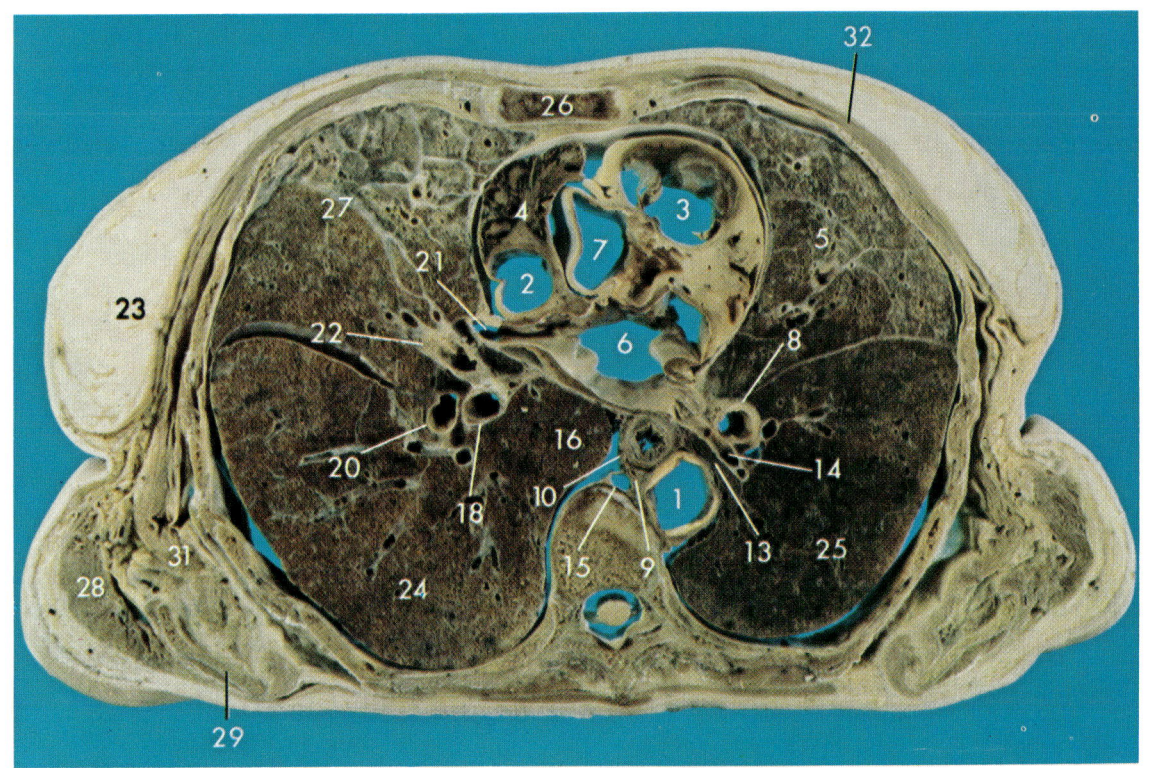

10. Esophagus
13. Left lower lobe of lung (preaortic)
14. Left inferior pulmonary vein
15. Azygos vein
16. Right lower lobe of lung in azygoesophageal recess
17. Superior segmental bronchus, right lower lobe
18. Right lower lobe bronchus
20. Right interlobar pulmonary artery
21. Right superior pulmonary vein
22. Right middle lobe bronchus
23. Breast
24. Right lower lobe of lung
25. Left lower lobe of lung
26. Sternum
27. Right middle lobe of lung
28. Latissimus dorsi muscle
29. Scapula
31. Serratus anterior muscle
32. Pectoralis major muscle

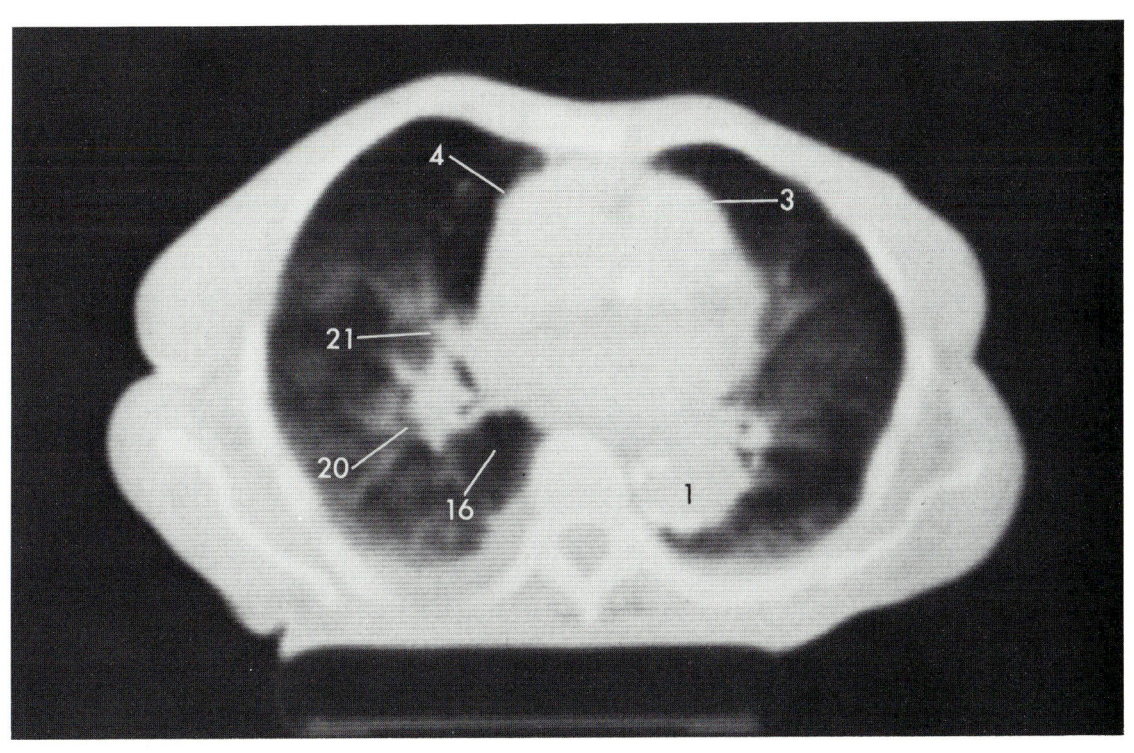

119

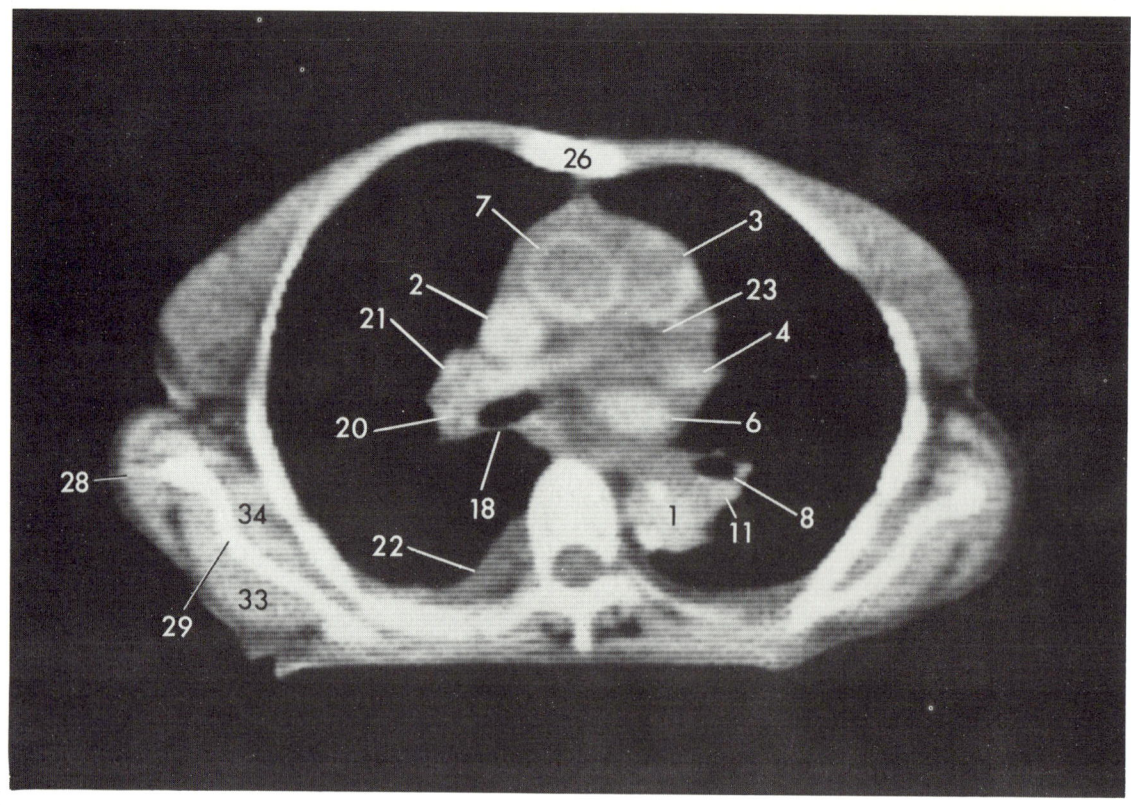

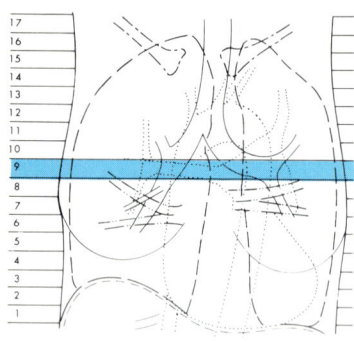

1. Descending thoracic aorta
2. Superior vena cava
3. Main pulmonary artery
4. Left atrial appendage
5. Lingular bronchus
6. Left atrium
7. Ascending thoracic aorta
8. Left lower lobe bronchus
9. Thoracic duct
10. Esophagus
11. Left interlobar pulmonary artery
14. Superior segmental bronchus, left lower lobe
15. Azygos vein

CHEST

Level 9

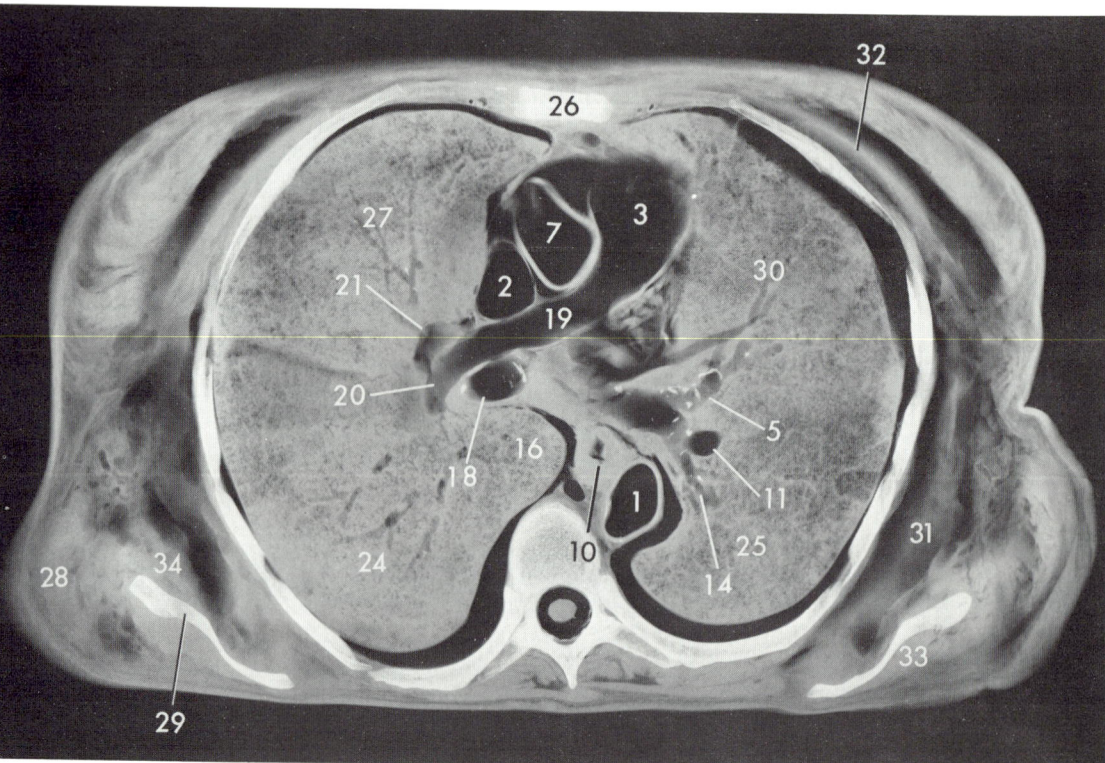

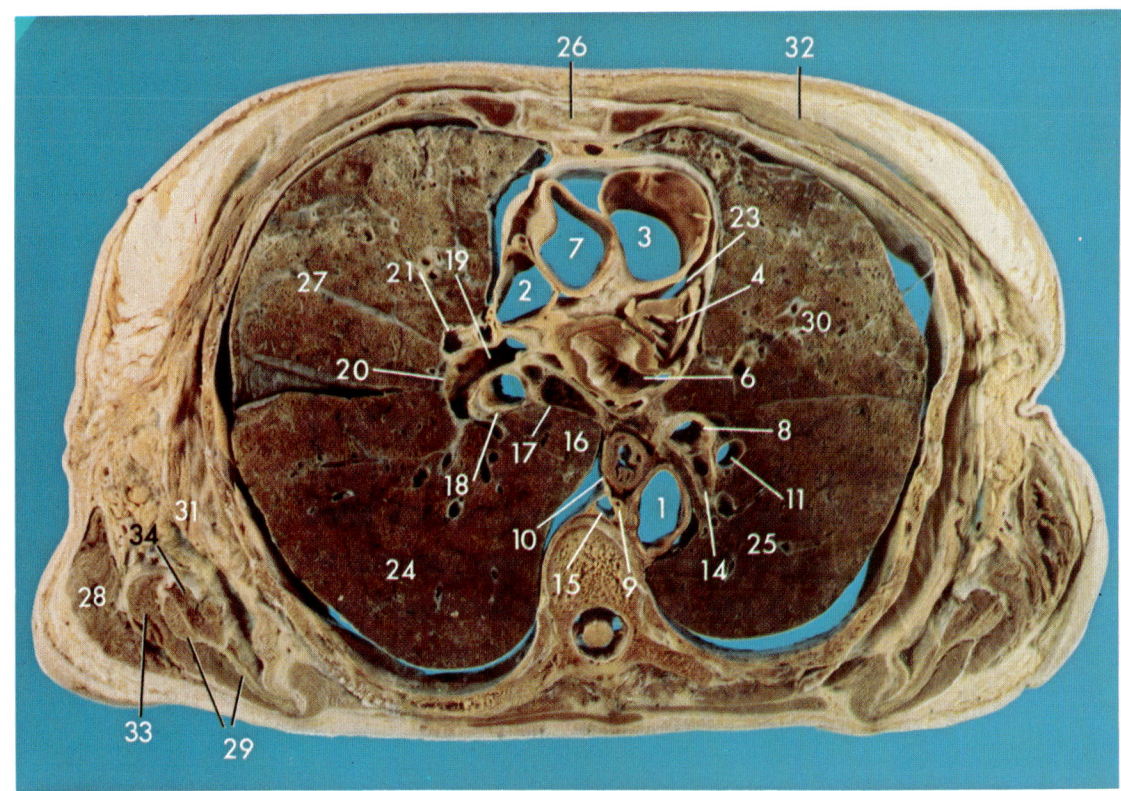

16. Right lower lobe in azygoesophageal recess
17. Subcarinal lymph nodes
18. Bronchus intermedius
19. Right pulmonary artery
20. Right interlobar pulmonary artery
21. Right superior pulmonary vein
22. Fluid in pleural cavity
23. Transverse pericardial sinus
24. Right lower lobe of lung
25. Left lower lobe of lung
26. Sternum
27. Right middle lobe of lung
28. Latissimus dorsi muscle
29. Scapula
30. Lingula of left lung
31. Serratus anterior muscle
32. Pectoralis major muscle
33. Teres major muscle
34. Subscapularis muscle

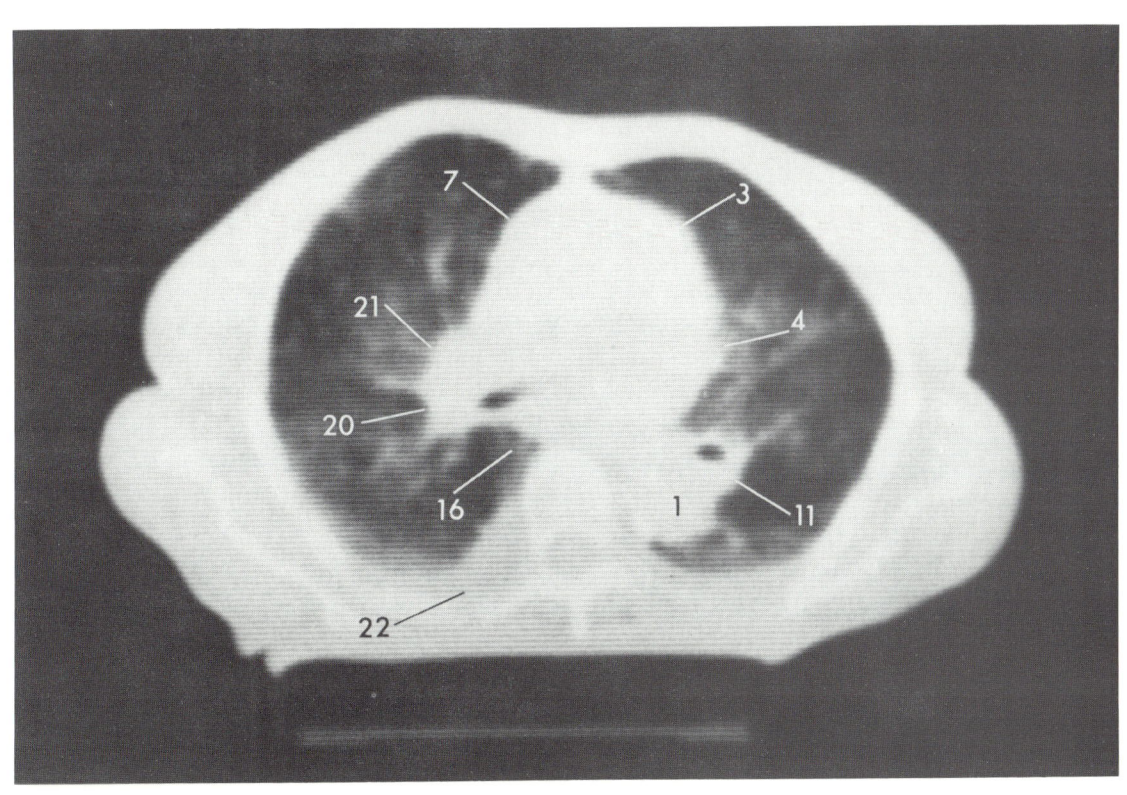

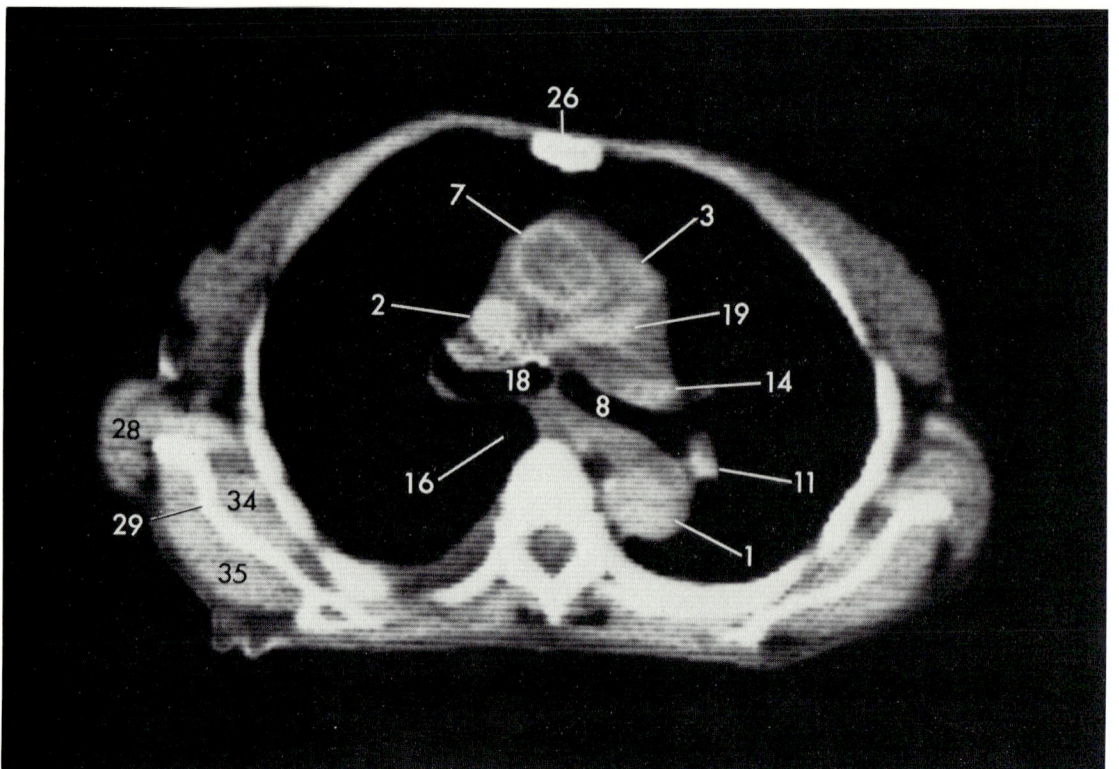

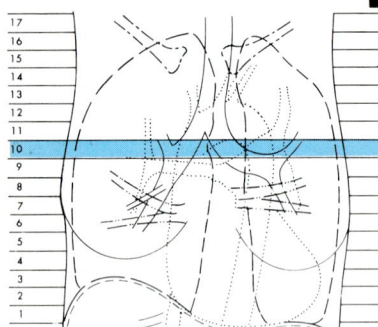

1. Descending thoracic aorta
2. Superior vena cava
3. Main pulmonary artery
4. Left superior pulmonary vein
5. Lingular bronchus
6. Left upper lobe bronchus
7. Ascending thoracic aorta
8. Left main bronchus
9. Thoracic duct
10. Esophagus
11. Left interlobar pulmonary artery
14. Left pulmonary artery
15. Azygos vein
16. Right lower lobe of lung in azygoesophageal recess
17. Subcarinal lymph nodes

CHEST

Level 10

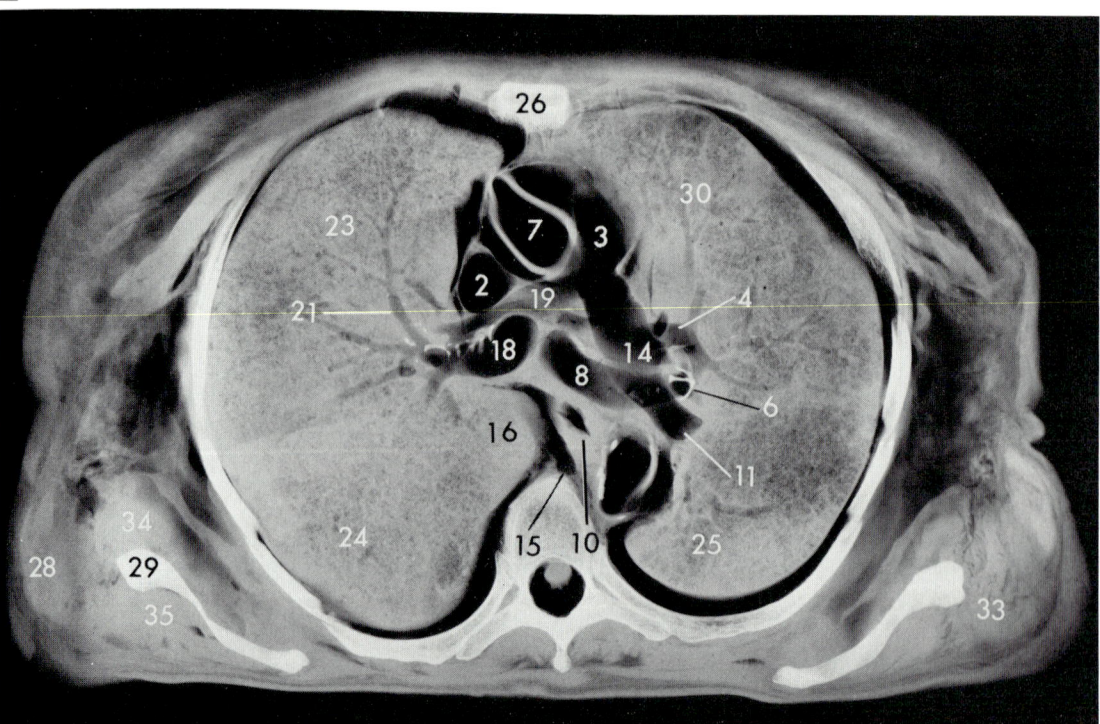

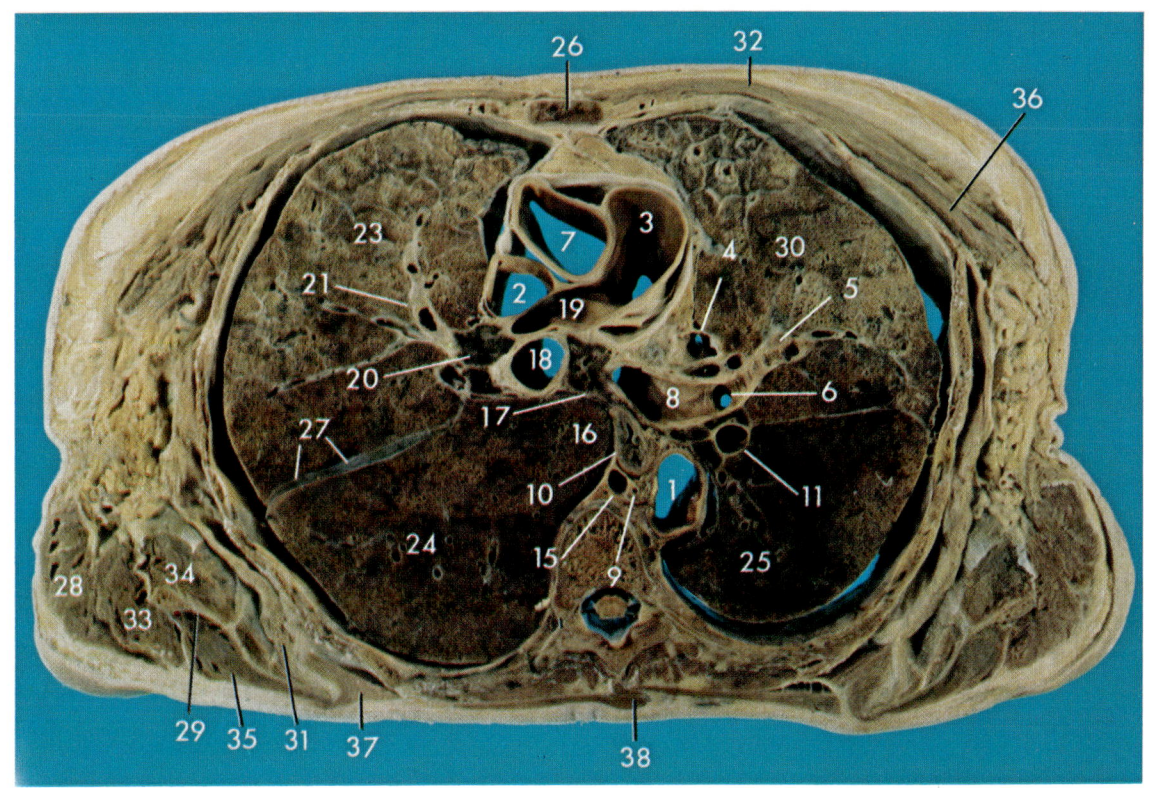

18. Right main bronchus
19. Right pulmonary artery
20. Right hilar lymph nodes
21. Anterior segmental bronchus, right upper lobe
23. Right upper lobe of lung
24. Right lower lobe of lung
25. Left lower lobe of lung
26. Sternum
27. Right major fissure
28. Latissimus dorsi muscle
29. Scapula
30. Left upper lobe of lung
31. Serratus anterior muscle
32. Pectoralis major muscle
33. Teres major muscle
34. Subscapularis muscle
35. Infraspinatus muscle
36. Pectoralis minor muscle
37. Rhomboideus major muscle
38. Trapezius muscle

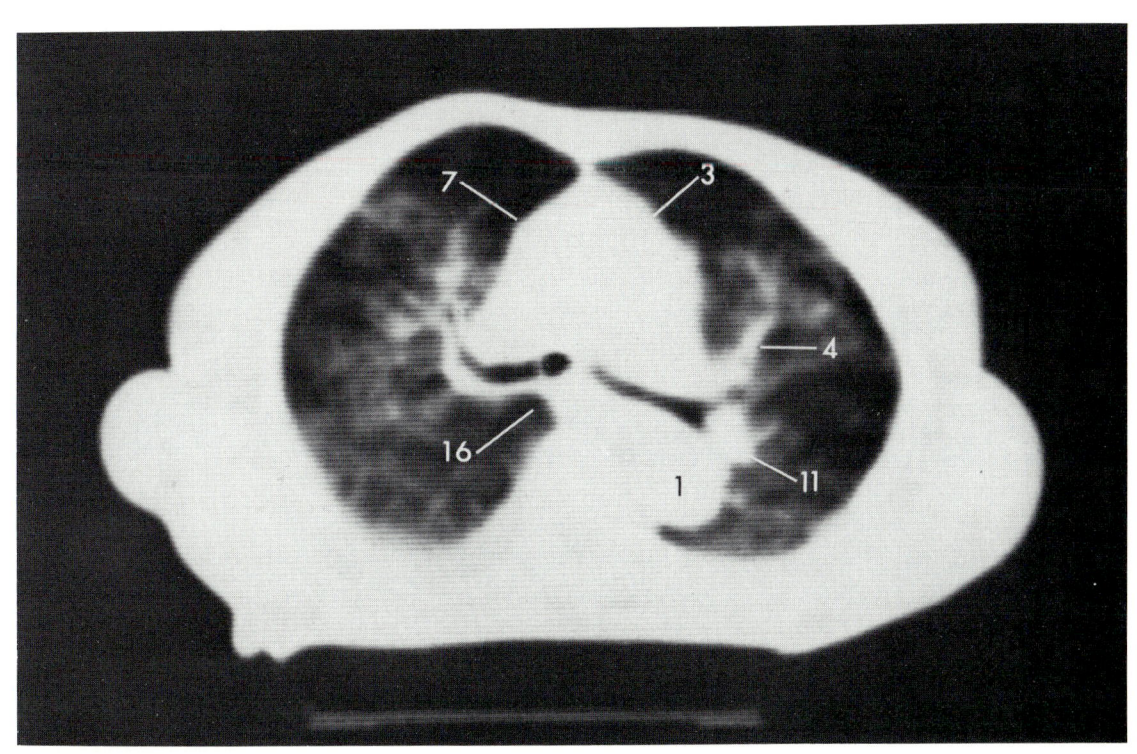

123

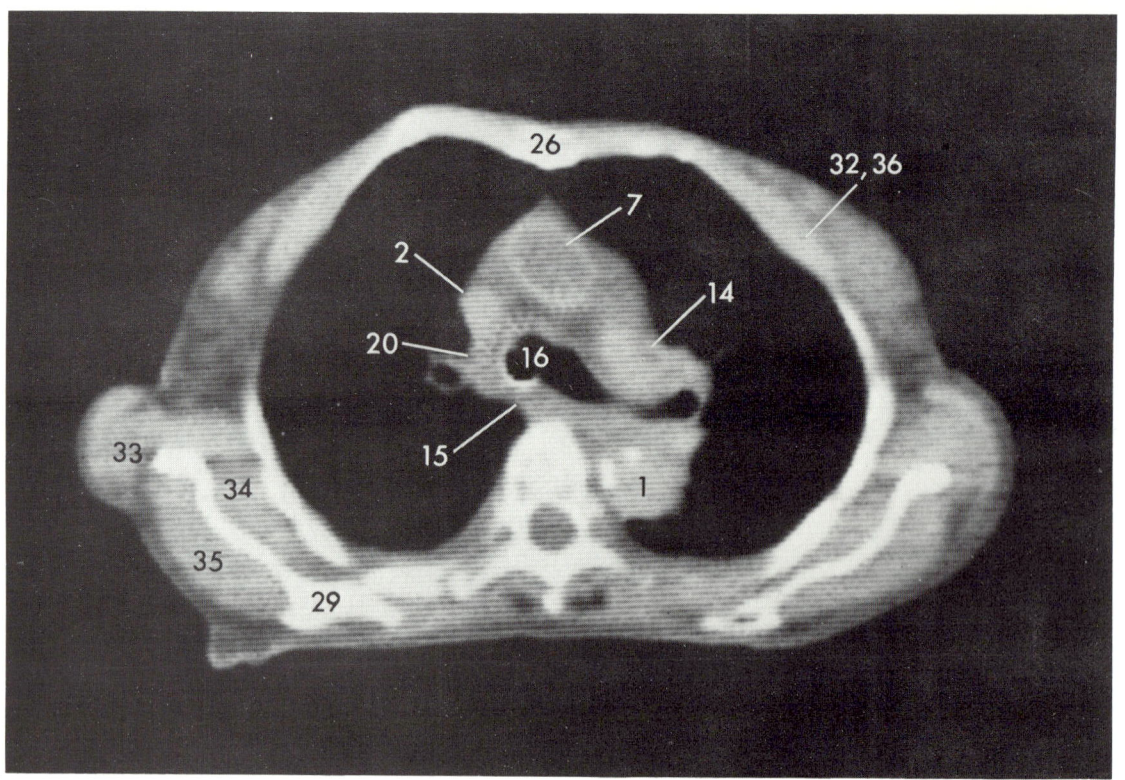

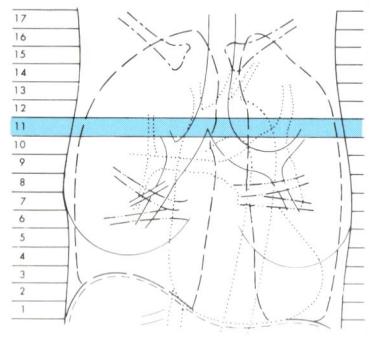

1. Descending thoracic aorta
2. Superior vena cava
3. Pericardial cavity (superior extent)
6. Anterior junction line area (anterior mediastinal fat)
7. Ascending thoracic aorta
8. Lymph nodes at the medial aspect of the aortic-pulmonic window
10. Esophagus
11. Anterior segmental pulmonary artery, left upper lobe
12. Accessory hemiazygos vein
13. Anterior segmental bronchus, left upper lobe
14. Left pulmonary artery
15. Azygos vein arch, posterior portion

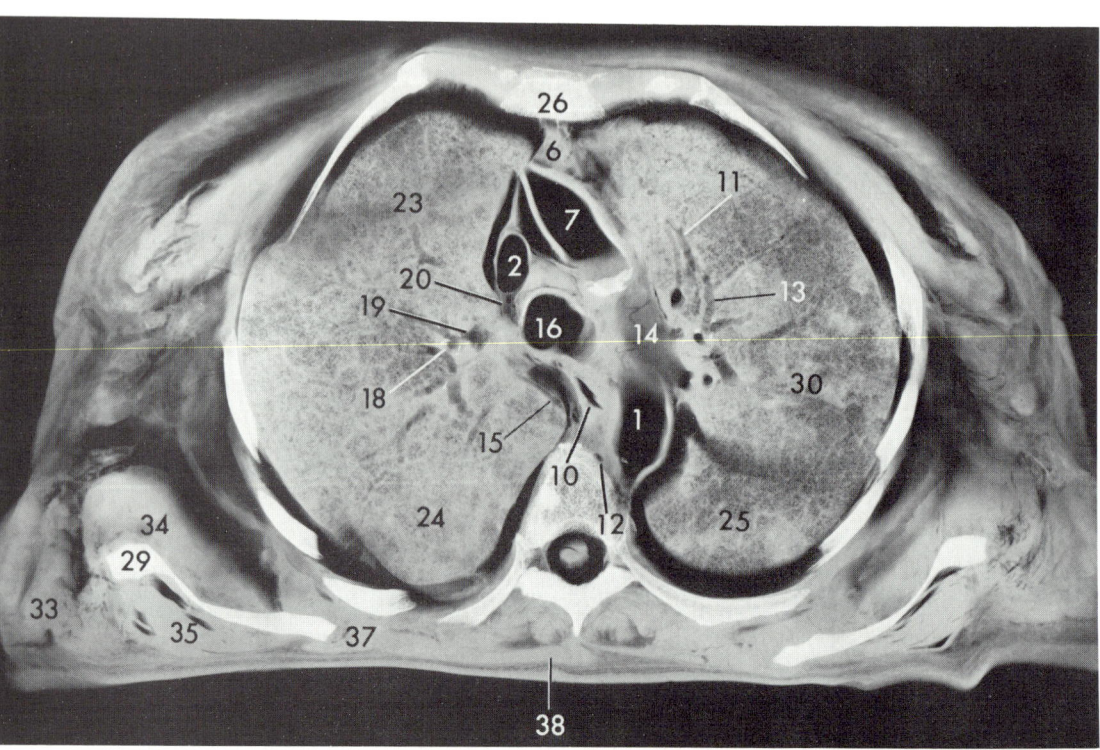

CHEST

Level 11

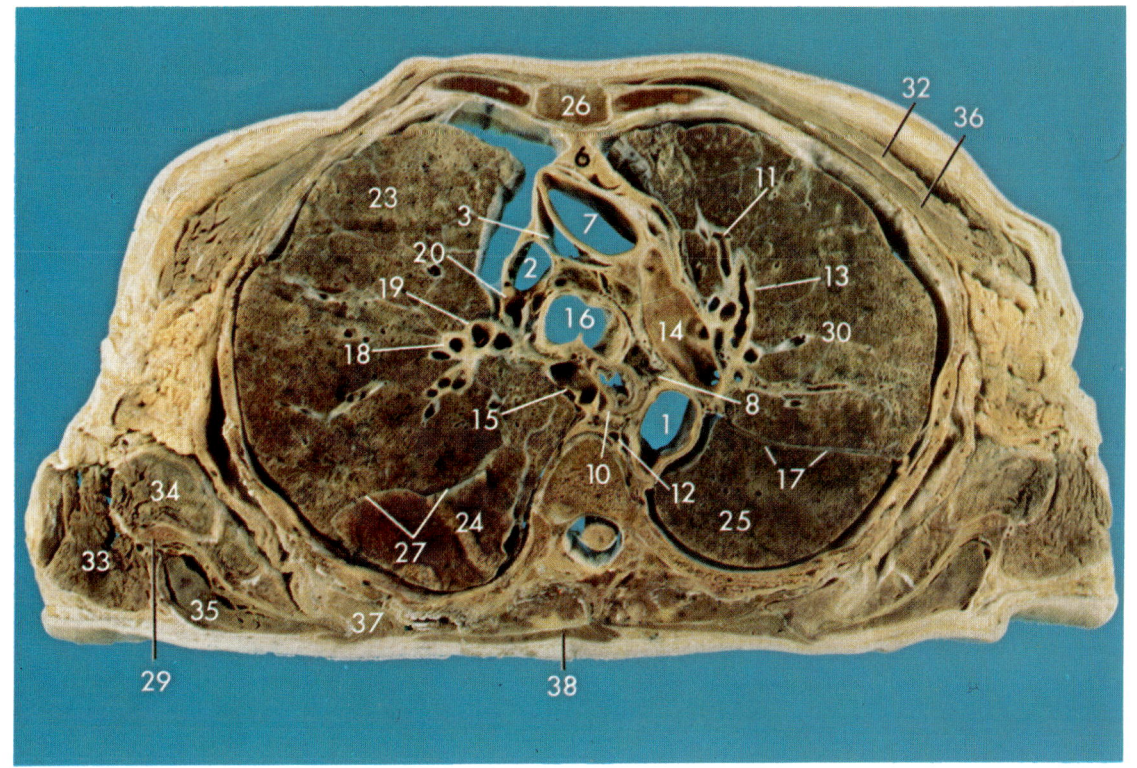

16. Bifurcation of trachea (carina)
17. Left major fissure
18. Apical segmental bronchus, right upper lobe
19. Truncus anterior of right pulmonary artery
20. Azygos vein arch, anterior portion
23. Right upper lobe of lung
24. Right lower lobe of lung
25. Left lower lobe of lung
26. Sternum
27. Right major fissure
29. Scapula
30. Left upper lobe of lung
32. Pectoralis major muscle
33. Teres major muscle
34. Subscapularis muscle
35. Infraspinatus muscle
36. Pectoralis minor muscle
37. Rhomboideus major muscle
38. Trapezius muscle

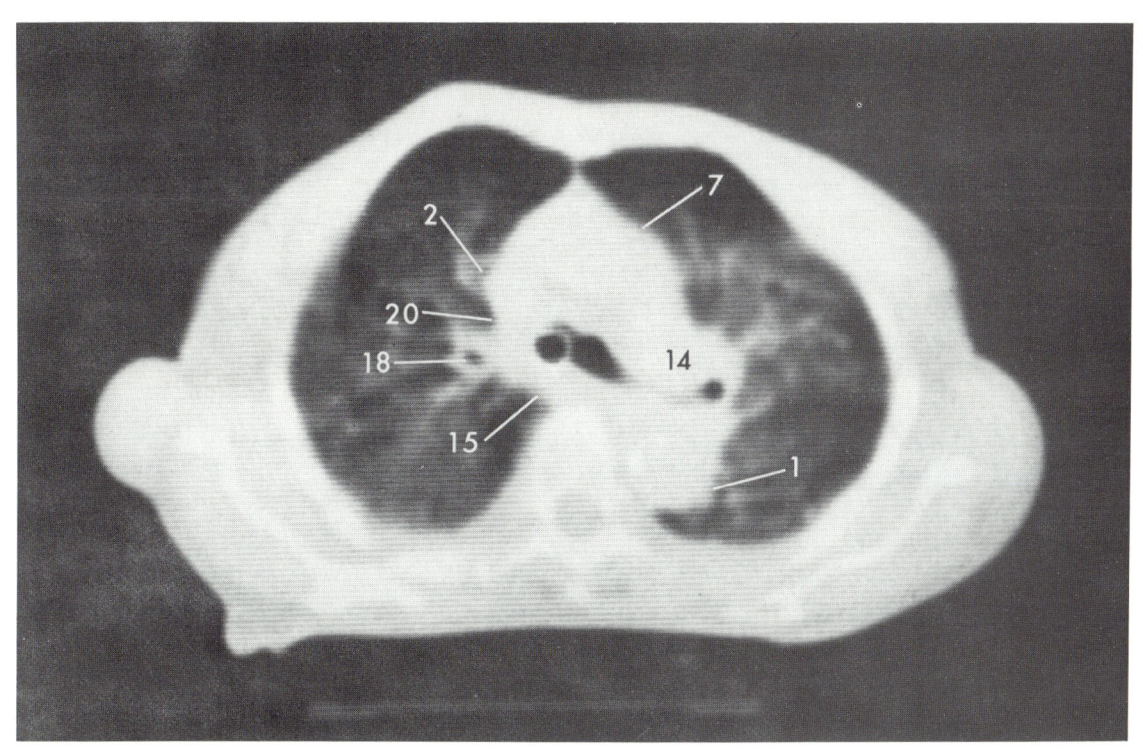

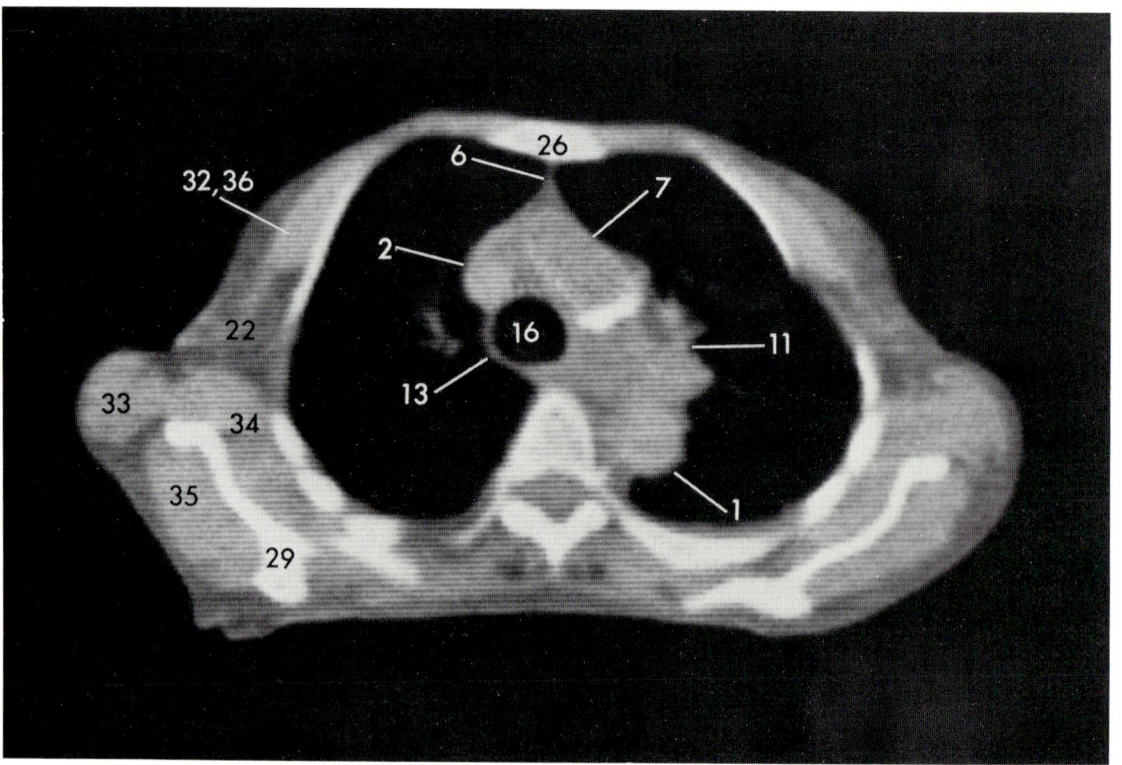

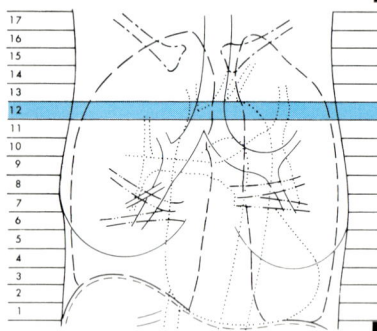

1. Aortic arch, posterior portion
2. Superior vena cava
3. Precaval lymph nodes
4. Internal mammary artery
5. Internal mammary vein
6. Anterior junction line area (anterior mediastinal fat)
7. Aortic arch, anterior portion
8. Lymph node at medial aspect of aortic–pulmonic window
9. Thoracic duct
10. Esophagus
11. Aortic–pulmonic window
12. Accessory hemiazygos vein

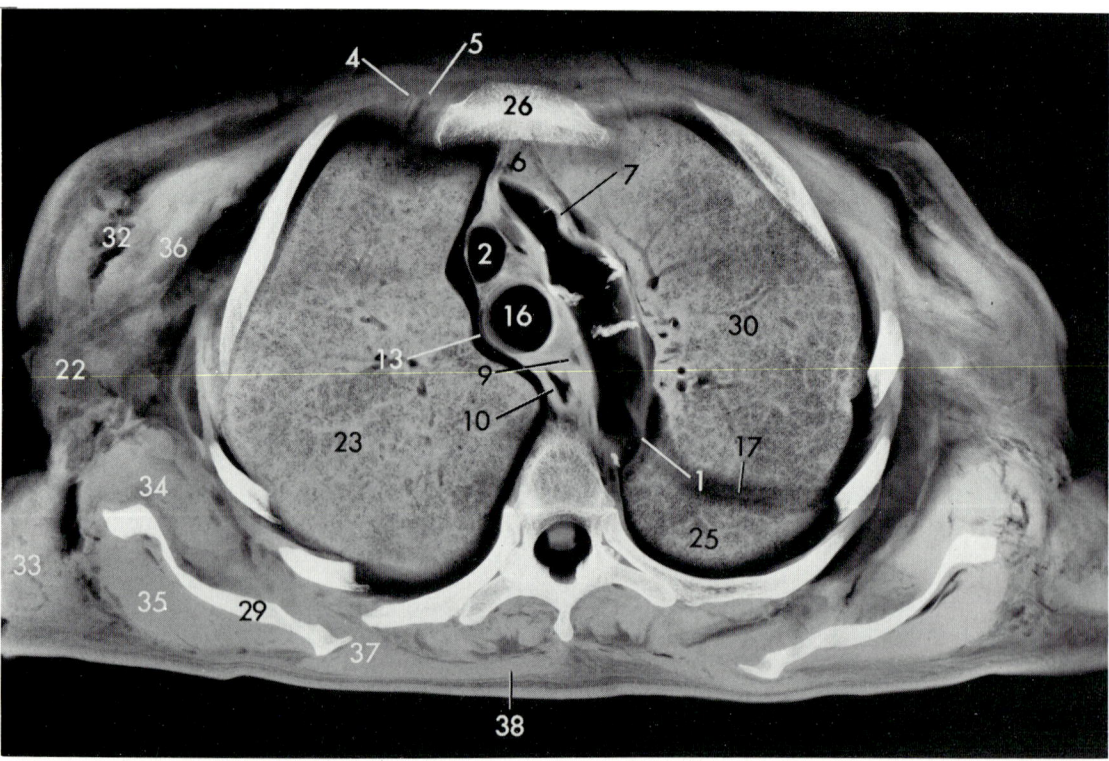

CHEST

Level 12

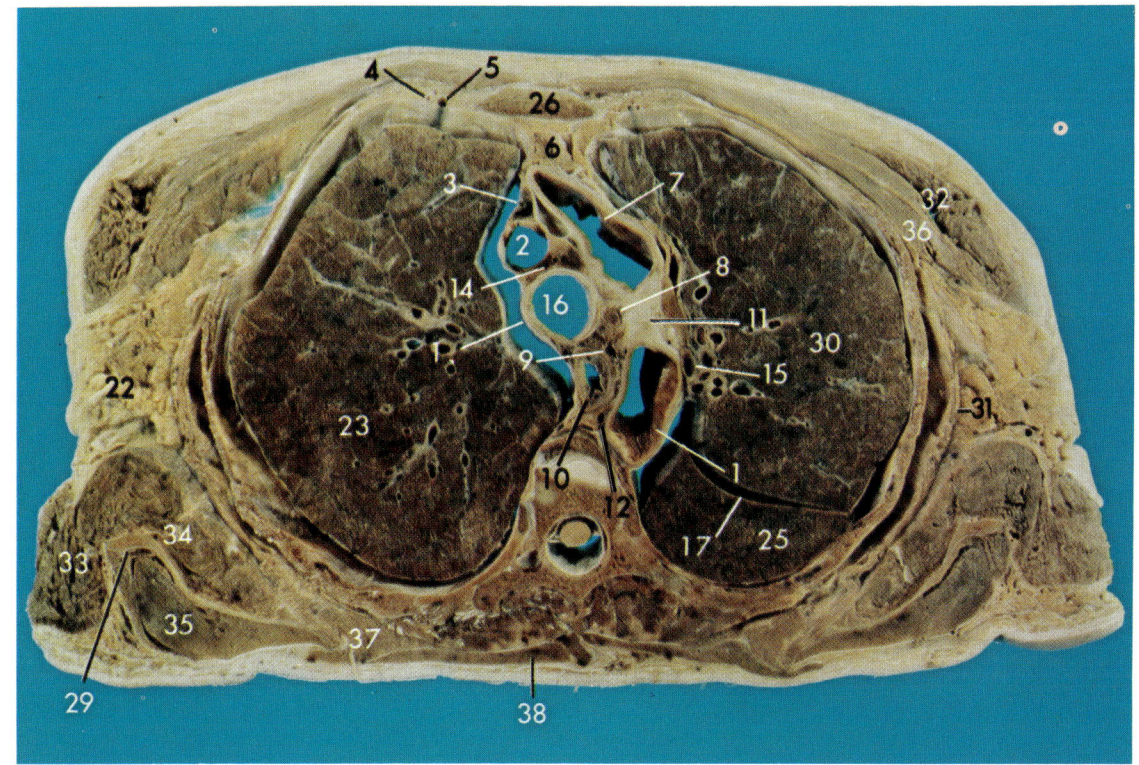

13. Right paratracheal stripe
14. Pretracheal lymph nodes
15. Lymph node at lateral aspect of aortic–pulmonic window (ductus node)
16. Trachea
17. Left major fissure
22. Axillary space (fat)
23. Right upper lobe of lung
25. Left lower lobe of lung
26. Sternum
29. Scapula
30. Left upper lobe of lung
31. Serratus anterior muscle
32. Pectoralis major muscle
33. Teres major muscle
34. Subscapularis muscle
35. Infraspinatus muscle
36. Pectoralis minor muscle
37. Rhomboideus major muscle
38. Trapezius muscle

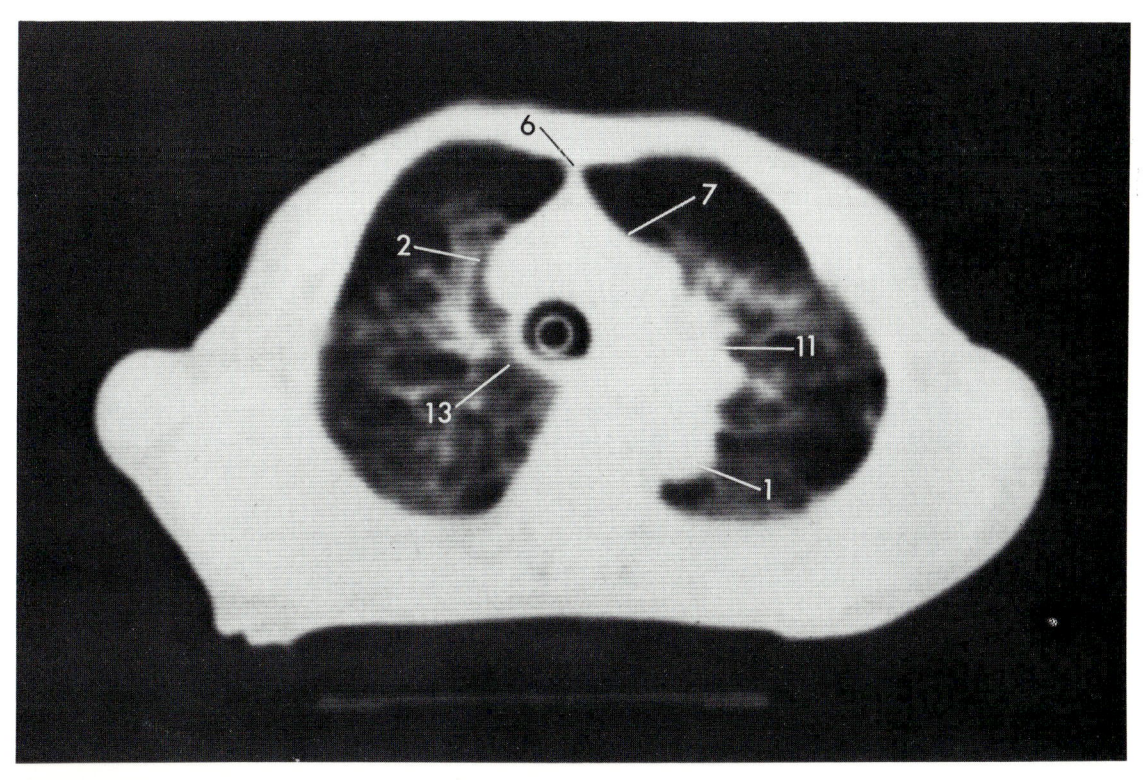

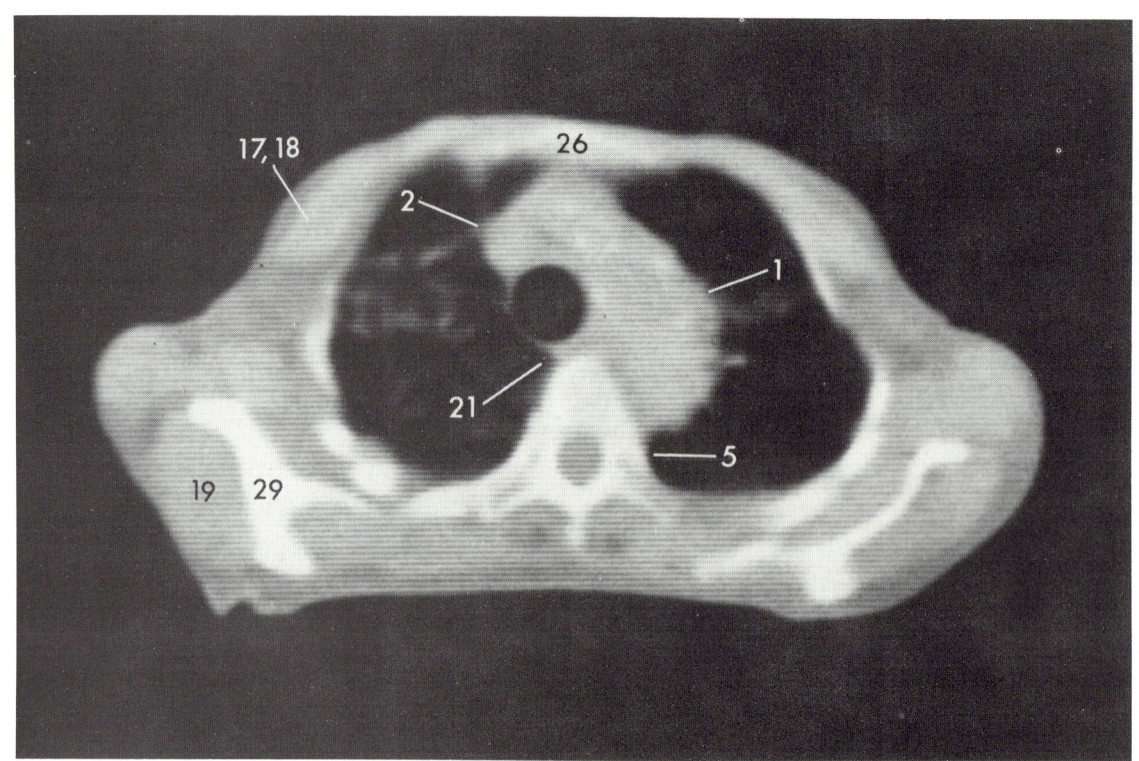

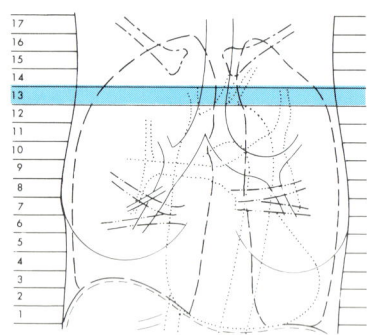

1. Aortic arch
2. Superior vena cava
3. Left common carotid artery
5. Left lower lobe of lung (retroaortic)
7. Left subclavian artery (orifice)
8. Left major fissure
10. Esophagus
11. Innominate artery

CHEST

Level 13

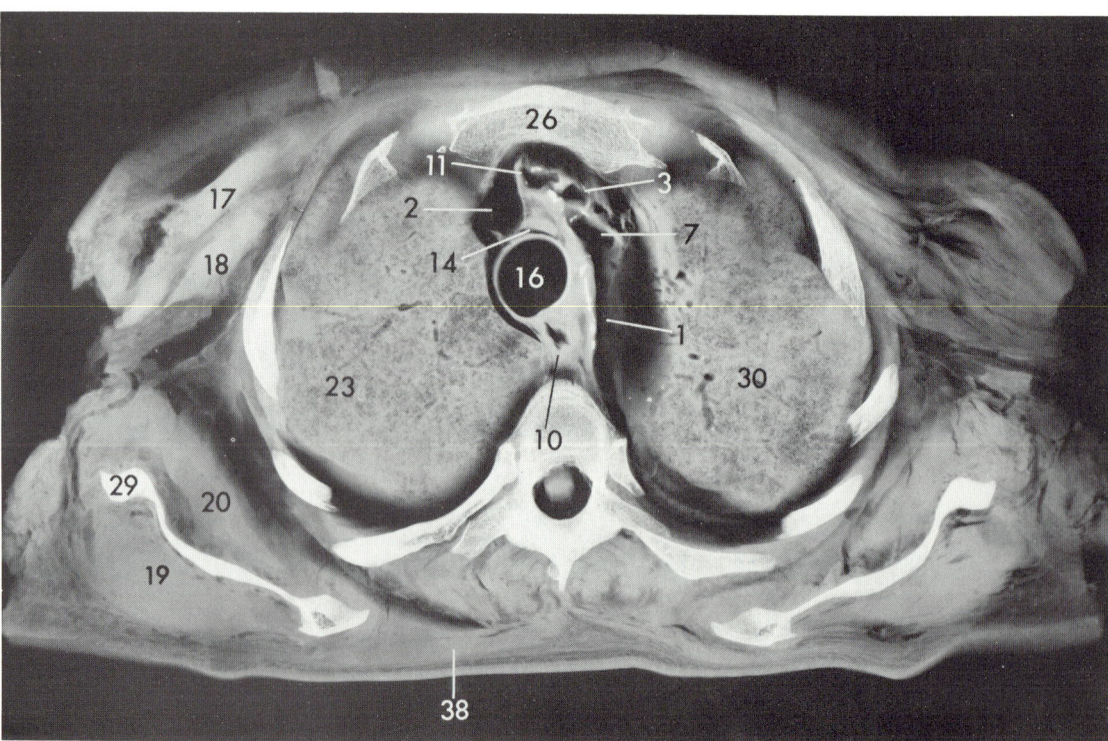

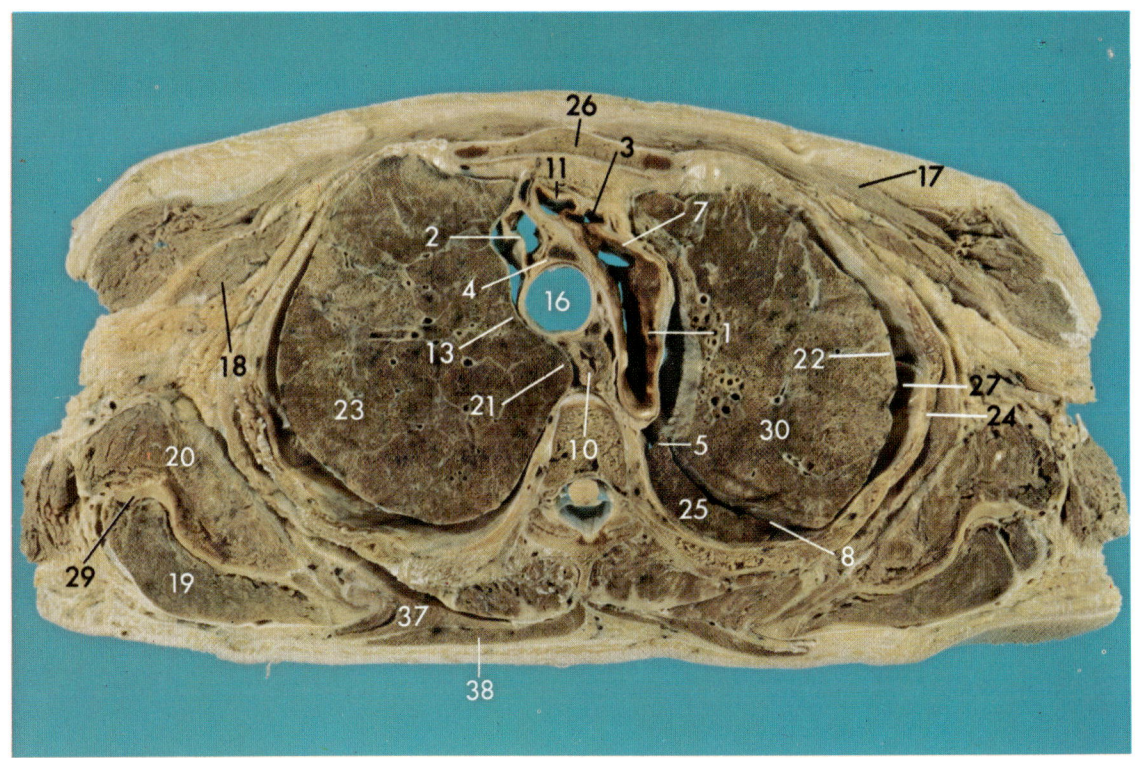

13. Right upper lobe of lung (paratracheal)
14. Pretracheal lymph nodes
16. Trachea (with endotracheal tube on CT)
17. Pectoralis major muscle
18. Pectoralis minor muscle
19. Infraspinatus muscle
20. Subscapularis muscle
21. Right upper lobe of lung (retrotracheal)
22. Visceral pleura
23. Right upper lobe of lung
24. Parietal pleura
25. Left lower lobe of lung
26. Sternum
27. Pleural cavity
29. Scapula
30. Left upper lobe of lung
37. Rhomboideus major muscle
38. Trapezius muscle

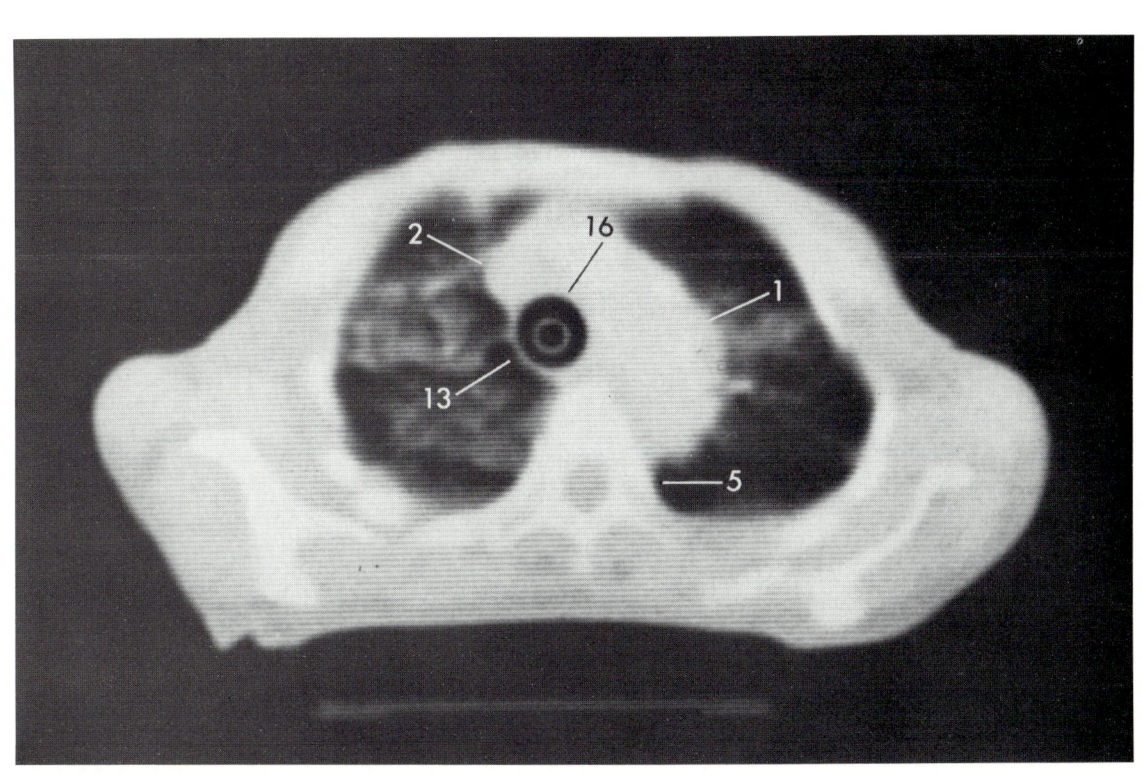

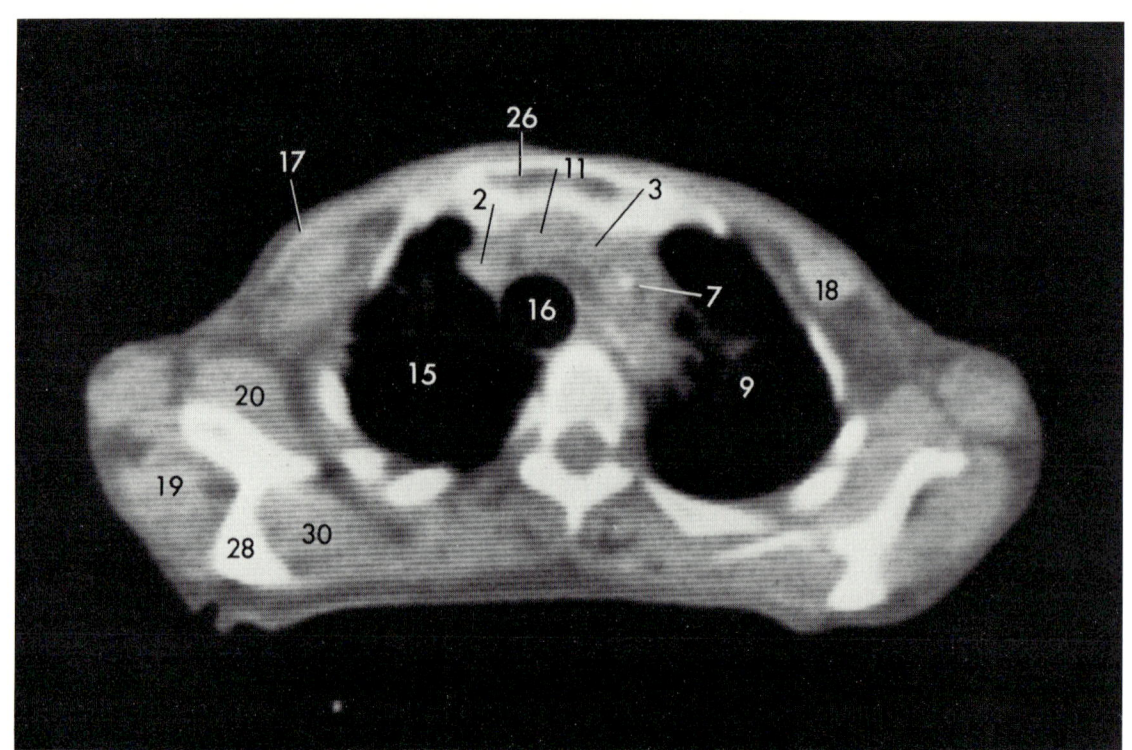

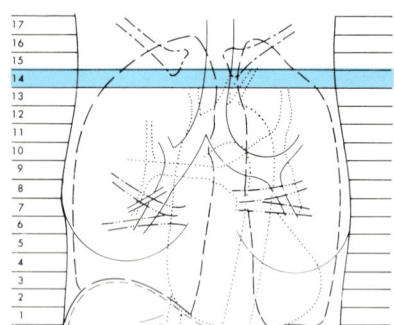

1. Costal cartilage of first rib
2. Right brachiocephalic (innominate) vein
3. Left comon carotid artery
4. Left brachiocephalic (innominate) vein (crossing midline to meet right brachiocephalic vein)
7. Left subclavian artery
8. Left axillary artery

CHEST

Level 14

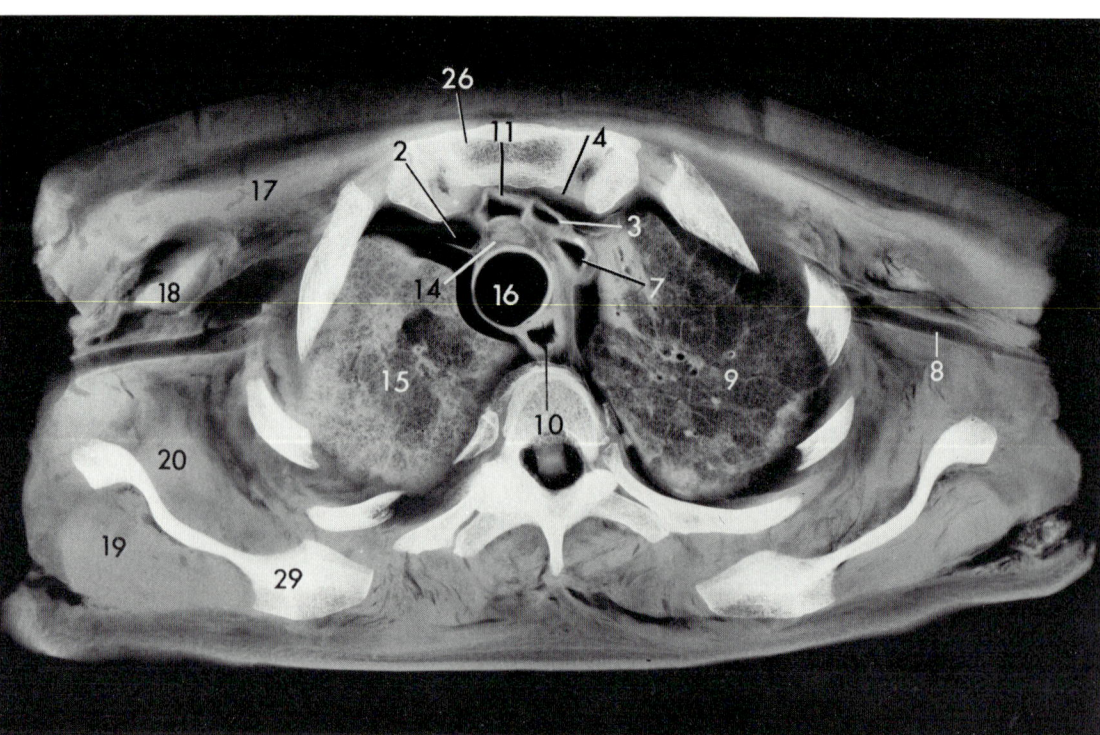

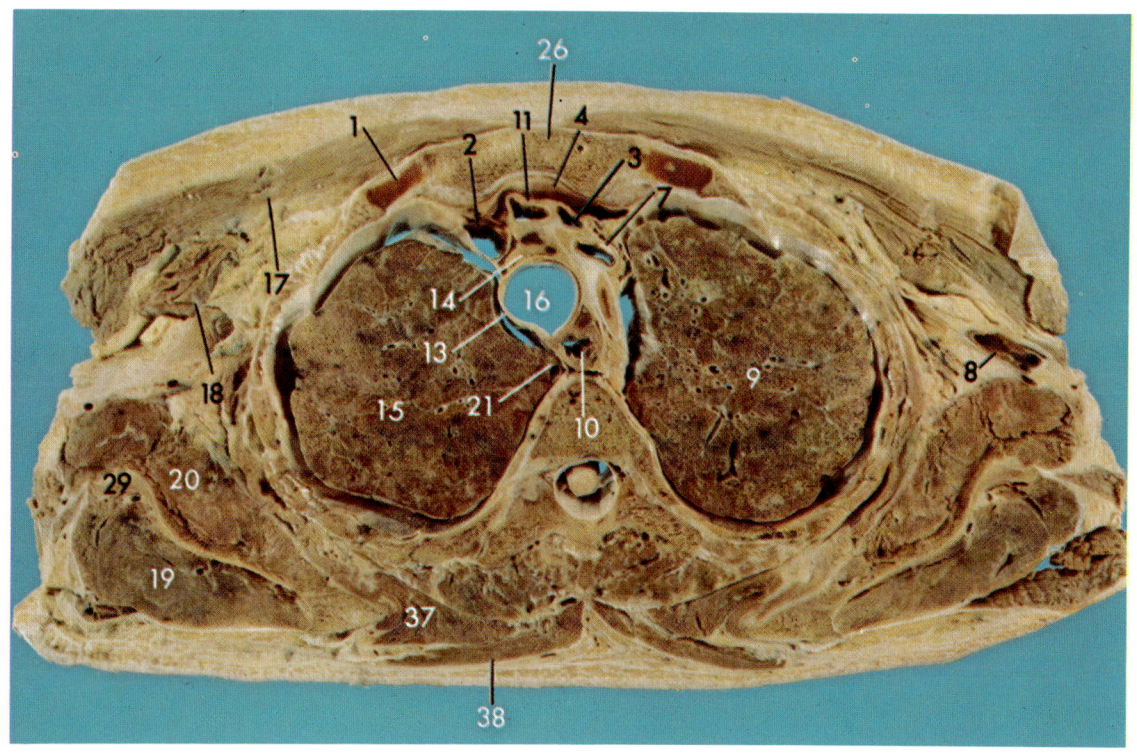

9. Left upper lobe of lung
10. Esophagus
11. Innominate artery
13. Right paratracheal stripe
14. Pretracheal lymph nodes
15. Right upper lobe of lung
16. Trachea (with endotracheal tube on CT)
17. Pectoralis major muscle
18. Pectoralis minor muscle
19. Infraspinatus muscle
20. Subscapularis muscle
21. Right upper lobe of lung (retrotracheal)
26. Manubrium of sternum
28. Spine of scapula
29. Scapula
30. Supraspinatus muscle
37. Rhomboideus major muscle
38. Trapezius muscle

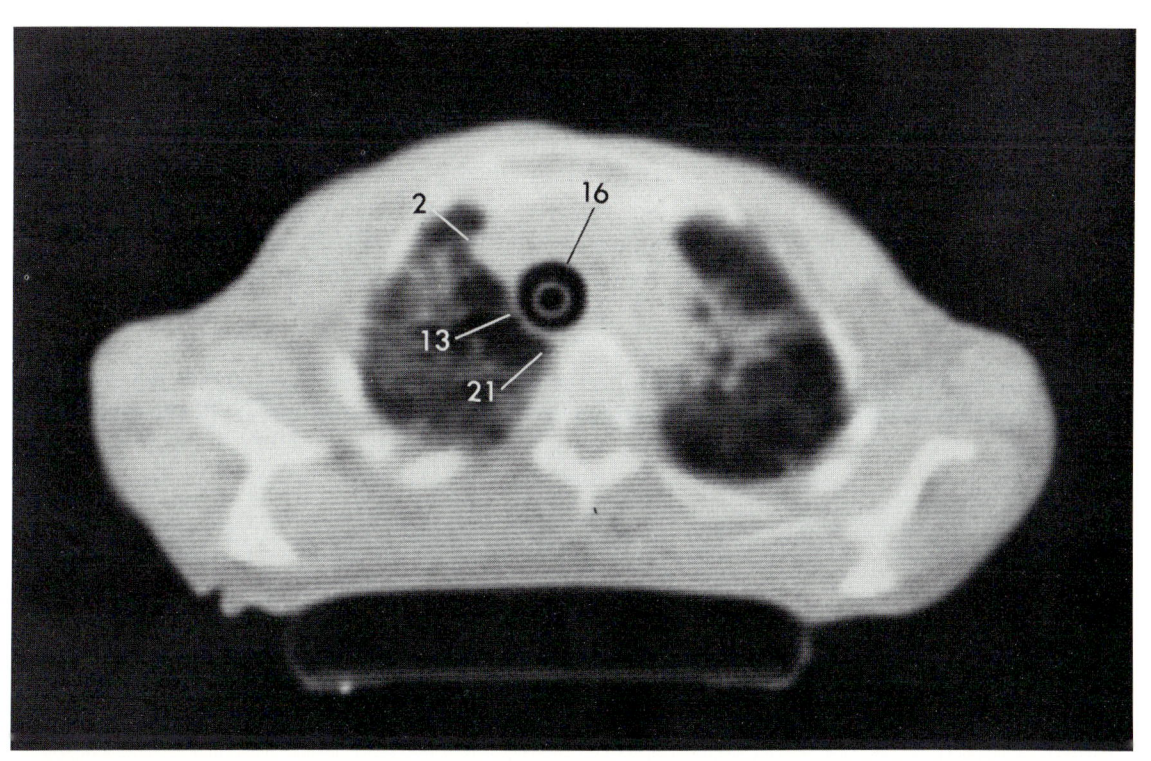

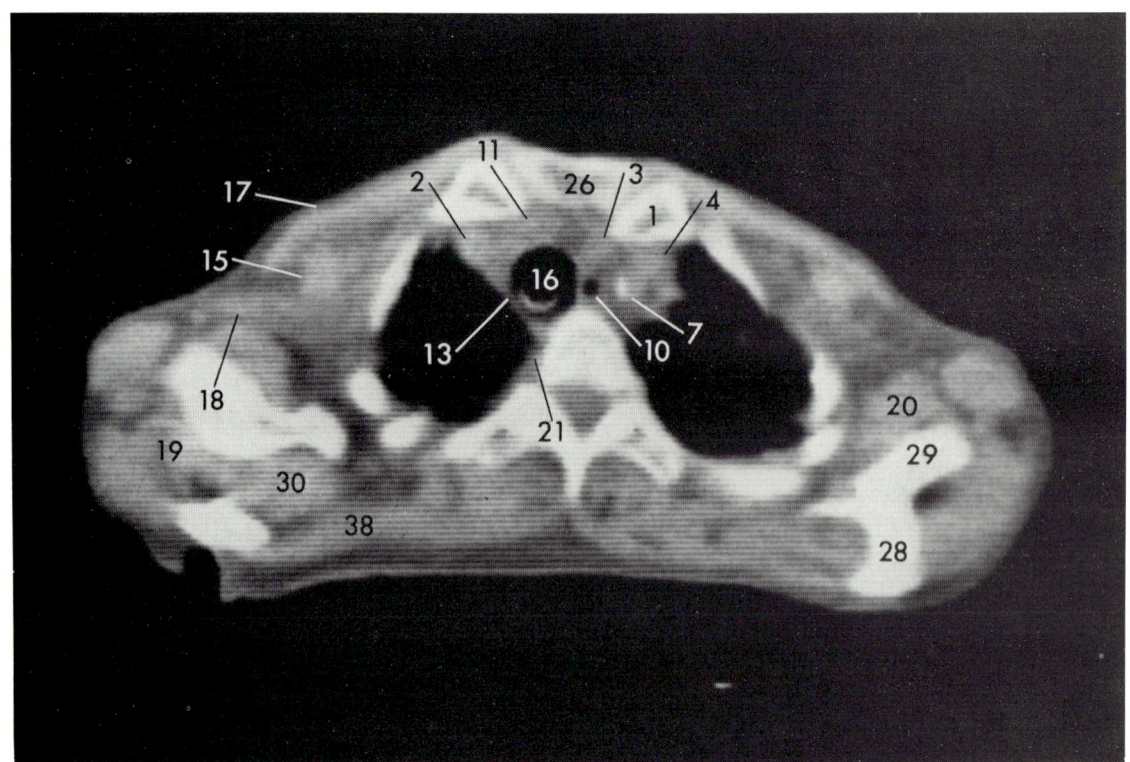

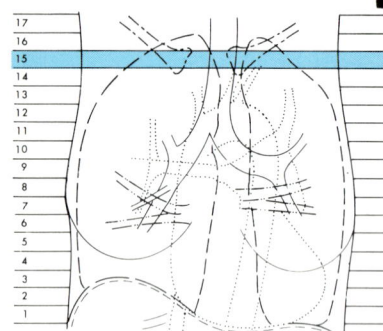

1. Clavicle
2. Right brachiocephalic (innominate) vein
3. Left common carotid artery
4. Left brachiocephalic (innominate) vein
5. Left axillary vein
6. Serratus anterior muscle

CHEST

Level 15

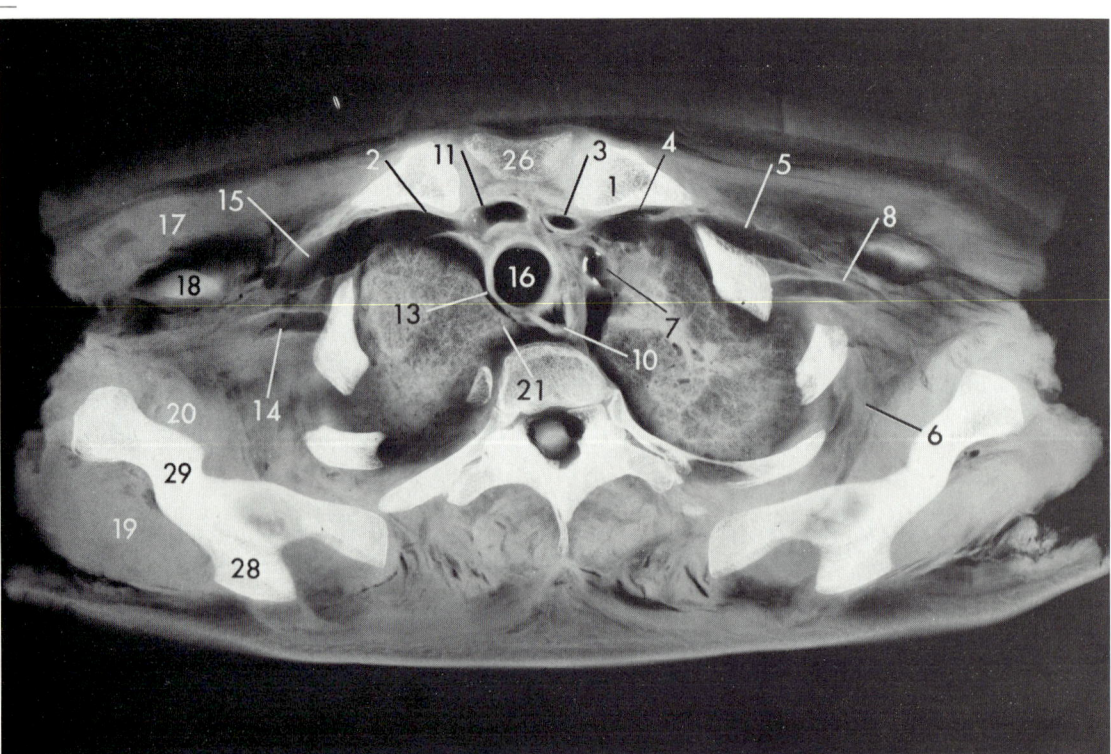

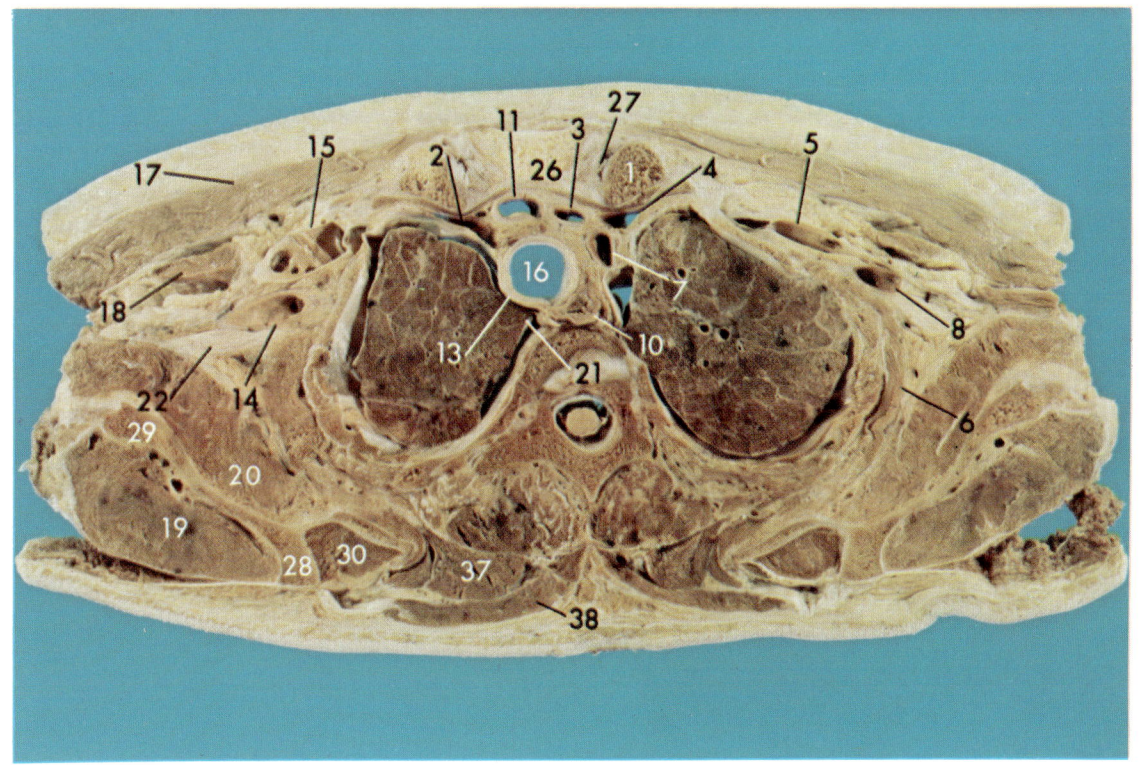

7. Left subclavian artery
8. Left axillary artery
10. Esophagus (with gas on CT images)
11. Innominate artery
13. Right paratracheal stripe
14. Right axillary artery
15. Right axillary vein
16. Trachea
17. Pectoralis major muscle
18. Pectoralis minor muscle
19. Infraspinatus muscle
20. Subscapularis muscle
21. Right upper lobe of lung (retrotracheal)
22. Brachial plexus, inferior trunk
26. Manubrium of sternum
27. Sternoclavicular joint
28. Spine of scapula
29. Scapula
30. Supraspinatus muscle
37. Rhomboideus major muscle
38. Trapezius muscle

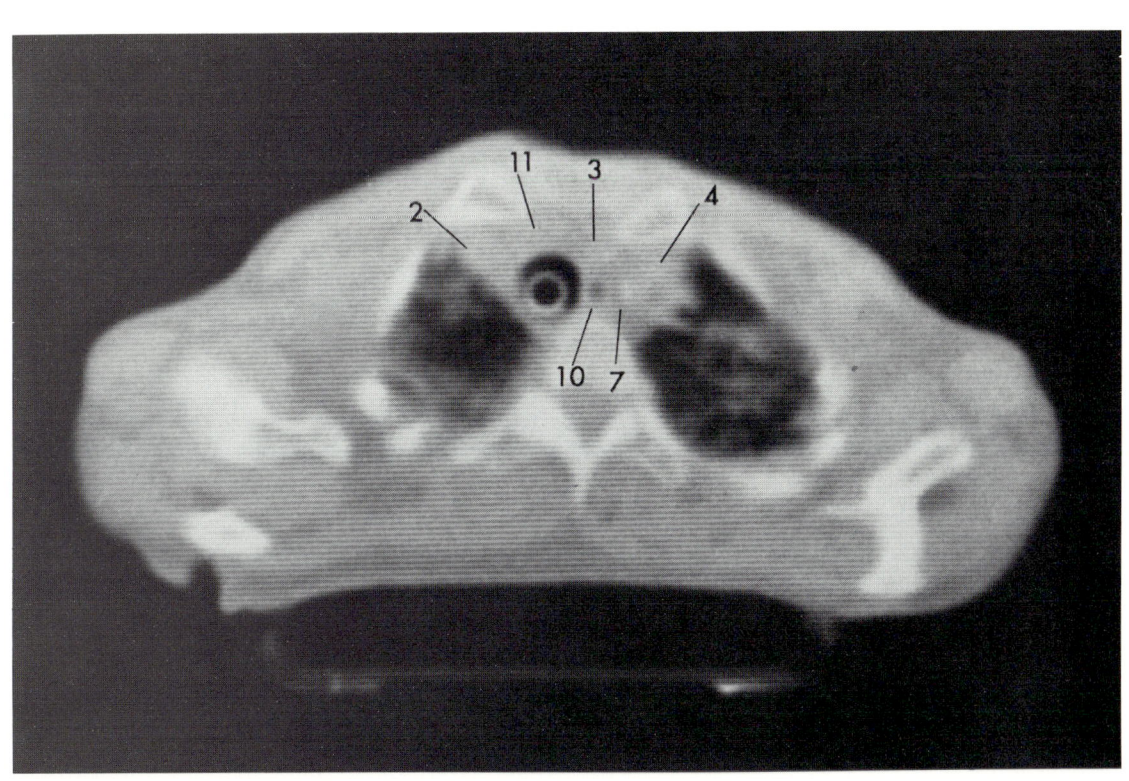

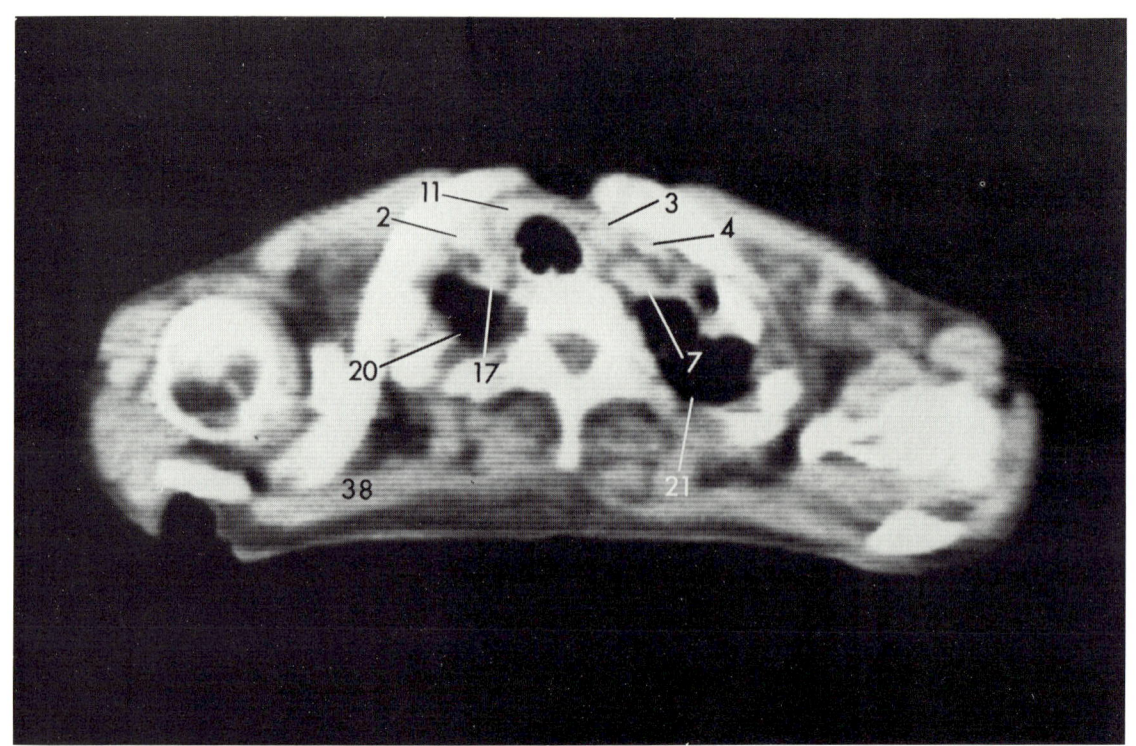

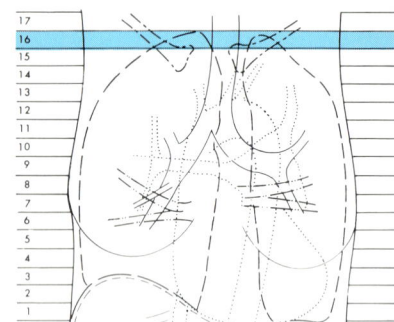

1. Subclavius muscle
2. Right brachiocephalic (innominate) vein
3. Left common carotid artery
4. Left brachiocephalic (innominate) vein
5. Left subclavian vein
6. Scalenus anterior muscle

CHEST

Level 16

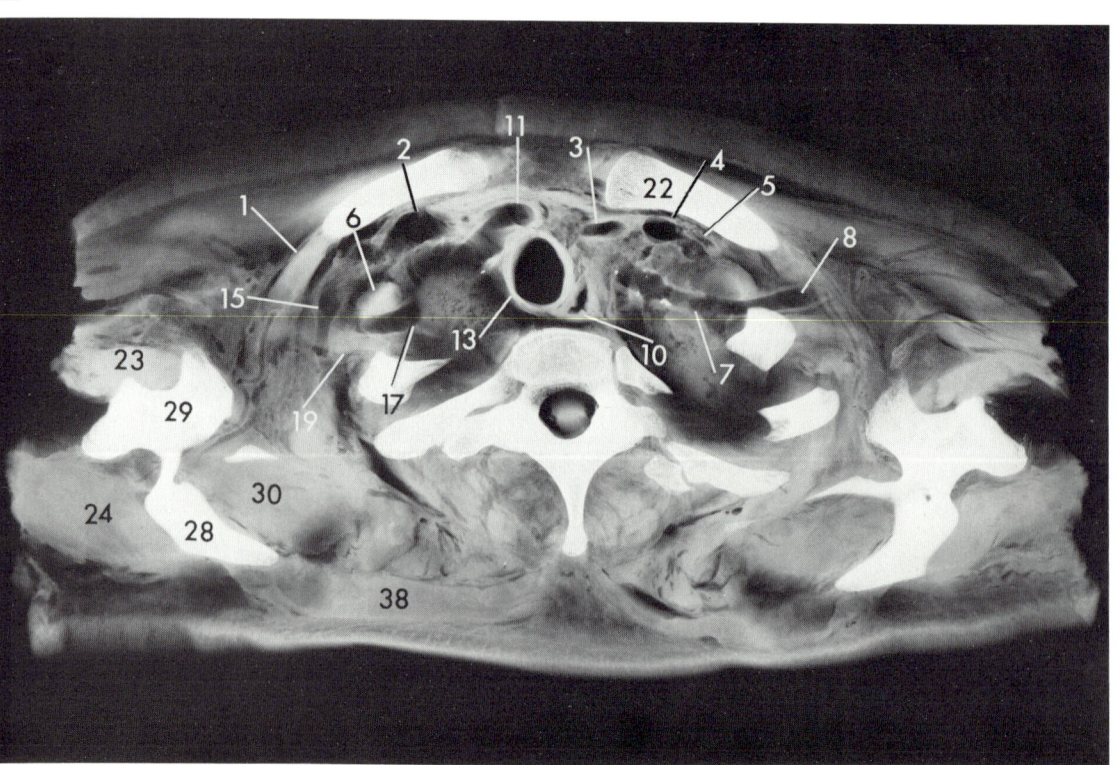

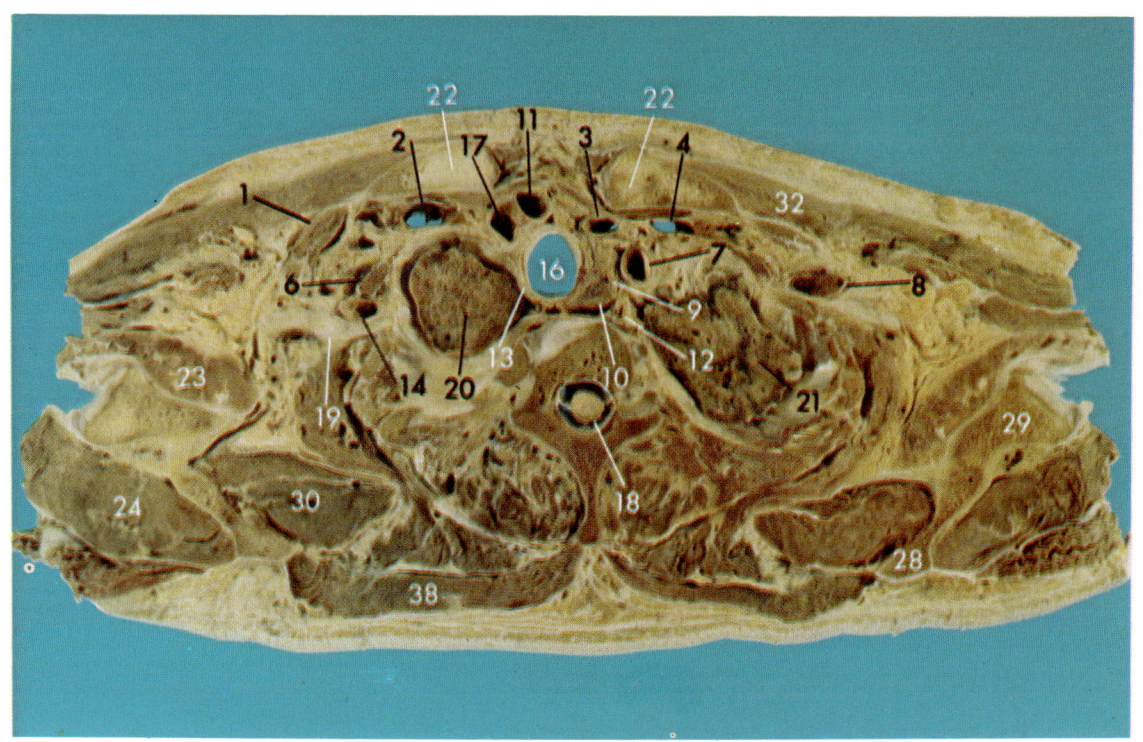

7. Left subclavian artery
8. Left axillary artery
9. Thoracic duct
10. Esophagus
11. Right common carotid artery
12. Left superior intercostal vein
13. Right paratracheal stripe
14. Right axillary artery
15. Right axillary vein
16. Trachea
17. Right subclavian artery
18. Spinal cord
19. Brachial plexus
20. Right lung apex
21. Left lung apex
22. Clavicle
23. Subscapularis muscle
24. Infraspinatus muscle
28. Spine of scapula
29. Scapula
30. Supraspinatus muscle
32. Pectoralis major muscle
38. Trapezius muscle

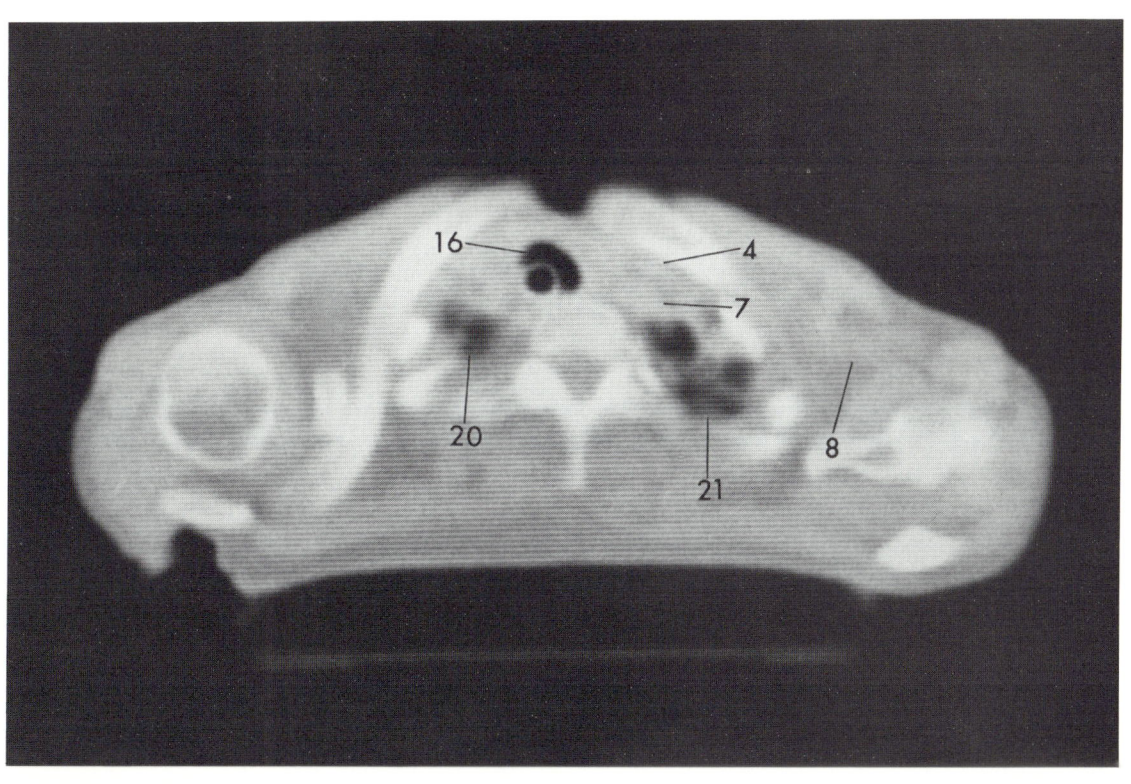

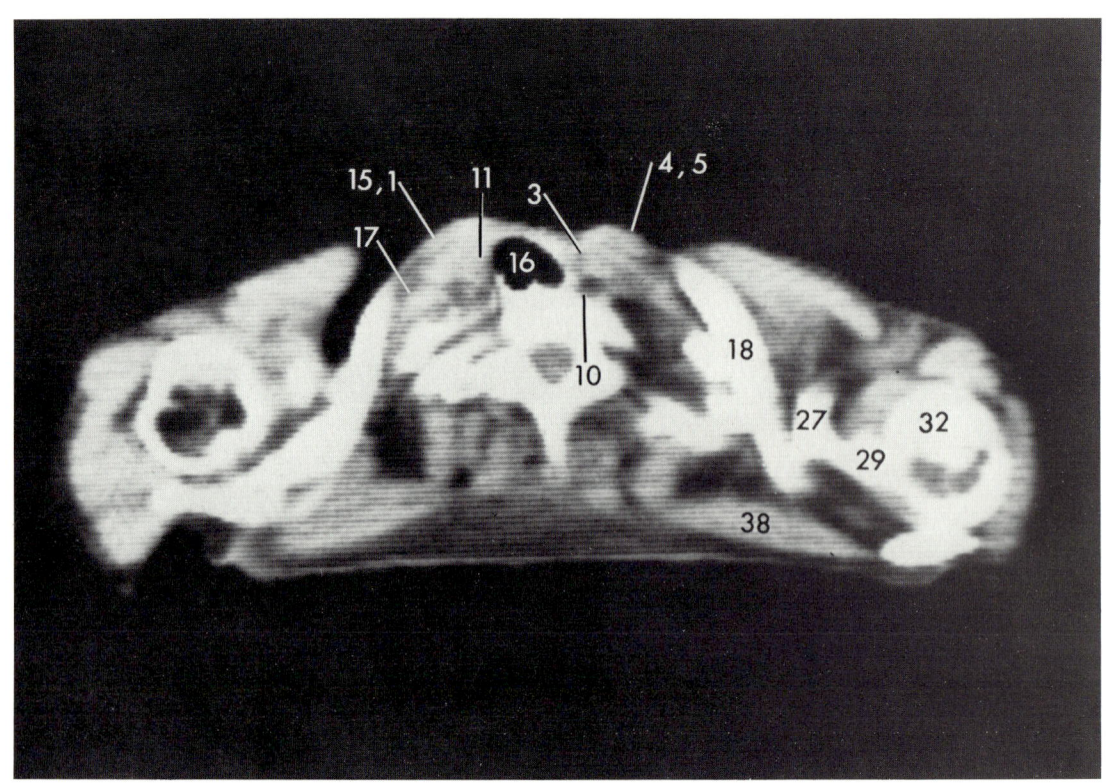

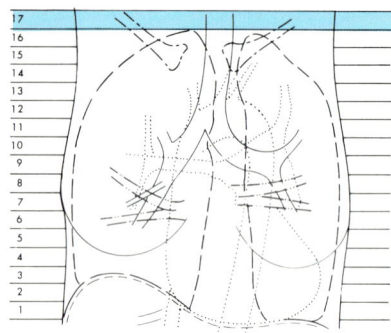

CHEST

Level 17

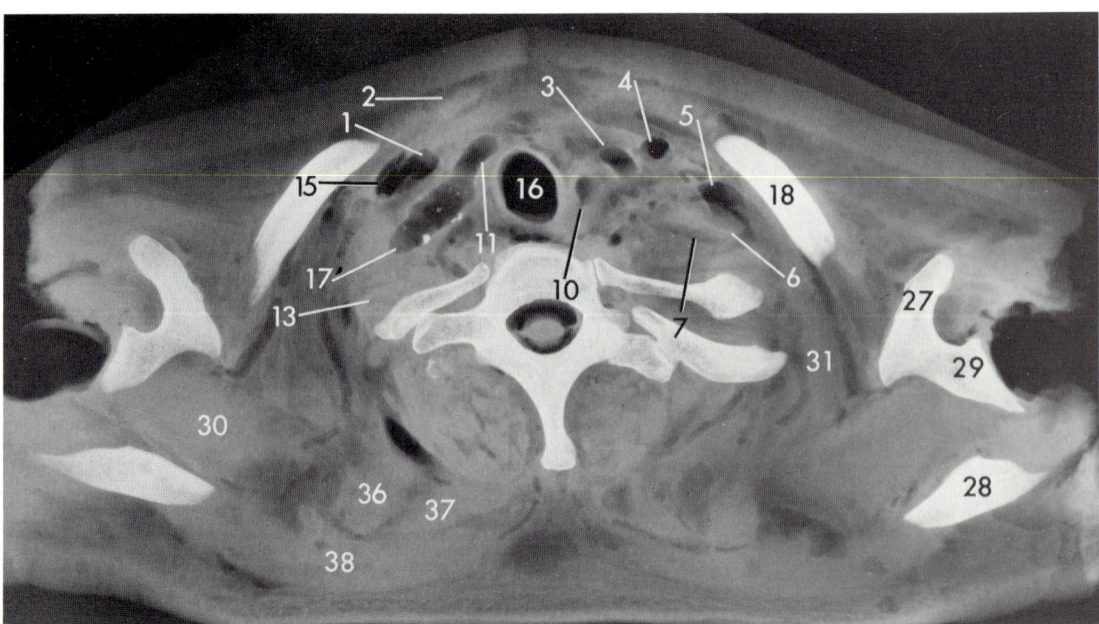

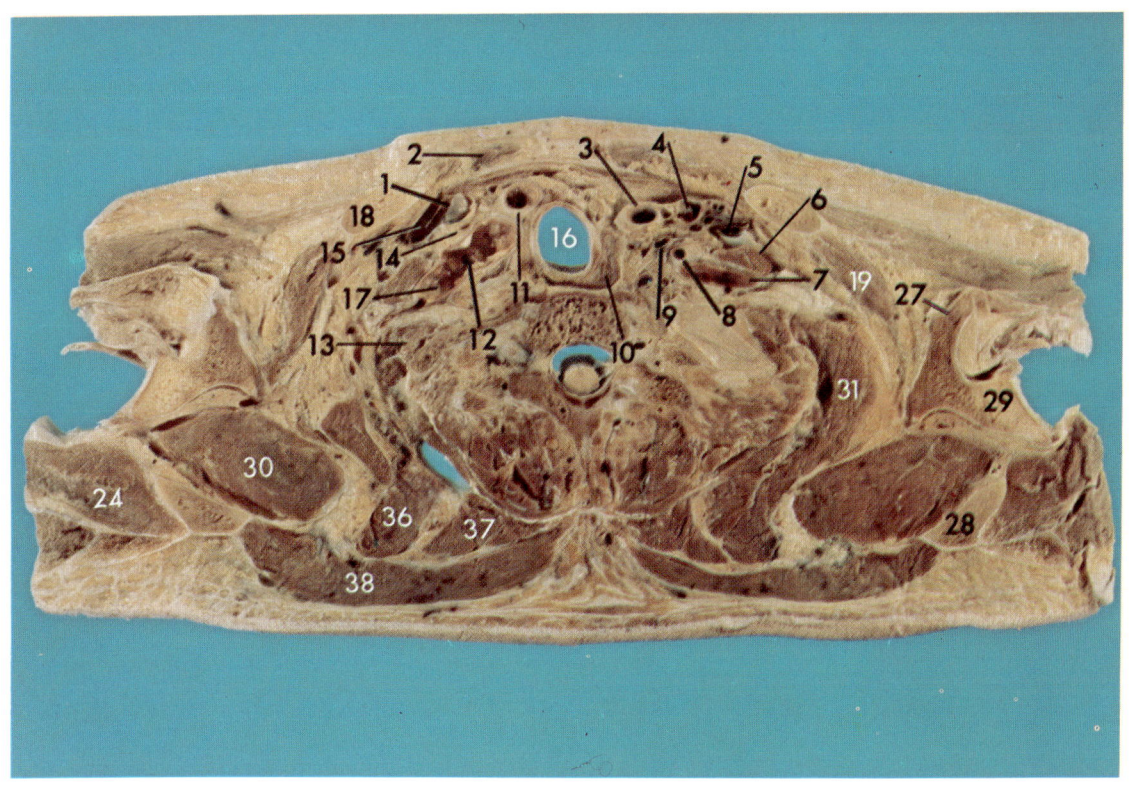

1. Right internal jugular vein
2. Sternocleidomastoid muscle
3. Left common carotid artery
4. Left internal jugular vein
5. Left subclavian vein
6. Scalenus anterior muscle
7. Left subclavian artery
8. Left vertebral artery
9. Thoracic duct
10. Esophagus (with gas on CT images)
11. Right common carotid artery
12. Right vertebral artery (orifice)
13. Scalenus medius and scalenus posterior muscles
14. Right lymphatic duct
15. Right subclavian vein
16. Trachea
17. Right subclavian artery
18. Clavicle
19. Subclavius muscle
24. Infraspinatus muscle
27. Coracoid process of scapula
28. Spine of scapula
29. Scapula
30. Supraspinatus muscle
31. Serratus anterior muscle
32. Head of humerus
36. Rhomboideus minor muscle
37. Rhomboideus major muscle
38. Trapezius muscle

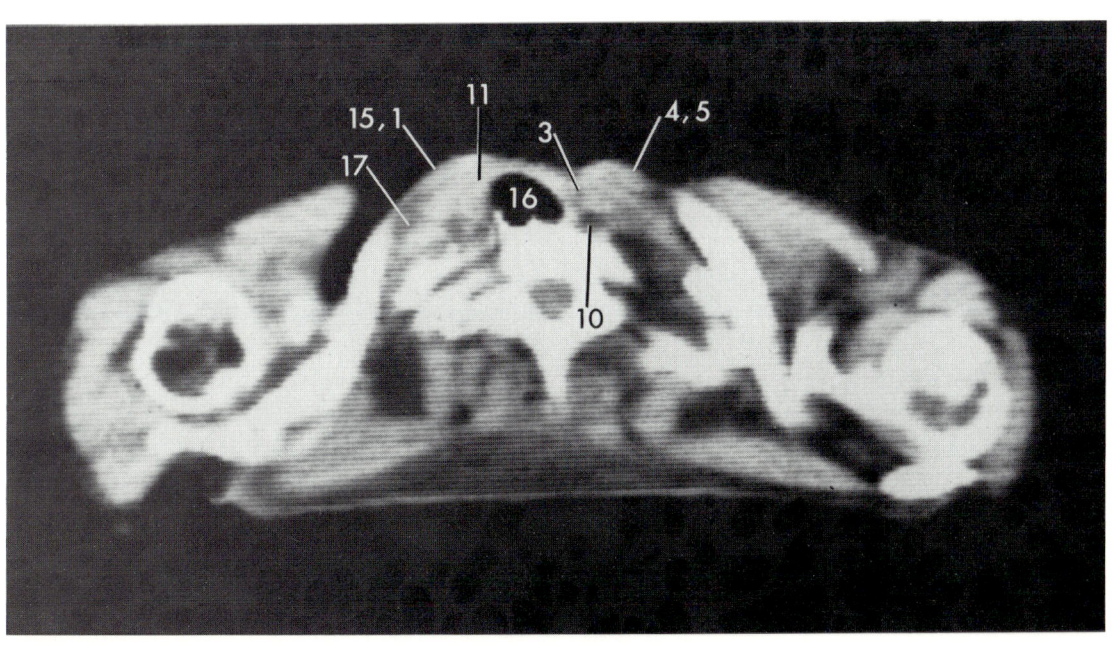

137

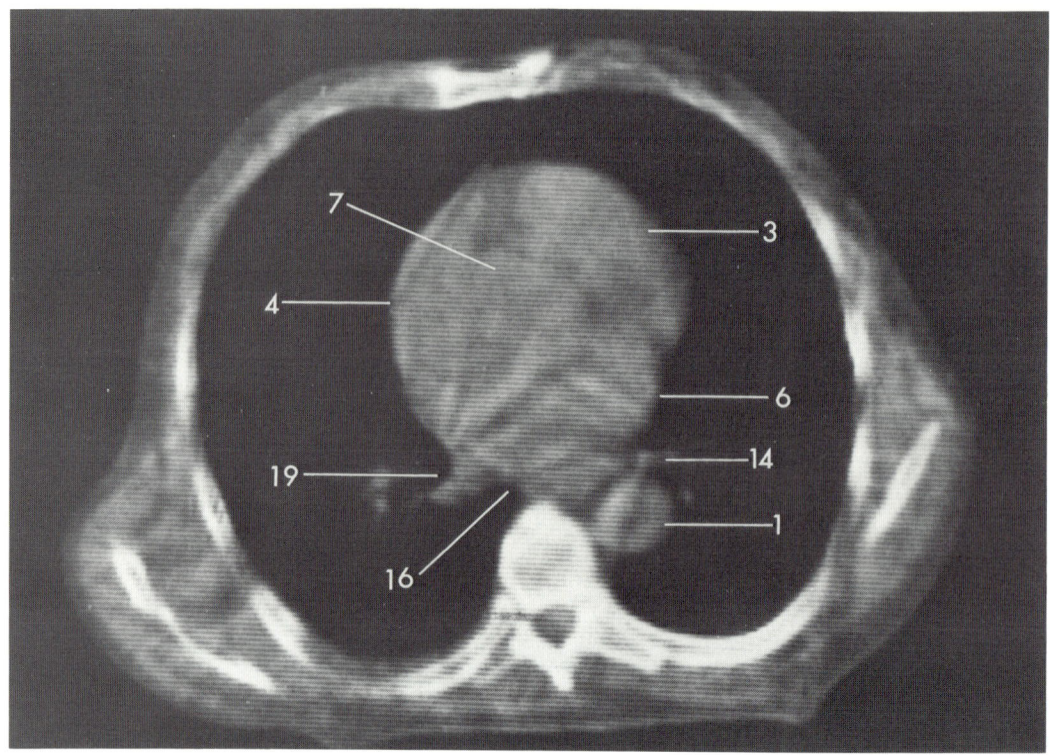

Fig. 5-1. Level of inferior pulmonary veins.
1. Descending thoracic aorta
3. Right ventricular outflow tract
4. Right atrium
6. Left atrium
7. Root of aorta
14. Left inferior pulmonary vein
16. Right lower lobe of lung in azygoesophageal recess
19. Right inferior pulmonary vein

Fig. 5-2. Level of right pulmonary artery.
1. Descending thoracic aorta
2. Superior vena cava
3. Main pulmonary artery
6. Left upper lobe bronchus
7. Ascending thoracic aorta
11. Left interlobar pulmonary artery
18. Right upper lobe bronchus
19. Right pulmonary artery

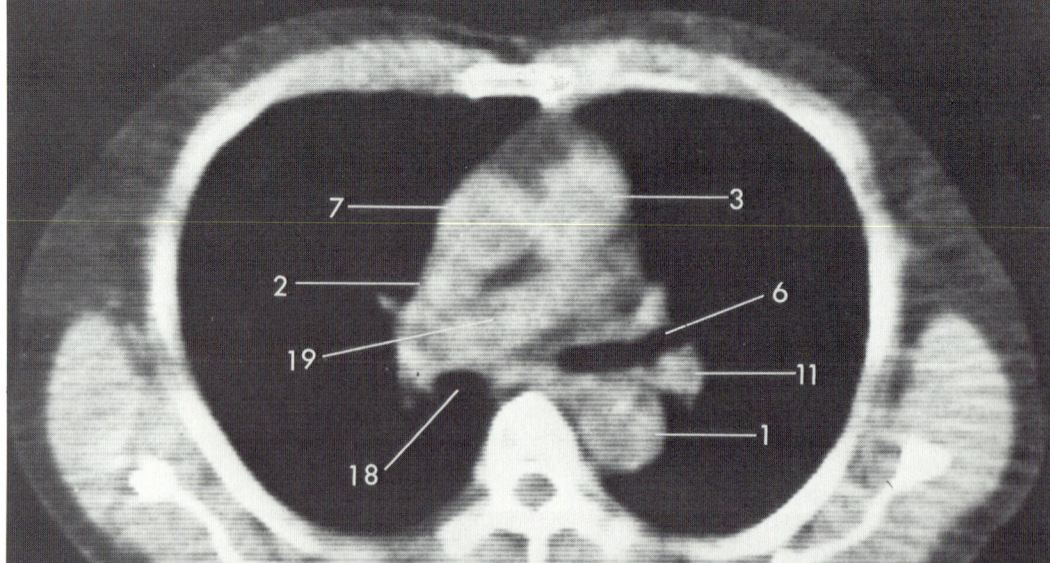

CHEST

Normal *In Vivo* Computed Tomographic Studies

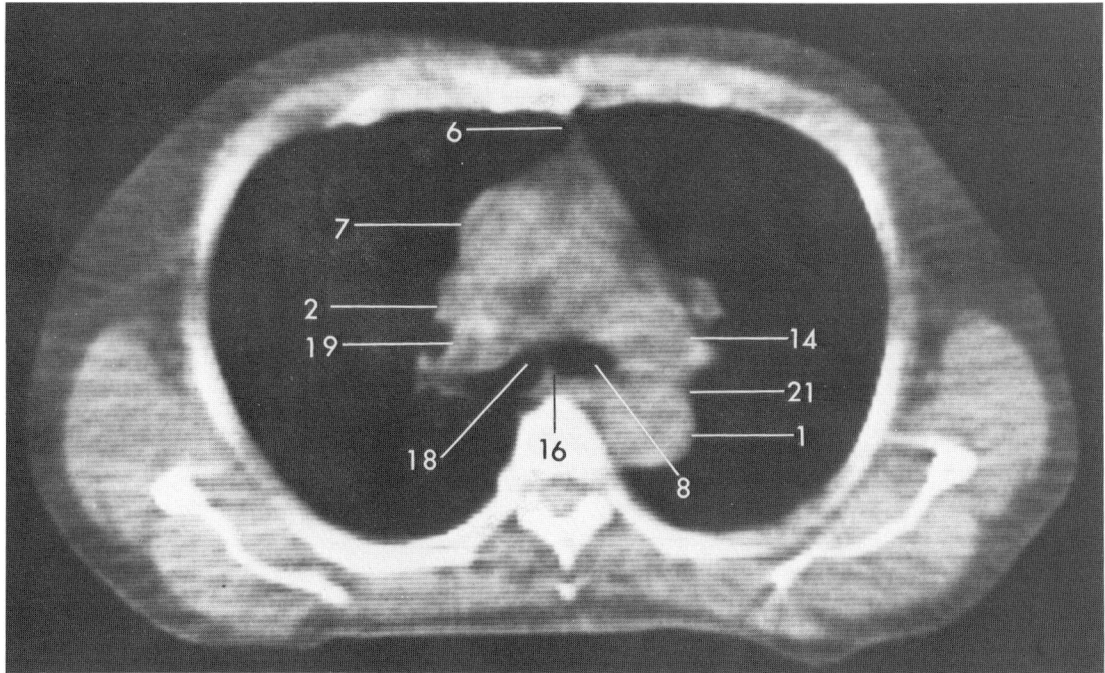

Fig. 5-3. Level of left pulmonary artery.
1. Descending thoracic aorta
2. Superior vena cava
6. Anterior junction line
7. Ascending thoracic aorta
8. Left main bronchus
14. Left pulmonary artery
16. Carina of trachea
18. Right main bronchus
19. Right pulmonary artery
21. Left lower lobe of lung in posterior aspect of aortic-pulmonic window

Fig. 5-4. Level of aortic arch.
1. Aortic arch, posterior portion
2. Superior vena cava
3. Mediastinal fat
7. Aortic arch, anterior portion
13. Azygos vein arch
16. Trachea

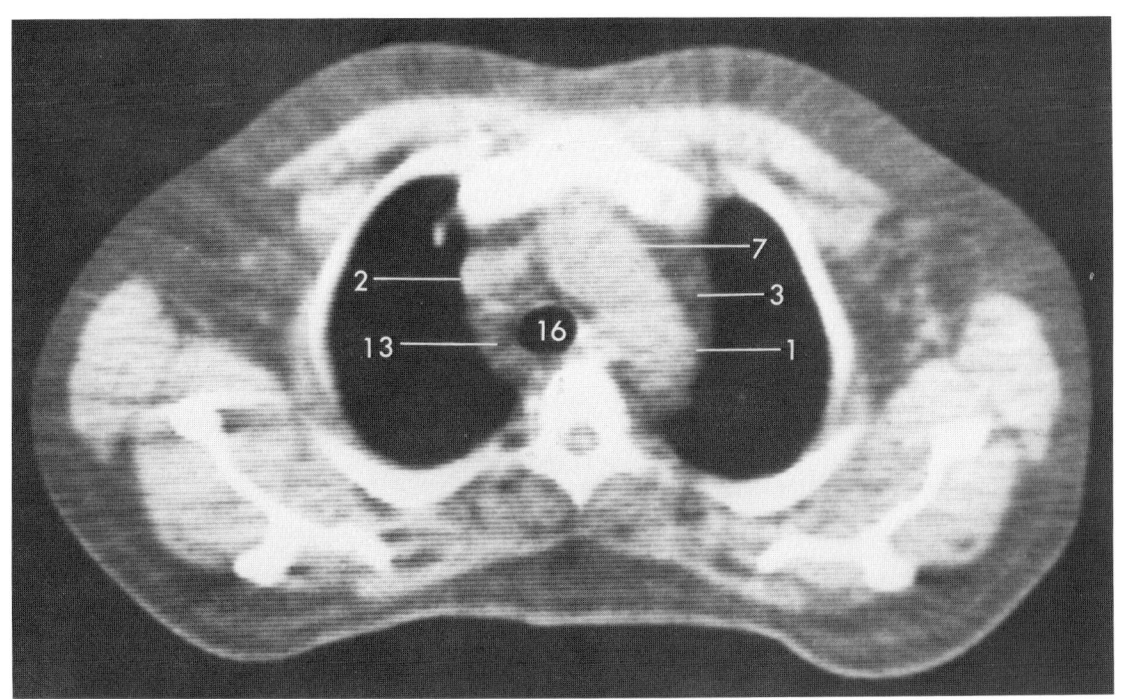

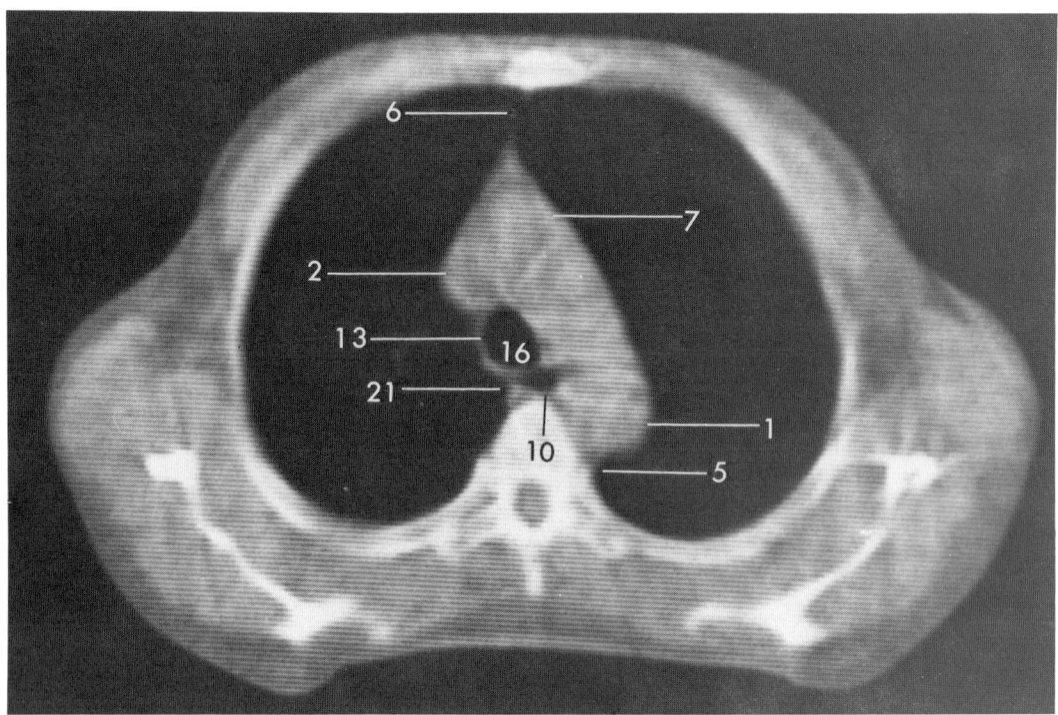

Fig. 5-5. Level of aortic arch.
1. Aortic arch, posterior portion
2. Superior vena cava
5. Left upper lobe of lung (retroaortic)
6. Anterior junction line
7. Aortic arch, anterior portion
10. Esophagus (containing air)
13. Right paratracheal stripe
16. Trachea
21. Right upper lobe of lung (retrotracheal)

Fig. 5-6. Azygos lobe.
1. Aortic arch, posterior portion
2. Superior vena cava
3. Azygos fissure
4. Parietal trigone
7. Aortic arch, anterior portion
10. Esophagus (containing barium)
13. Right paratracheal stripe

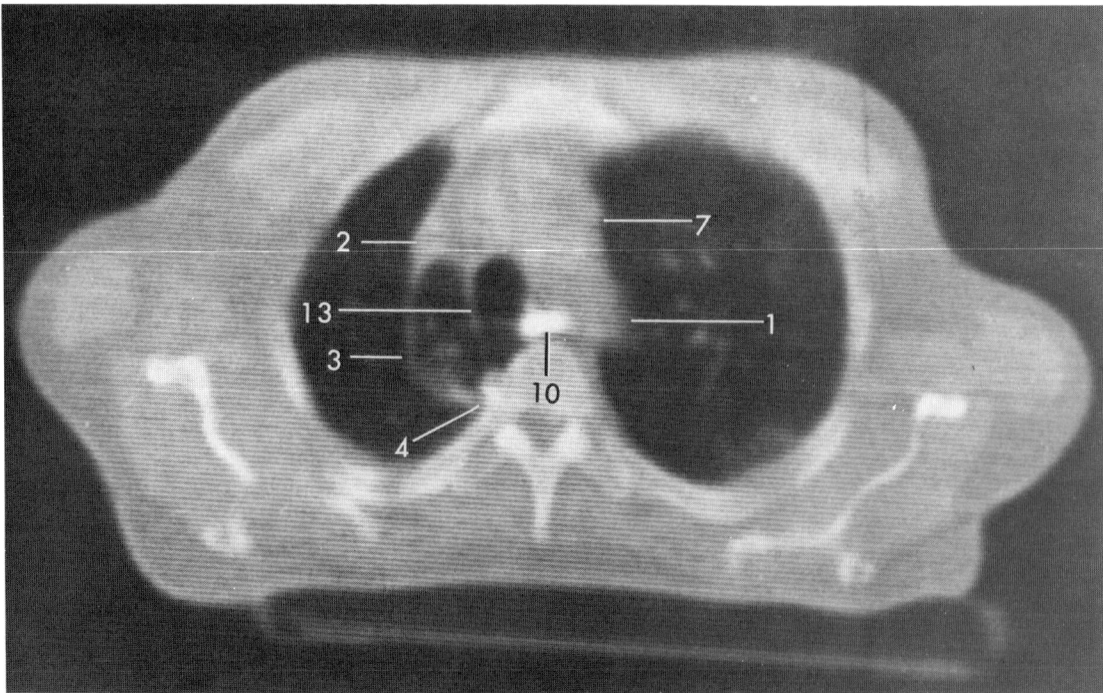

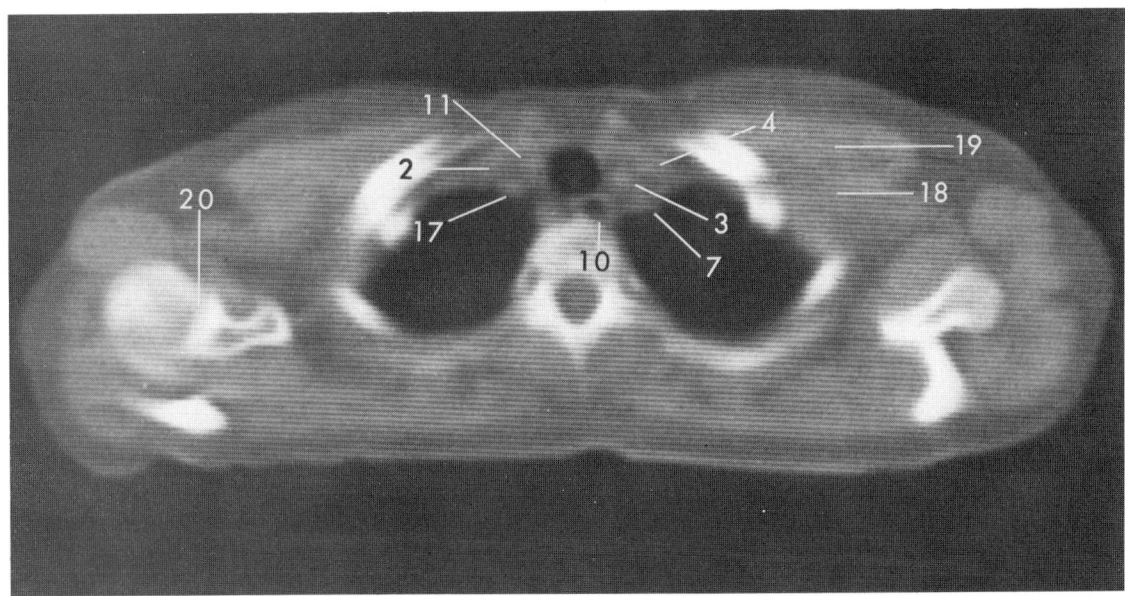

Fig. 5-7. Level of pulmonary apices.
2. Right brachiocephalic (innominate) vein
3. Left common carotid artery
4. Left brachiocephalic (innominate) vein
7. Left subclavian artery
10. Esophagus (containing air)
11. Right common carotid artery
17. Right subclavian artery
18. Pectoralis minor muscle
19. Pectoralis major muscle
20. Right glenohumeral joint

6
Abdomen and Pelvis

PATRICK J. BRYAN
WILLIAM N. COHEN
JERRY BROWN
FRANK E. SEIDELMANN
W. MARTIN DINN

The anatomy of the abdomen lends itself particularly well to examination by computed tomography in the transaxial plane. The presence of fat in fascial planes in the retroperitoneal space allows the precise delineation of muscular and visceral relationships in cross section. Similarly, the considerable fat in the mesentery enables clear delineation of intraperitoneal visceral anatomy.

This chapter consists of four parts. The first and largest part (Levels 1–35) demonstrates the cross-sectional anatomy in the female from the level of the perineum up to the diaphragm; in the midabdomen, a few levels have been omitted in which the anatomy essentially duplicated that of adjacent levels. The second part of the chapter (Levels M1–M3) includes three cross-sectional levels of the male pelvis and demonstrates the male lower genitourinary tract. This is followed by a short third portion (Figs. 6–1 to 6–6) demonstrating normal cross-sectional computed tomographic and sonographic anatomy of the abdomen as seen in living subjects. The final part of the chapter (Levels L1–6) includes several key longitudinal sections in the sagittal plane which are correlated with sonograms at approximately the same levels from living patients.

A few small metastatic deposits are present in the sacrum, lumbar spine, and liver of the cadaver used in the first and major portion of this chapter, but these do not in any way distort the normal anatomy on the computed tomogram.

In the lower abdomen, the levels of the computed tomograms and the sonograms correspond closely to the gross anatomic sections. In the upper abdomen, the plane of the computed tomographic and sonographic studies is slightly oblique, creating a slight discrepancy between these images and the gross anatomy; the correspondence between the various images at these levels is still sufficiently close to provide good roentgen–anatomic correlation.

The sonographic characteristics of tissues are altered significantly within a relatively short period after death. Thus, a number of the ultrasound studies of the cadaver were not technically satisfactory, and examples with corresponding anatomy are substituted from studies of living patients. The sonograms and computed tomograms from living patients (*in vivo* studies) are indicated in this chapter by a large asterisk (✱).

Several anatomic variants are present in the cadaver used in the first part of this chapter:

1. The left renal vein courses posterior to the aorta on Level 23, 24, and 25. A section from another cadaver is included (Level 25A) to demonstrate the usual course of the left renal vein anterior to the aorta and posterior to the superior mesenteric artery.
2. The pyramidalis muscle is absent in this cadaver but is present on the sections of the male pelvis.

The portion of the pancreas which lies anterior to the upper pole of the left kidney and the left adrenal gland is labeled as a part of the body of the pancreas. This is at variance with common radiologic usage which refers to this segment as the tail of the pancreas. However, *Gray's Anatomy, 29th American Edition* restricts the definition of the tail of the pancreas to that portion of the gland lying within the two layers of the lienorenal ligament; this definition has been used in this atlas.

A shortage of cadaver material necessitated the use of gross specimens from the files of the Department of Anatomy of the Upstate Medical Center for the cross sections of the male pelvis and the longitudinal sections of the abdomen. It was not possible to obtain radiographic, computed tomographic, or sonographic studies of these sections, and comparable images from living patients are included in their stead. Owing to their prolonged immersion in formalin, these gross specimens show considerable variation in color from the anatomic sections displayed elsewhere in this atlas.

Technical factors for computed tomography of the abdomen included center settings in the range of 50–80 Hounsfield units and window widths of 300–400 Hounsfield units. A scanning circle 45 cm in diameter was employed for all computed tomographic studies in this chapter.

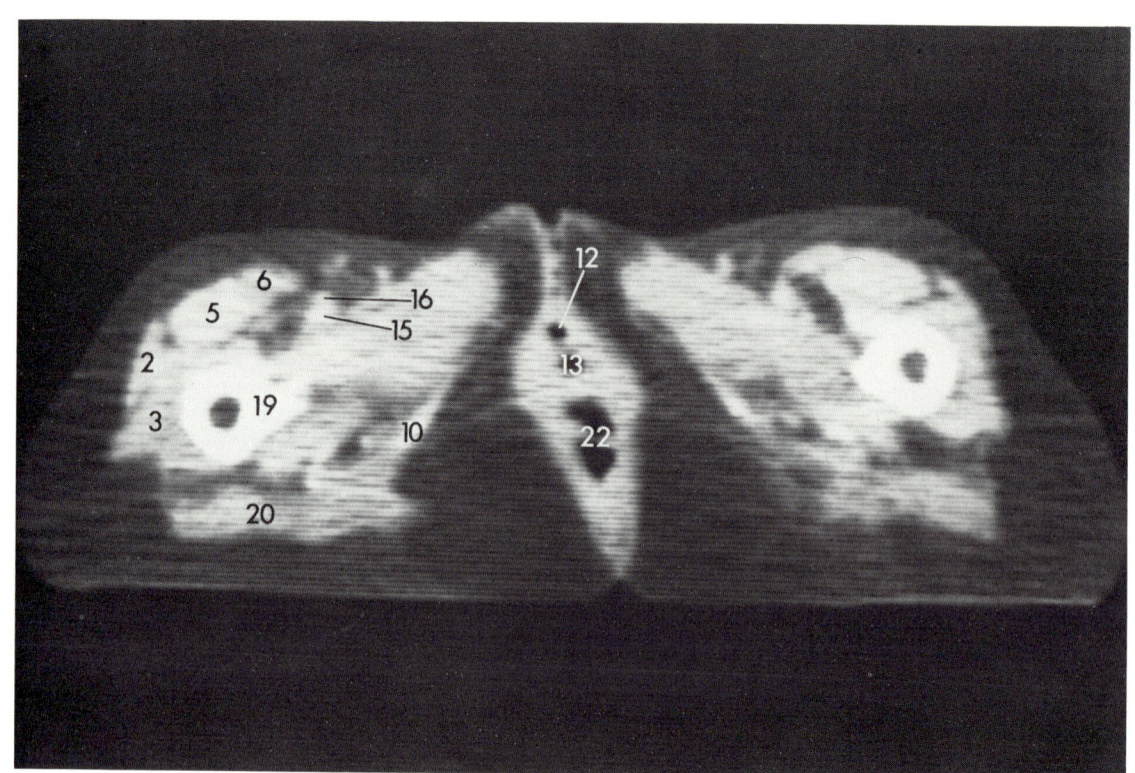

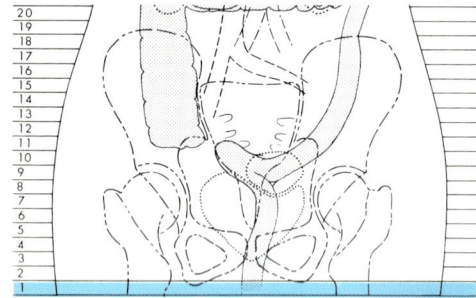

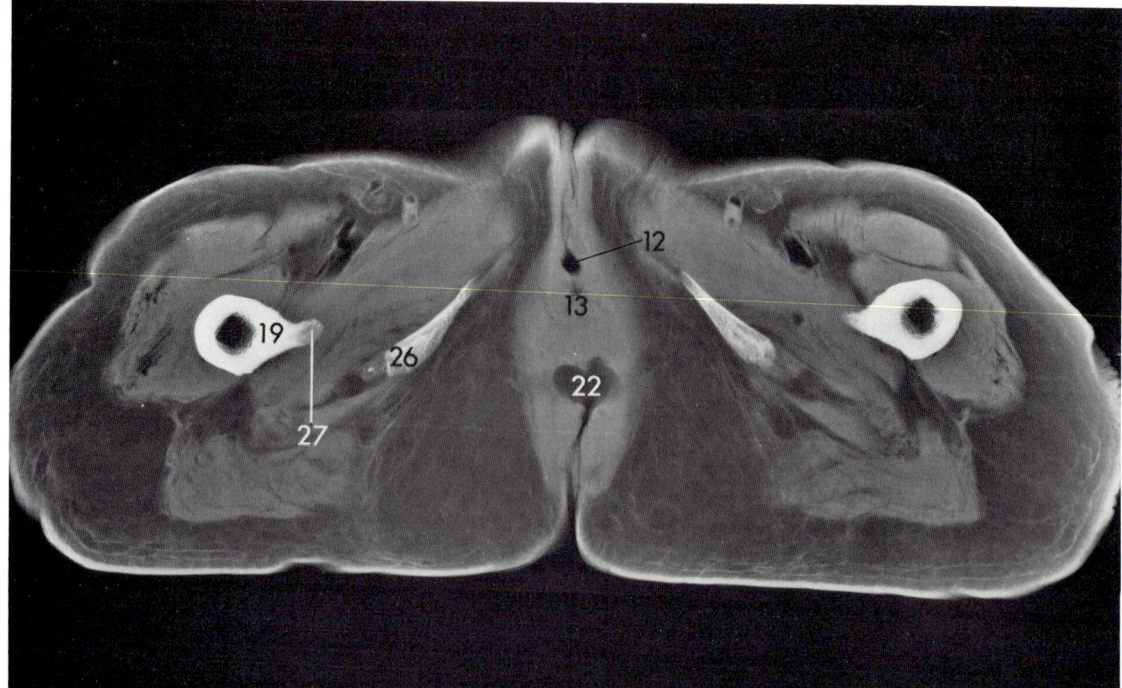

ABDOMEN AND PELVIS

Level 1

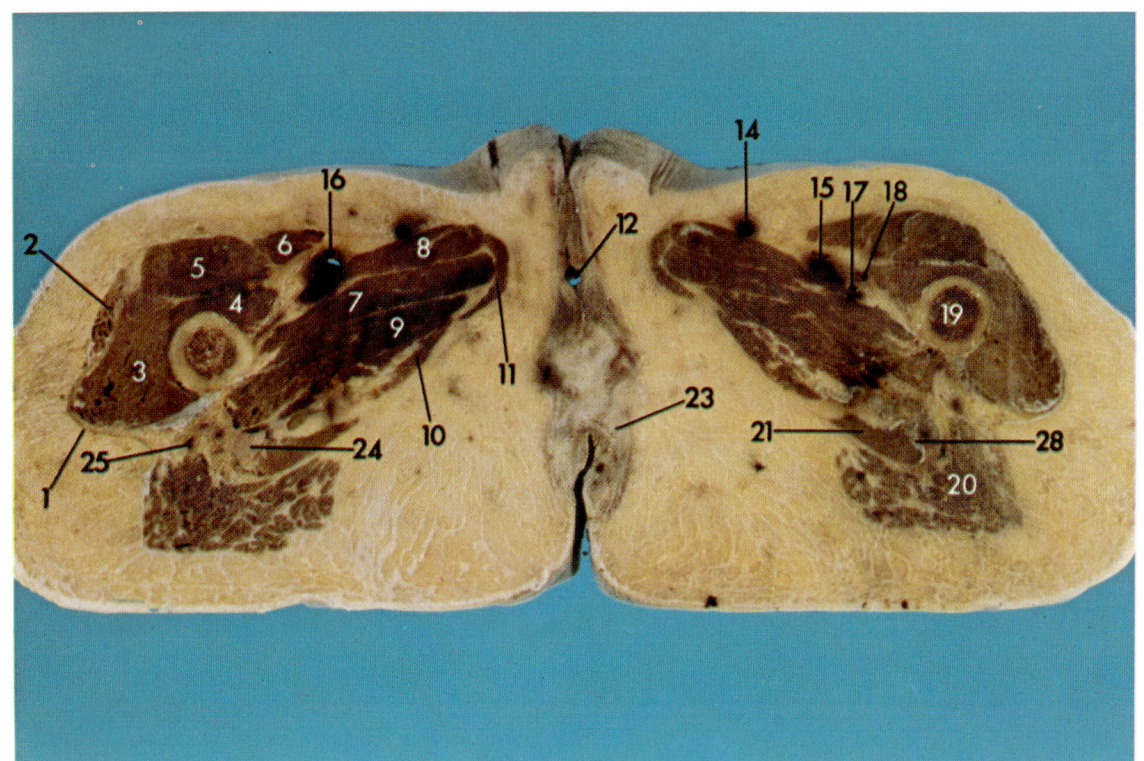

1. Fascia lata
2. Tensor fasciae latae muscle
3. Vastus lateralis muscle
4. Vastus intermedius and vastus medialis muscles
5. Rectus femoris muscle
6. Sartorius muscle
7. Adductor brevis muscle
8. Adductor longus muscle
9. Adductor minimus muscle
10. Adductor magnus muscle
11. Gracilis muscle
12. Urethra
13. Vaginal introitus
14. Saphenous vein
15. Femoral vein
16. Superficial femoral artery
17. Deep femoral artery
18. Femoral nerve
19. Femur
20. Gluteus maximus muscle
21. Biceps femoris muscle (long head)
22. Anus
23. Anal sphincter
24. Sciatic nerve
25. Circumflex femoral vessels
26. Inferior pubic ramus
27. Lesser trochanter
28. Semitendinosus tendon

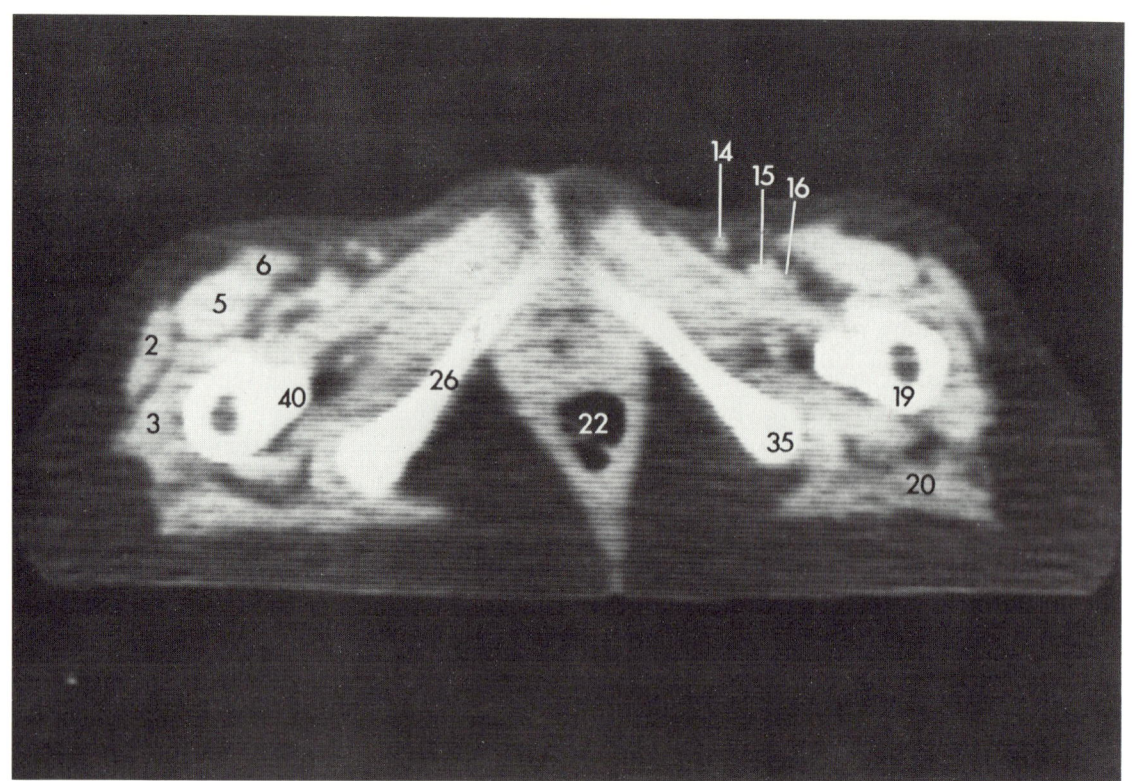

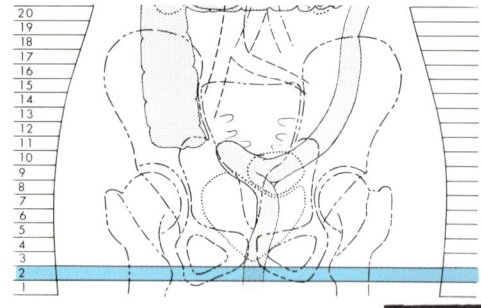

ABDOMEN AND PELVIS

Level 2

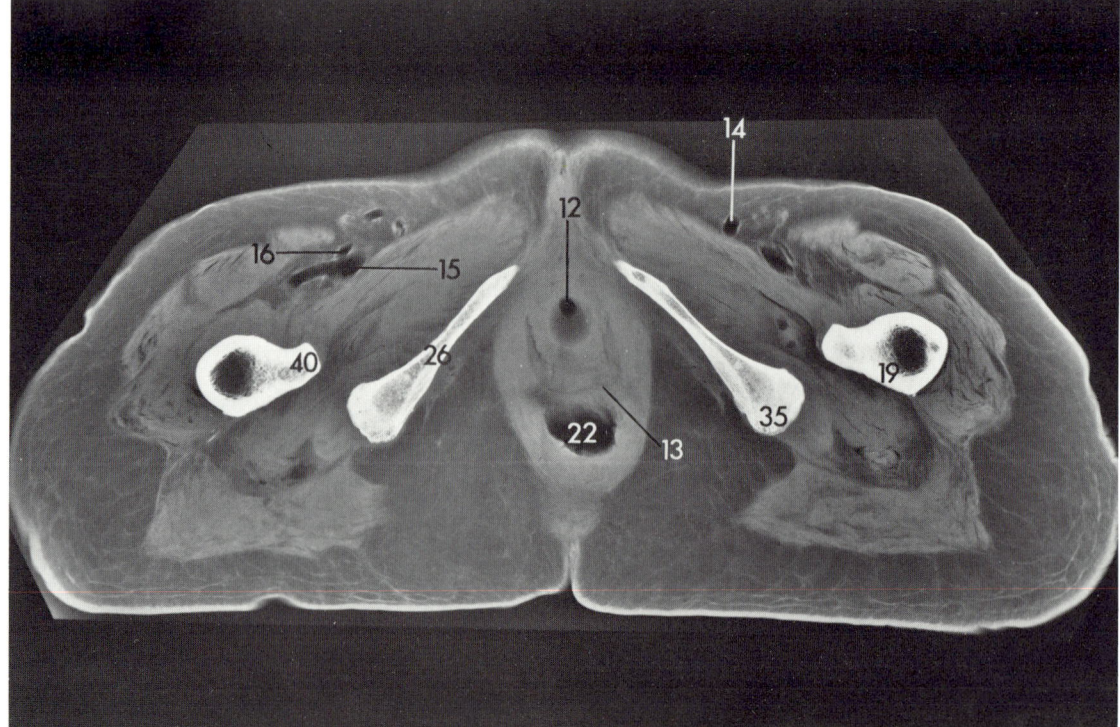

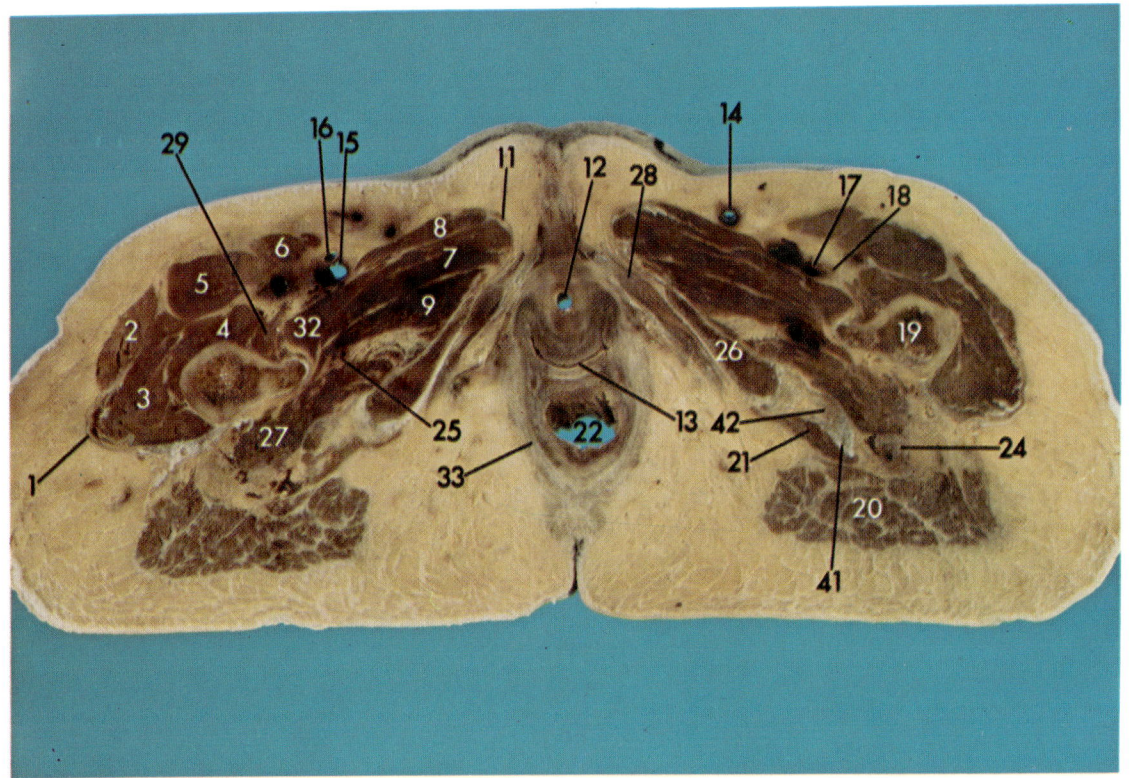

1. Fascia lata
2. Tensor fasciae latae muscle
3. Vastus lateralis muscle
4. Vastus intermedius muscle
5. Rectus femoris muscle
6. Sartorius muscle
7. Adductor brevis muscle
8. Adductor longus muscle
9. Adductor minimus muscle
11. Gracilis muscle
12. Urethra
13. Vagina
14. Saphenous vein
15. Femoral vein
16. Superficial femoral artery
17. Deep femoral artery
18. Femoral nerve
19. Femur
20. Gluteus maximus muscle
21. Biceps femoris muscle (long head)
22. Rectum
24. Sciatic nerve
25. Circumflex femoral vessels
26. Inferior pubic ramus
27. Quadratus femoris muscle
28. Ischiocavernosus muscle
29. Iliopsoas muscle
32. Pectineus muscle
33. Levator ani muscle
35. Ischial tuberosity
40. Lesser trochanter
41. Semitendinosus tendon
42. Semimembranosus tendon

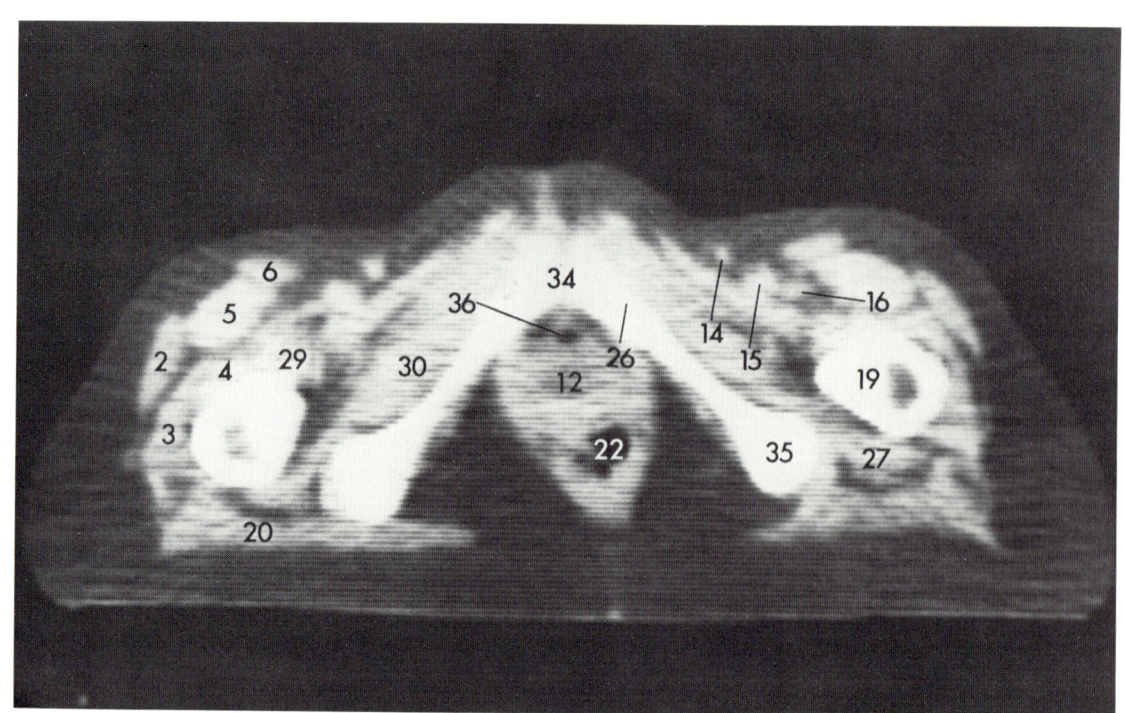

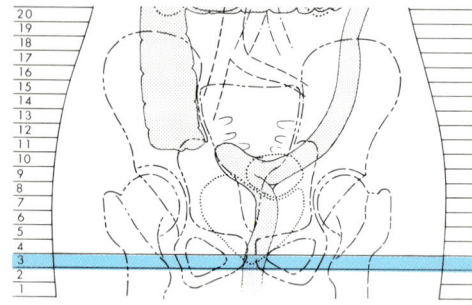

ABDOMEN AND PELVIS

Level 3

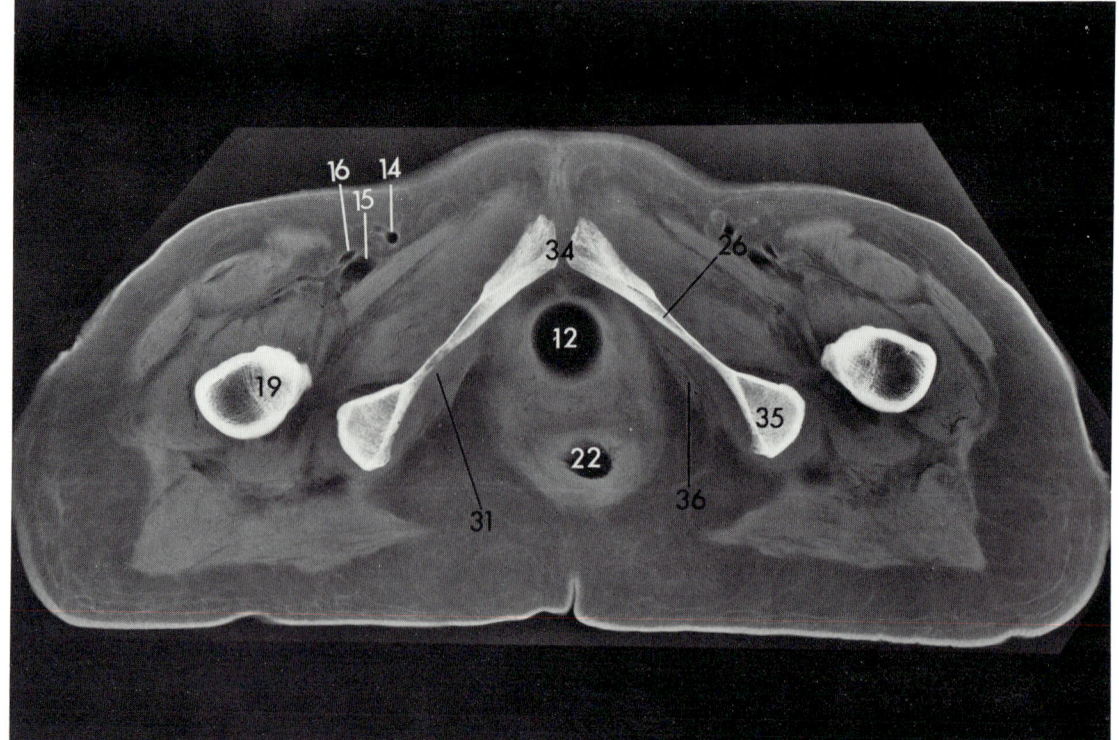

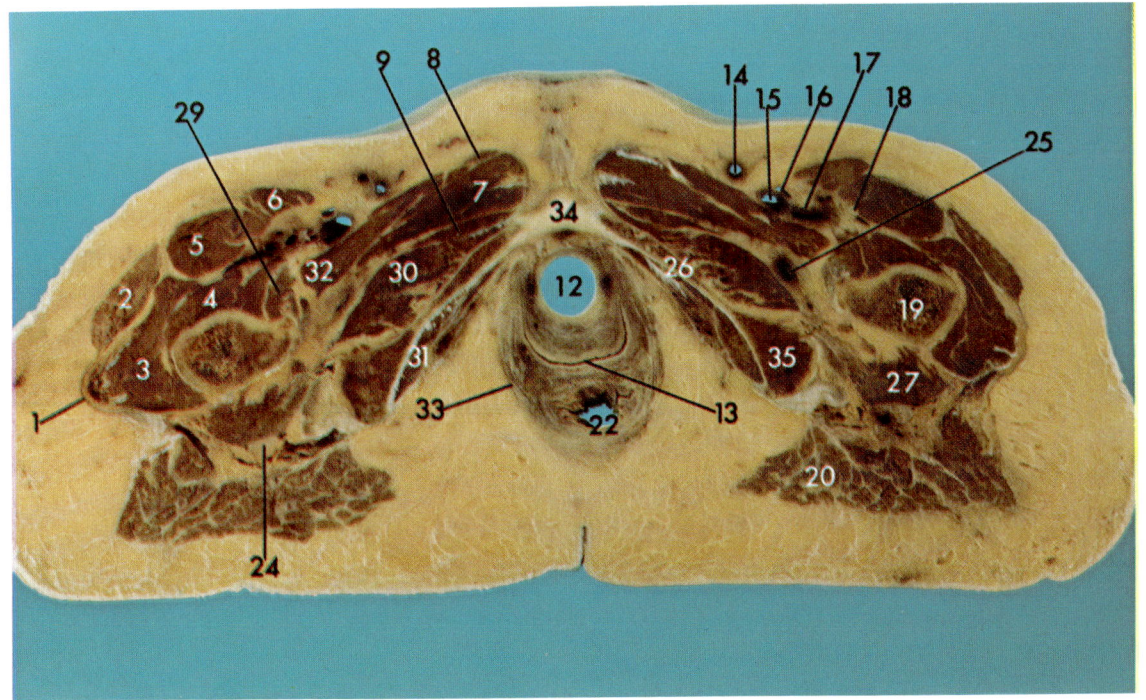

1. Fascia lata
2. Tensor fasciae latae muscle
3. Vastus lateralis muscle
4. Vastus intermedius muscle
5. Rectus femoris muscle
6. Sartorius muscle
7. Adductor brevis muscle
8. Adductor longus muscle
9. Adductor minimus muscle
12. Bladder
13. Vagina
14. Saphenous vein
15. Femoral vein
16. Superficial femoral artery
17. Deep femoral artery
18. Femoral nerve
19. Femur
20. Gluteus maximus muscle
22. Rectum
24. Sciatic nerve
25. Circumflex femoral vessels
26. Inferior pubic ramus
27. Quadratus femoris muscle
29. Iliopsoas muscle
30. Obturator externus muscle
31. Obturator internus muscle
32. Pectineus muscle
33. Levator ani muscle
34. Pubic symphysis
35. Ischial tuberosity
36. Catheter (containing air) in bladder

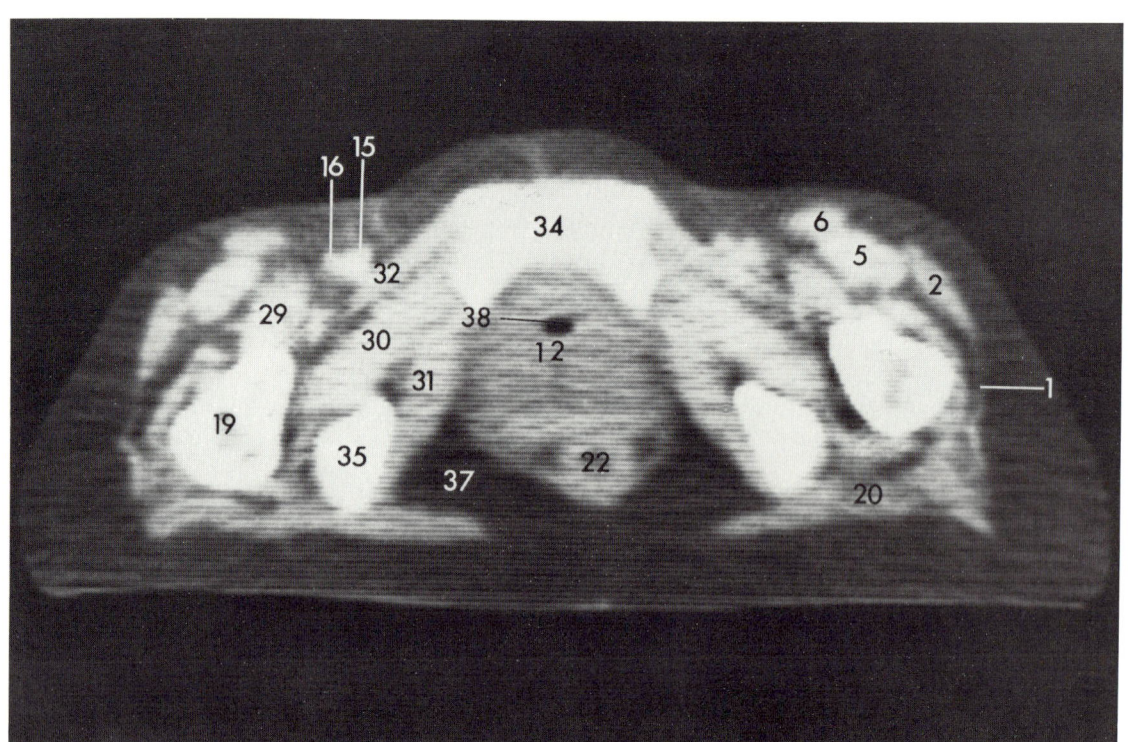

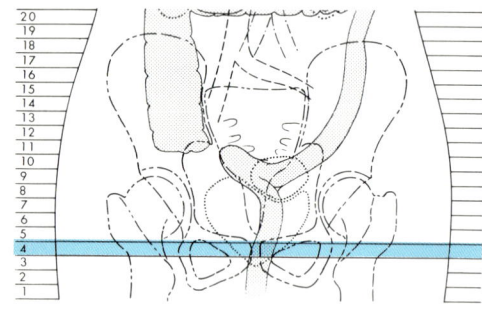

ABDOMEN AND PELVIS

Level 4

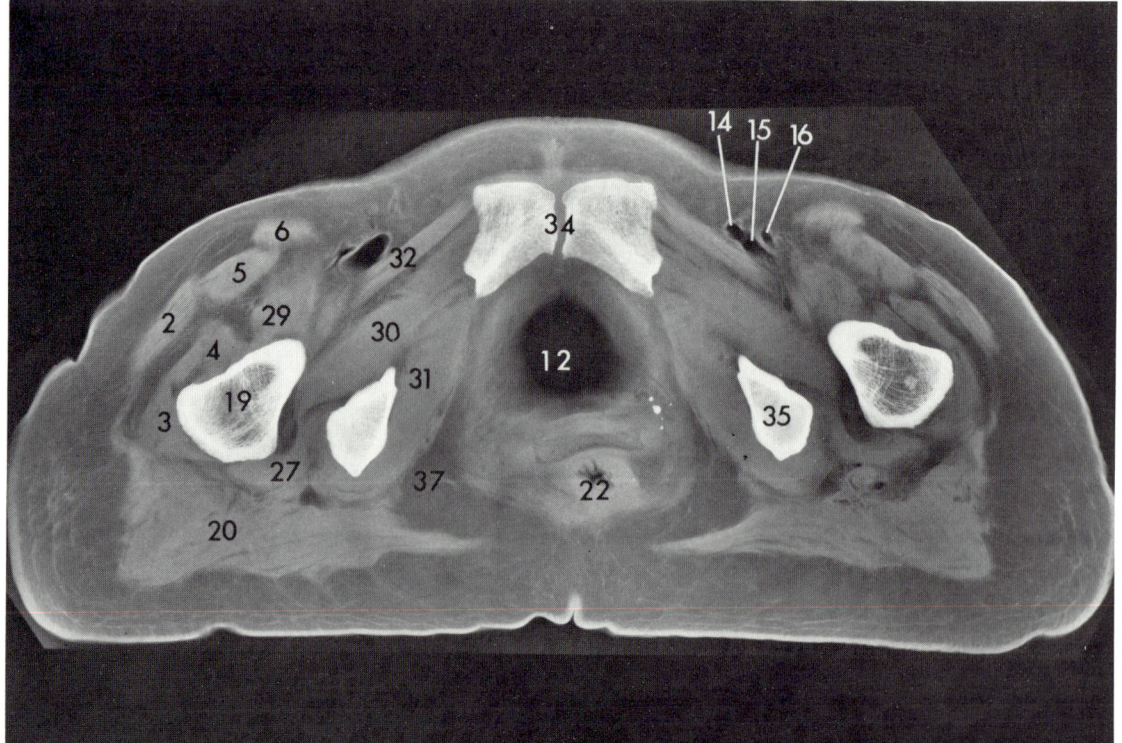

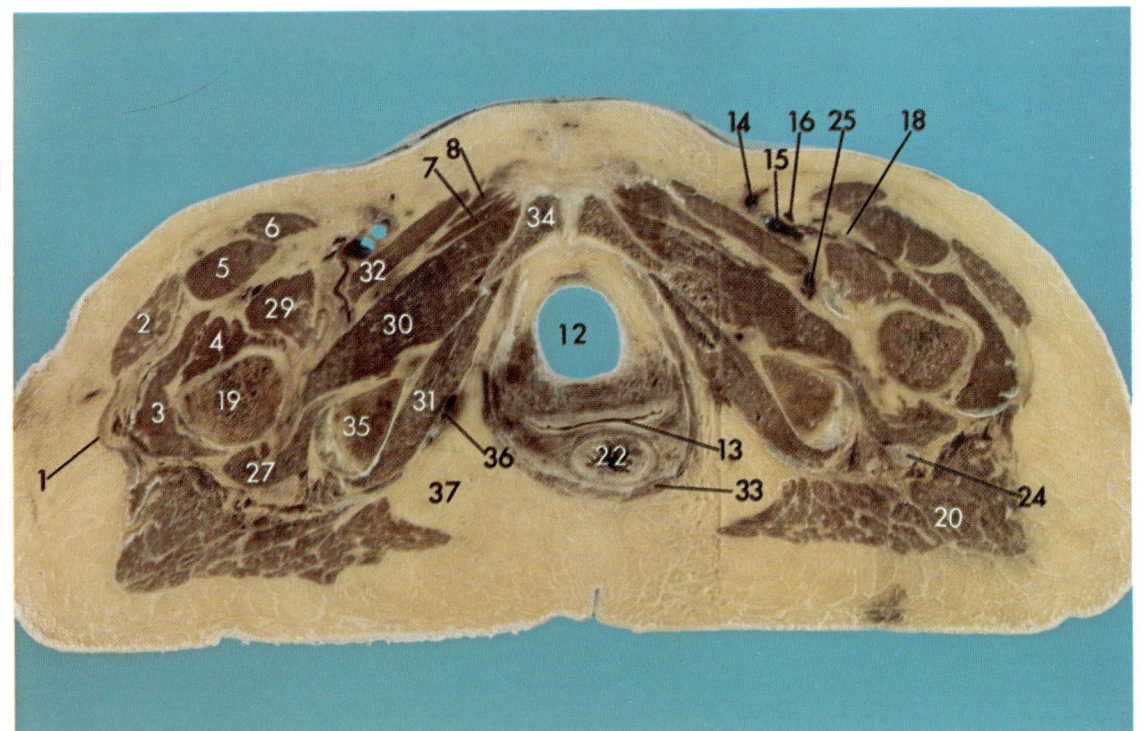

1. Fascia lata
2. Tensor fasciae latae muscle
3. Vastus lateralis muscle
4. Vastus intermedius muscle
5. Rectus femoris muscle
6. Sartorius muscle
7. Adductor brevis muscle
8. Adductor longus muscle
12. Bladder
13. Vagina
14. Saphenous vein
15. Femoral vein
16. Femoral artery
18. Femoral nerve
19. Femur
20. Gluteus maximus muscle
22. Rectum
24. Sciatic nerve
25. Circumflex femoral vessels
27. Quadratus femoris muscle
29. Iliopsoas muscle
30. Obturator externus muscle
31. Obturator internus muscle
32. Pectineus muscle
33. Levator ani
34. Pubic symphysis
35. Ischial tuberosity
36. Internal pudendal vessels
37. Ischiorectal fossa
38. Catheter (containing air) in bladder

153

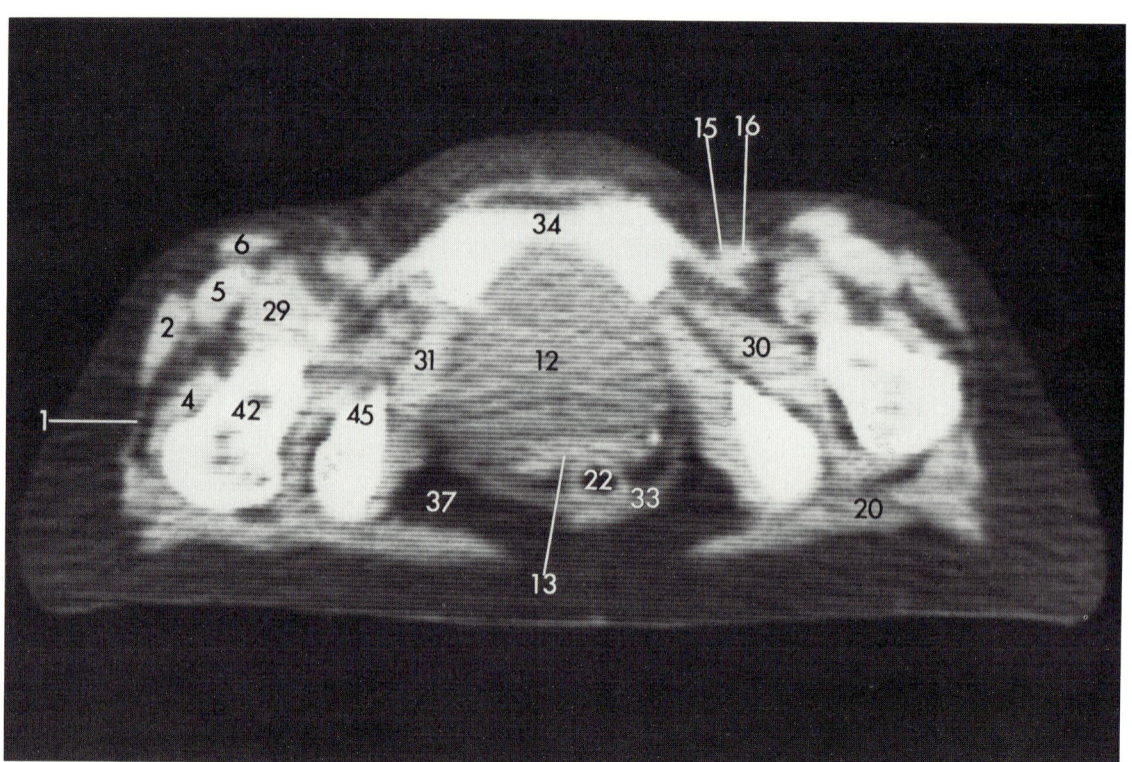

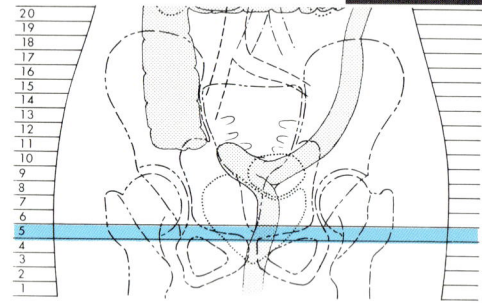

ABDOMEN AND PELVIS

Level 5

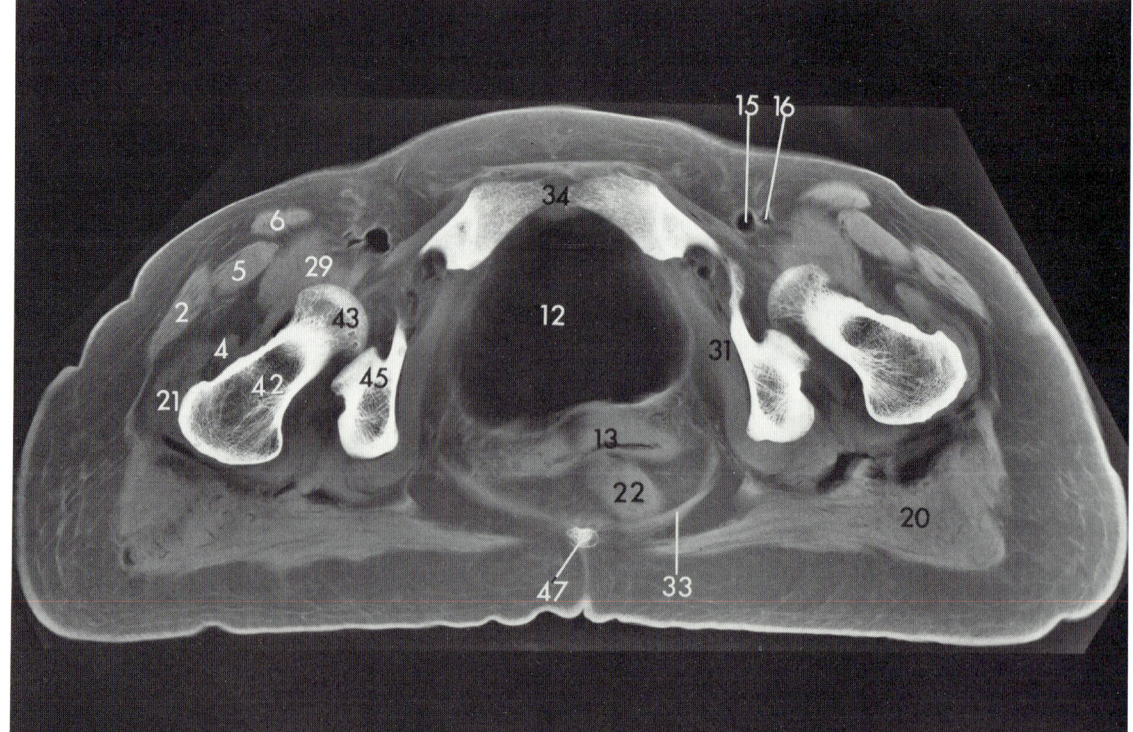

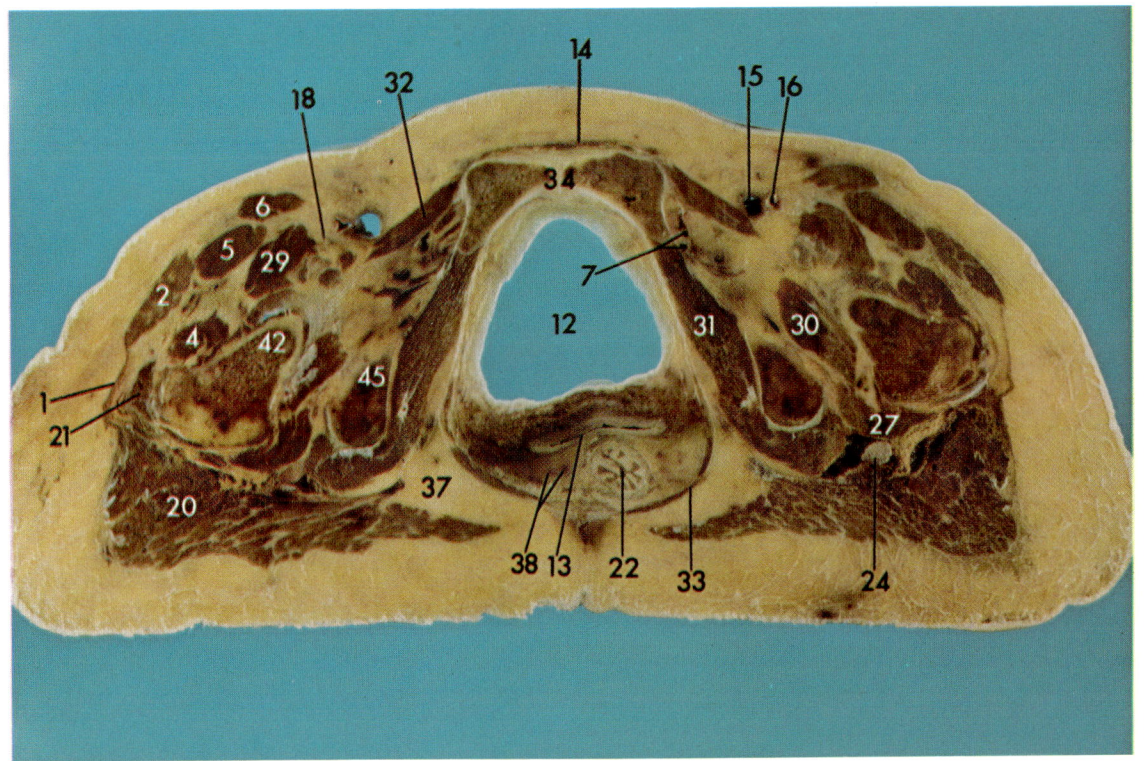

1. Fascia lata
2. Tensor fasciae latae muscle
4. Vastus intermedius muscle
5. Rectus femoris muscle
6. Sartorius muscle
7. Obturator vessels
12. Bladder
13. Vagina
14. Rectus abdominis muscle
15. Femoral vein
16. Femoral artery
18. Femoral nerve
20. Gluteus maximus muscle
21. Gluteus medius muscle
22. Rectum
24. Sciatic nerve
27. Quadratus femoris muscle
29. Iliopsoas muscle
30. Obturator externus muscle
31. Obturator internus muscle
32. Pectineus muscle
33. Levator ani muscle
34. Pubic symphysis
37. Ischiorectal fossa
38. Superior hemorrhoidal vessels
42. Neck of femur
43. Head of femur
45. Acetabulum (medial surface)
47. Coccyx

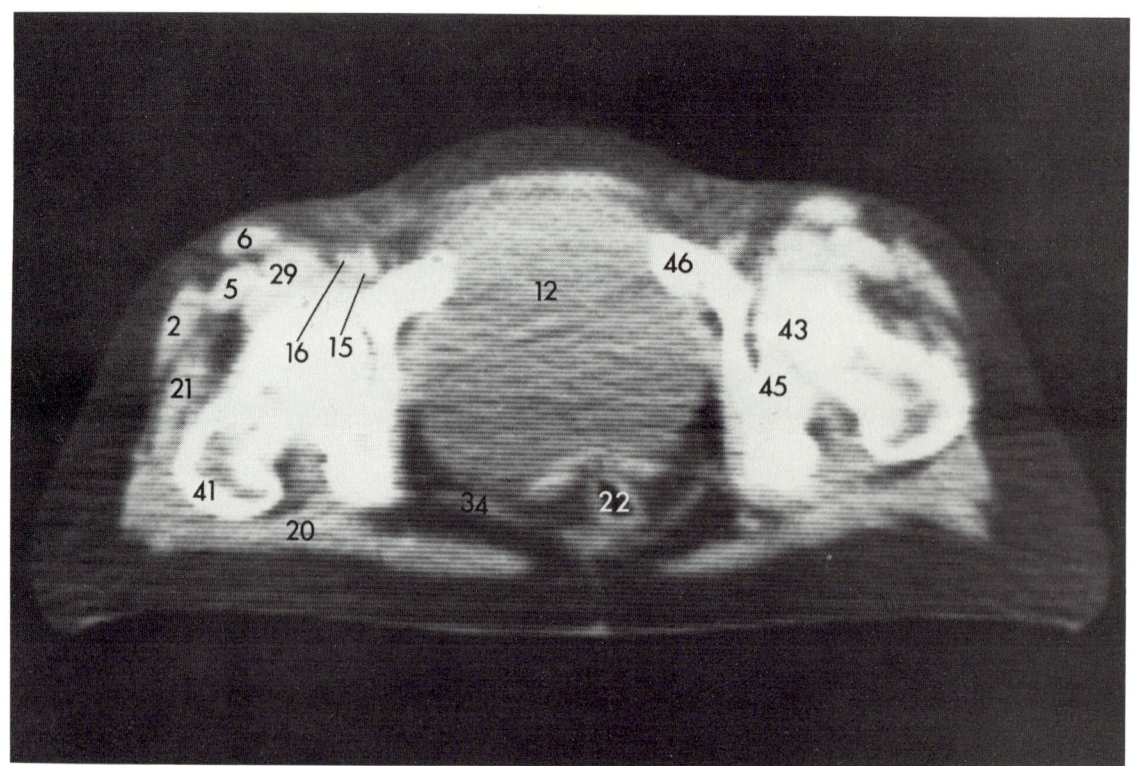

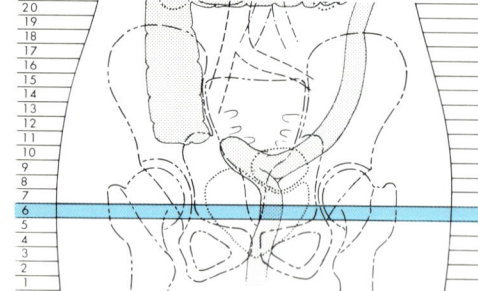

1. Fascia lata
2. Tensor fasciae latae muscle
3. Ureter
5. Rectus femoris muscle
6. Sartorius muscle
7. Obturator vessels
8. Capsule of hip joint
11. Anterior lip of cervix (with dilated glands)
12. Bladder

ABDOMEN AND PELVIS

Level 6

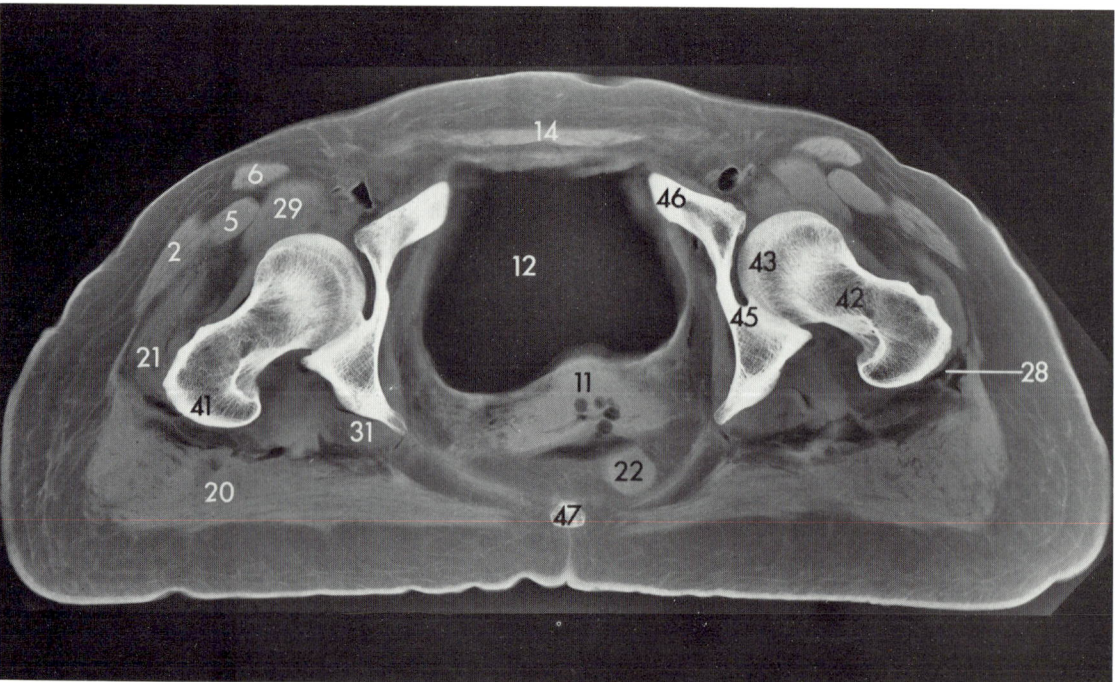

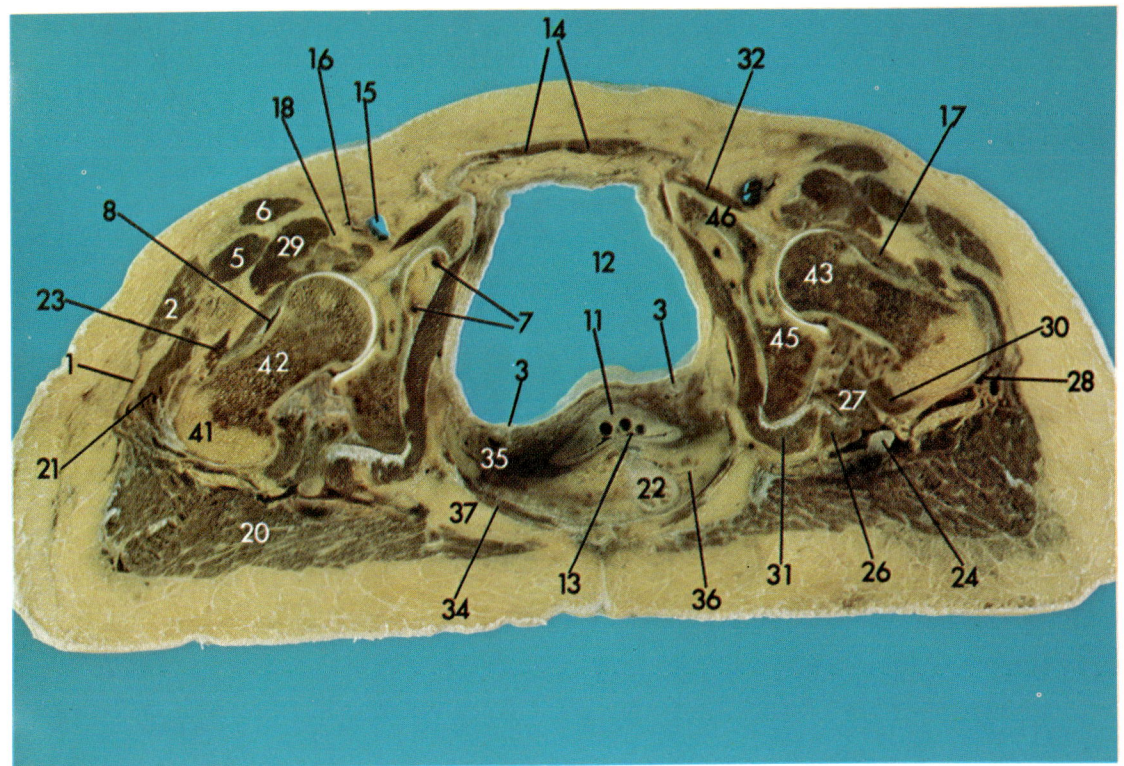

13. Vagina	24. Sciatic nerve	36. Superior hemorrhoidal vessels
14. Rectus abdominis muscle	26. Gemellus inferior muscle	37. Ischiorectal fossa
15. Femoral vein	27. Quadratus femoris muscle	41. Greater trochanter of femur
16. Femoral artery	28. Trochanteric bursa	42. Neck of femur
17. Iliofemoral ligament	29. Iliopsoas muscle	43. Head of femur
18. Femoral nerve	30. Obturator externus muscle	45. Acetabulum
20. Gluteus maximus muscle	31. Obturator internus muscle	46. Superior ramus of pubis
21. Gluteus medius muscle	32. Pectineus muscle	47. Coccyx
22. Rectum	34. Coccygeus muscle	
23. Gluteus minimus muscle	35. Uterovaginal vascular plexus	

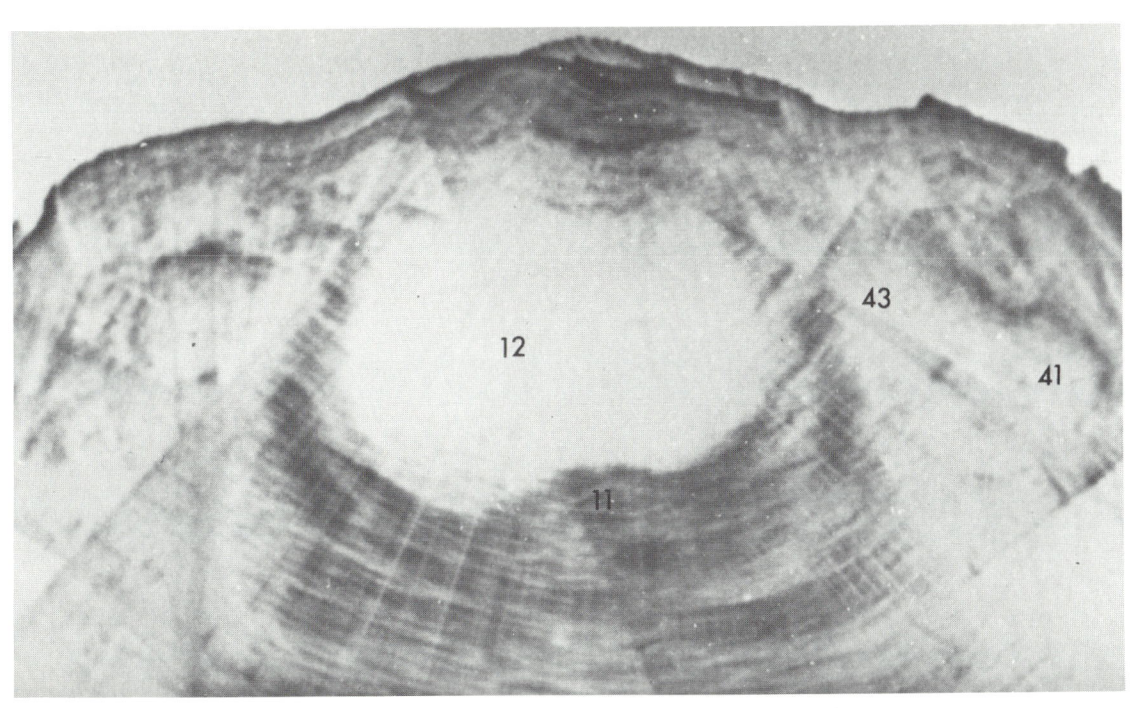

157

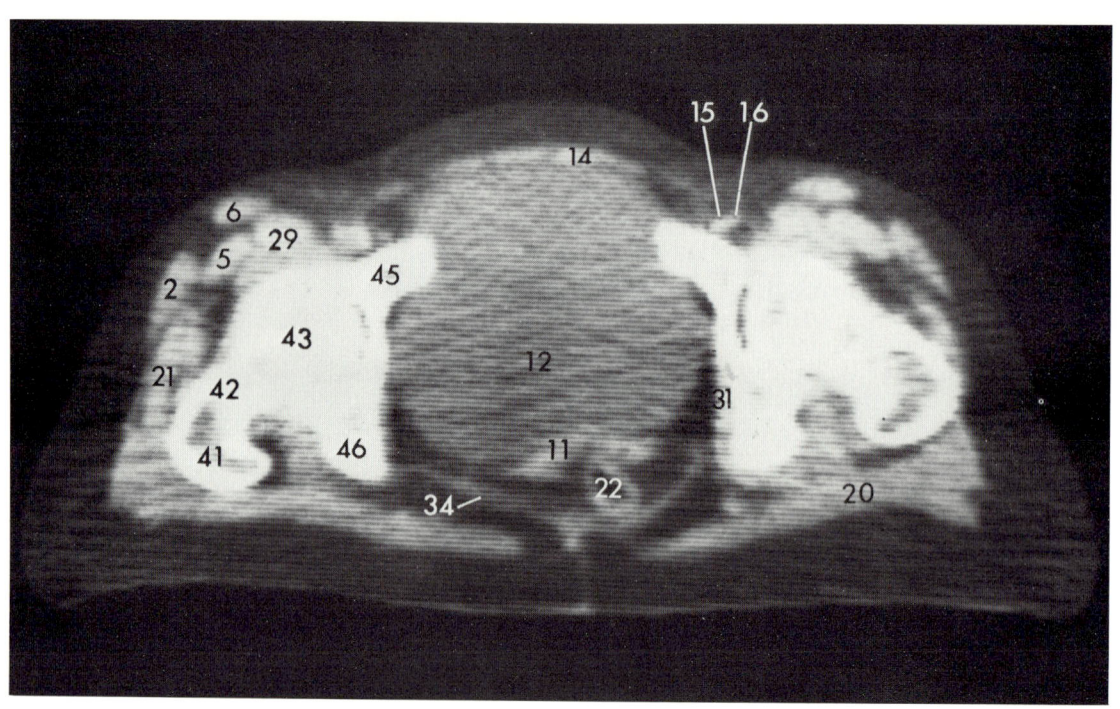

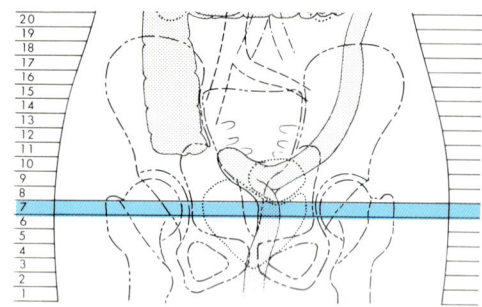

ABDOMEN AND PELVIS

Level 7

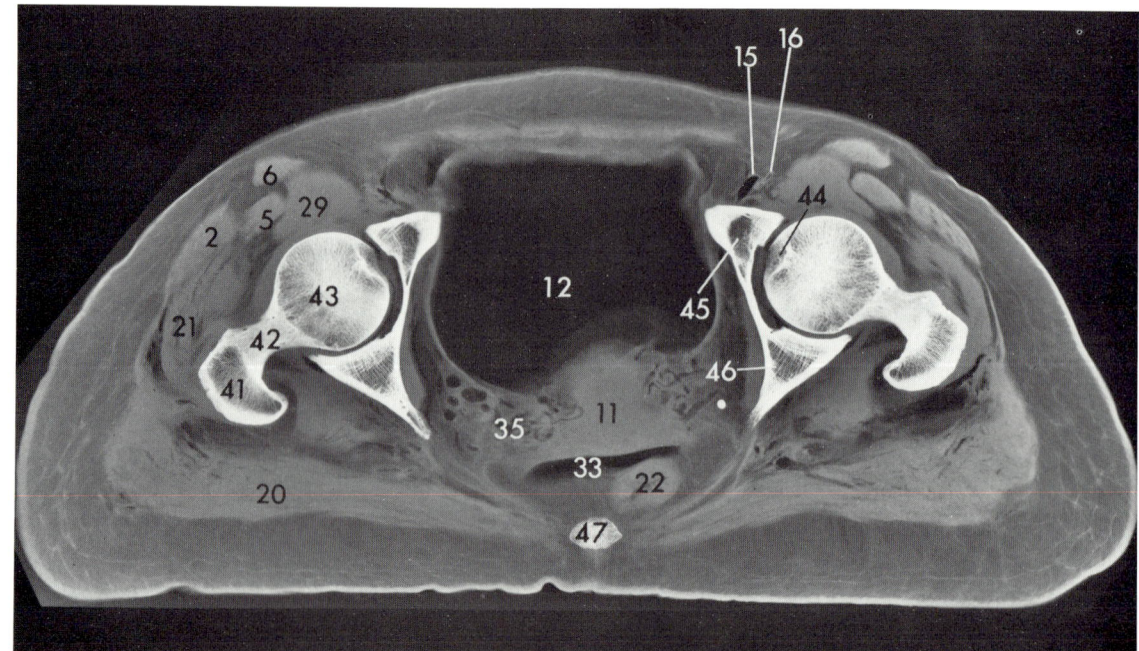

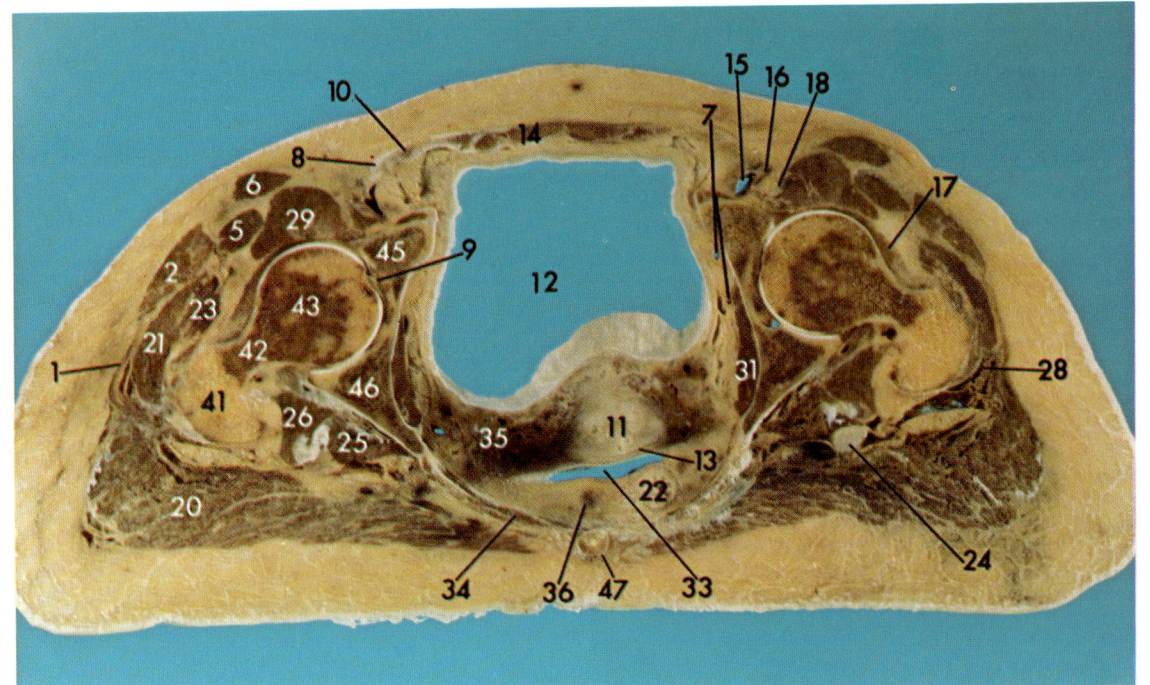

1. Fascia lata
2. Tensor fasciae latae muscle
5. Rectus femoris muscle
6. Sartorius muscle
7. Obturator vessels
8. Inguinal ligament
9. Ligamentum teres femoris
10. Round ligament
11. Cervix
12. Bladder
13. Posterior fornix of vagina
14. Rectus abdominis muscle
15. Femoral vein
16. Femoral artery
17. Iliofemoral ligament
18. Femoral nerve
20. Gluteus maximus muscle
21. Gluteus medius muscle
22. Rectum
23. Gluteus minimus muscle
24. Sciatic nerve
25. Gemellus superior muscle
26. Gemellus inferior muscle
28. Trochanteric bursa
29. Iliopsoas muscle
31. Obturator internus muscle
33. Rectouterine pouch (Douglas) of peritoneal cavity
34. Coccygeus muscle
35. Uterovaginal vascular plexus
36. Superior hemorrhoidal vessels
41. Greater trochanter
42. Neck of femur
43. Head of femur
44. Fovea of head of femur
45. Pubis
46. Ischium
47. Coccyx

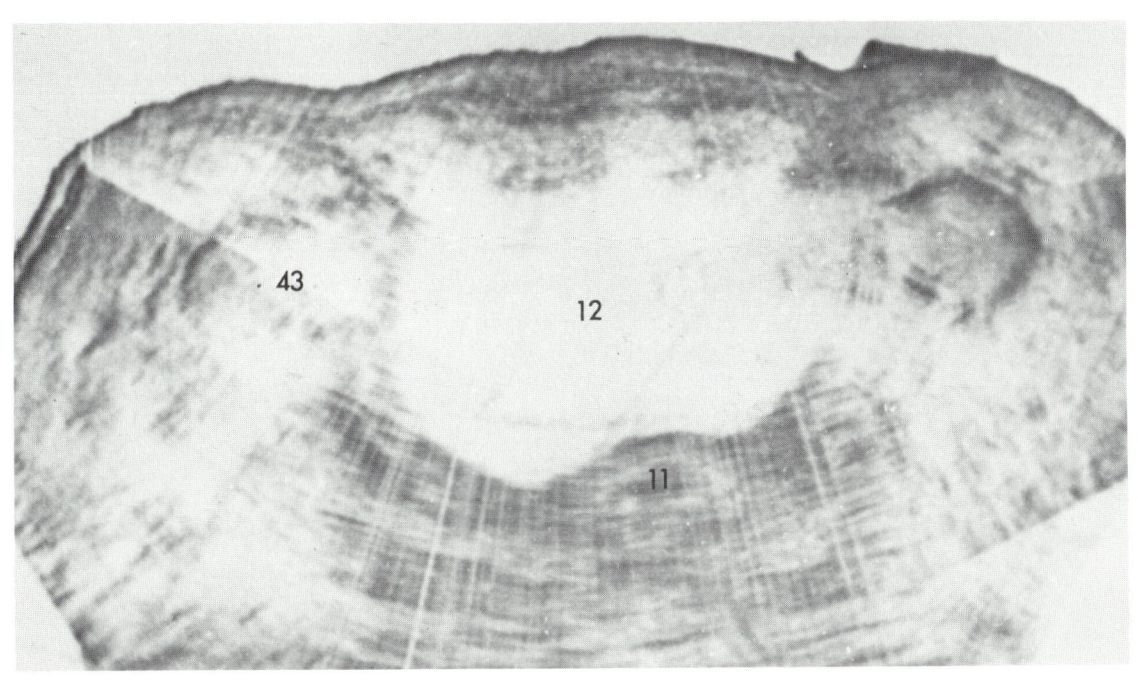

159

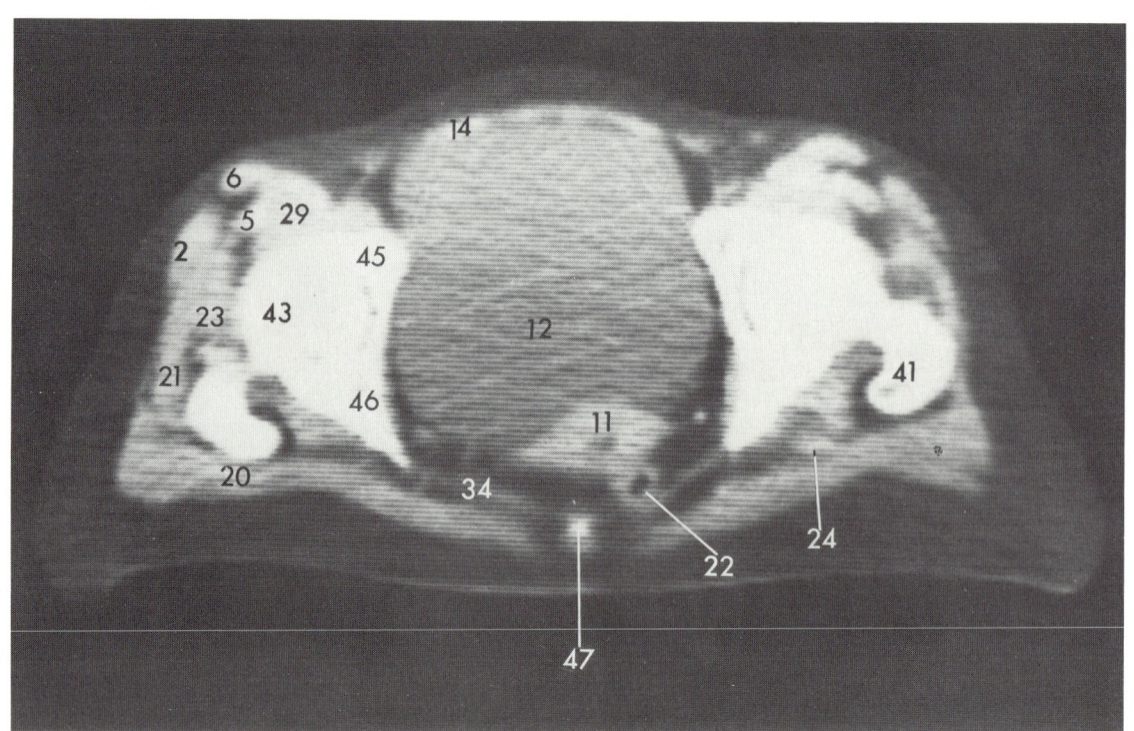

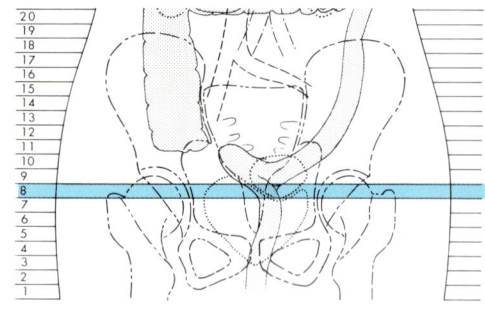

ABDOMEN AND PELVIS

Level 8

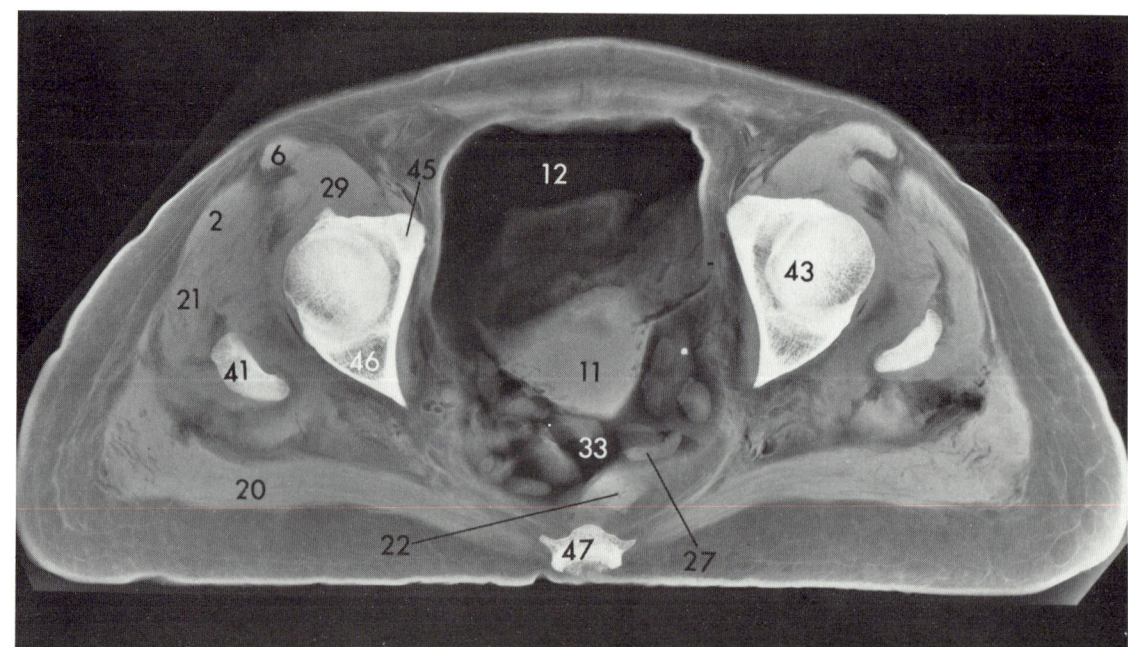

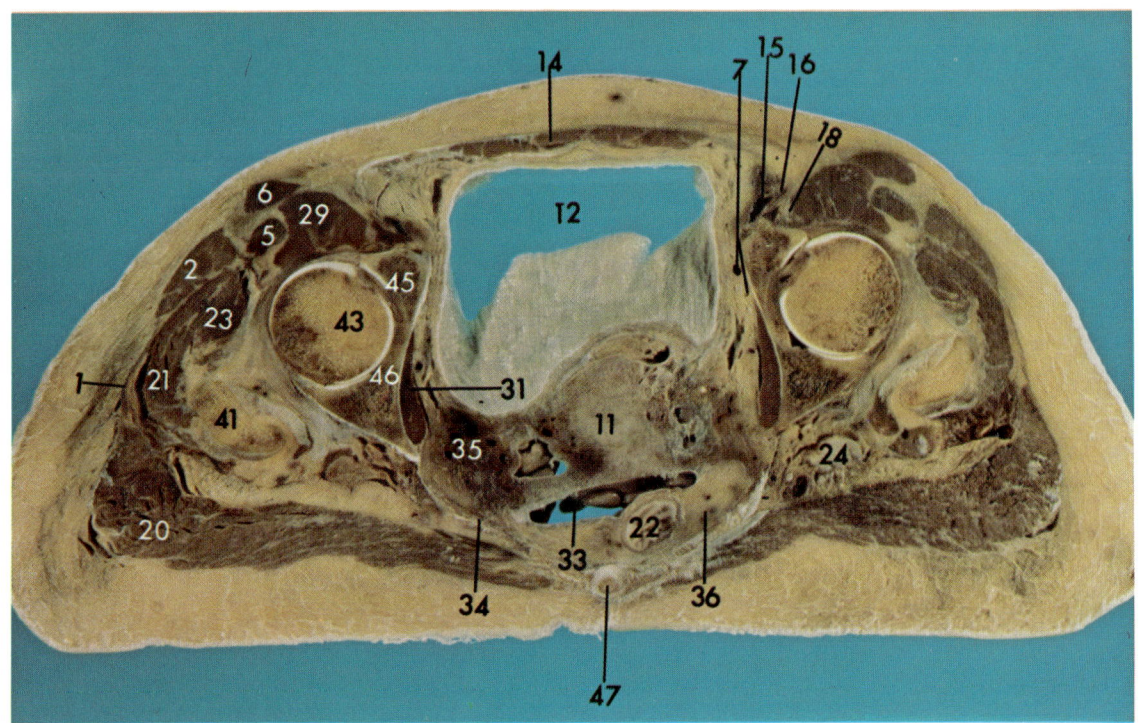

1. Fascia lata
2. Tensor fasciae latae muscle
5. Rectus femoris muscle
6. Sartorius muscle
7. Obturator vessels
11. Uterus
12. Bladder
14. Rectus abdominis muscle
15. Femoral vein
16. Femoral artery
18. Femoral nerve
20. Gluteus maximus muscle
21. Gluteus medius muscle
22. Rectum
23. Gluteus minimus muscle
24. Sciatic nerve
27. Appendices epiploicae of sigmoid colon
29. Iliopsoas muscle
31. Obturator internus muscle
33. Rectouterine pouch (Douglas) of peritoneal cavity
34. Coccygeus muscle
35. Uterovaginal vascular plexus
36. Superior hemorrhoidal vessels
41. Greater trochanter
43. Head of femur
45. Pubis
46. Ischium
47. Coccyx

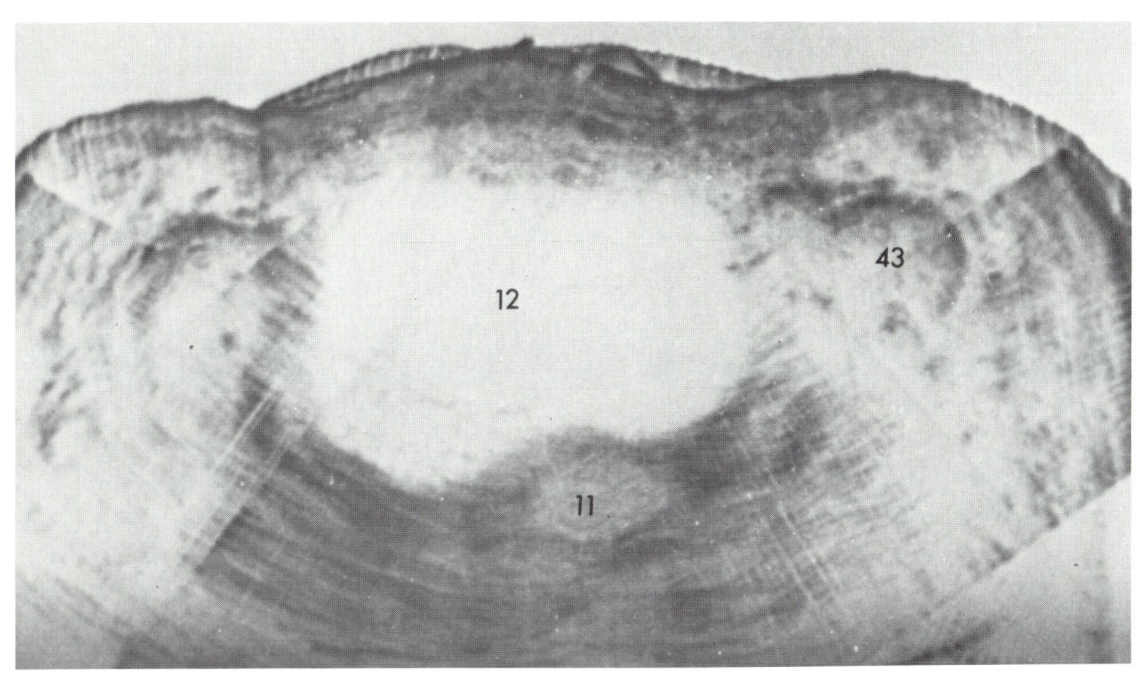

161

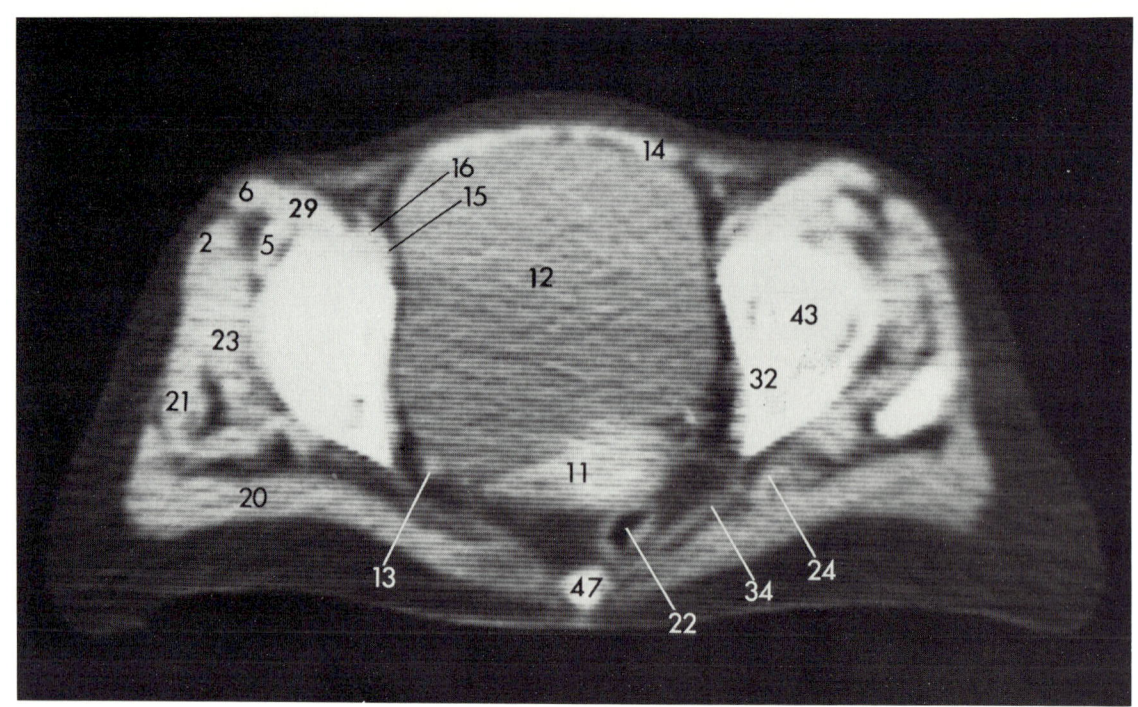

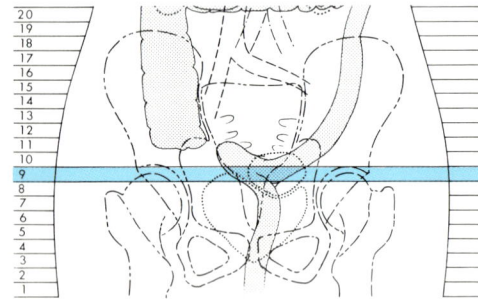

ABDOMEN AND PELVIS

Level 9

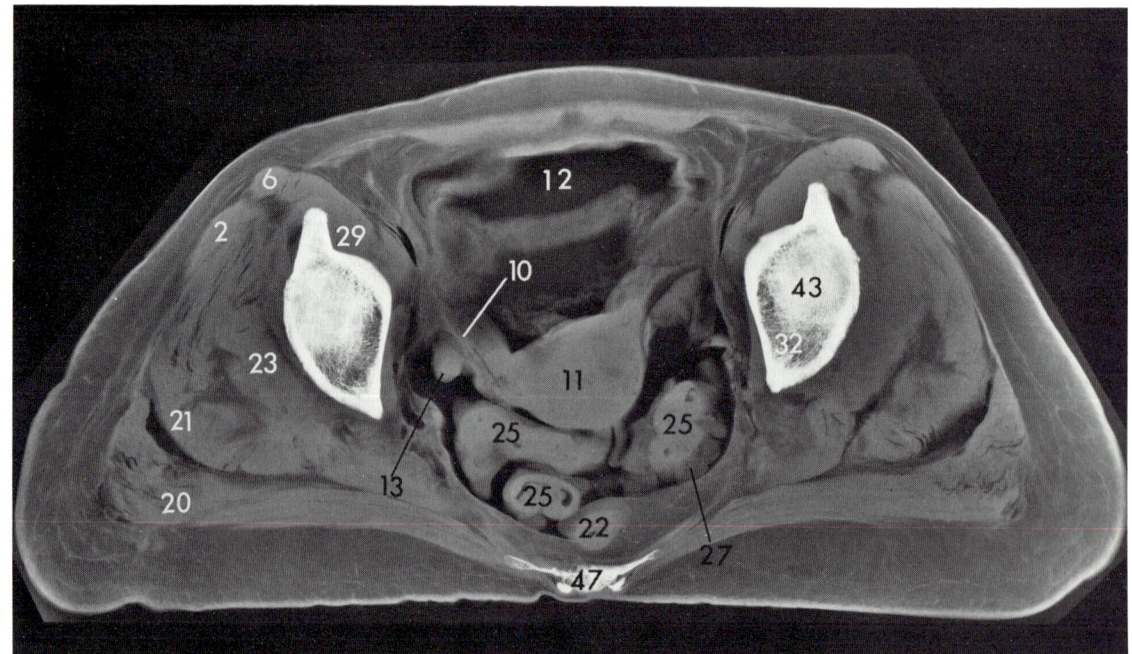

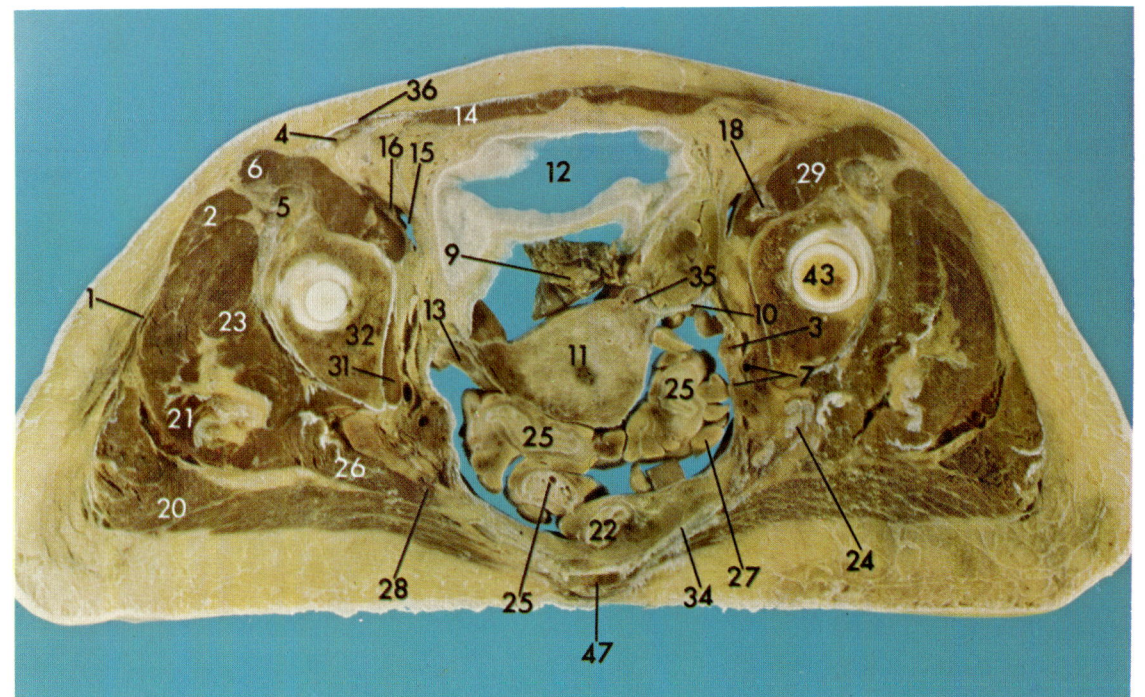

1. Fascia lata
2. Tensor fasciae latae muscle
3. Ureter
4. Internal oblique muscle
5. Rectus femoris tendon
6. Sartorius muscle
7. Obturator vessels
8. Inferior epigastric artery
9. Ileum
10. Broad ligament of uterus
11. Uterus
12. Bladder
13. Ovary
14. Rectus abdominis muscle
15. External iliac vein
16. External iliac artery
18. Femoral nerve
20. Gluteus maximus muscle
21. Gluteus medius muscle
22. Rectum
23. Gluteus minimus muscle
24. Sciatic nerve
25. Loop of sigmoid colon in rectouterine pouch (Douglas) of peritoneal cavity
26. Piriformis muscle
27. Appendices epiploicae of sigmoid colon
28. Pudendal nerve
29. Iliopsoas muscle
31. Obturator internus muscle
32. Ilium
34. Coccygeus muscle
35. Uterovaginal vascular plexus
36. Aponeurosis of external oblique muscle
43. Head of femur
47. Coccyx

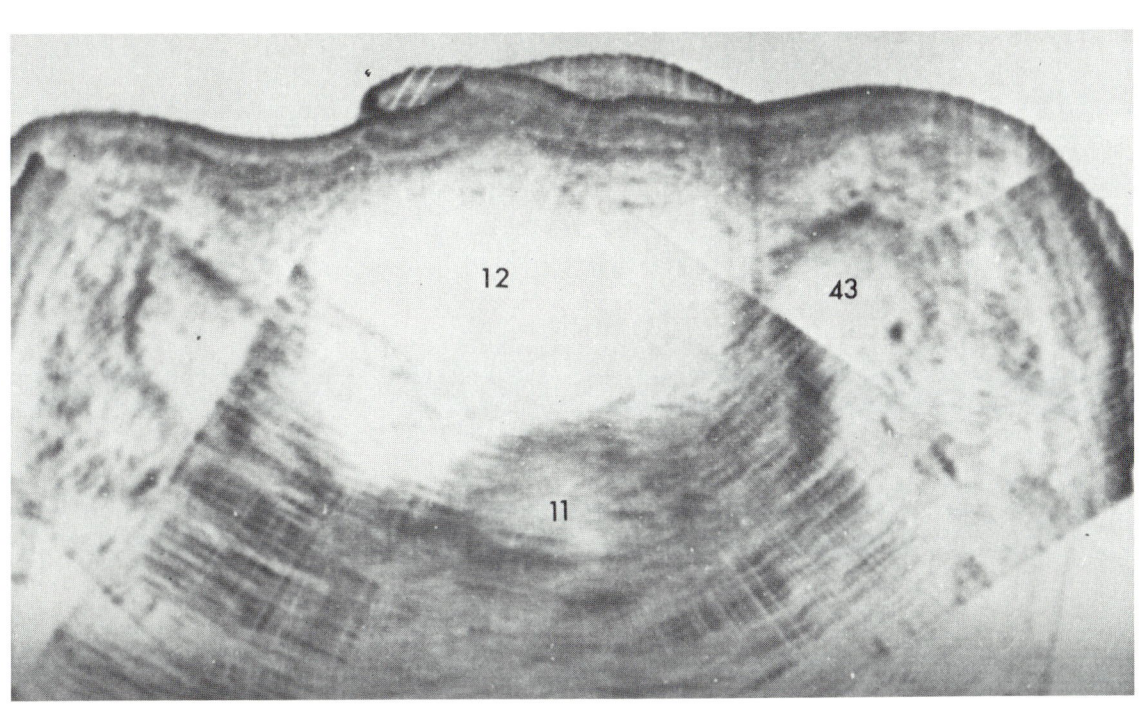

163

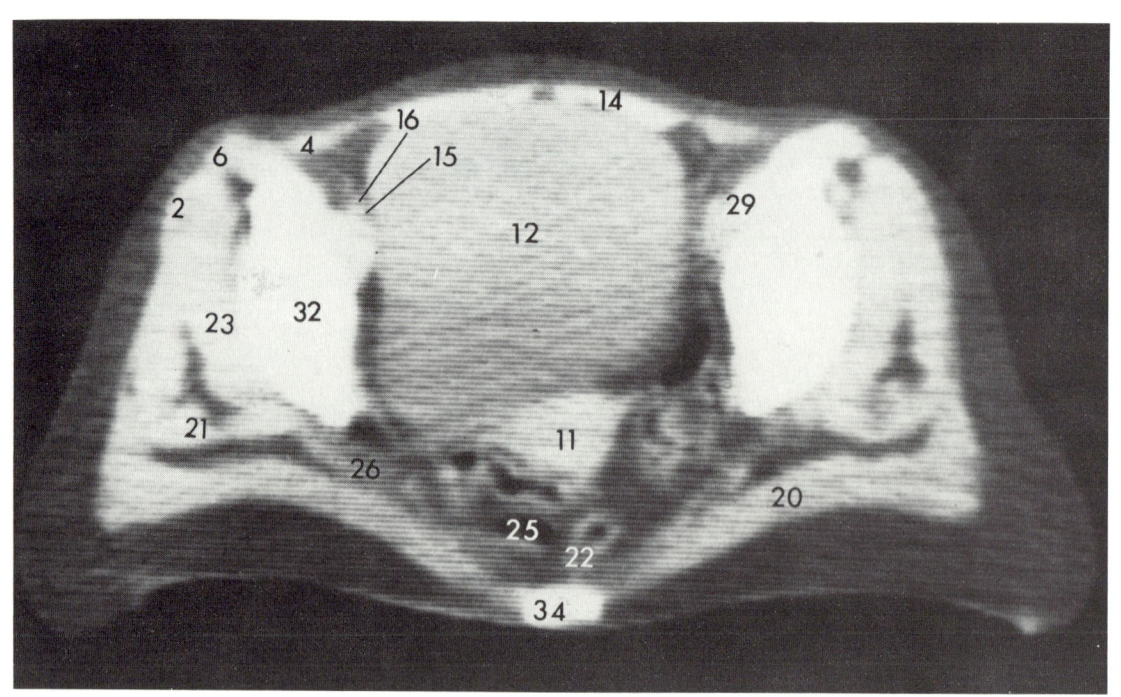

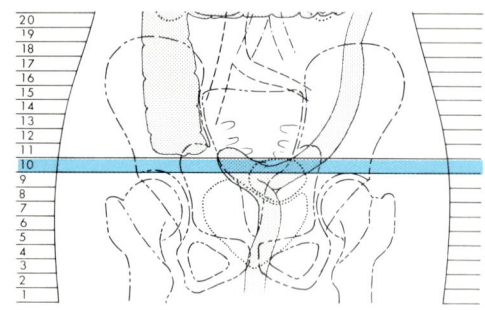

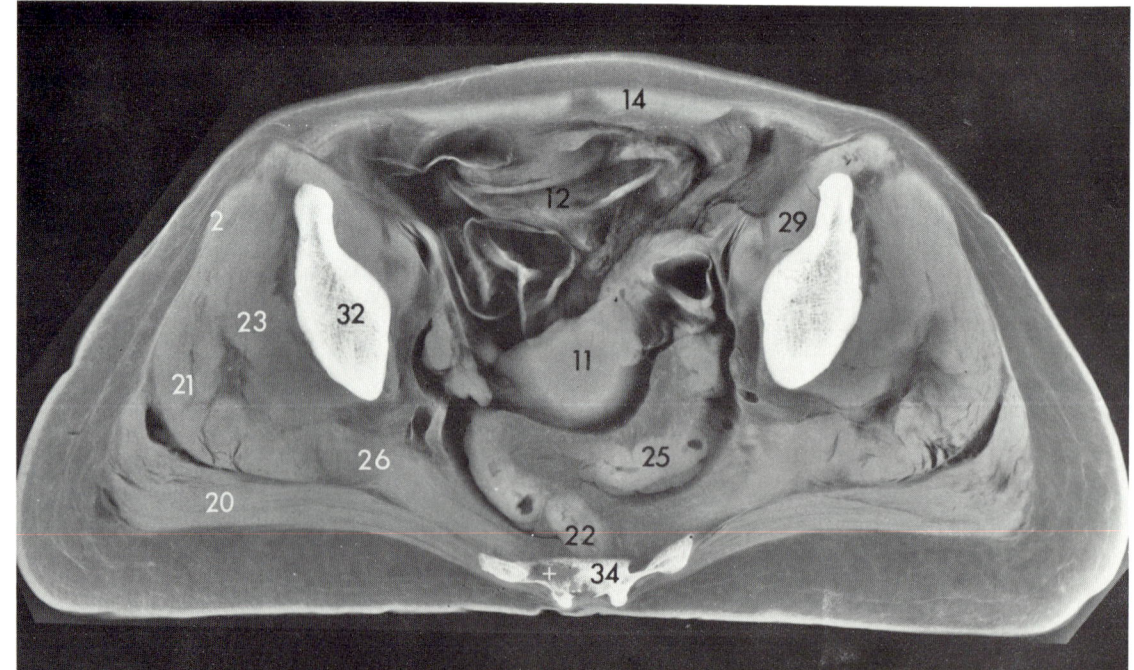

ABDOMEN AND PELVIS

Level 10

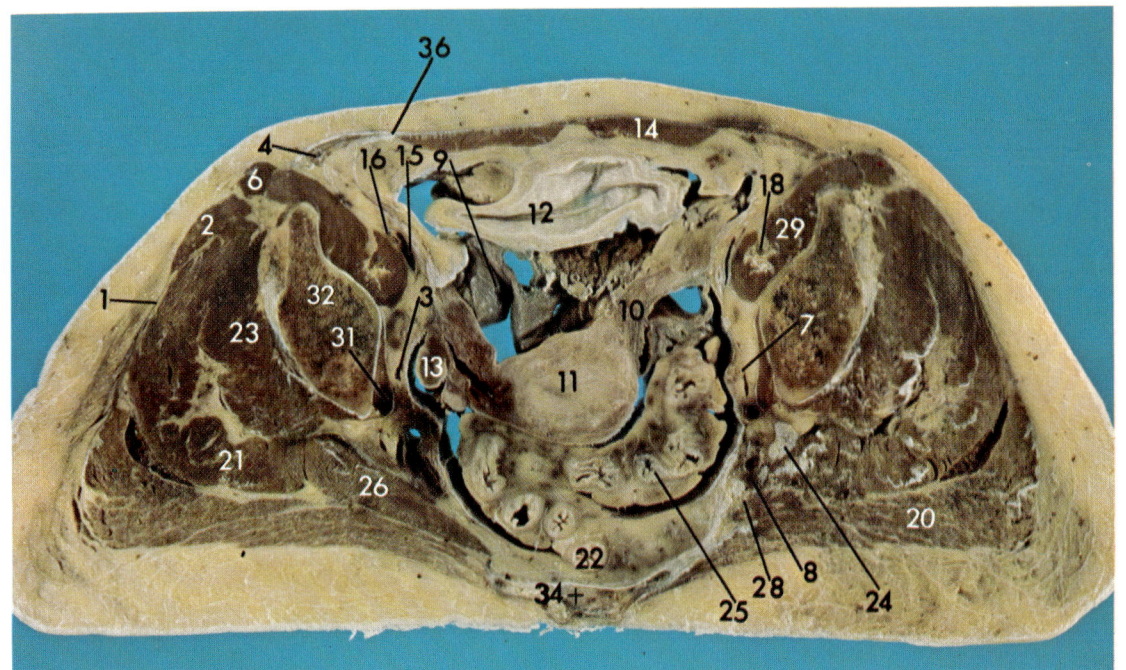

1. Fascia lata
2. Tensor fasciae latae muscle
3. Ureter
4. Internal oblique muscle
5. Inferior epigastric artery
6. Sartorius muscle
7. Obturator vessels
8. Inferior gluteal vessels
9. Ileum
10. Broad ligament of uterus
11. Uterus
12. Dome of bladder
13. Ovary
14. Rectus abdominis muscle
15. External iliac vein
16. External iliac artery
18. Femoral nerve
20. Gluteus maximus muscle
21. Gluteus medius muscle
22. Rectum
23. Gluteus minimus muscle
24. Sciatic nerve
25. Sigmoid colon
26. Piriformis muscle
28. Pudendal nerve
29. Iliopsoas muscle
31. Obturator internus muscle
32. Ilium
34. Sacrum
36. Aponeurosis of external oblique muscle
+ Metastasis in sacrum

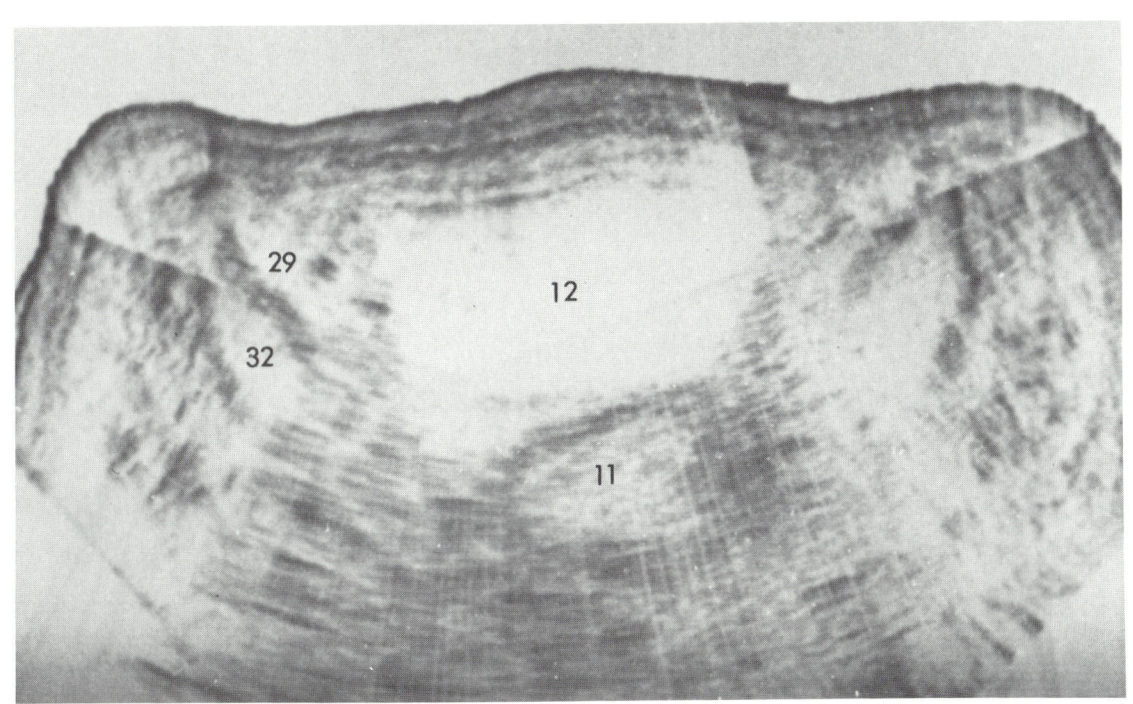

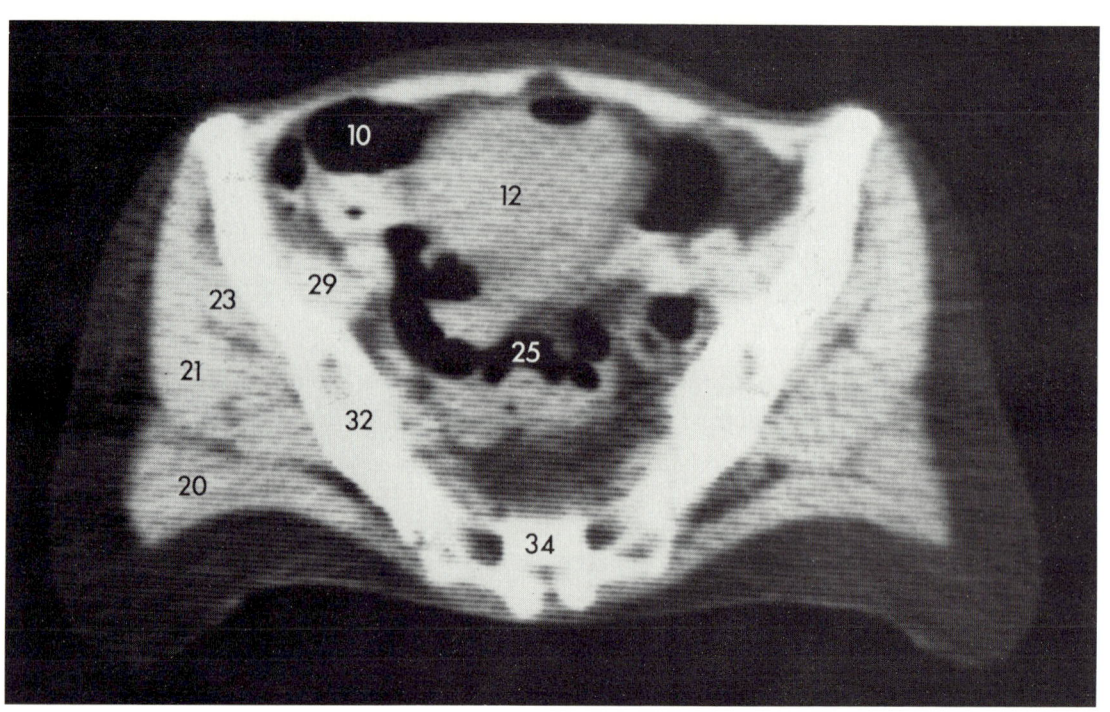

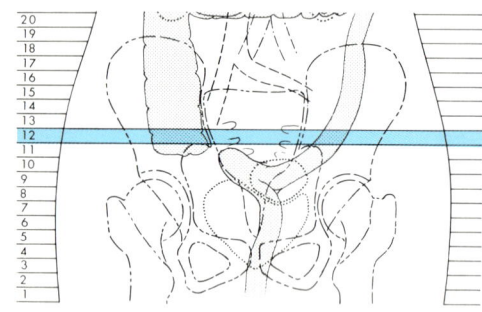

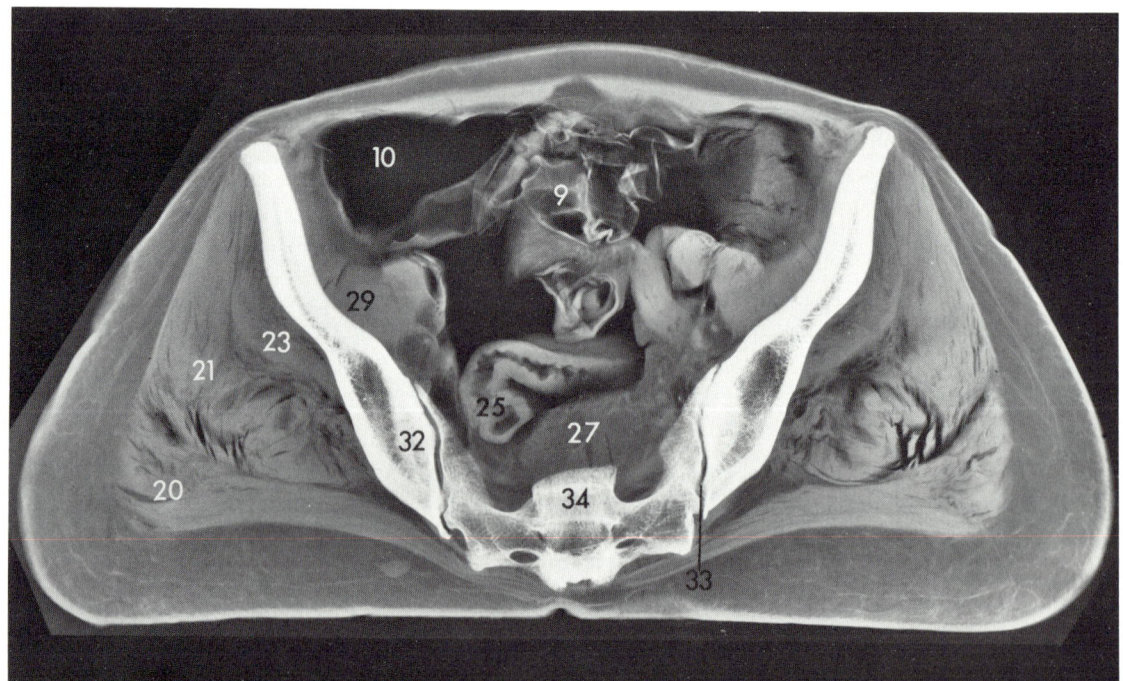

ABDOMEN AND PELVIS

Level 12

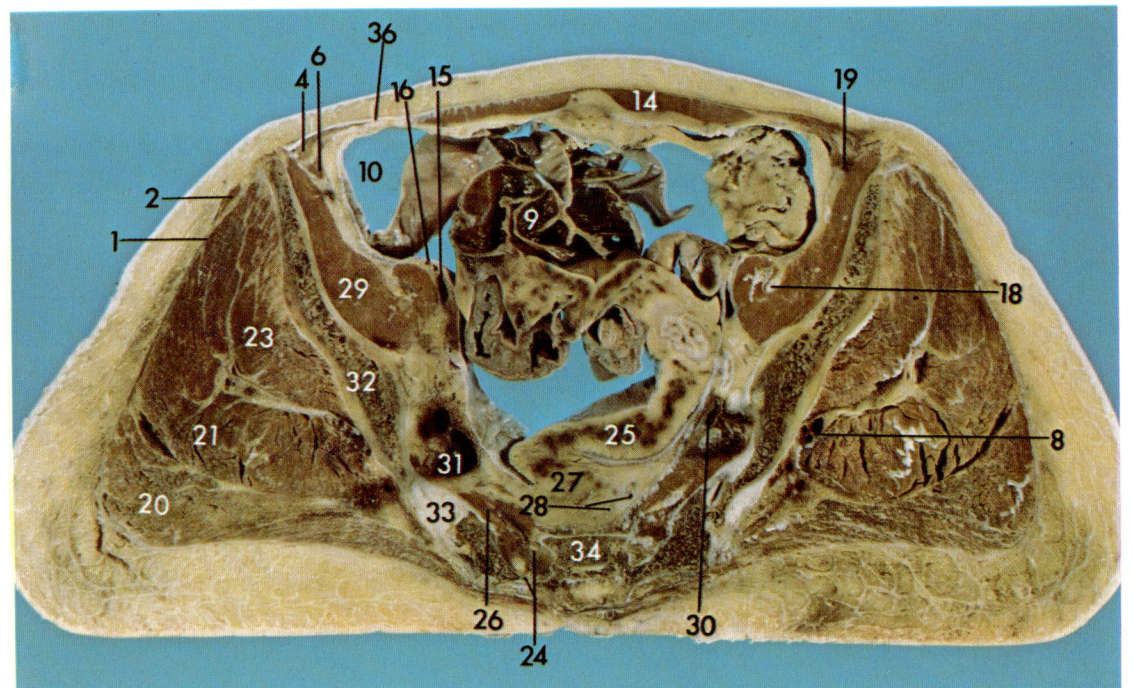

1. Fascia lata
2. Tensor fasciae latae muscle
4. Internal oblique muscle
5. Inferior epigastric artery
6. Transversus abdominis muscle
8. Superior gluteal vessels
9. Ileum
12. Bladder
14. Rectus abdominis muscle
15. External iliac vein
16. External iliac artery
18. Femoral nerve
19. Deep circumflex iliac vessels
20. Gluteus maximus muscle
21. Gluteus medius muscle
23. Gluteus minimus muscle
24. Sacral nerves
25. Sigmoid colon
26. Piriformis muscle
27. Mesentery of sigmoid colon
28. Superior hemorrhoidal vessels
29. Iliopsoas muscle
30. Internal iliac artery
31. Internal iliac vein
32. Ilium
33. Sacroiliac joint
34. Sacrum
36. Aponeurosis of external oblique muscle

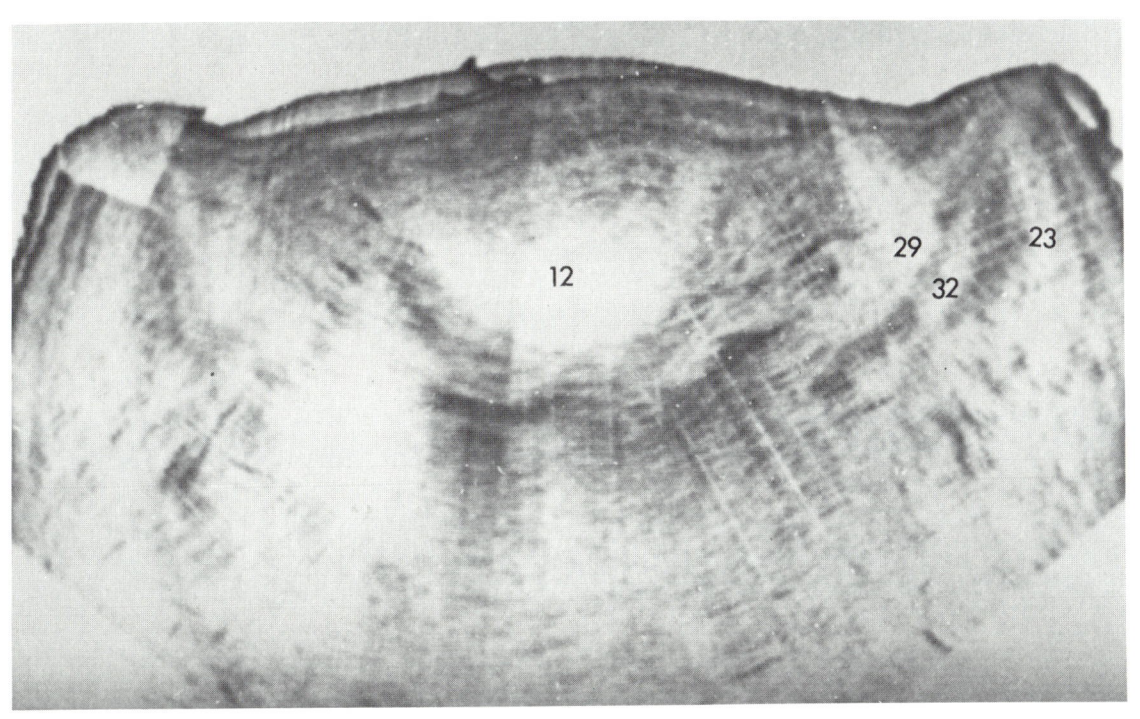

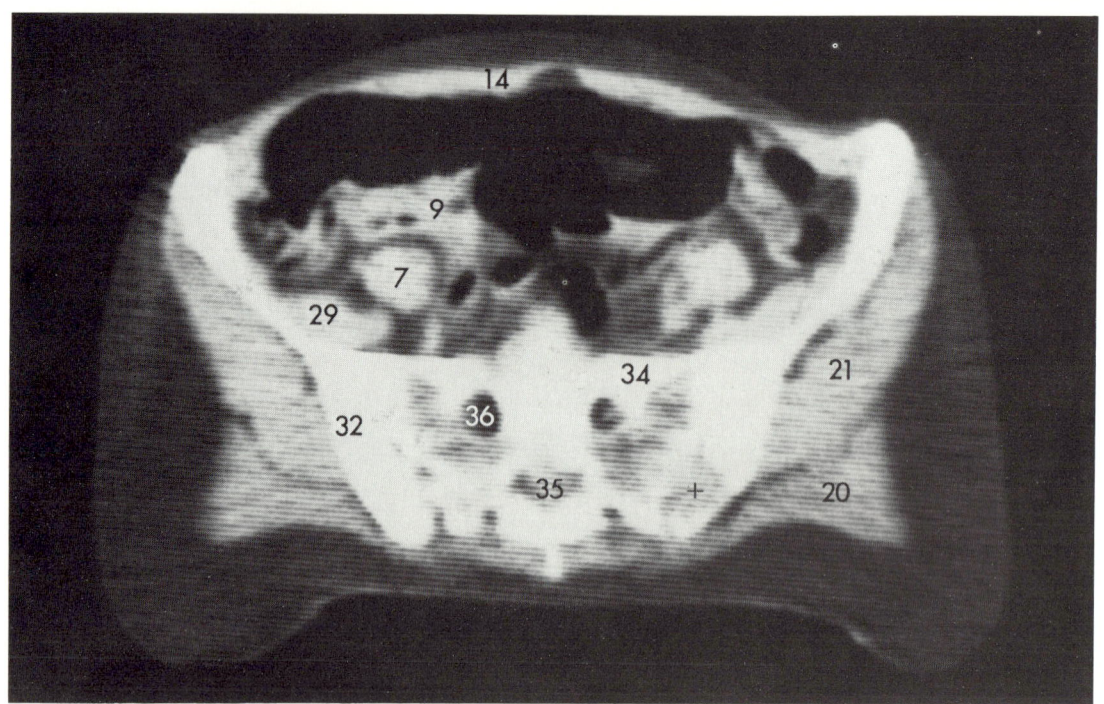

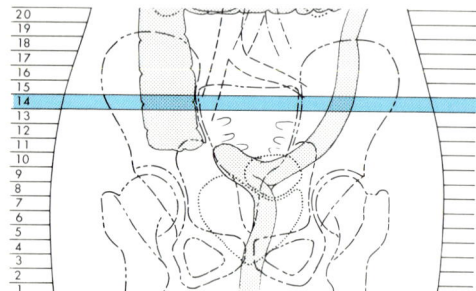

3. Ureter
4. Internal oblique muscle
5. Inferior epigastric artery
6. Transversus abdominis muscle
7. Psoas muscle
8. Superior gluteal vessels
9. Small intestine
10. Cecum

ABDOMEN AND PELVIS

Level 14

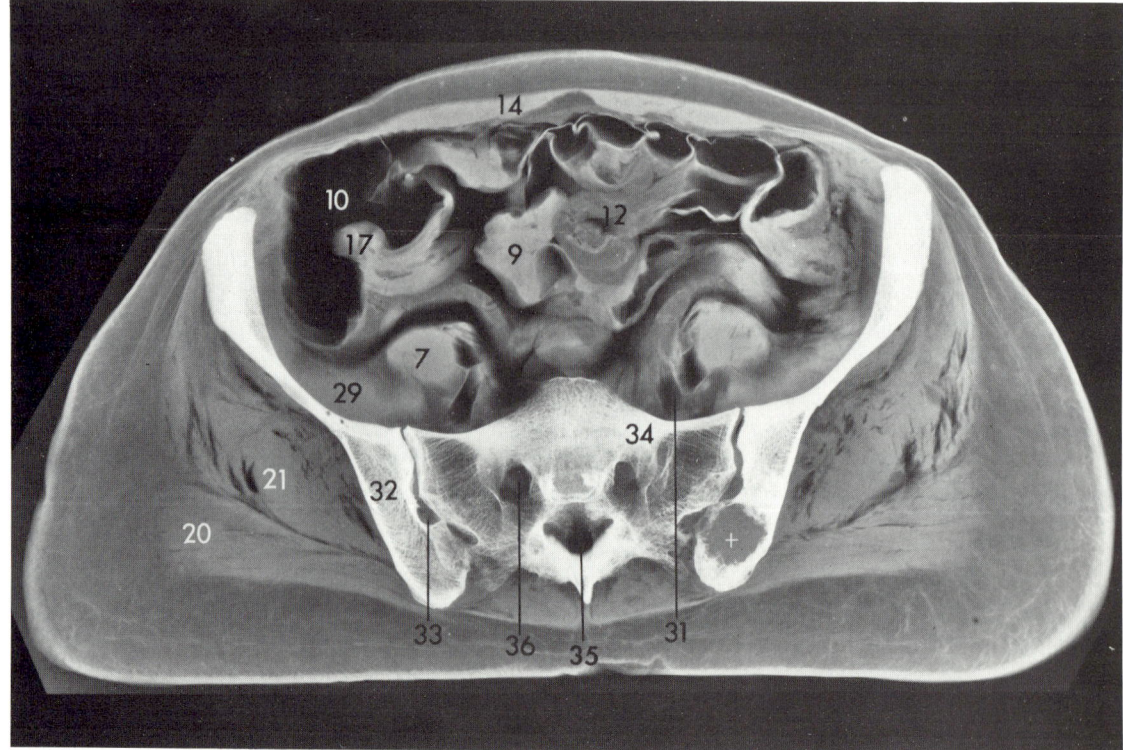

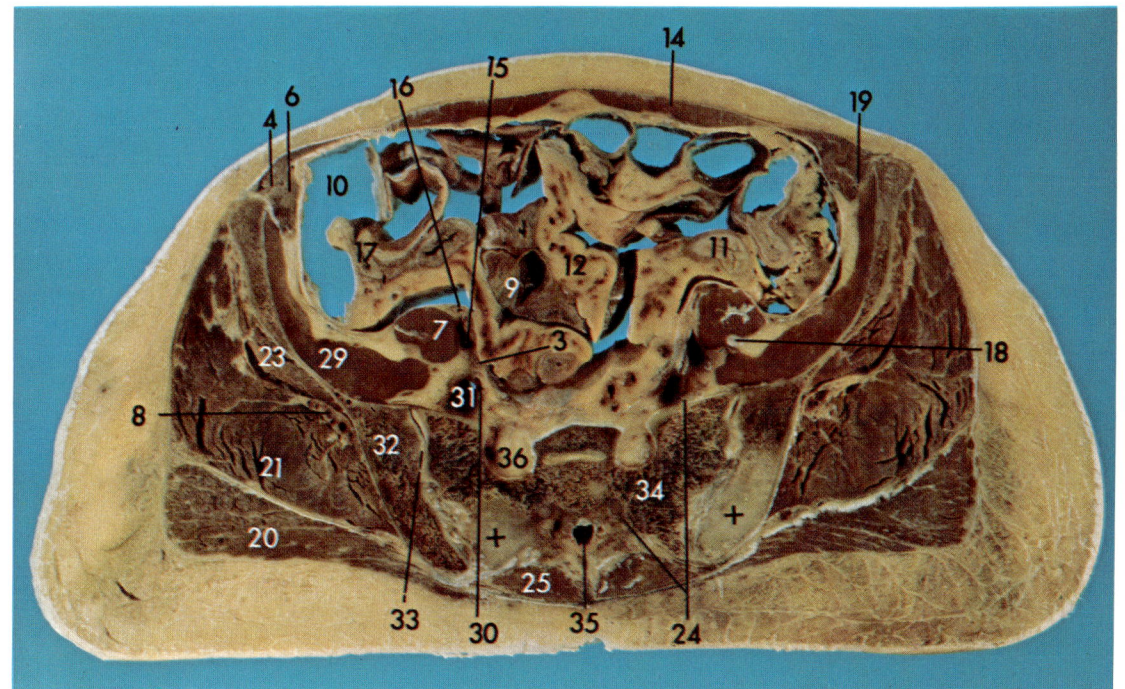

11. Descending colon
12. Mesentery of small intestine
14. Rectus abdominis muscle
15. External iliac vein
16. External iliac artery
17. Iliocecal valve
18. Femoral nerve
19. Deep circumflex iliac vessels
20. Gluteus maximus muscle
21. Gluteus medius muscle
23. Gluteus minimus muscle
24. Sacral nerve
25. Multifidus and erector spinae muscles
29. Iliacus muscle
30. Internal iliac artery
31. Internal iliac vein
32. Ilium
33. Sacroiliac joint
34. Second sacral vertebra
35. Sacral canal
36. Anterior sacral foramen
+ Metastases in left ilium and right sacral ala

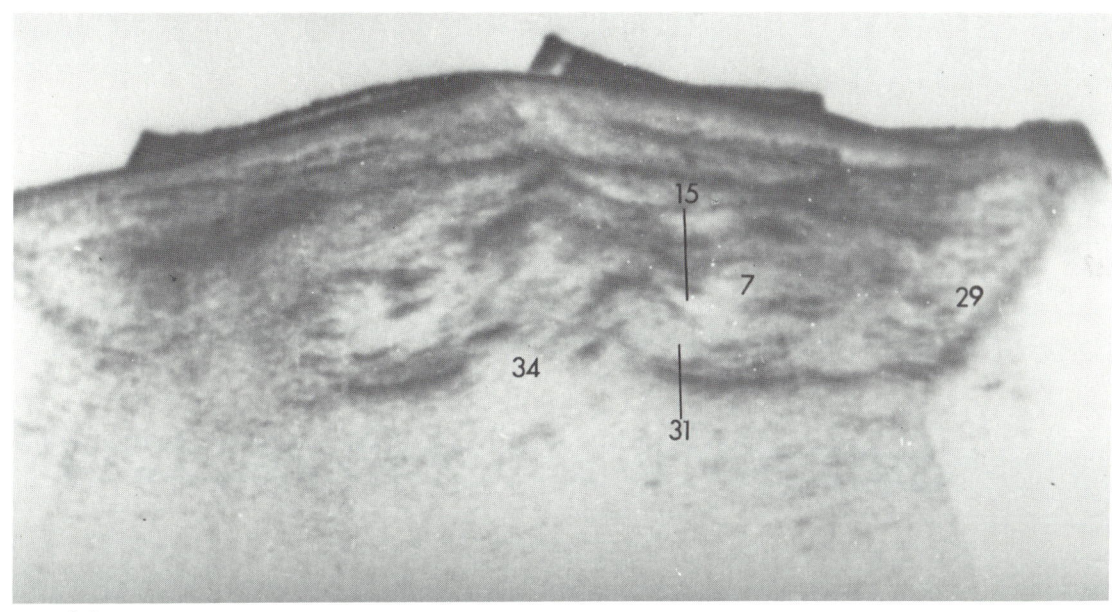

169

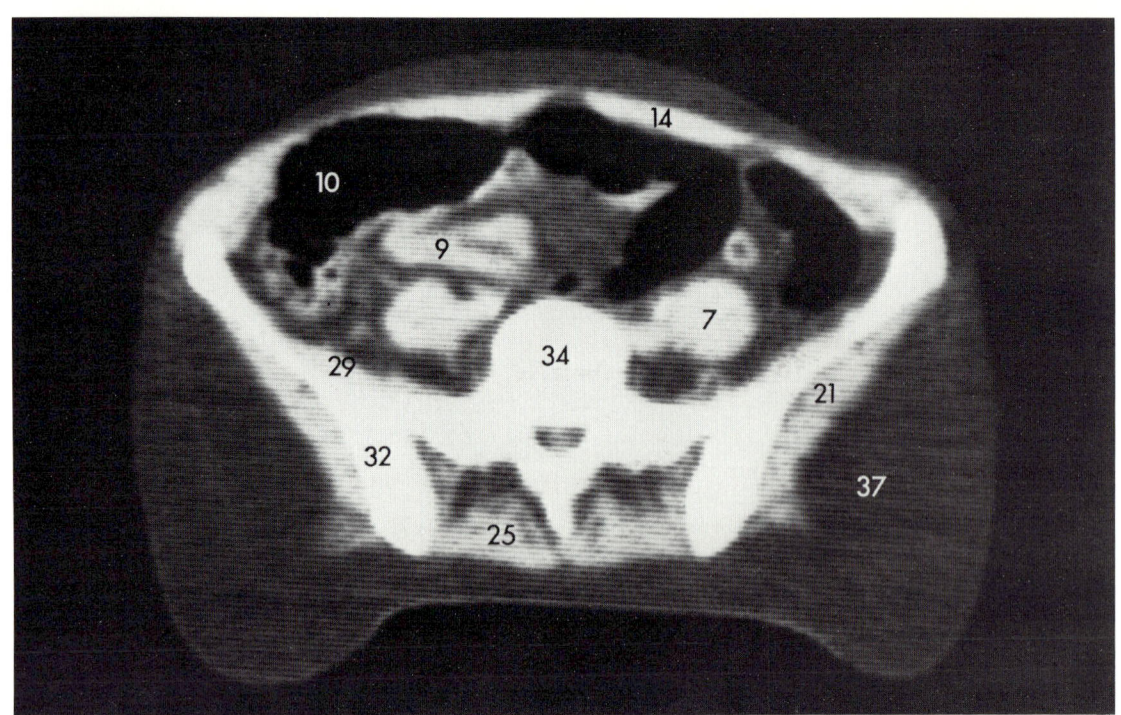

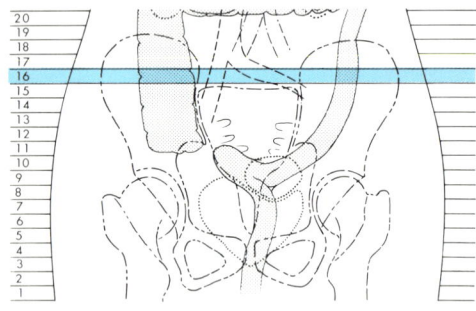

ABDOMEN AND PELVIS

Level 16

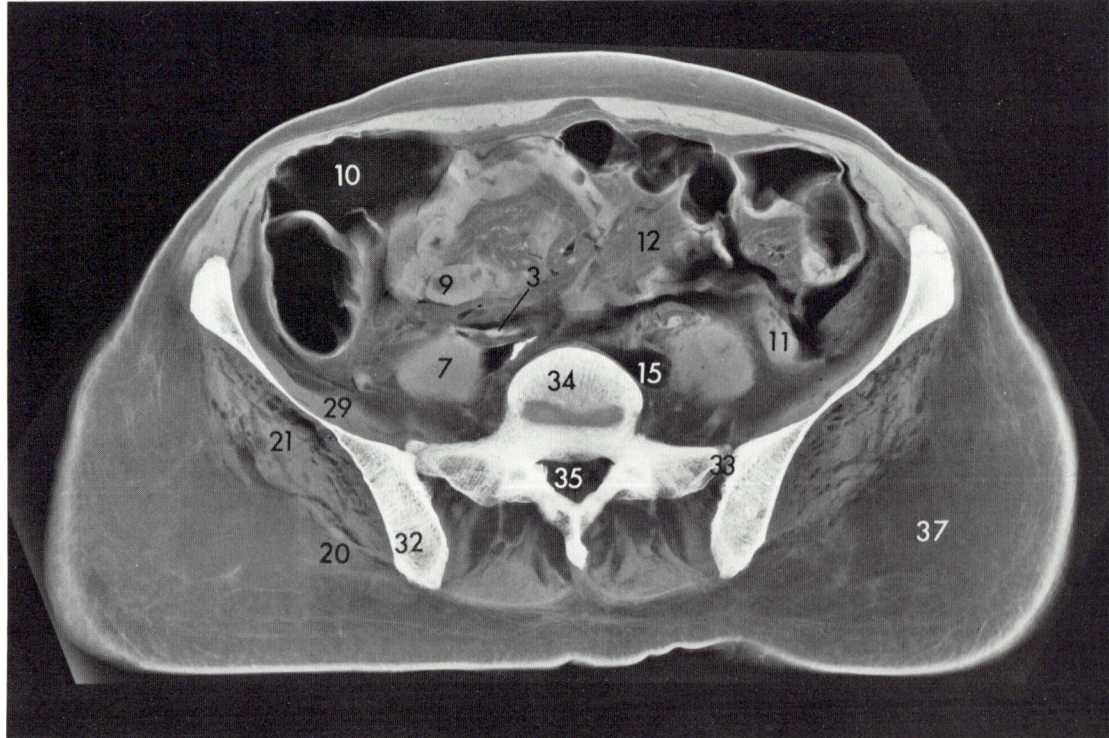

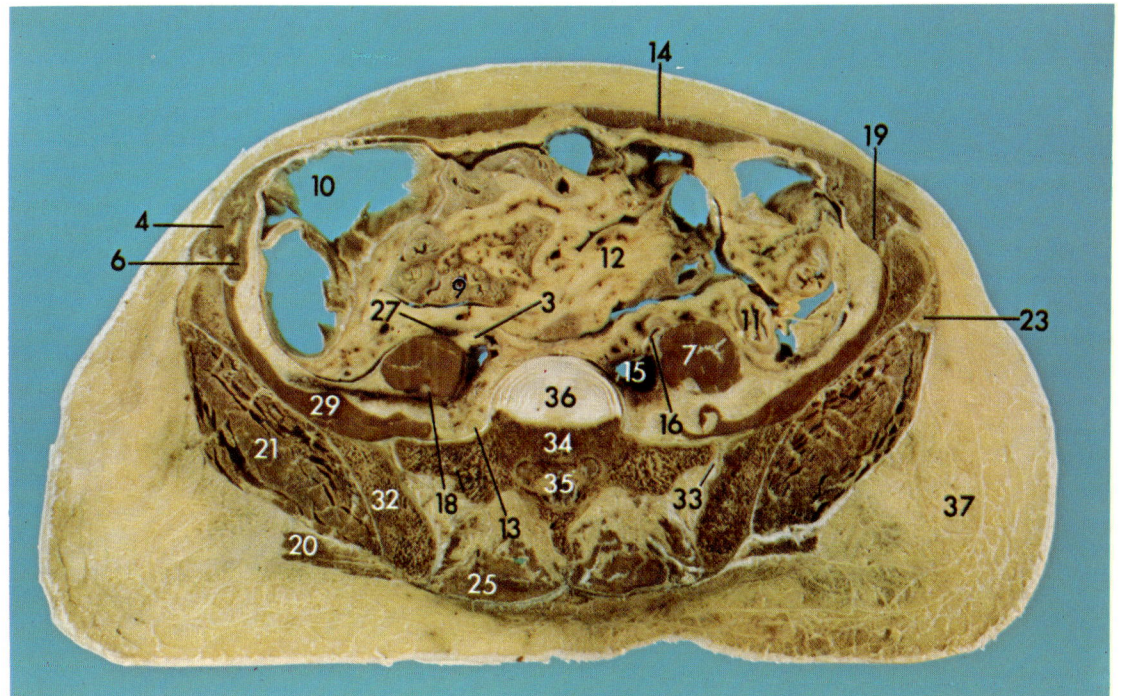

3. Ureter
4. Internal oblique muscle
6. Transversus abdominis muscle
7. Psoas muscle
8. Inferior epigastric artery
9. Small intestine
10. Ascending colon
11. Descending colon
12. Mesentery of small intestine
13. Lumbar nerve
14. Rectus abdominis muscle
15. Common iliac vein
16. Common iliac artery
18. Femoral nerve
19. Deep circumflex iliac vessels
20. Gluteus maximus muscle
21. Gluteus medius muscle
23. Gluteus minimus muscle
25. Multifidus and erector spinae muscles
27. Ovarian vessels
29. Iliacus muscle
32. Ilium
33. Sacroiliac joint
34. Body of first sacral vertebra
35. Sacral canal
36. L5–S1 intervertebral disc
37. Subcutaneous fat

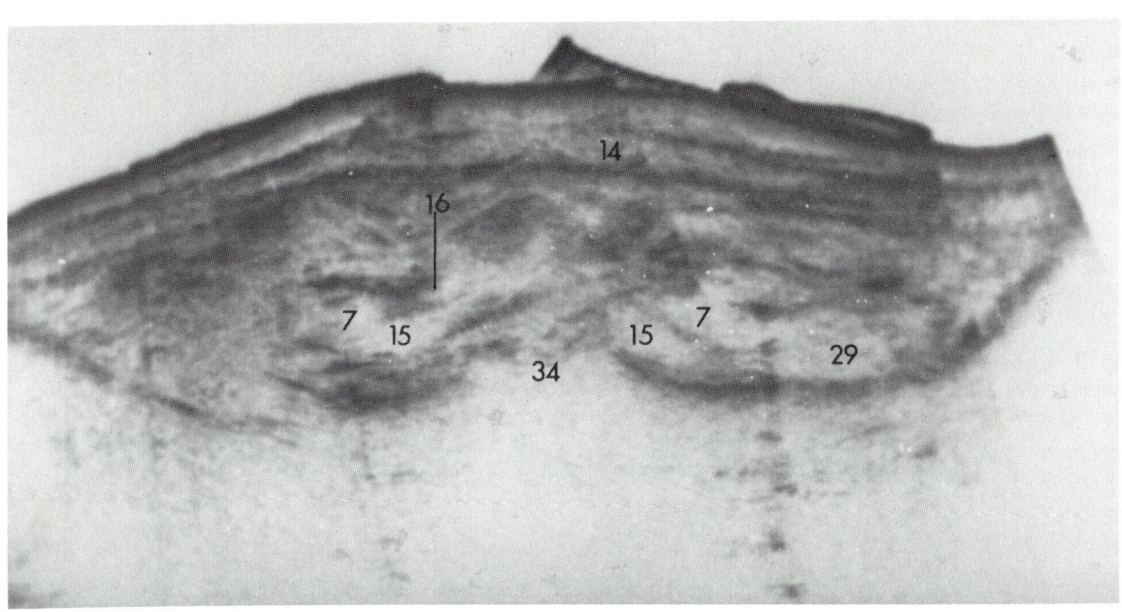

171

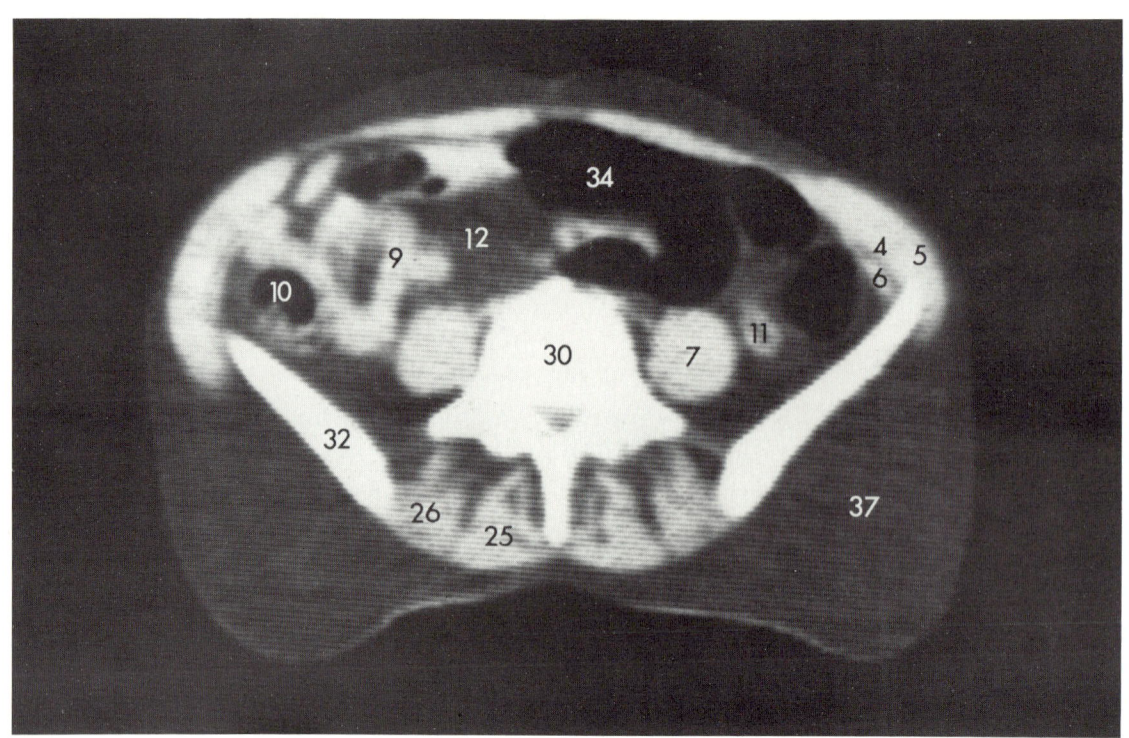

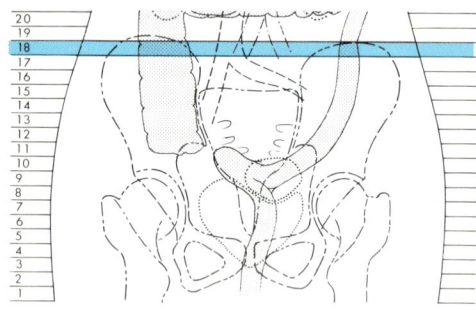

ABDOMEN AND PELVIS

Level 18

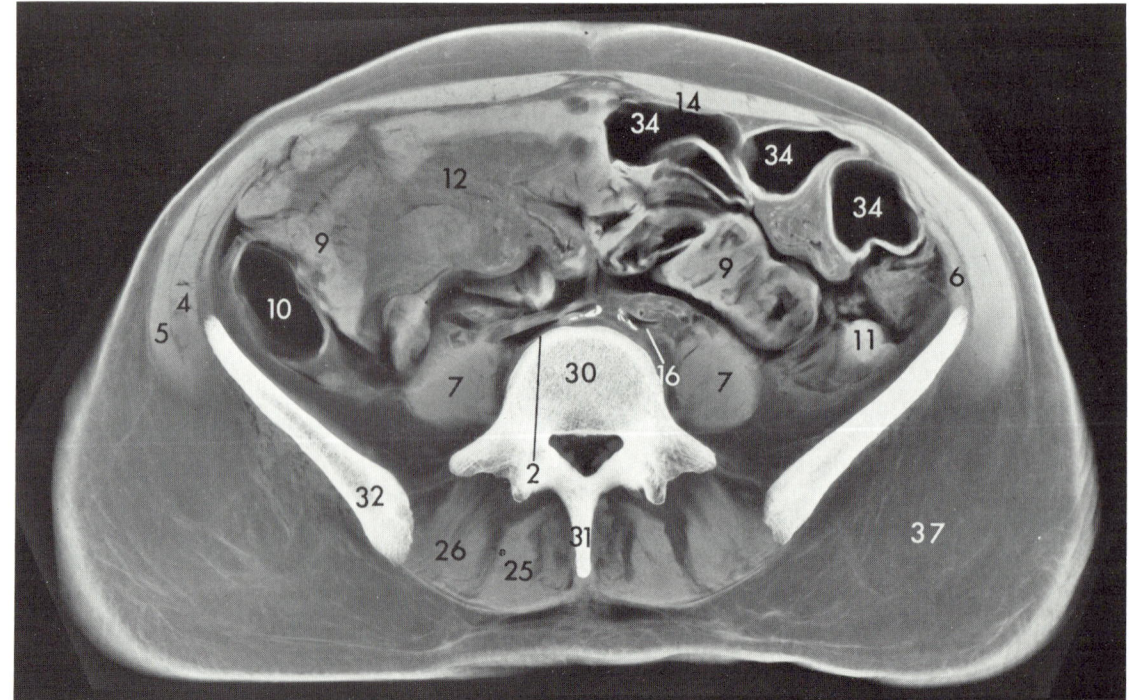

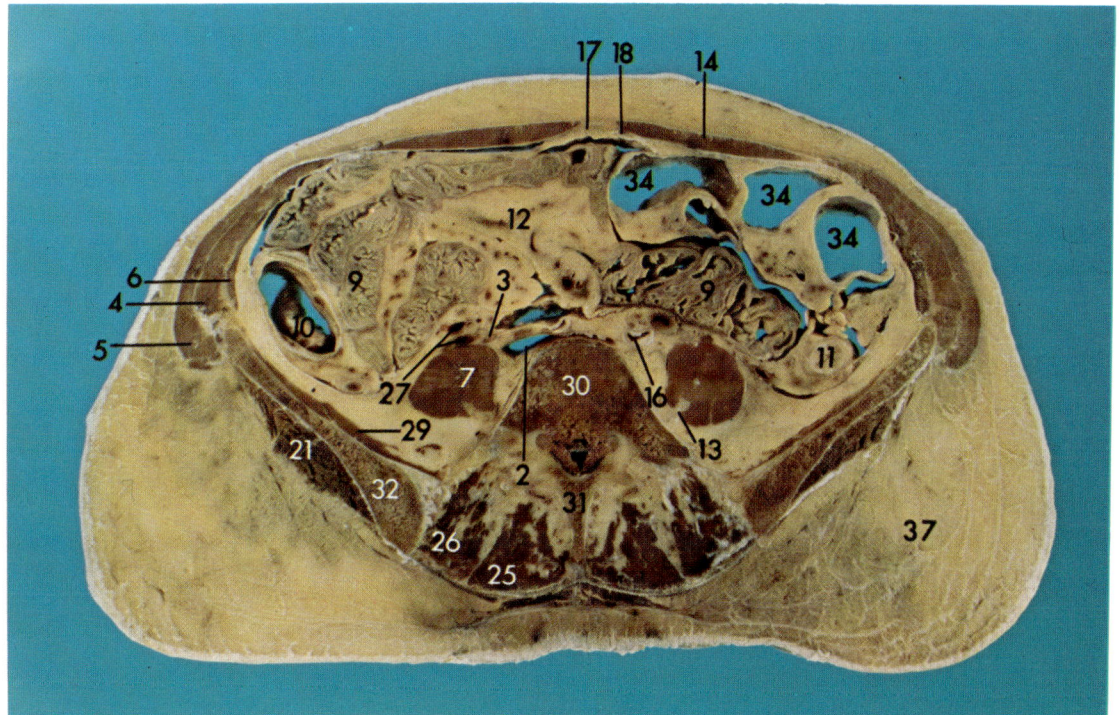

2. Inferior vena cava
3. Ureter
4. Internal oblique muscle
5. External oblique muscle
6. Transversus abdominis muscle
7. Psoas muscle
8. Inferior epigastric artery
9. Jejunum
10. Ascending colon
11. Descending colon
12. Mesentery of small intestine
13. Femoral nerve
14. Rectus abdominis muscle
16. Common iliac artery
17. Median umbilical ligament (urachus)
18. Medial umbilical ligament (umbilical artery)
21. Gluteus medius muscle
25. Multifidus muscle
26. Erector spinae muscle
27. Ovarian vessels
29. Iliacus muscle
30. Body of fifth lumbar vertebra
31. Spinous process of fourth lumbar vertebra
32. Ilium
34. Ileum
37. Subcutaneous fat

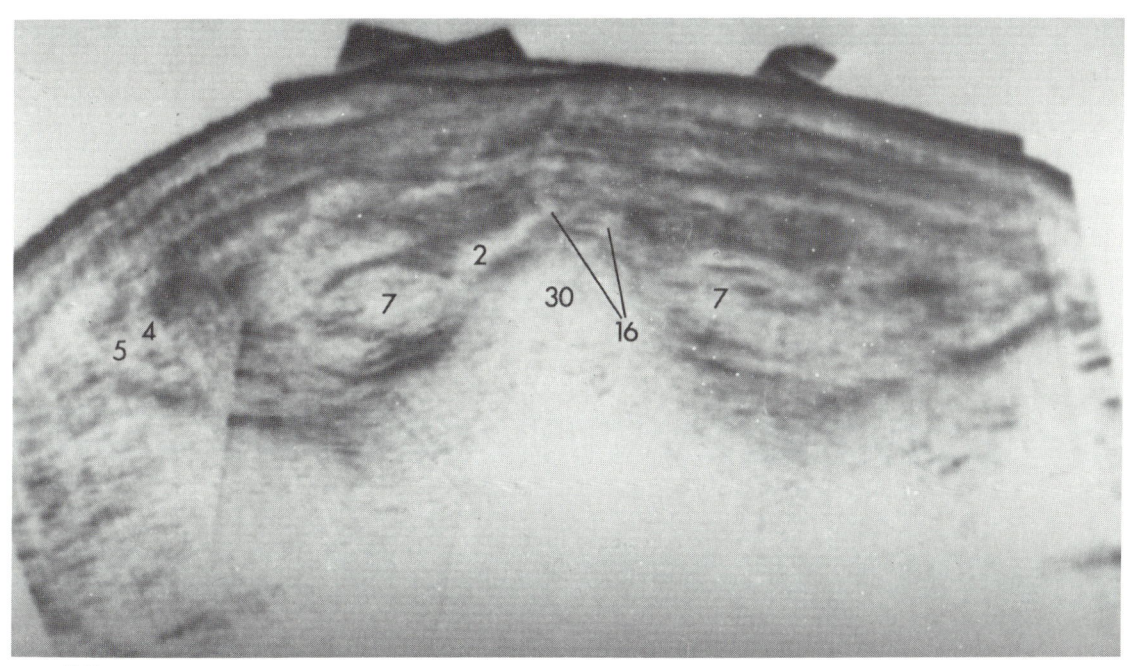

173

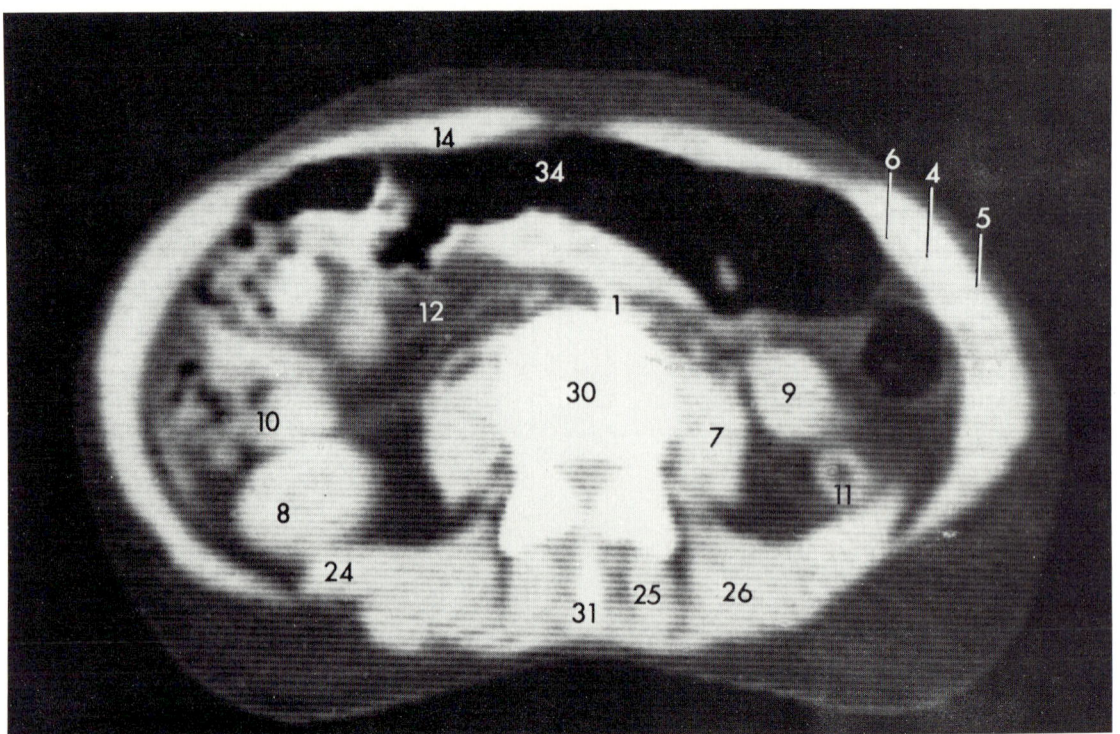

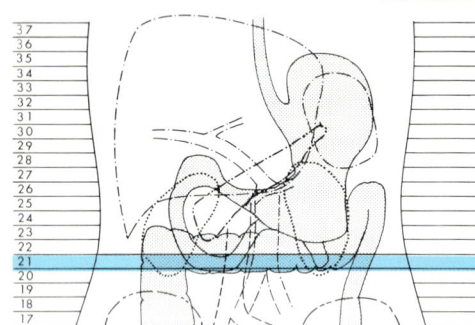

1. Aorta
2. Inferior vena cava
3. Ureter
4. Internal oblique muscle
5. External oblique muscle
6. Transversus abdominis muscle
7. Psoas muscle
8. Lower pole of kidney
9. Small intestine
10. Ascending colon

ABDOMEN AND PELVIS

Level 21

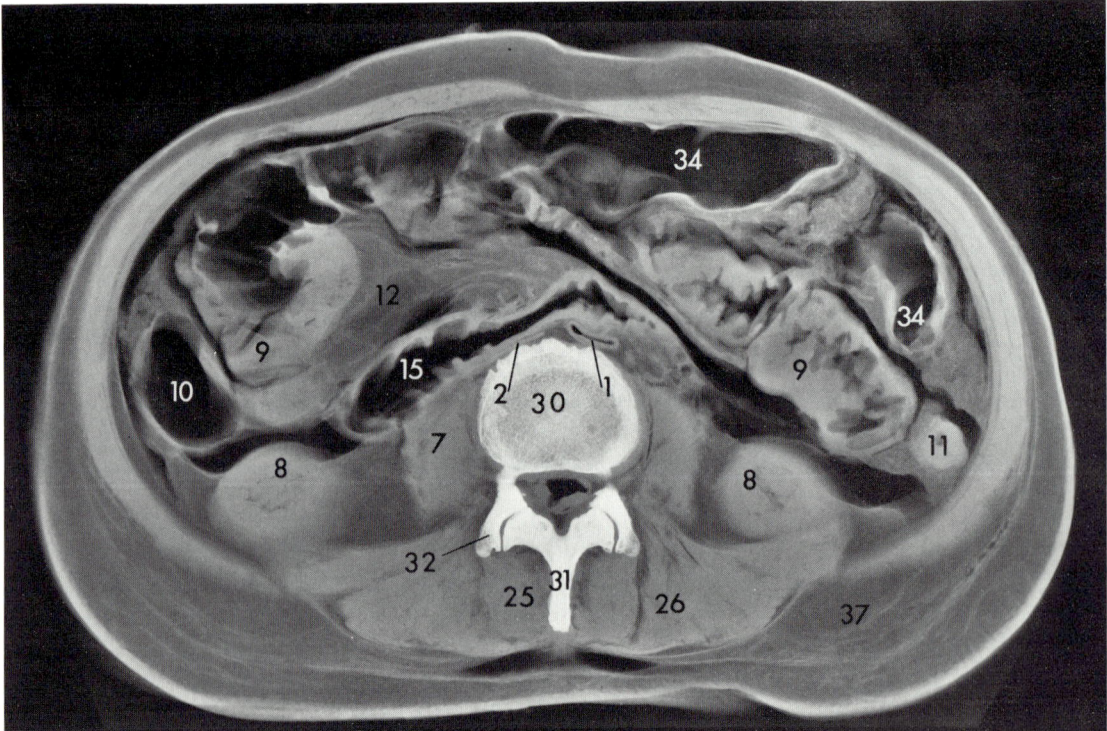

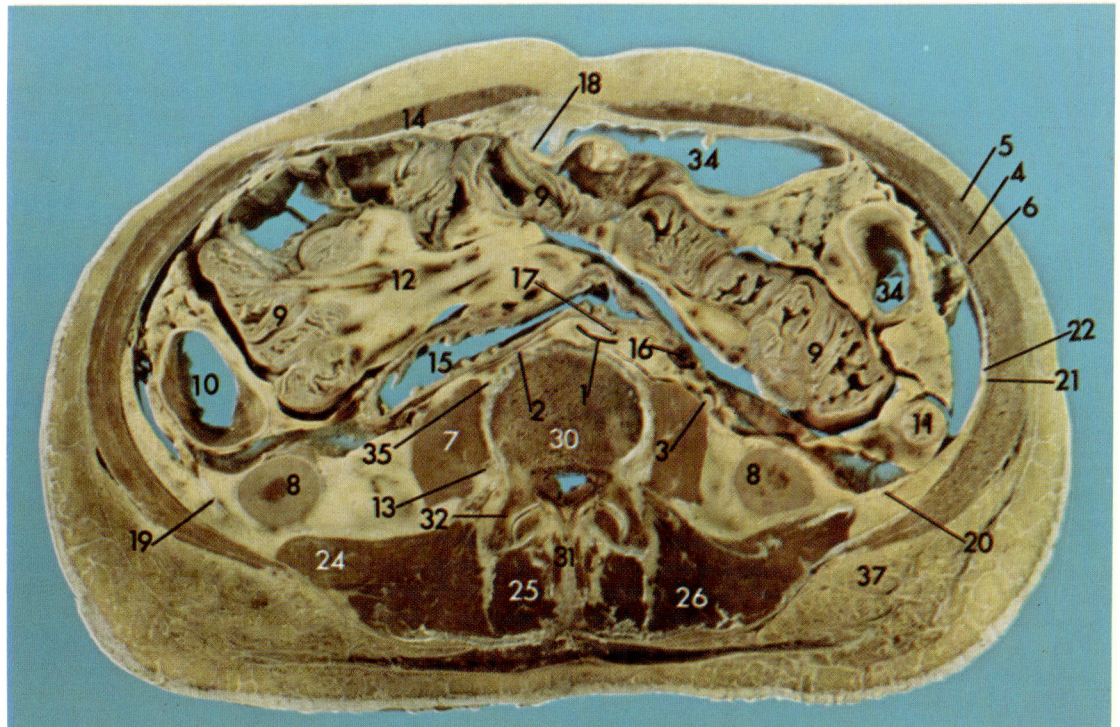

11. Descending colon
12. Mesentery of small intestine
13. Lumbar nerve
14. Rectus abdominis muscle
15. Third portion of duodenum
16. Inferior mesenteric vein
17. Inferior mesenteric artery
18. Falciform ligament
19. Renal fascia (Gerota)
20. Lateroconal fascia
21. Transversalis fascia
22. Parietal peritoneum
24. Quadratus lumborum muscle
25. Multifidus muscle
26. Erector spinae muscle
30. Body of third lumbar vertebra
31. Spinous process of second lumbar vertebra
32. Superior articular facet of third lumbar vertebra
34. Transverse colon
35. Sympathetic trunk
37. Subcutaneous fat

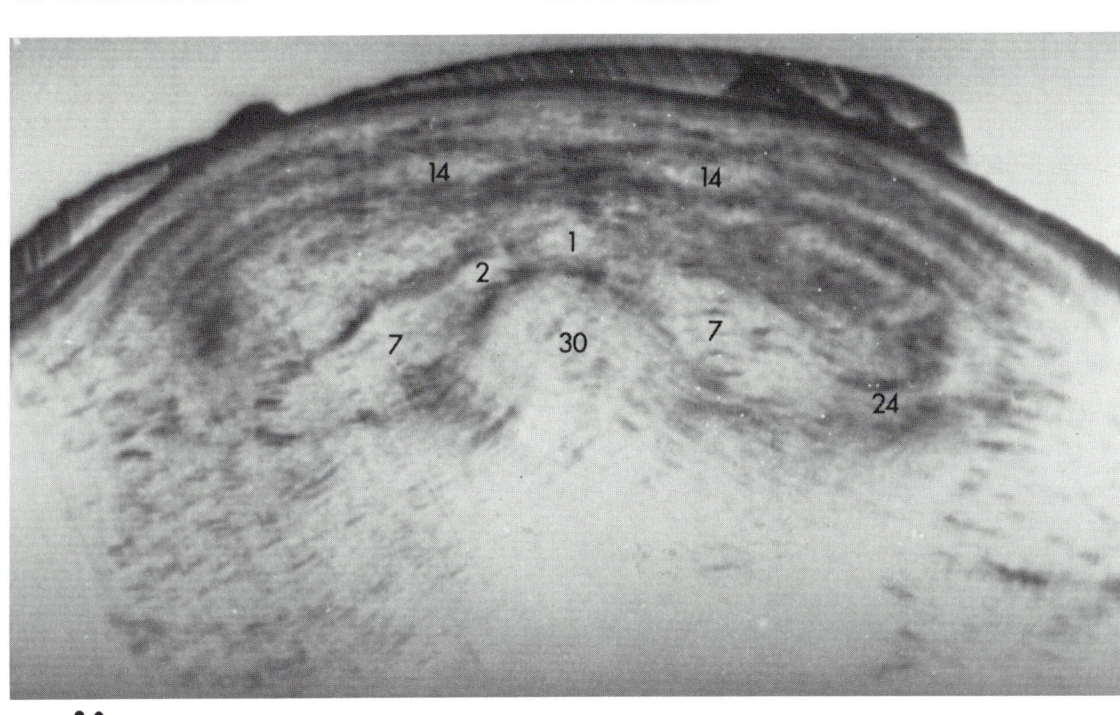

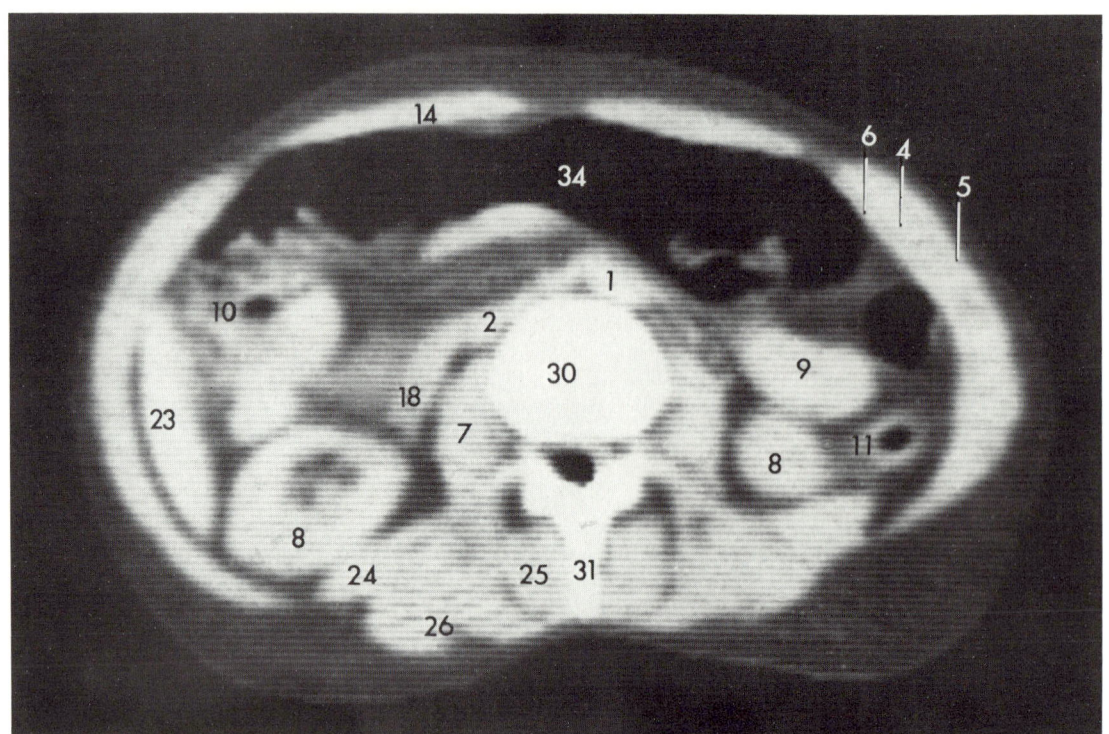

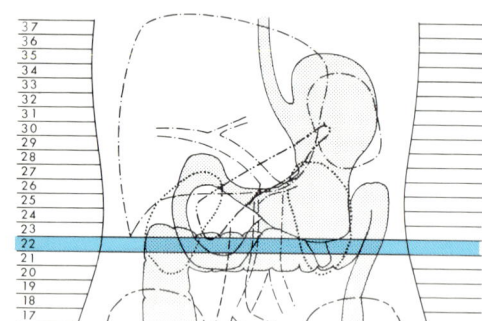

1. Aorta
2. Inferior vena cava
3. Ureter
4. Internal oblique muscle
5. External oblique muscle
6. Transversus abdominis muscle
7. Psoas muscle
8. Kidney
9. Small intestine

ABDOMEN AND PELVIS

Level 22

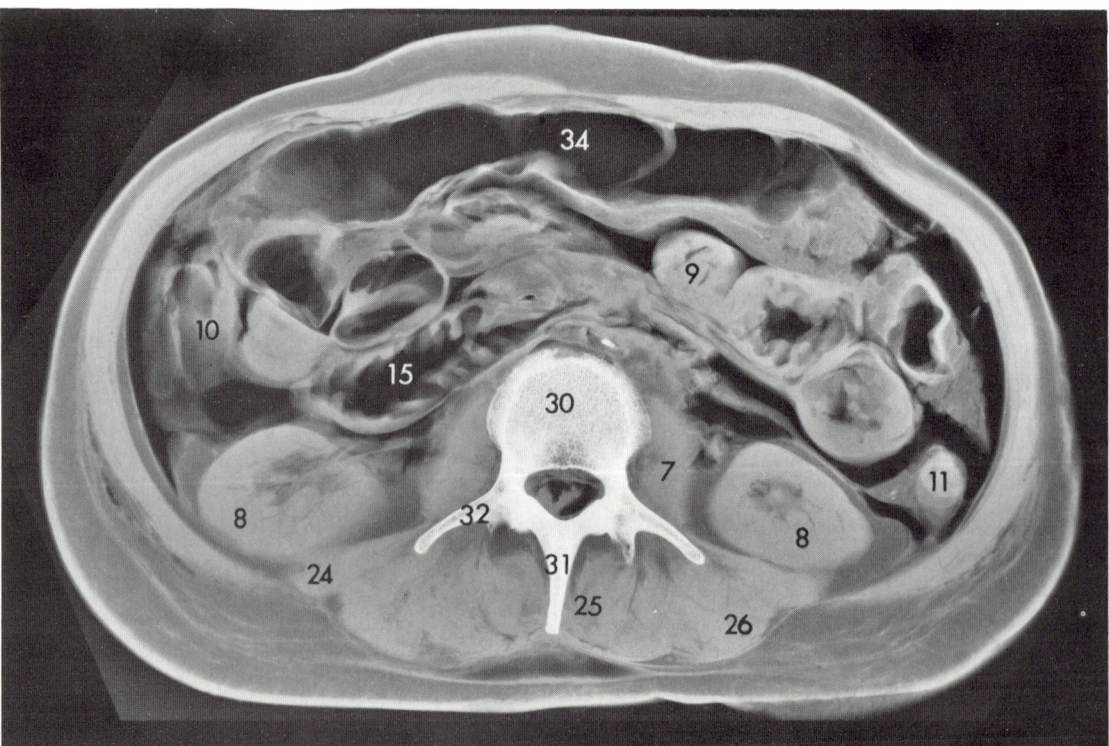

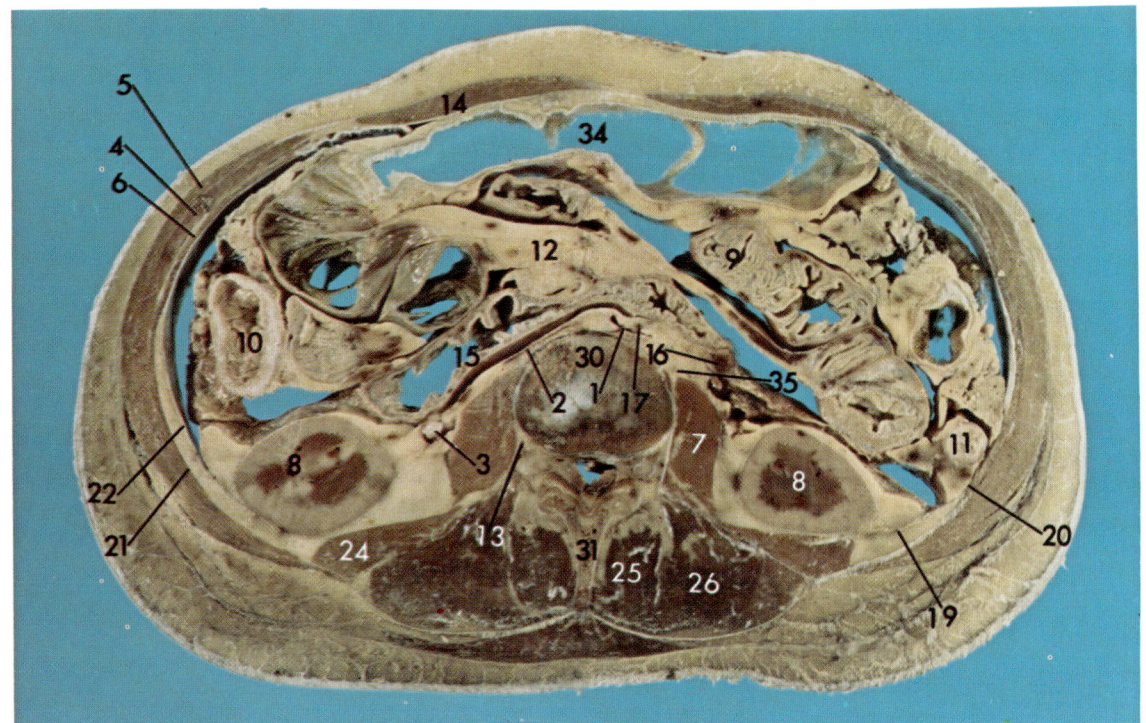

10. Ascending colon
11. Descending colon
12. Mesentery of small intestine
13. Lumbar nerve
14. Rectus abdominis muscle
15. Third portion of duodenum
16. Inferior mesenteric vein
17. Inferior mesenteric artery
18. Right renal vein
19. Renal fascia (Gerota)
20. Lateroconal fascia
21. Transversalis fascia
22. Parietal peritoneum
23. Right lobe of liver
24. Quadratus lumborum muscle
25. Multifidus muscle
26. Erector spinae muscle
30. Body of second lumbar vertebra
31. Spinous process of second lumbar vertebra
32. Transverse process of second lumbar vertebra
34. Transverse colon
35. Sympathetic trunk

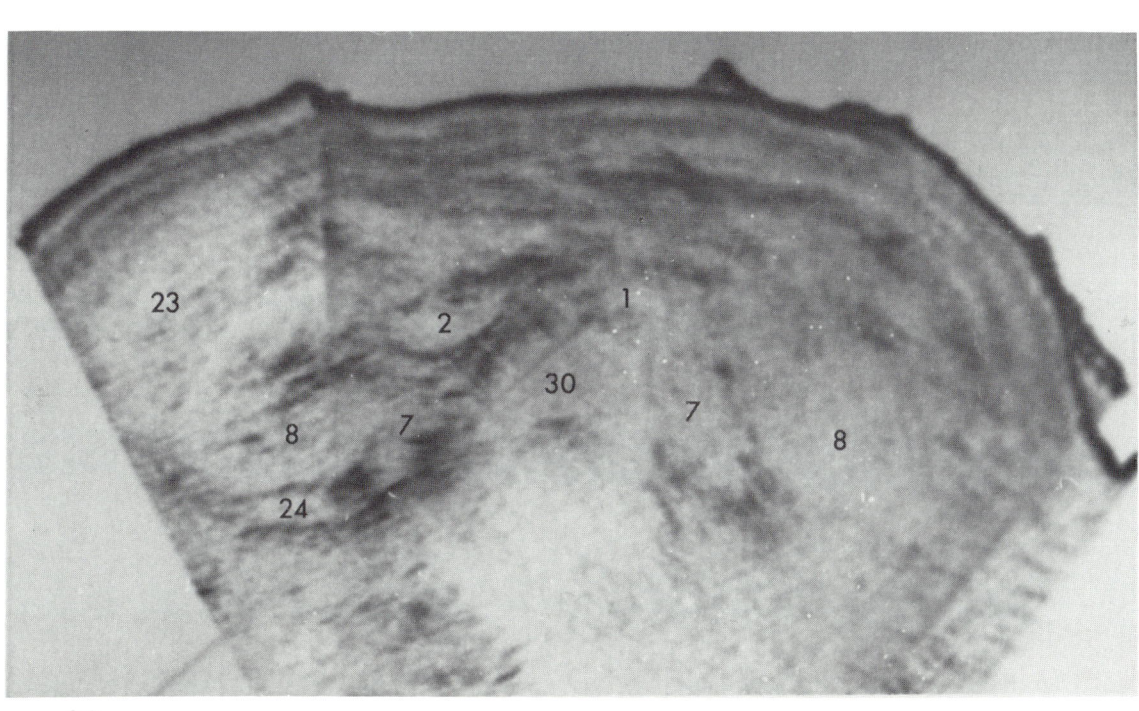

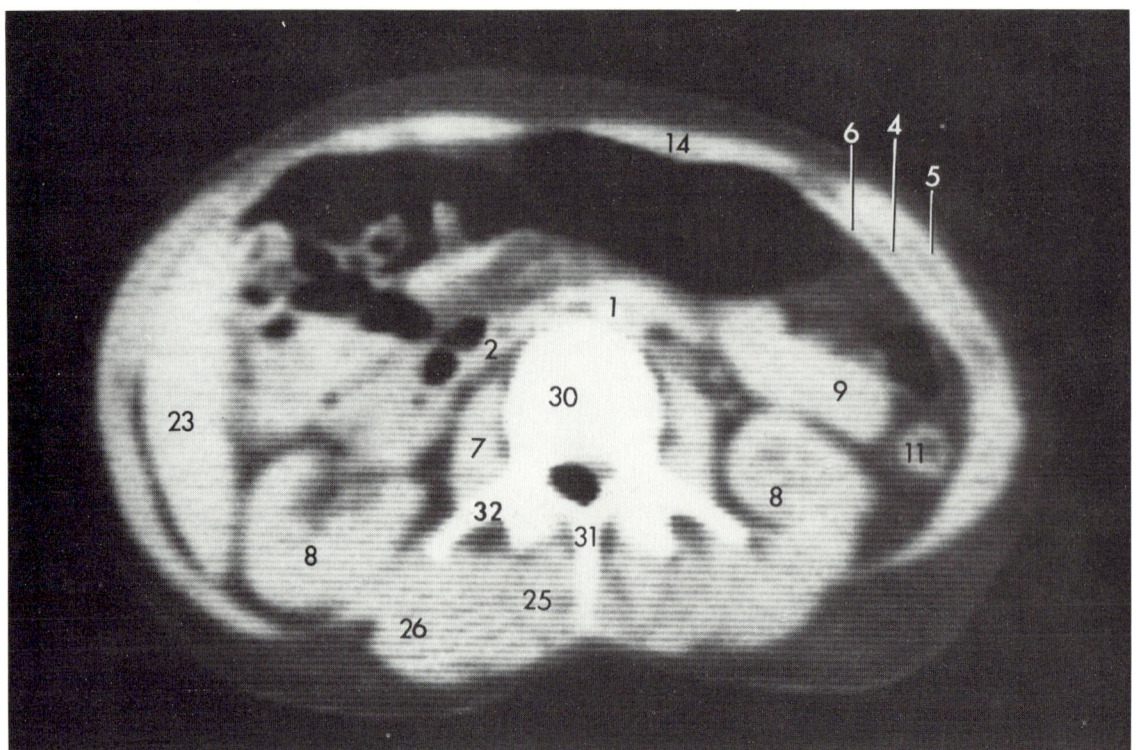

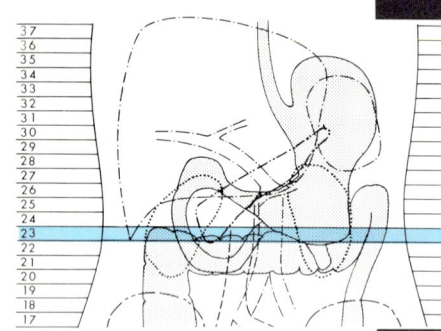

1. Aorta
2. Inferior vena cava
4. Internal oblique muscle
5. External oblique muscle
6. Transversus abdominis muscle
7. Psoas muscle
8. Kidney
9. Jejunum

10. Hepatic flexure of colon
11. Descending colon
12. Linea alba
13. Renal pelvis
14. Rectus abdominis muscle
15. Junction of second and third portions of duodenum
16. Inferior mesenteric vein

ABDOMEN AND PELVIS

Level 23

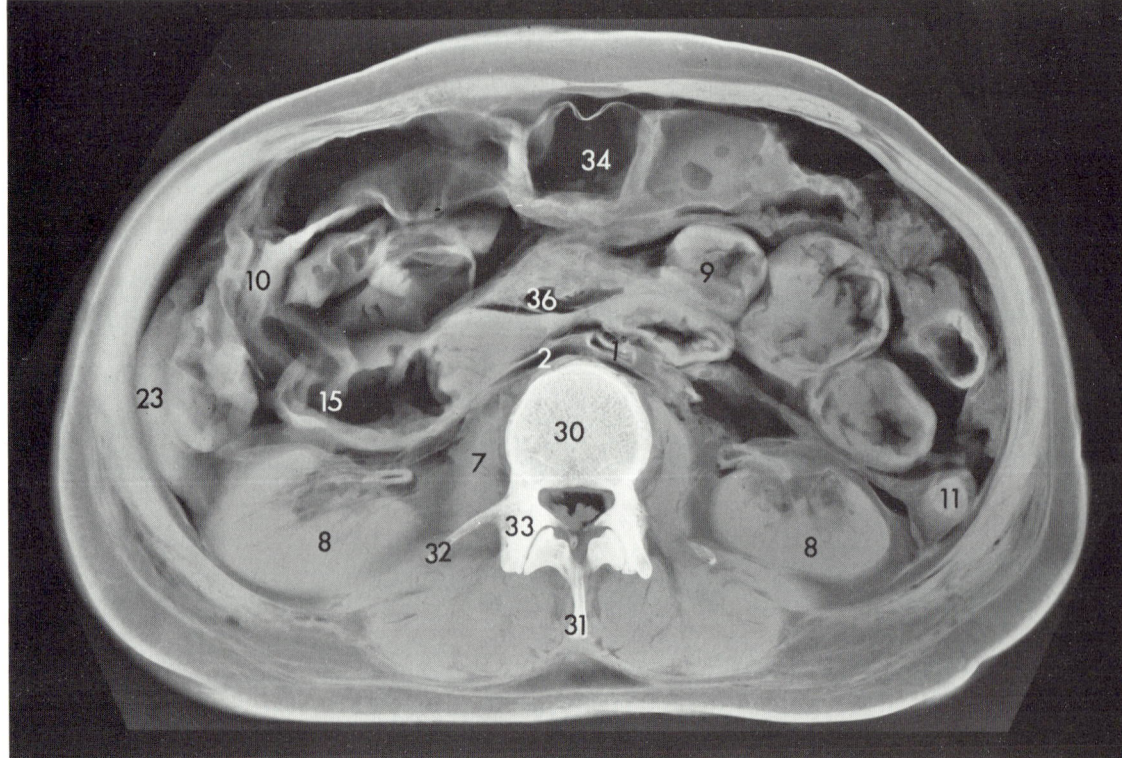

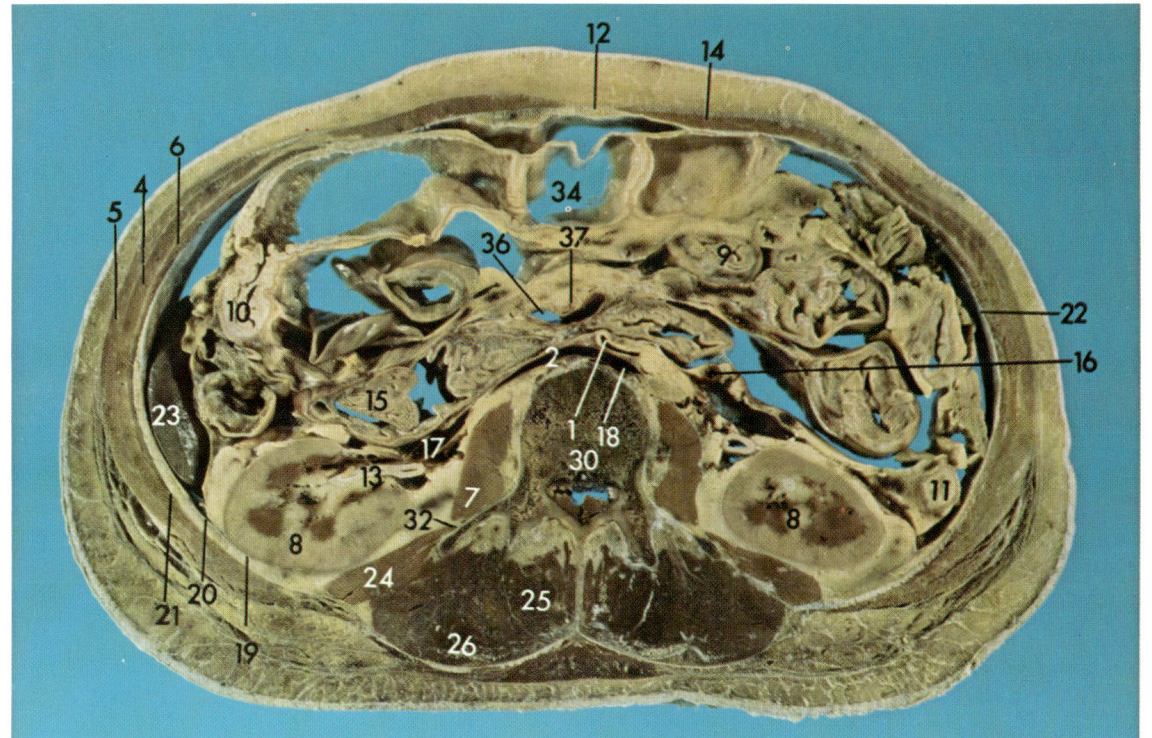

17. Right renal vein
18. Left renal vein (anomalous course posterior to aorta)†
19. Renal fascia (Gerota)
20. Lateroconal fascia
21. Transversalis fascia
22. Parietal peritoneum
23. Right lobe of liver
24. Quadratus lumborum muscle
25. Multifidus muscle
26. Erector spinae muscle
30. Body of second lumbar vertebra
31. Spinous process of first lumbar vertebra
32. Transverse process of second lumbar vertebra
33. Superior articular facet of second lumbar vertebra
34. Transverse colon
36. Superior mesenteric vein
37. Superior mesenteric artery

†The usual relationship of the left renal vein to the aorta is shown on Level 25A.

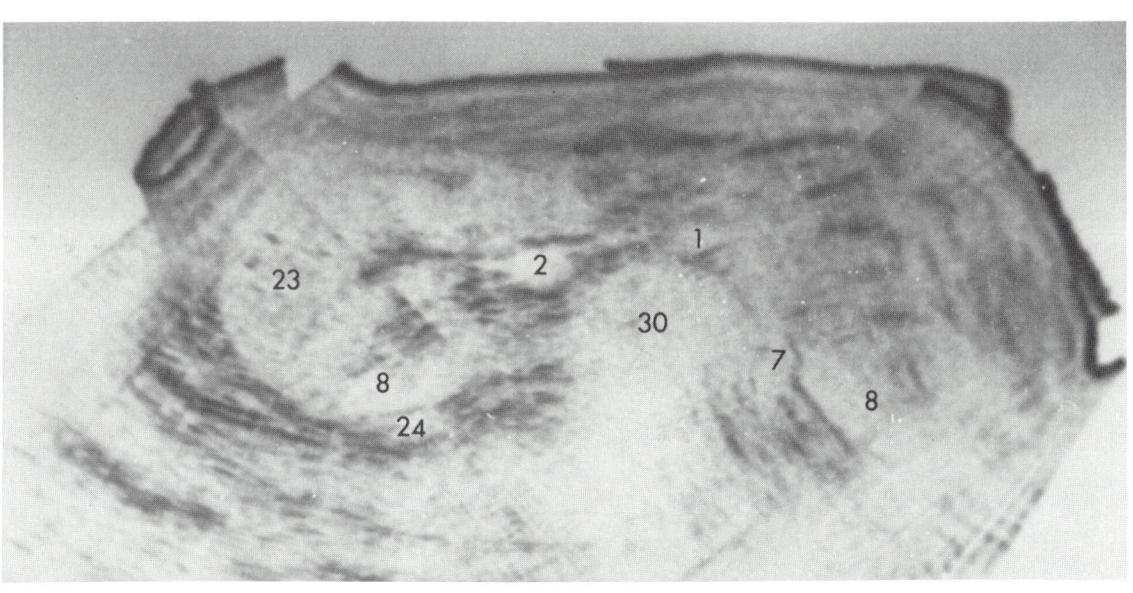

179

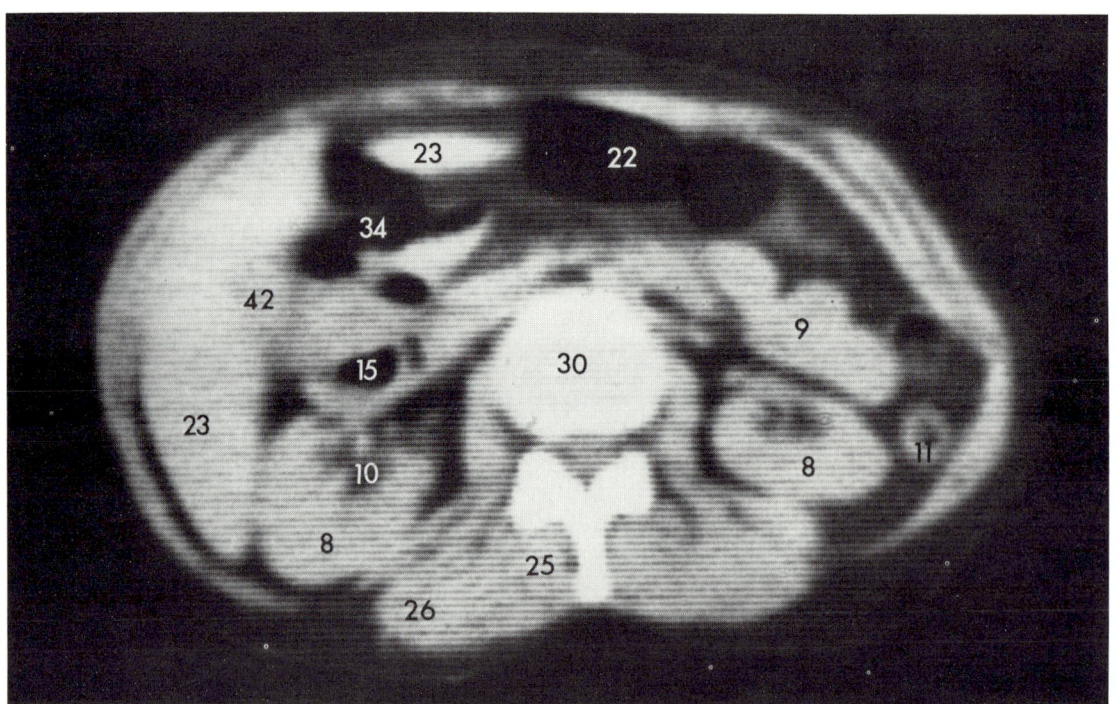

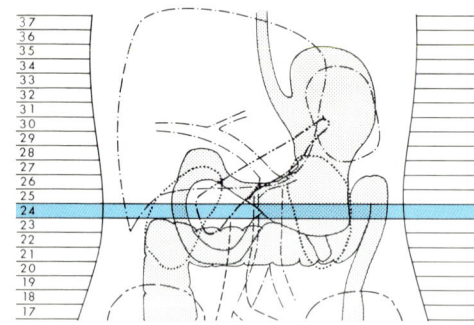

1. Aorta
2. Inferior vena cava
4. Internal oblique muscle
5. External oblique muscle
6. Transversus abdominis muscle
7. Psoas muscle
8. Kidney
9. Jejunum
10. Hepatic flexure of colon
11. Descending colon
12. Transverse mesocolon
13. Renal pelvis
14. Rectus abdominis muscle
15. Second portion of duodenum
16. Inferior mesenteric vein
17. Renal vein†
18. Renal artery
19. Renal fascia (Gerota)

ABDOMEN AND PELVIS

Level 24

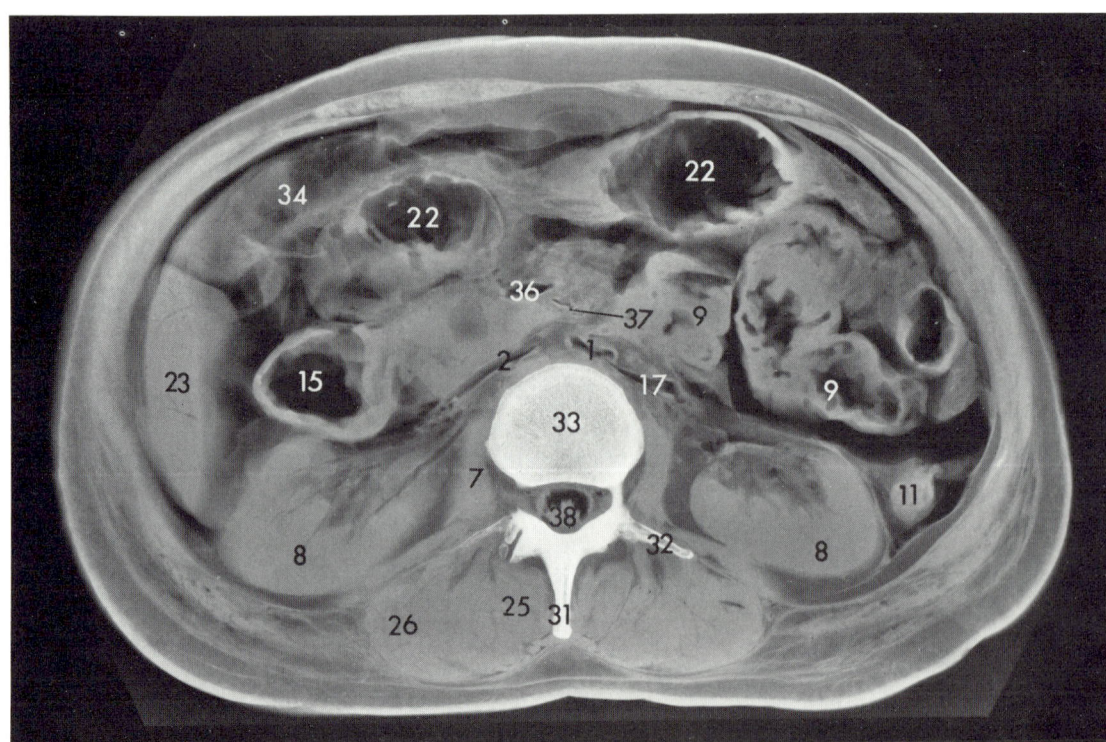

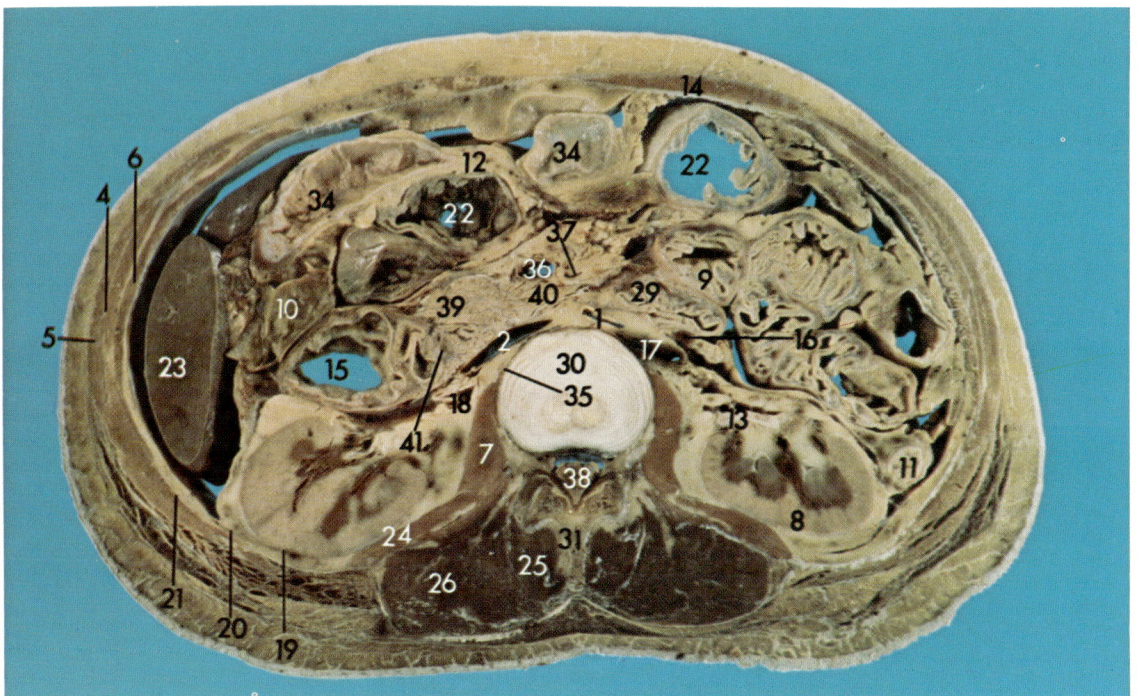

20. Lateroconal fascia
21. Transversalis fascia
22. Stomach
23. Right lobe of liver
24. Quadratus lumborum muscle
25. Multifidus muscle
26. Erector spinae muscle
29. Fourth portion of duodenum
30. L1–2 intervertebral disc
31. Spinous process of first lumbar vertebra
32. Transverse process of first lumbar vertebra
33. Body of first lumbar vertebra
34. Transverse colon
35. Sympathetic trunk
36. Superior mesenteric vein
37. Superior mesenteric artery
38. Cauda equina
39. Head of pancreas
40. Uncinate process of pancreas
42. Gall bladder

†The left renal vein in this cadaver follows an anomalous course posterior to the aorta. The usual relationship of the left renal vein to the aorta is shown on Level 25A.

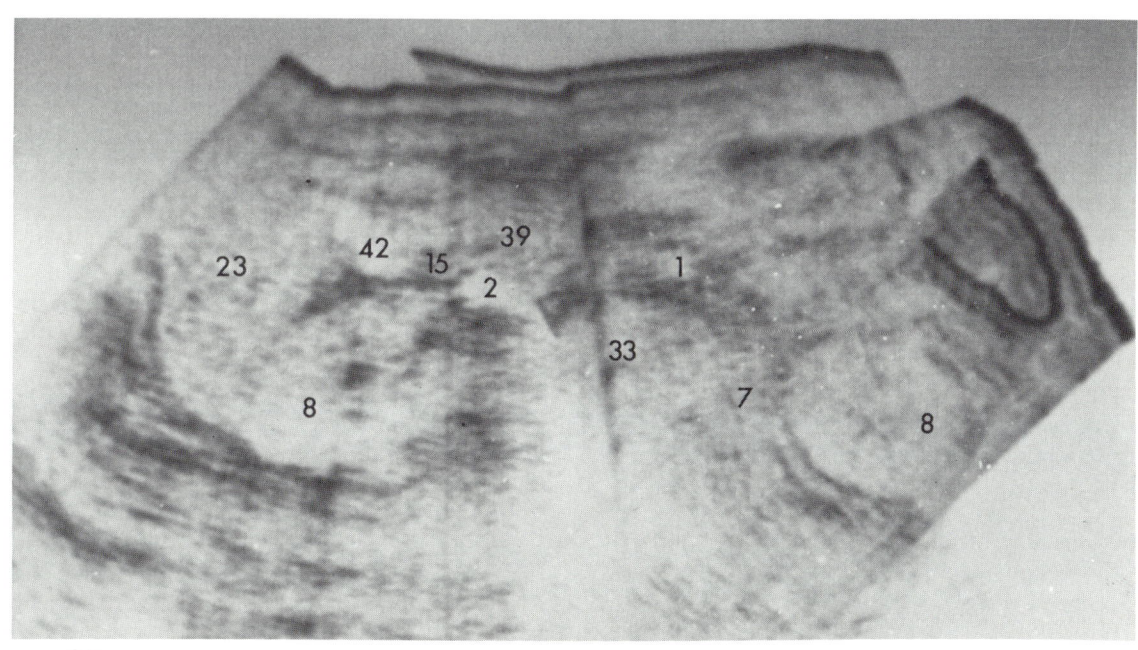

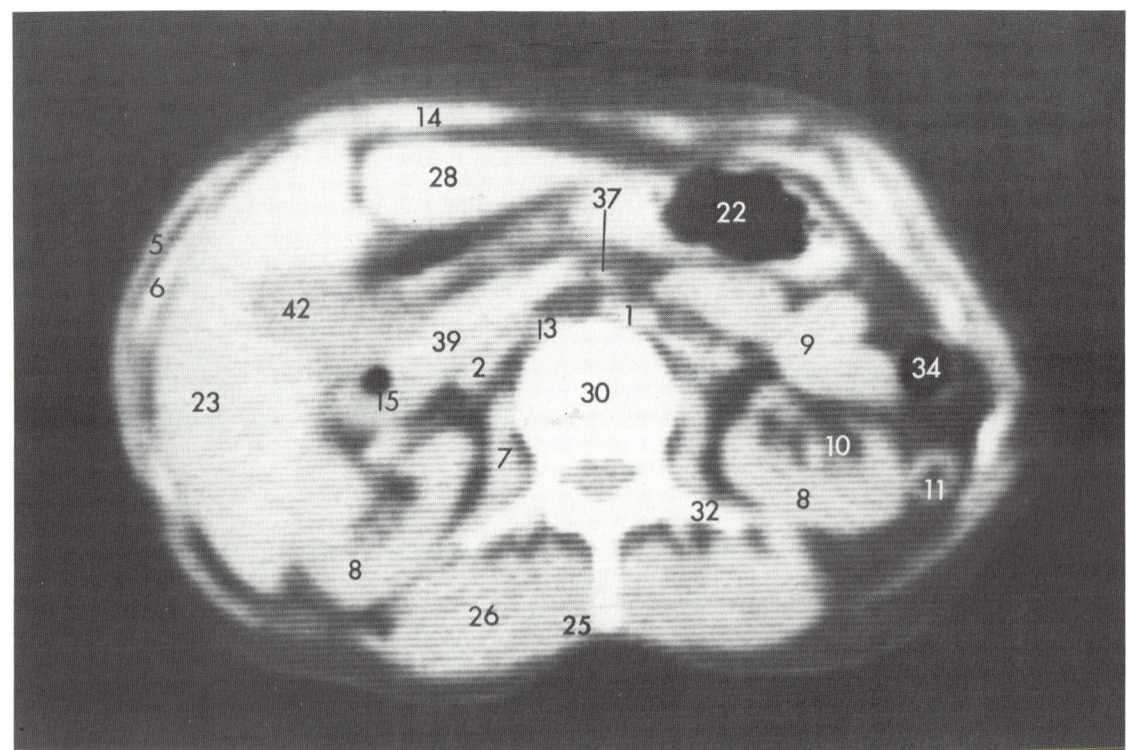

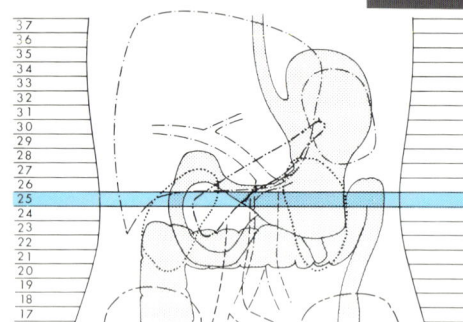

1. Aorta
2. Inferior vena cava
4. Internal oblique muscle
5. External oblique muscle
6. Transversus abdominis muscle
7. Psoas muscle
8. Kidney
9. Jejunum
10. Fat in renal sinus
11. Descending colon
12. Linea alba
13. Right crus of diaphragm
14. Rectus abdominis muscle
15. Second portion of duodenum
16. Inferior mesenteric vein
17. Left renal vein (anomalous course posterior to aorta)†
18. Renal artery
19. Renal fascia (Gerota)
20. Renal pelvis

ABDOMEN AND PELVIS

Level 25

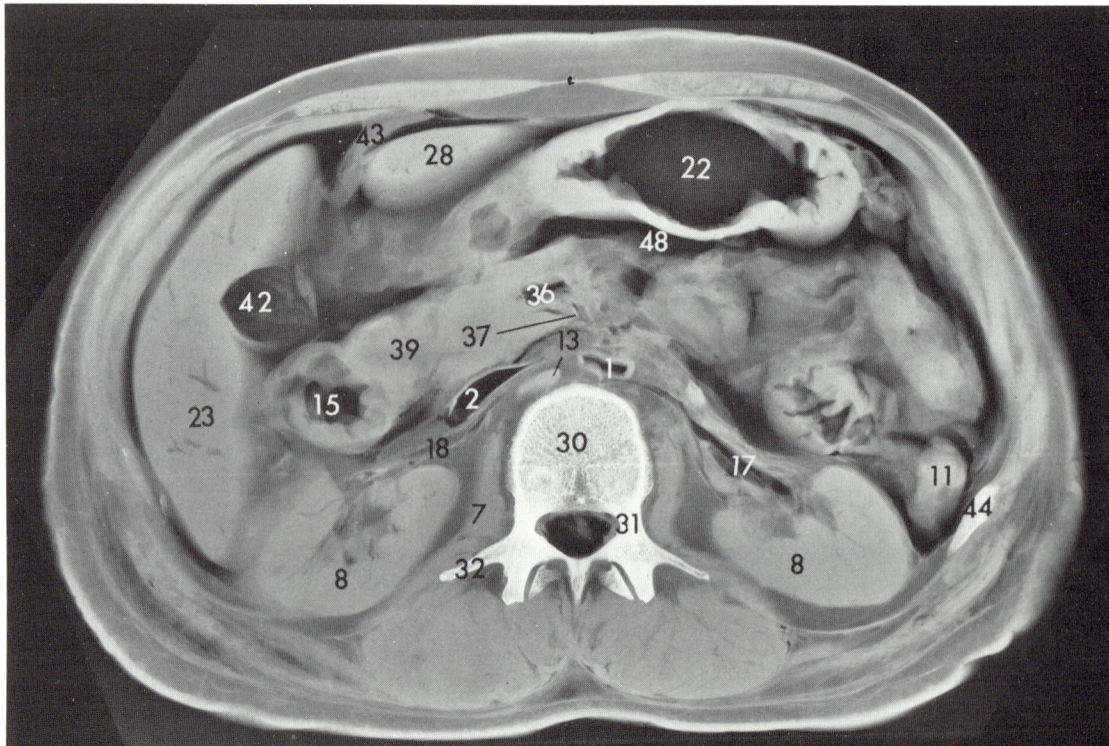

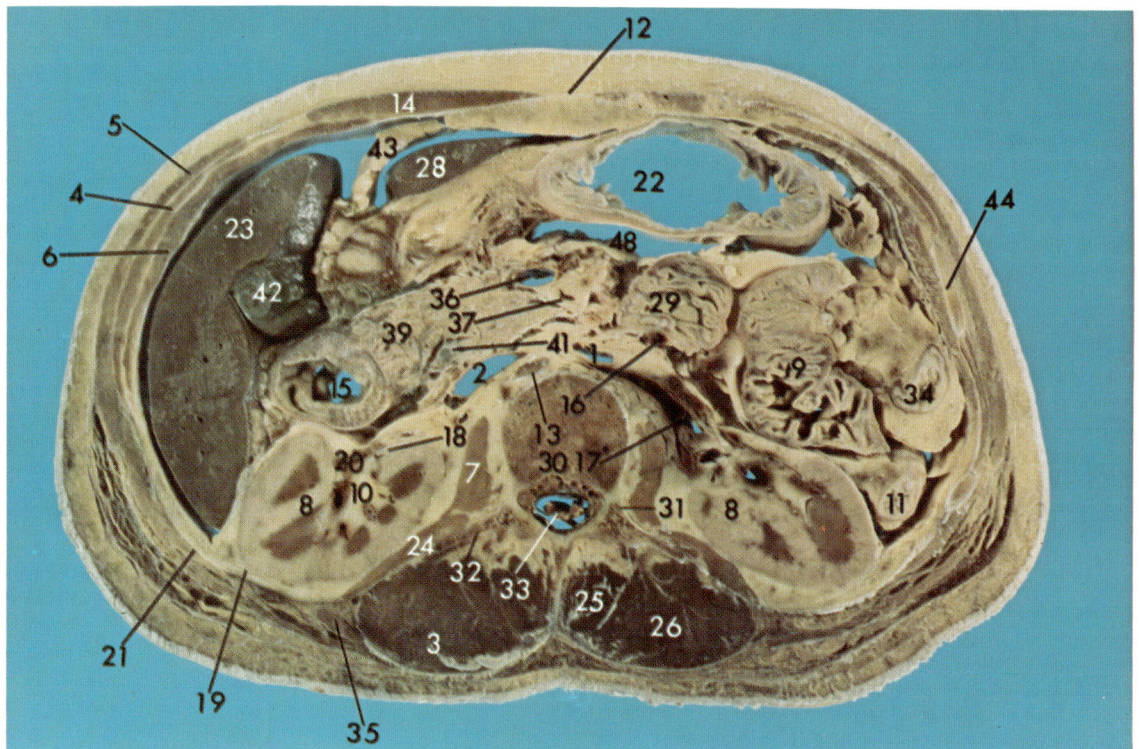

21. Transversalis fascia
22. Stomach
23. Right lobe of liver
24. Quadratus lumborum muscle
25. Multifidus muscle
26. Erector spinae muscle
28. Left lobe of liver
29. Fourth portion of duodenum
30. Body of first lumbar vertebra
31. Pedicle of first lumbar vertebra
32. Transverse process of first lumbar vertebra
33. Conus medullaris of spinal cord
34. Transverse colon
35. Latissimus dorsi muscle
36. Superior mesenteric vein
37. Superior mesenteric artery
39. Head of pancreas
40. Body of pancreas
41. Common bile duct
42. Gall bladder
43. Falciform ligament
44. Rib
48. Lesser peritoneal sac

†The usual relationship of the left renal vein to the aorta is shown on Level 25A.

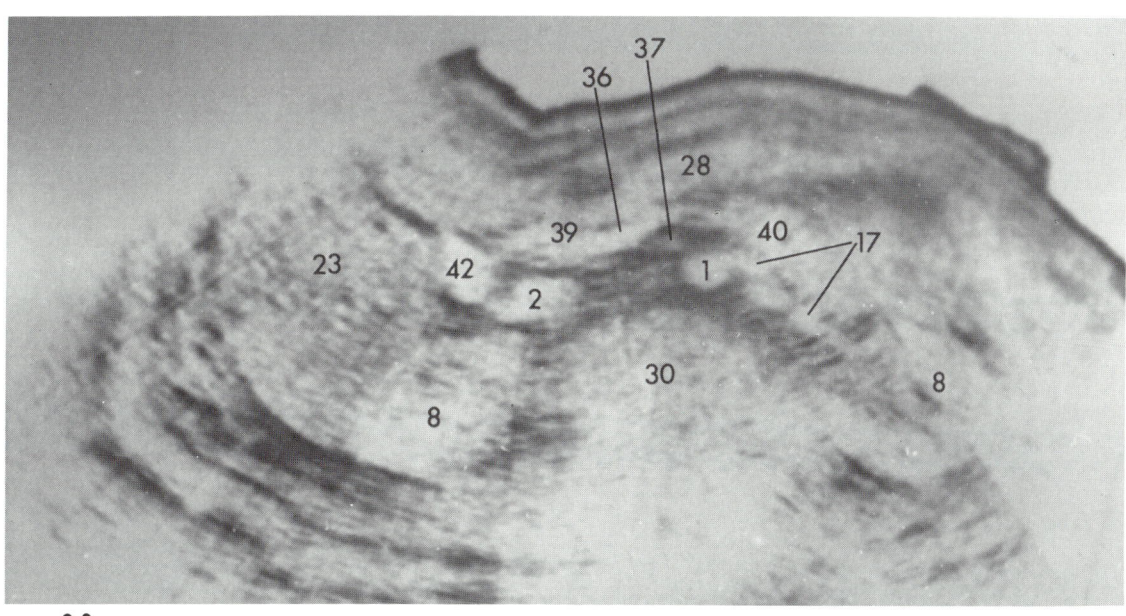

183

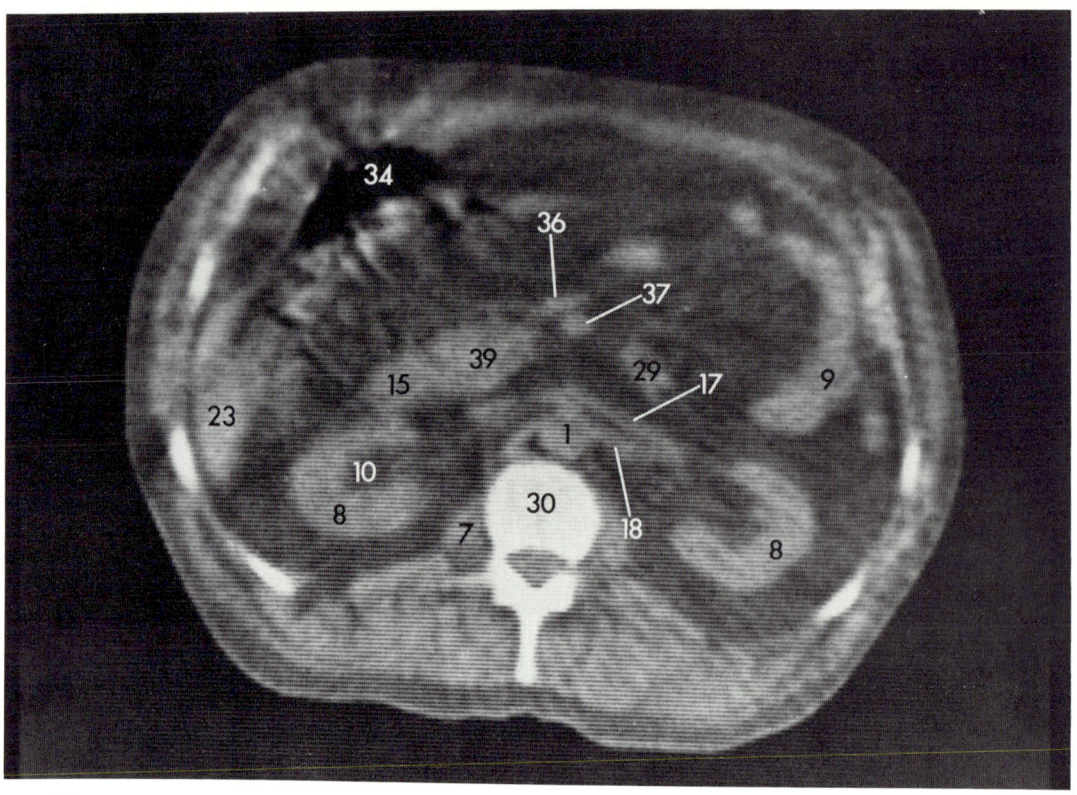

*

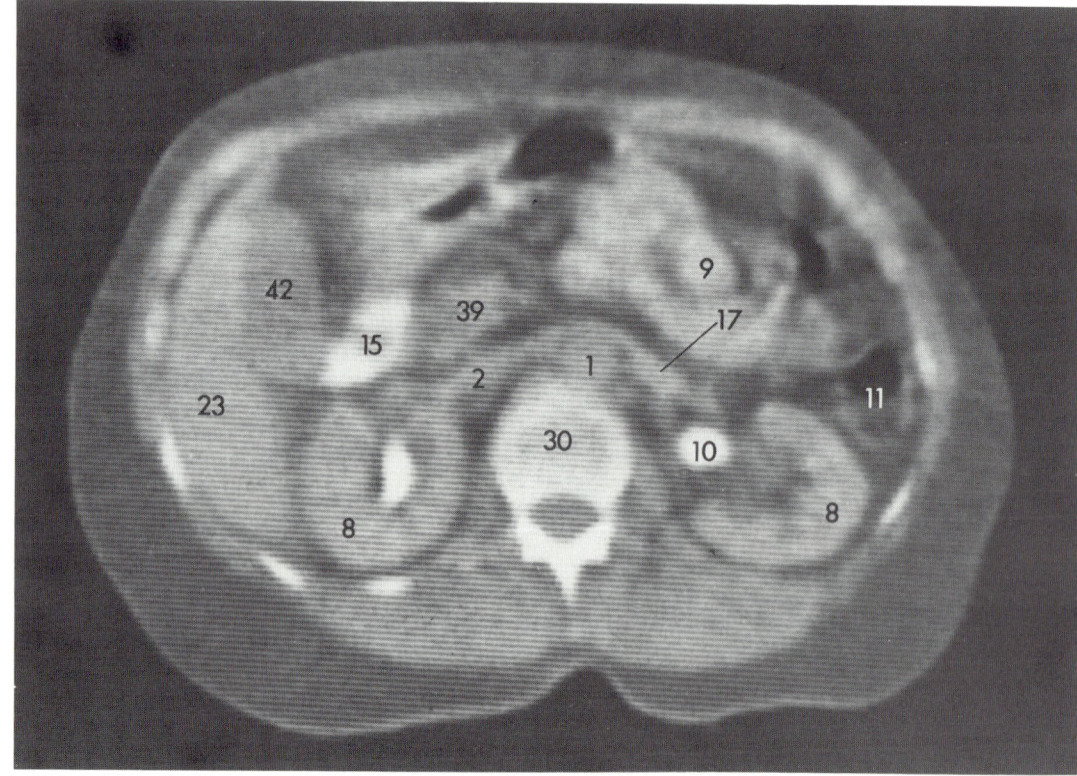

ABDOMEN AND PELVIS

Level 25A

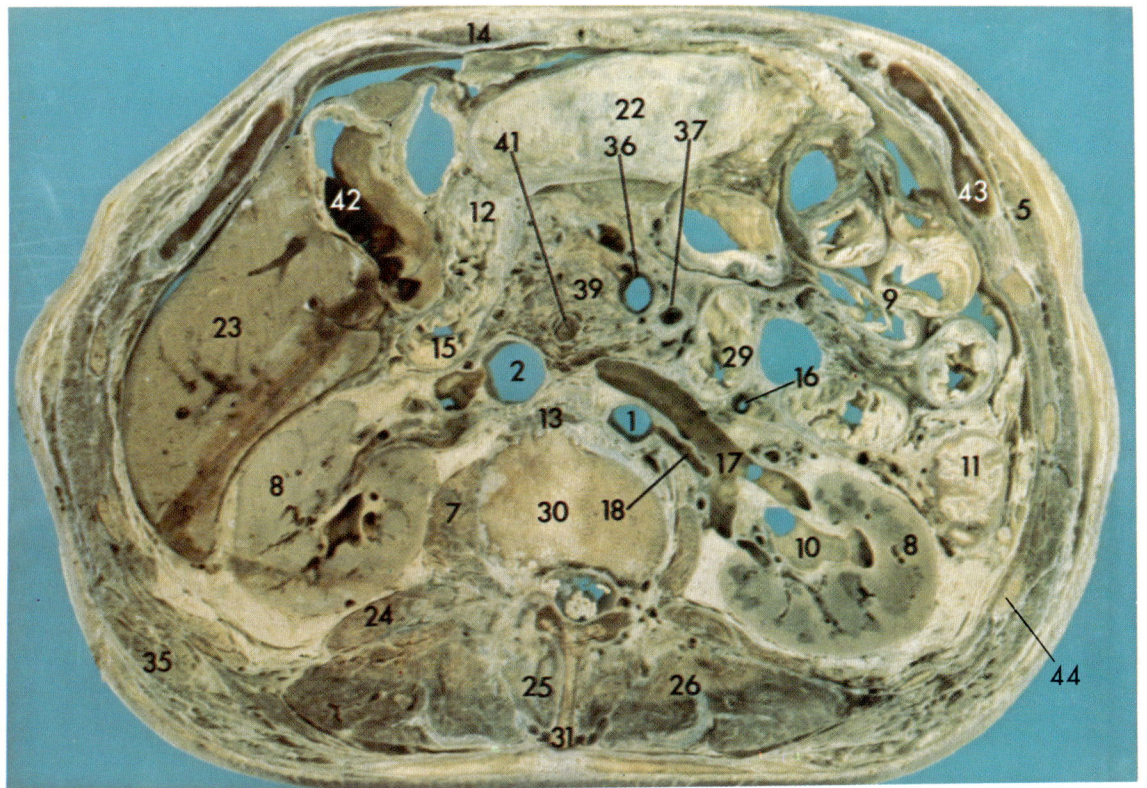

1. Aorta
2. Inferior vena cava
3. Portal vein
4. Splenic vein
5. External oblique muscle
7. Psoas muscle
8. Kidney
9. Jejunum
10. Renal pelvis
11. Descending colon
12. Duodenal bulb
13. Right crus of diaphragm
14. Rectus abdominis muscle
15. Second portion of duodenum
16. Inferior mesenteric vein
17. Left renal vein
18. Renal artery
22. Stomach
23. Right lobe of liver
24. Quadratus lumborum muscle
25. Multifidus muscle
26. Erector spinae muscle
29. Fourth portion of duodenum
30. Body of first lumbar vertebra
31. Spinous process
34. Transverse colon
35. Latissimus dorsi muscle
36. Superior mesenteric vein
37. Superior mesenteric artery
38. Spleen
39. Head of pancreas
41. Common bile duct
42. Gall bladder
43. Costal cartilage
44. Rib

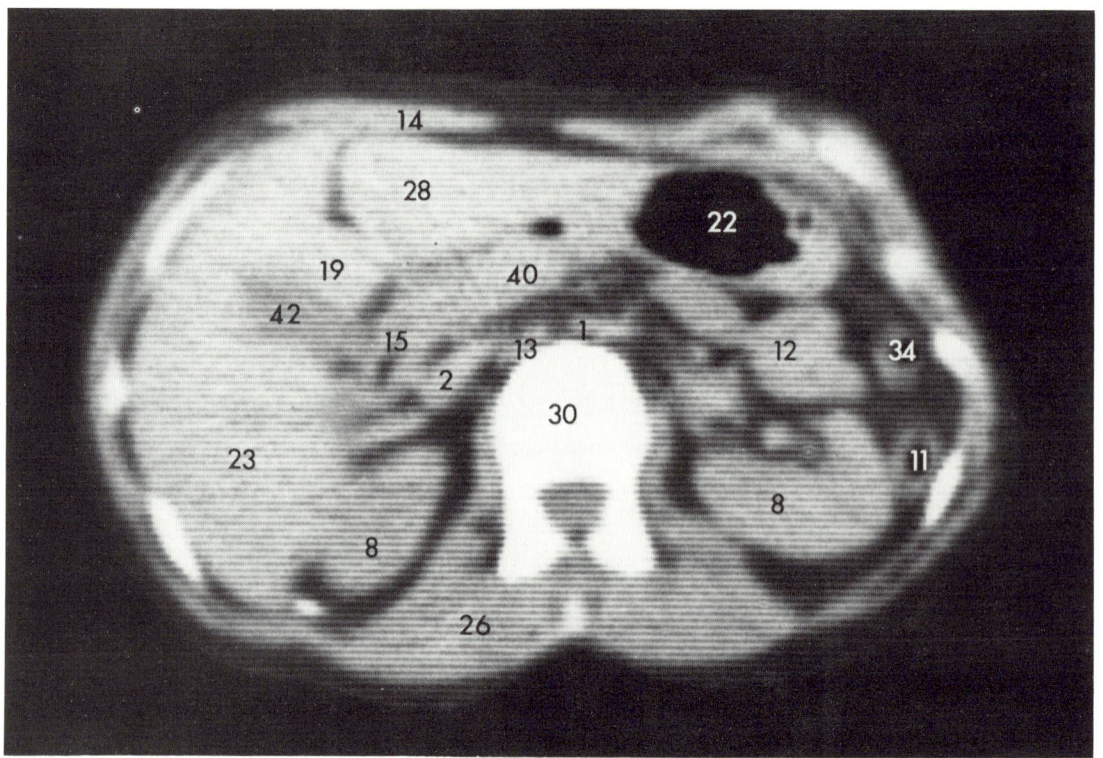

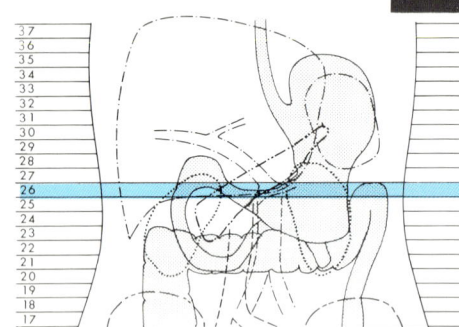

1. Aorta
2. Inferior vena cava
4. Splenic vein
5. External oblique muscle
6. Transversus abdominis muscle
7. Psoas muscle
8. Kidney
9. Gastroduodenal artery
10. Fat in renal sinus
11. Descending colon
12. Jejunum
13. Right crus of diaphragm
14. Rectus abdominis muscle
15. Second portion of duodenum
16. Inferior mesenteric vein
17. Renal vein
19. Quadrate lobe of liver
21. Transversalis fascia

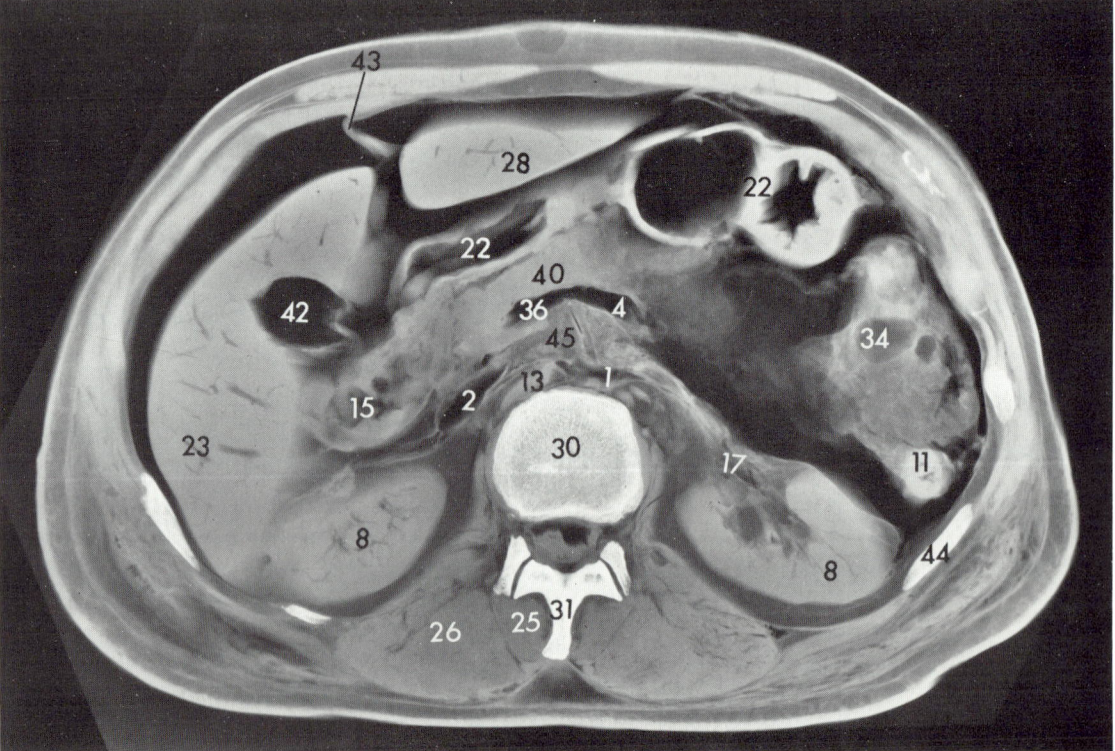

ABDOMEN AND PELVIS

Level 26

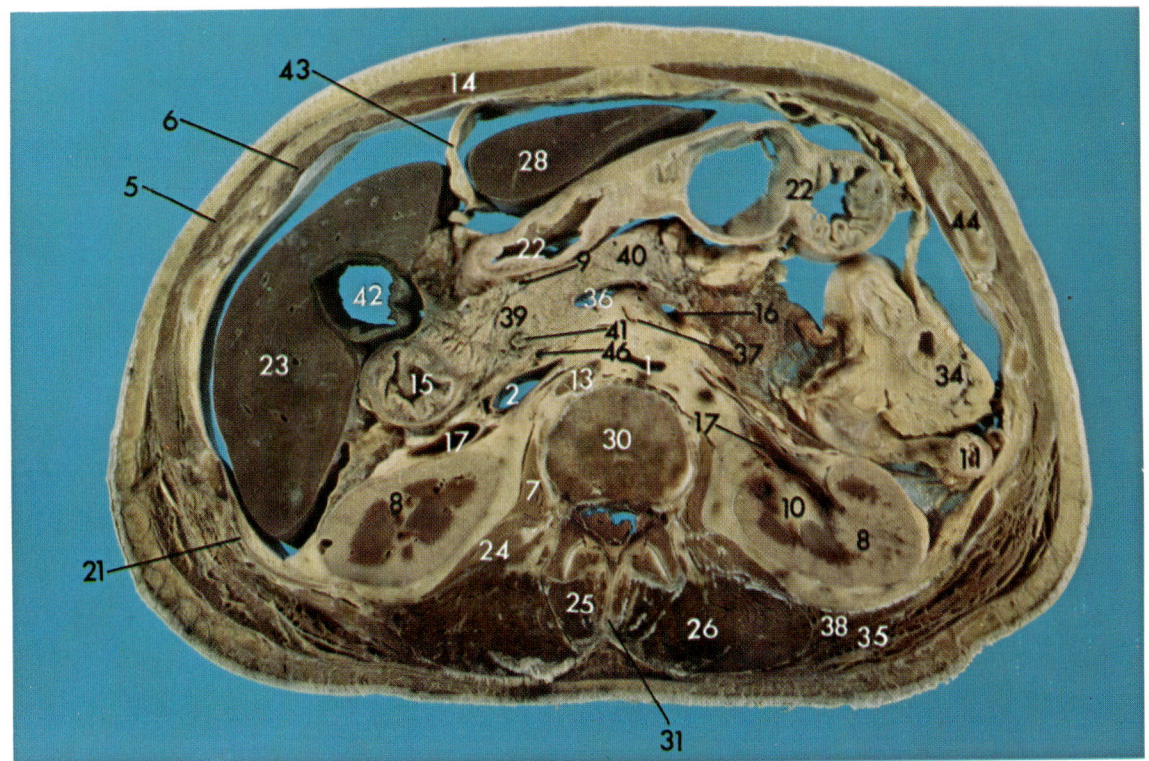

22. Stomach
23. Right lobe of liver
24. Quadratus lumborum muscle
25. Multifidus muscle
26. Erector spinae muscle
28. Left lobe of liver
30. Body of first lumbar vertebra
31. Spinous process of twelfth thoracic vertebra
34. Distal transverse colon
35. Latissimus dorsi muscle
36. Confluence of superior mesenteric and splenic veins
37. Superior mesenteric artery
38. Serratus posterior inferior muscle
39. Head of pancreas
40. Body of pancreas
41. Common bile duct
42. Gall bladder
43. Falciform ligament
44. Rib
45. Retropancreatic fat
46. Posterior superior pancreaticoduodenal vessel

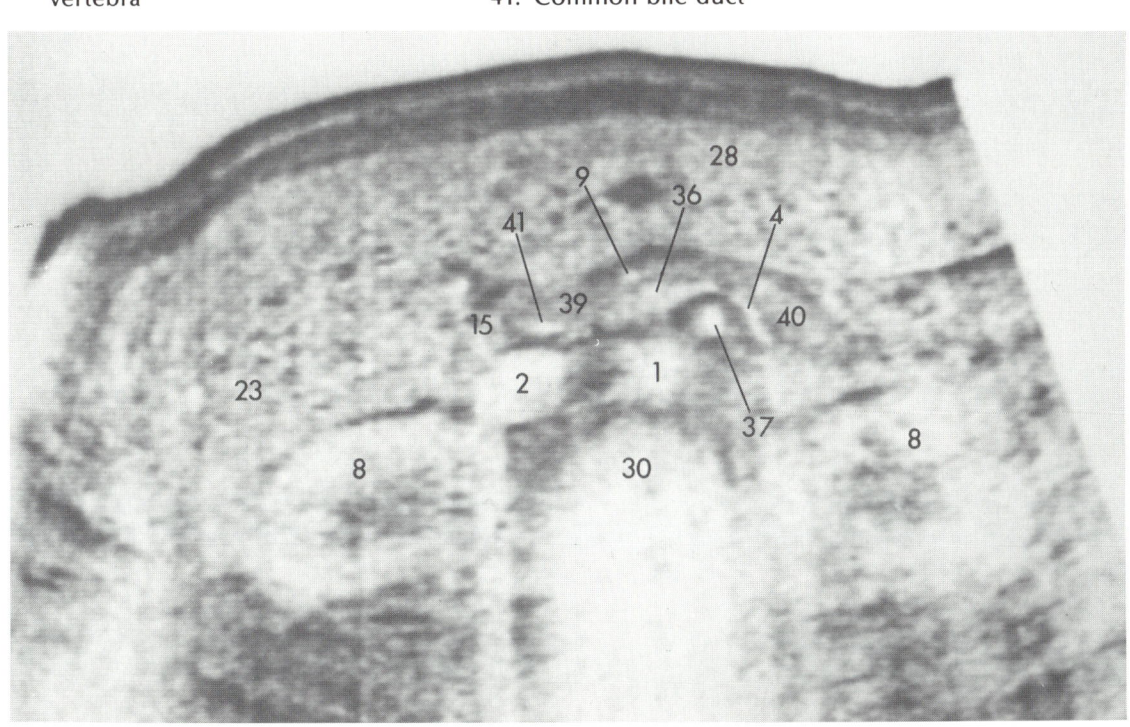

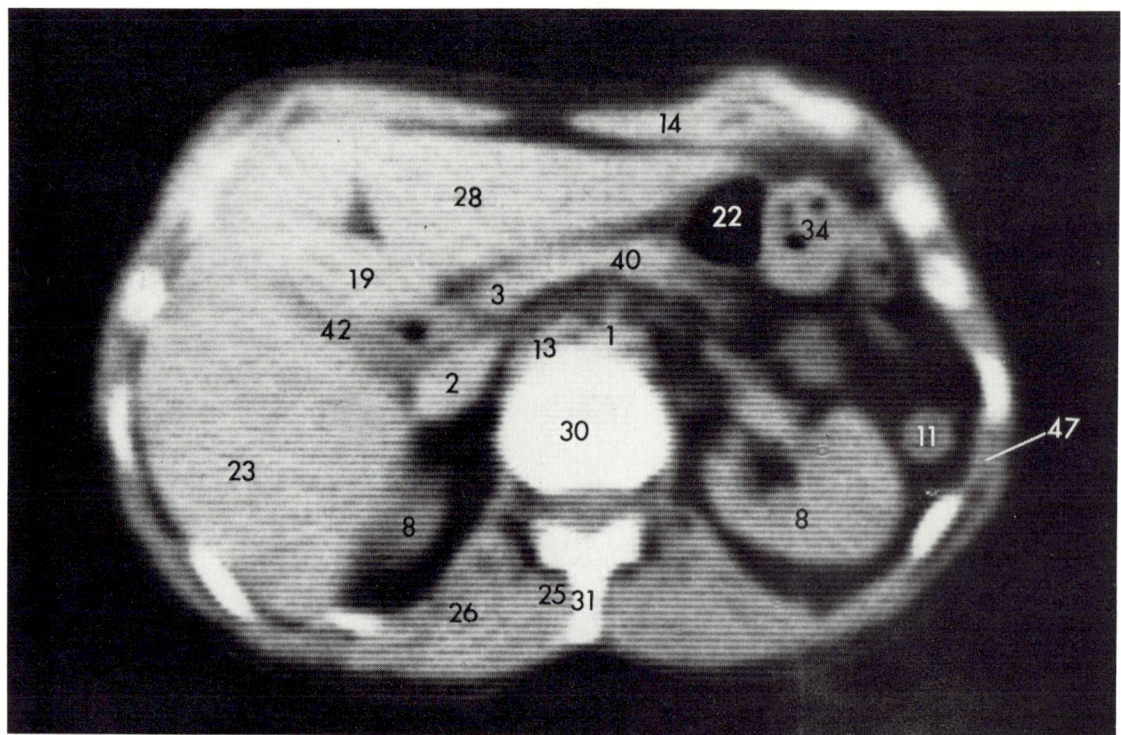

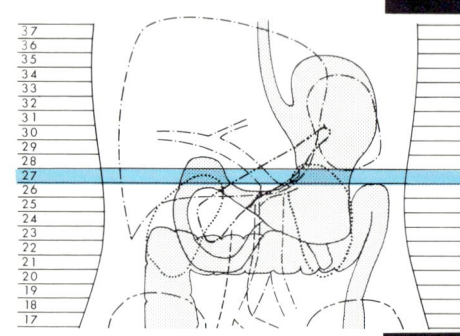

1. Aorta
2. Inferior vena cava
3. Portal vein
4. Splenic vein
5. External oblique muscle
6. Transversus abdominis muscle
7. Psoas muscle
8. Kidney
9. Gastroduodenal artery

11. Descending colon
12. Left crus of diaphragm
13. Right crus of diaphragm
14. Rectus abdominis muscle
15. Duodenal bulb
16. Left adrenal gland
17. Left renal artery
18. Parietal peritoneum
19. Quadrate lobe of liver

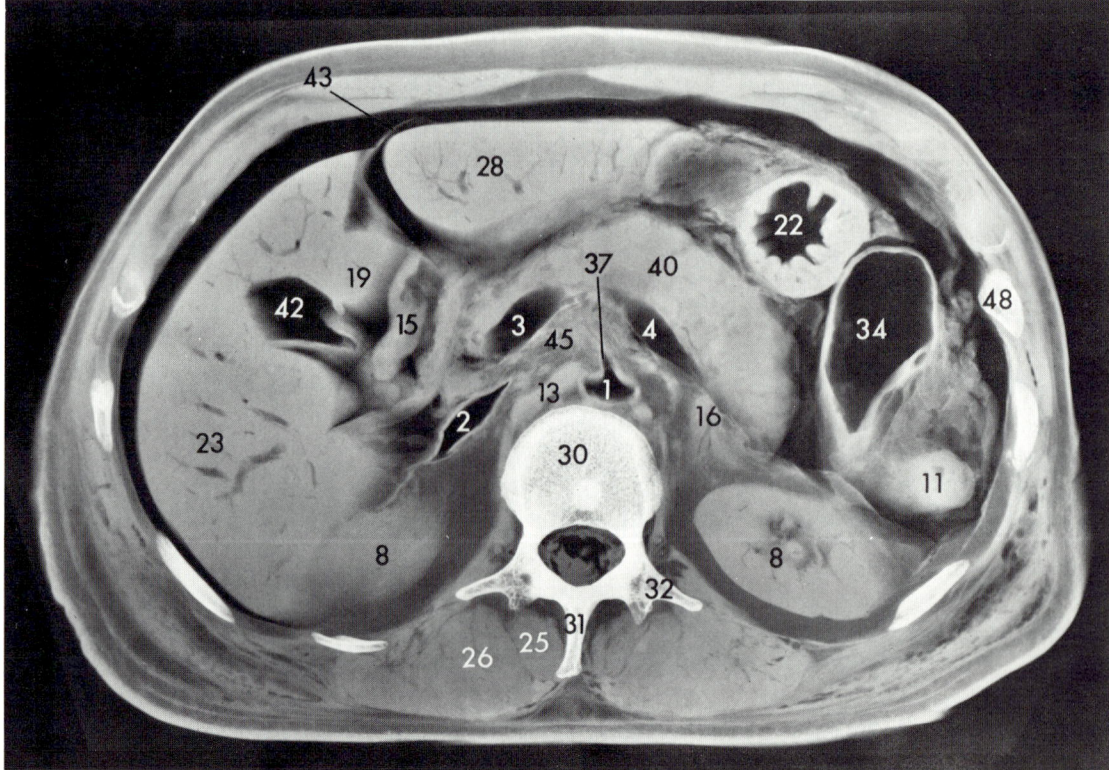

ABDOMEN AND PELVIS

Level 27

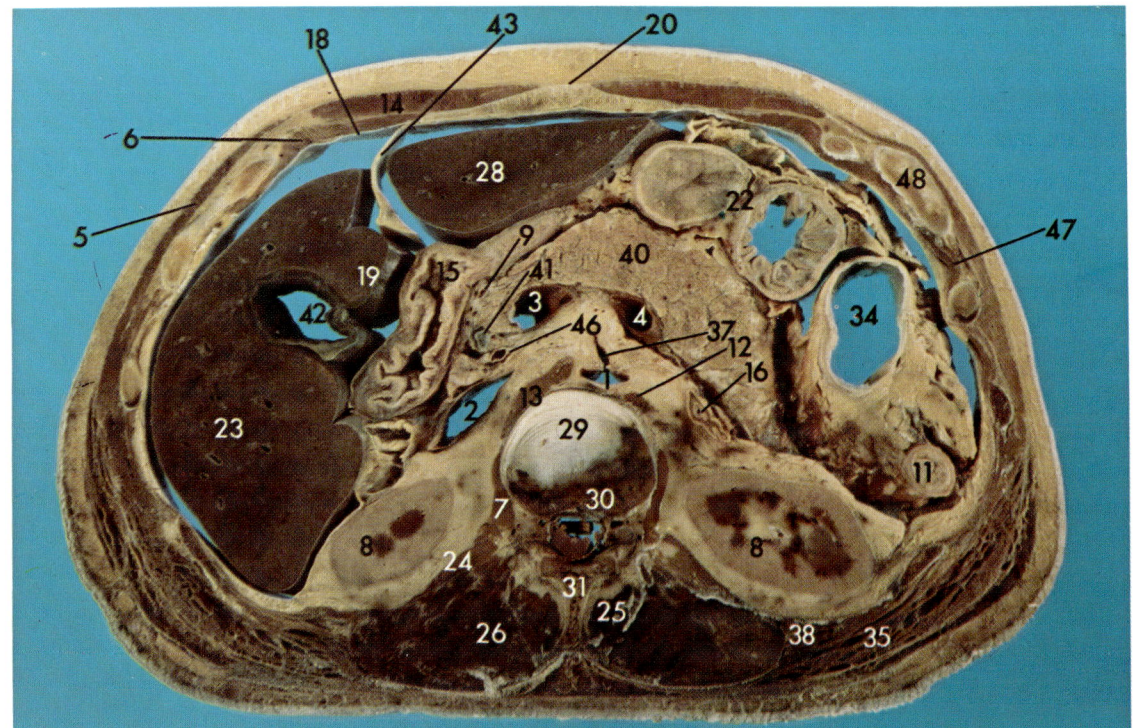

20. Linea alba	31. Spinous process of twelfth thoracic vertebra	39. Head of pancreas
22. Stomach		40. Body of pancreas
23. Right lobe of liver	32. Transverse process of twelfth thoracic vertebra	41. Common bile duct
24. Quadratus lumborum muscle		42. Gall bladder
25. Multifidus muscle	34. Distal transverse colon	43. Falciform ligament
26. Erector spinae muscle	35. Latissimus dorsi muscle	44. Ligamentum teres (umbilical vein)
28. Left lobe of liver	36. Superior mesenteric vein	45. Retropancreatic fat
29. T12–L1 intervertebral disc	37. Superior mesenteric artery	47. Intercostal muscle
30. Body of twelfth thoracic vertebra	38. Serratus posterior inferior muscle	48. Rib

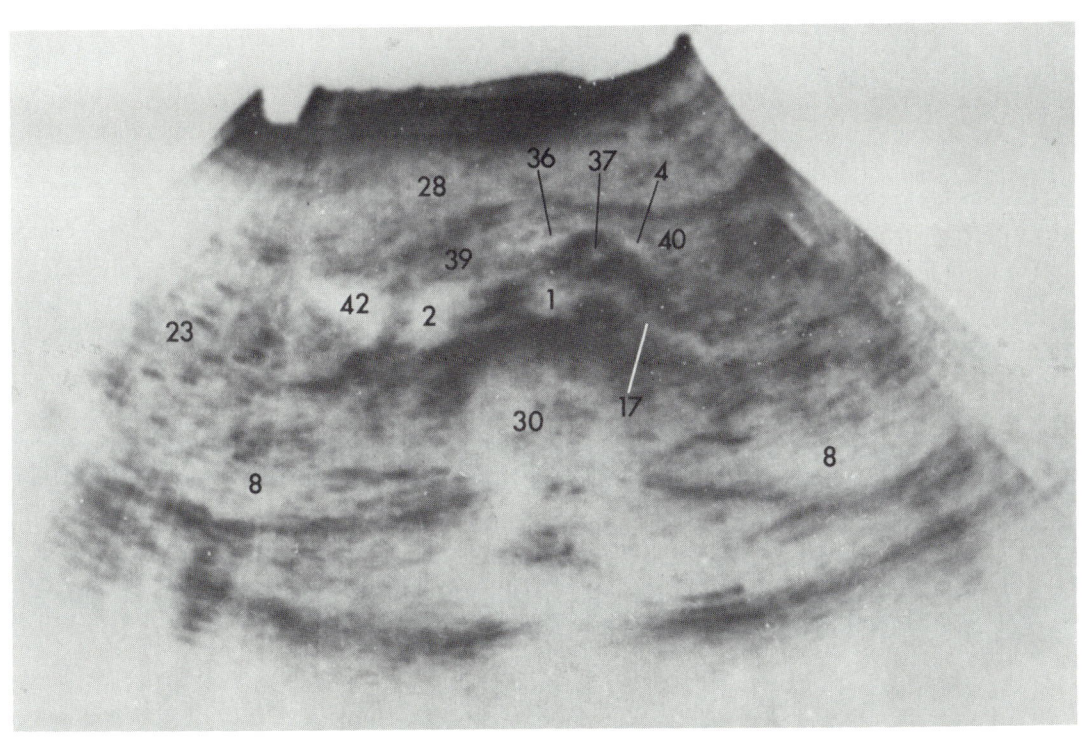

189

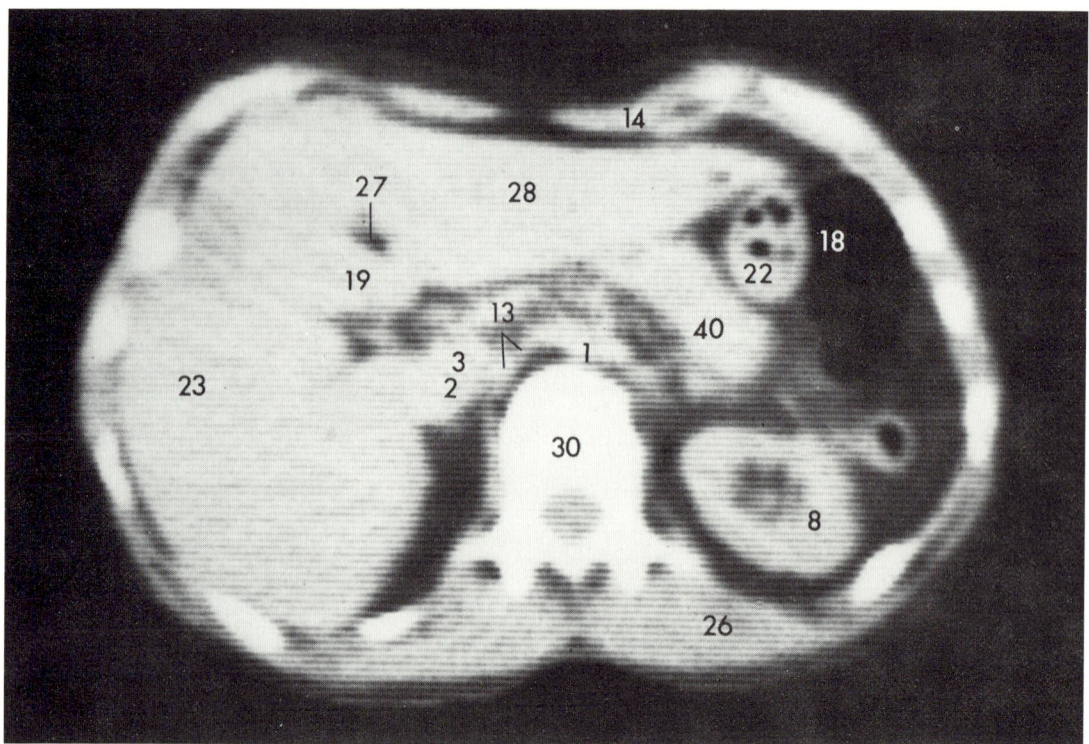

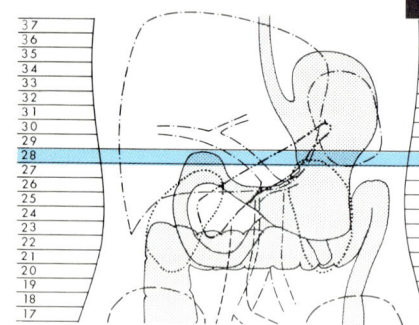

1. Aorta
2. Inferior vena cava
3. Portal vein
4. Splenic vein
5. External oblique muscle
6. Transversus abdominis muscle
7. Psoas muscle
8. Kidney
9. Hepatic artery
10. Celiac artery
11. Splenic artery
12. Left crus of diaphragm
13. Right crus of diaphragm
14. Rectus abdominis muscle
15. Duodenal bulb
16. Left adrenal gland
17. Lymph node
18. Splenic flexure of colon

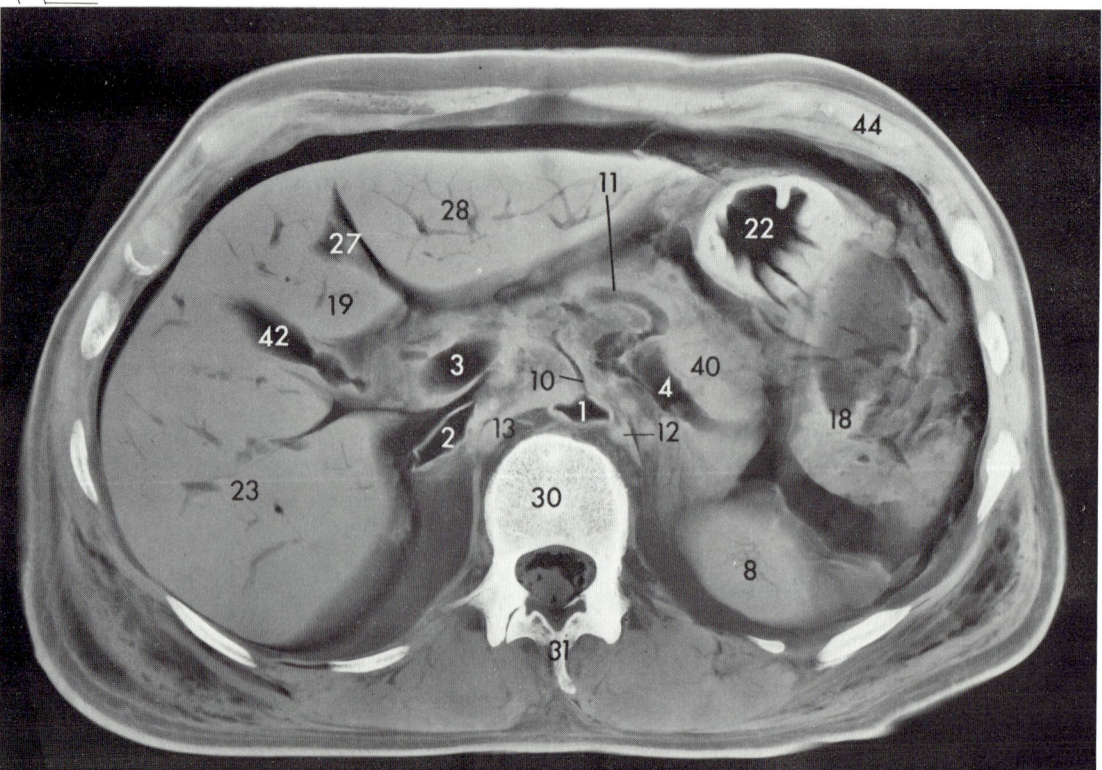

ABDOMEN AND PELVIS

Level 28

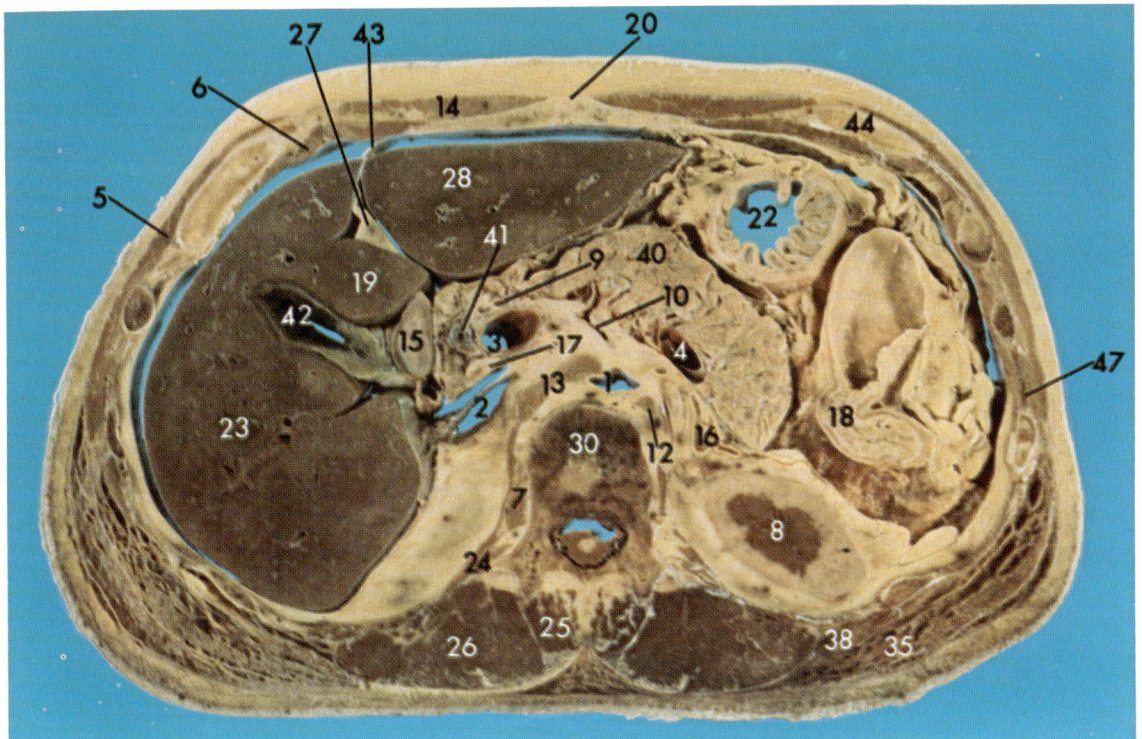

19. Quadrate lobe of liver
20. Linea alba
21. Inferior phrenic vein
22. Stomach
23. Right lobe of liver
24. Quadratus lumborum muscle
25. Multifidus muscle
26. Erector spinae muscle
27. Ligamentum teres with surrounding fat
28. Left lobe of liver
29. Spleen
30. Body of twelfth thoracic vertebra
31. Spinous process of twelfth thoracic vertebra
35. Latissimus dorsi muscle
38. Serratus posterior inferior muscle
40. Body of pancreas
41. Common bile duct
42. Gall bladder
43. Falciform ligament
44. Rib
47. Intercostal muscle

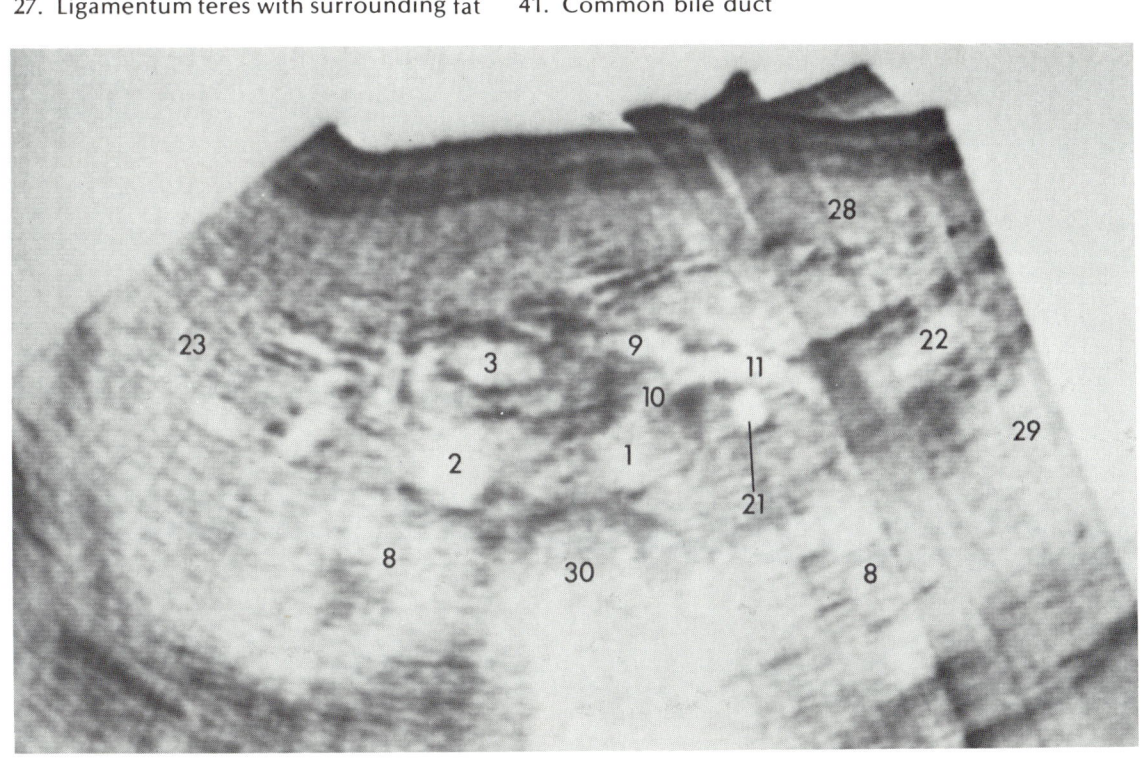

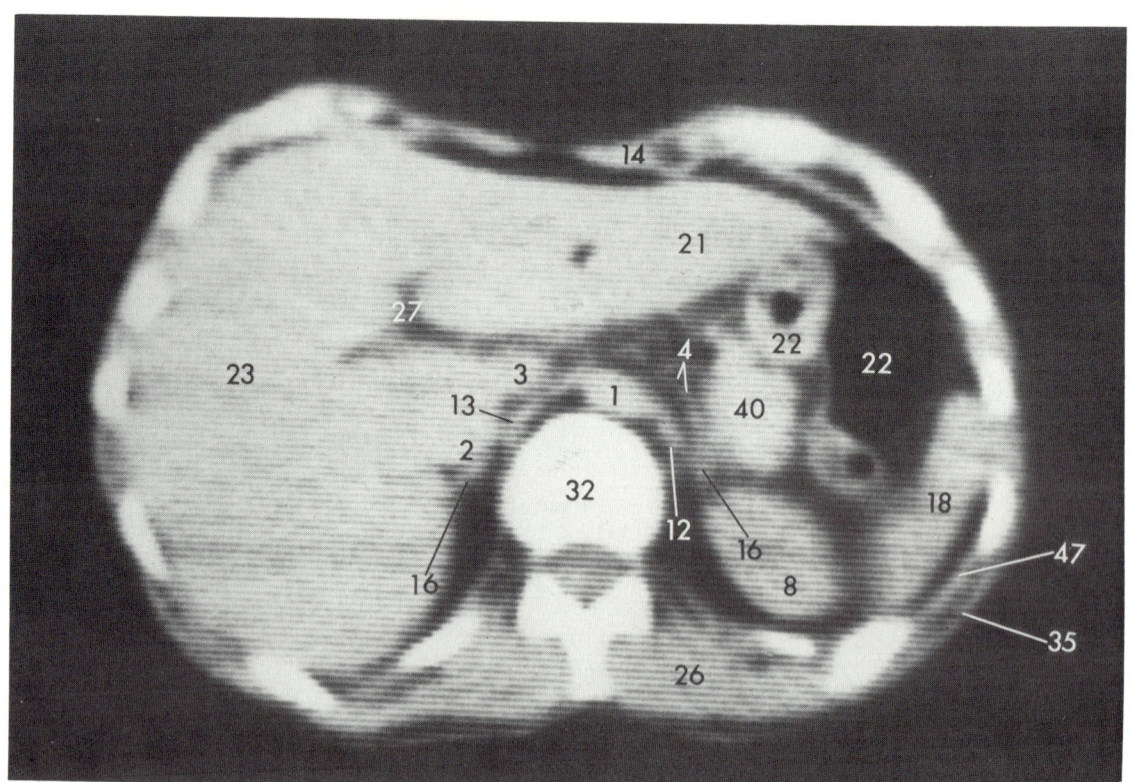

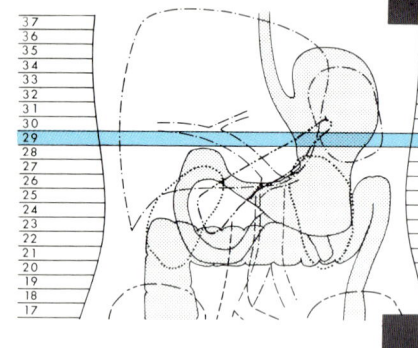

ABDOMEN AND PELVIS

Level 29

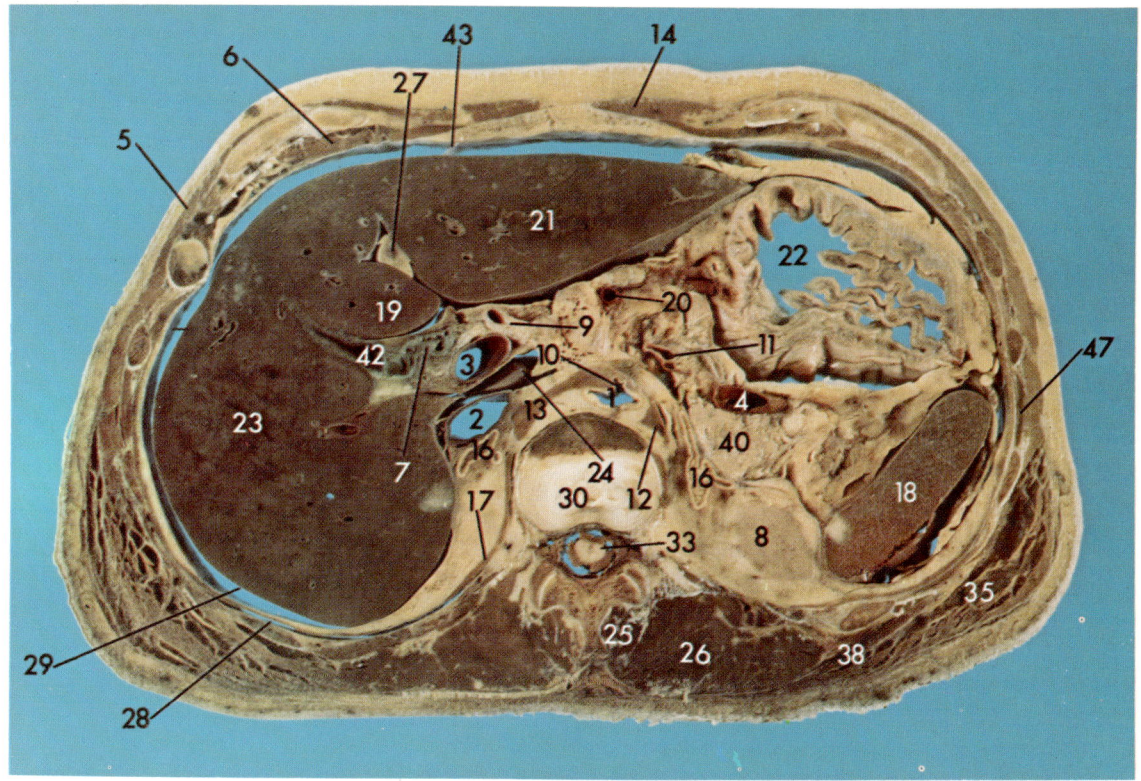

1. Aorta
2. Inferior vena cava
3. Portal vein
4. Splenic vein
5. External oblique muscle
6. Transversus abdominis muscle
7. Cystic duct
8. Upper pole of kidney
9. Hepatic artery
10. Celiac artery
11. Splenic artery
12. Left crus of diaphragm
13. Right crus of diaphragm
14. Rectus abdominis muscle
16. Adrenal gland
17. Diaphragm
18. Spleen
19. Quadrate lobe of liver
20. Left gastric vein
21. Left lobe of liver
22. Stomach
23. Right lobe of liver
24. Caudate lobe of liver
25. Multifidus muscle
26. Erector spinae muscle
27. Ligamentum teres with surrounding fat
28. Pleural cavity
29. Peritoneal cavity
30. T11–12 intervertebral disc
31. Spinous process of eleventh thoracic vertebra
32. Body of twelfth thoracic vertebra
33. Spinal cord
35. Latissimus dorsi muscle
38. Serratus posterior inferior muscle
40. Body of pancreas
42. Neck of gall bladder
43. Falciform ligament
44. Rib
47. Intercostal muscle

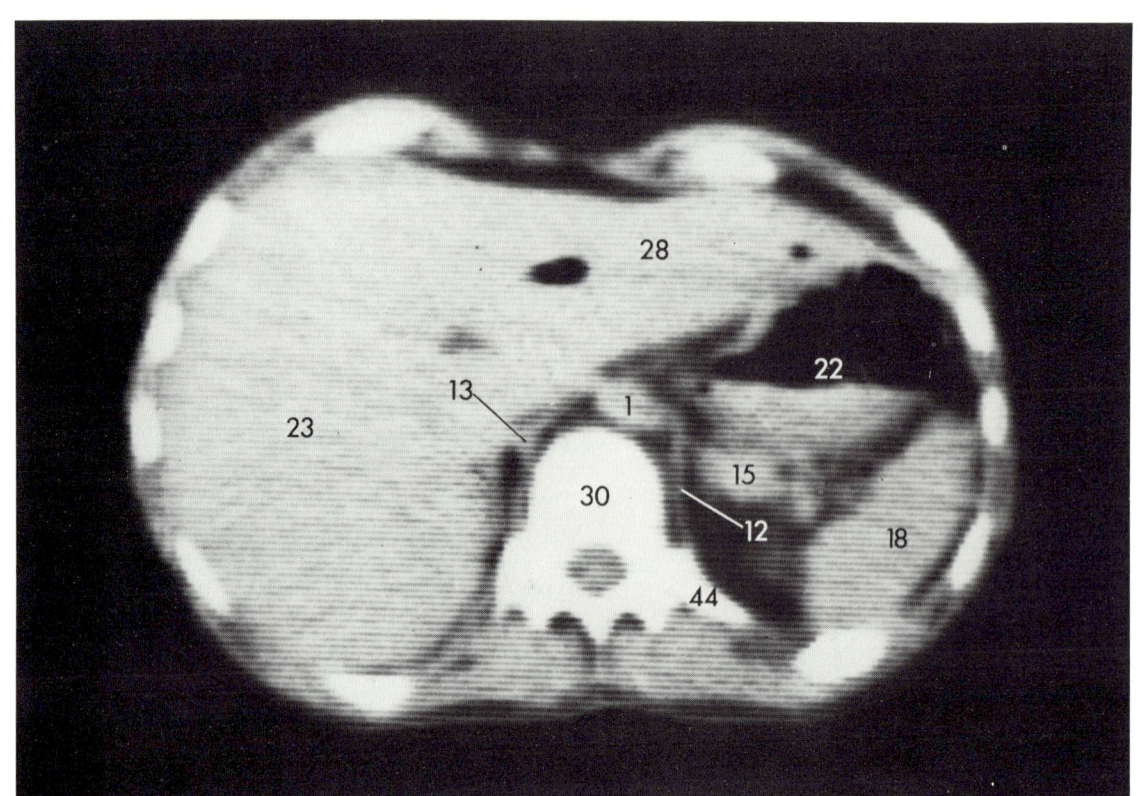

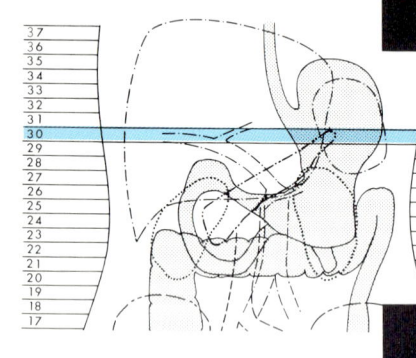

ABDOMEN AND PELVIS

Level 30

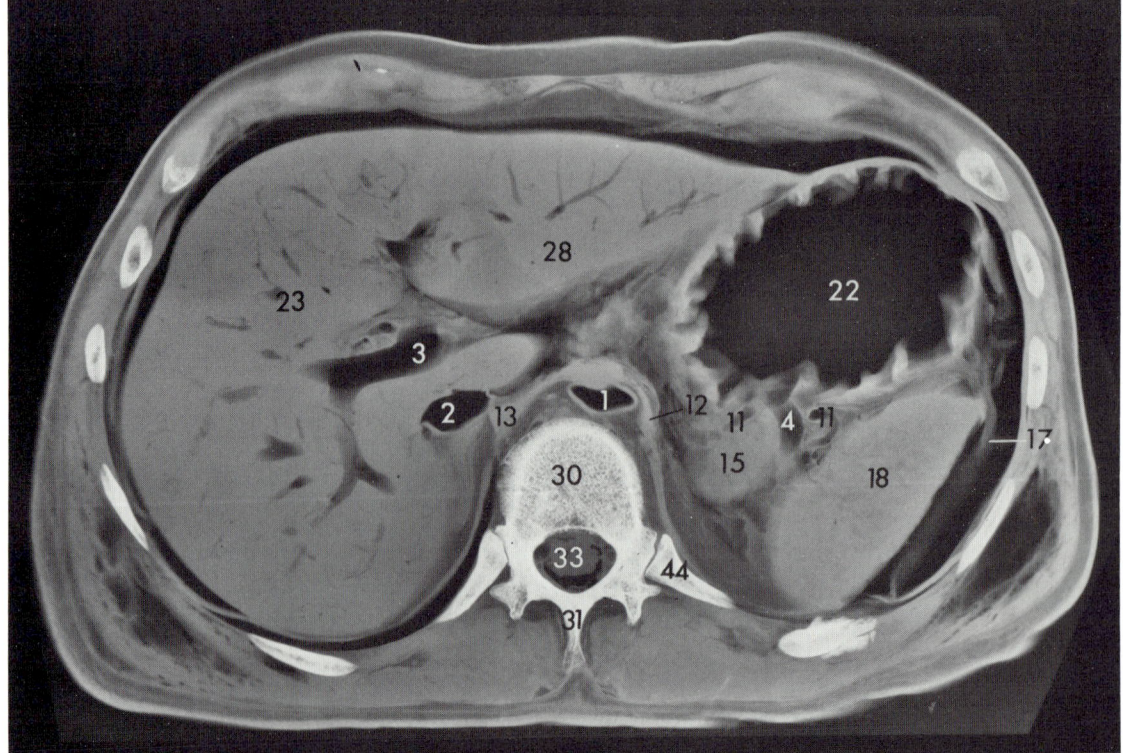

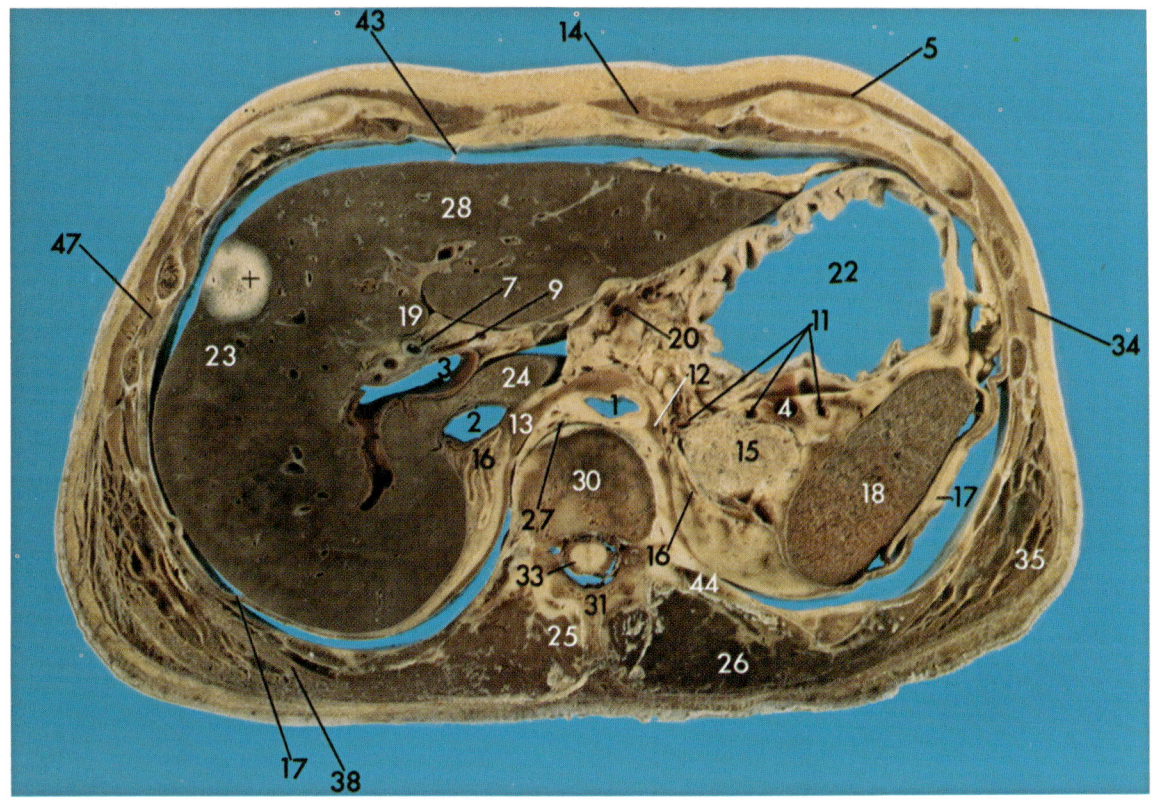

1. Aorta
2. Inferior vena cava
3. Portal vein
4. Splenic vein
5. External oblique muscle
7. Common hepatic duct
9. Hepatic artery
11. Splenic artery
12. Left crus of diaphragm
13. Right crus of diaphragm
14. Rectus abdominis muscle
15. Tail of pancreas
16. Adrenal gland
17. Diaphragm
18. Spleen
19. Quadrate lobe of liver
20. Left gastric vein
22. Stomach
23. Right lobe of liver
24. Caudate lobe of liver
25. Multifidus muscle
26. Erector spinae muscle
27. Azygos vein
28. Left lobe of liver
30. Body of eleventh thoracic vertebra
31. Spinous process of eleventh thoracic vertebra
33. Spinal cord
34. Serratus anterior muscle
35. Latissimus dorsi muscle
38. Serratus posterior inferior muscle
43. Falciform ligament
44. Eleventh rib
47. Intercostal muscle
+ Metastasis in liver

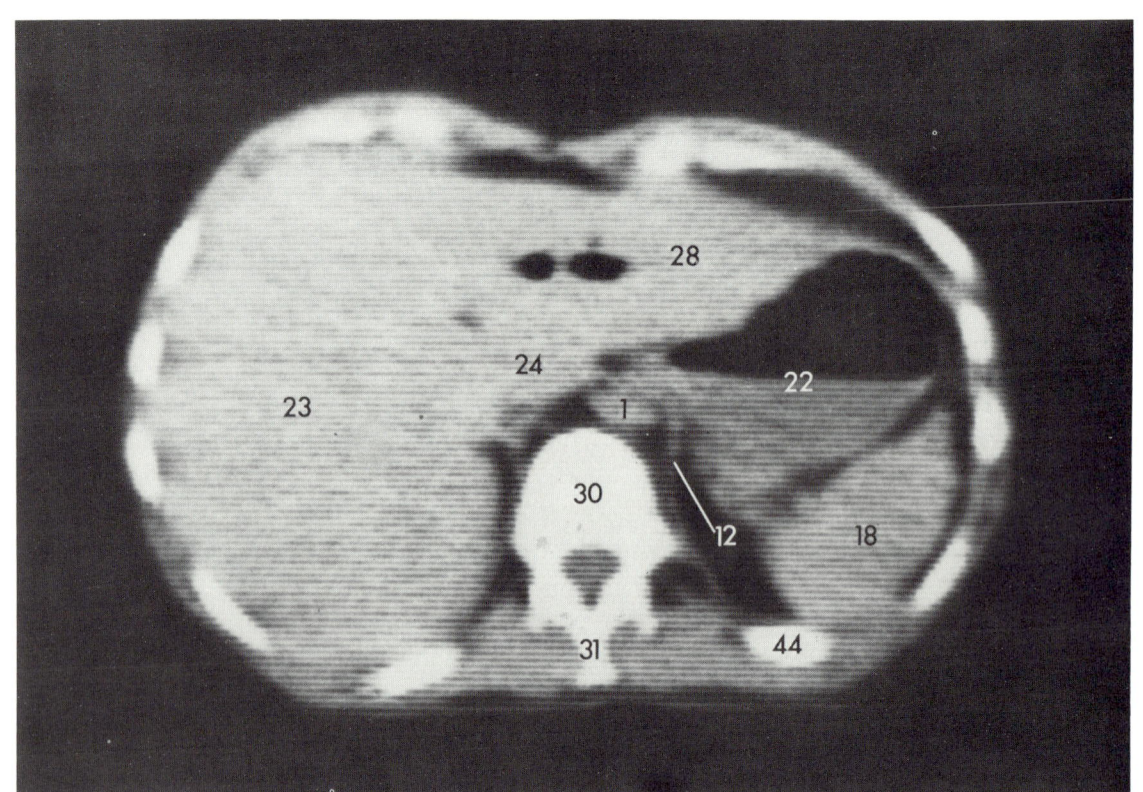

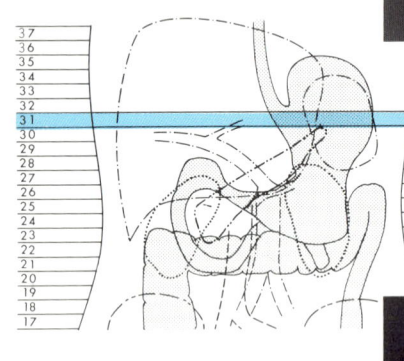

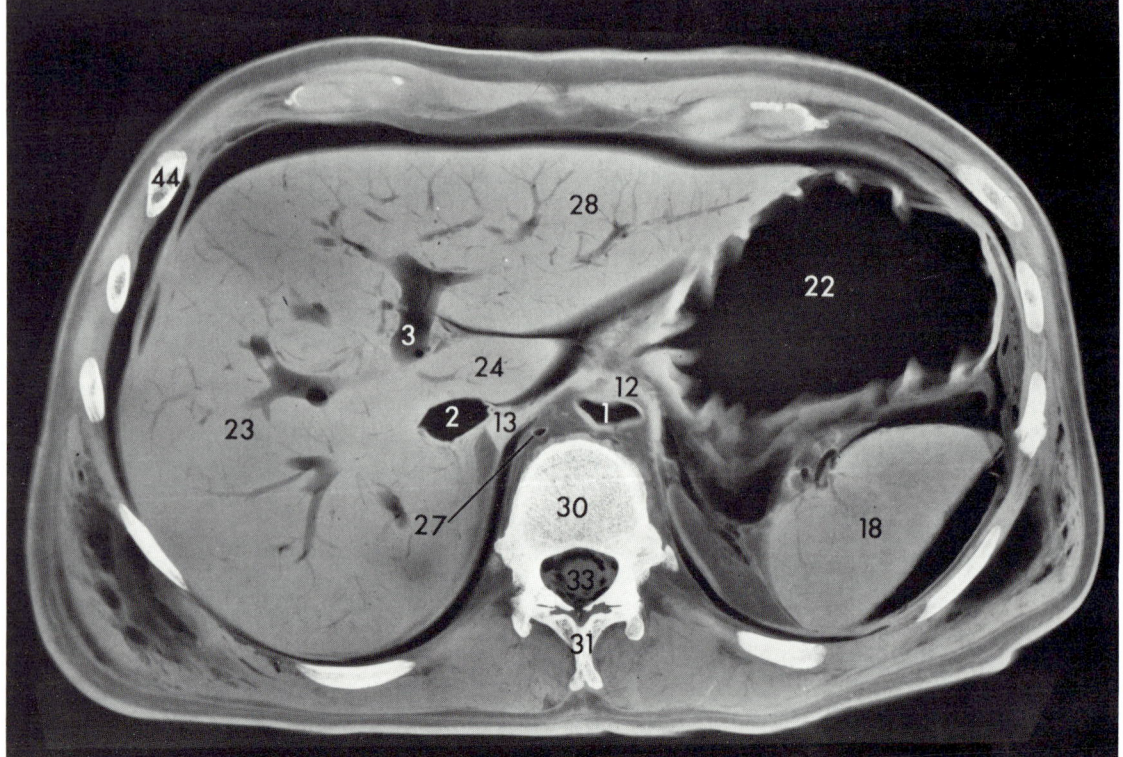

ABDOMEN AND PELVIS

Level 31

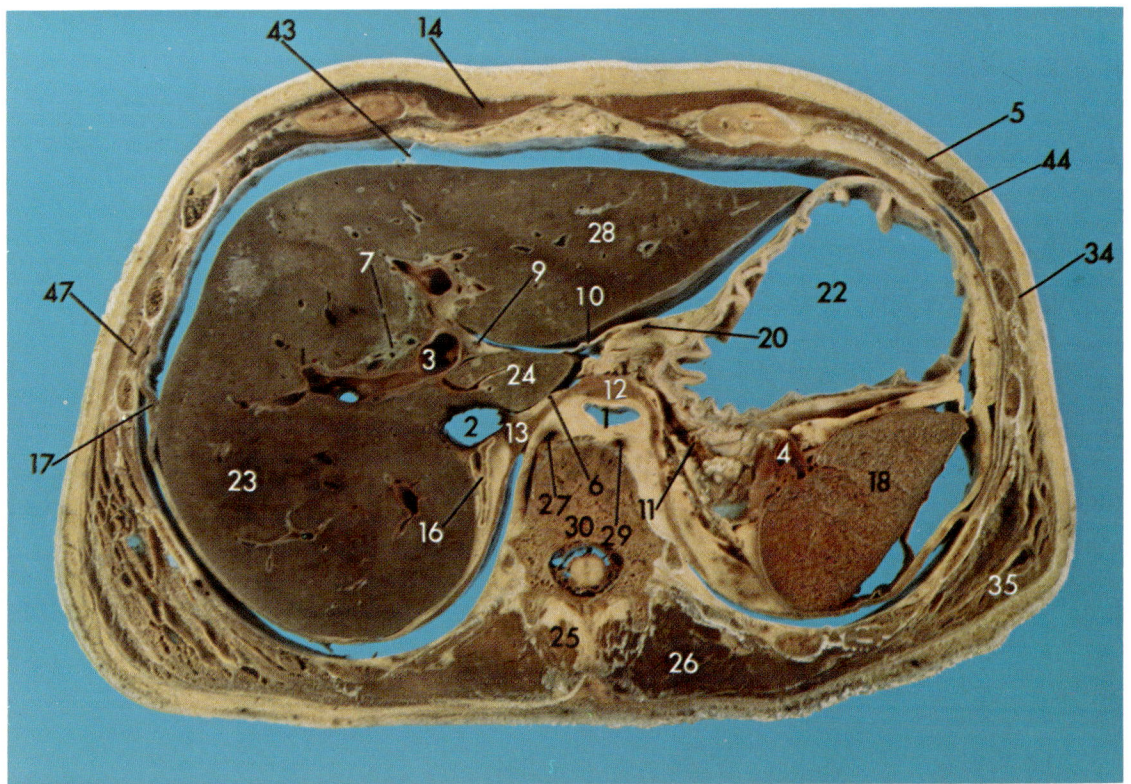

1. Aorta
2. Inferior vena cava
3. Portal vein at porta hepatis
4. Splenic vein
5. External oblique muscle
6. Inferior phrenic artery
7. Hepatic ducts
9. Hepatic artery
10. Lesser omentum
11. Short gastric vein
12. Left crus of diaphragm
13. Right crus of diaphragm
14. Rectus abdominis muscle
16. Adrenal gland
17. Diaphragm
18. Spleen
20. Left gastric vein
22. Stomach
23. Right lobe of liver
24. Caudate lobe of liver
25. Multifidus muscle
26. Erector spinae muscle
27. Azygos vein
28. Left lobe of liver
29. Hemiazygos vein
30. Body of eleventh thoracic vertebra
31. Spinous process of eleventh thoracic vertebra
33. Spinal cord
34. Serratus anterior muscle
35. Latissimus dorsi muscle
43. Falciform ligament
44. Rib
47. Intercostal muscle

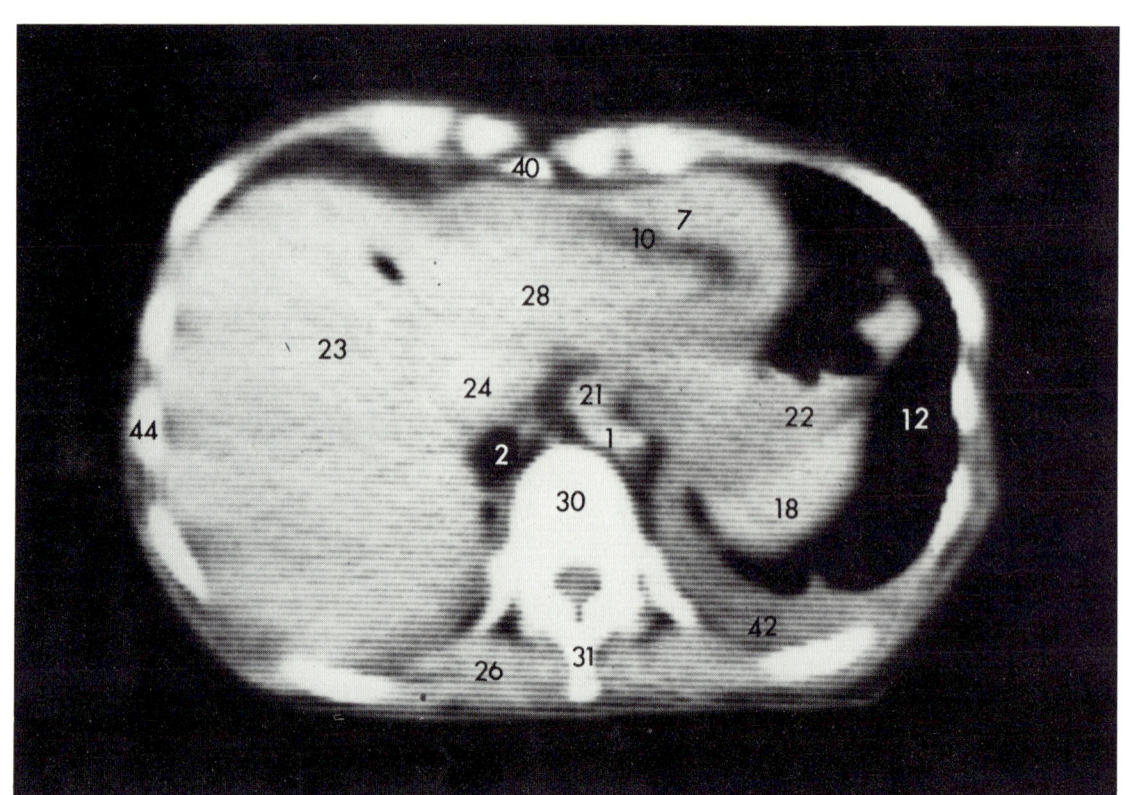

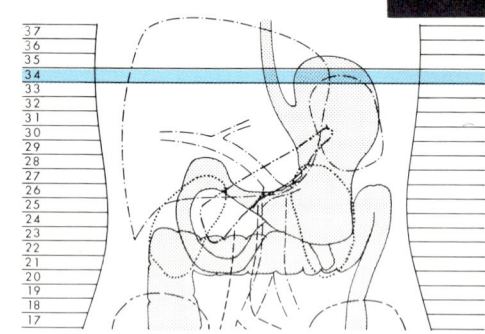

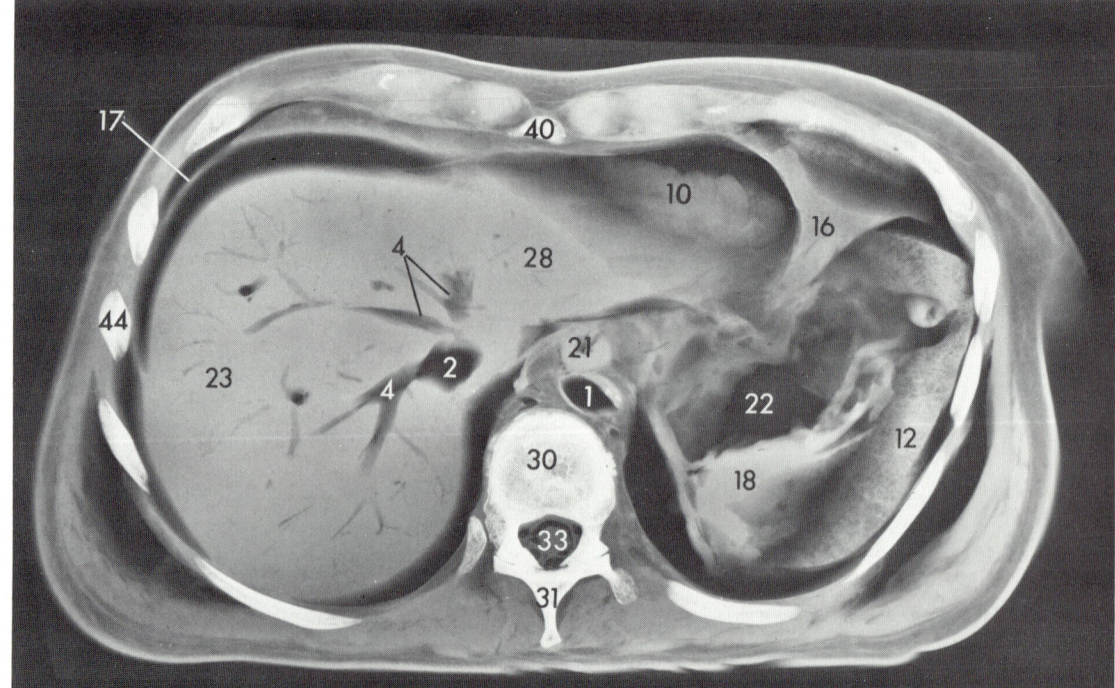

ABDOMEN AND PELVIS

Level 34

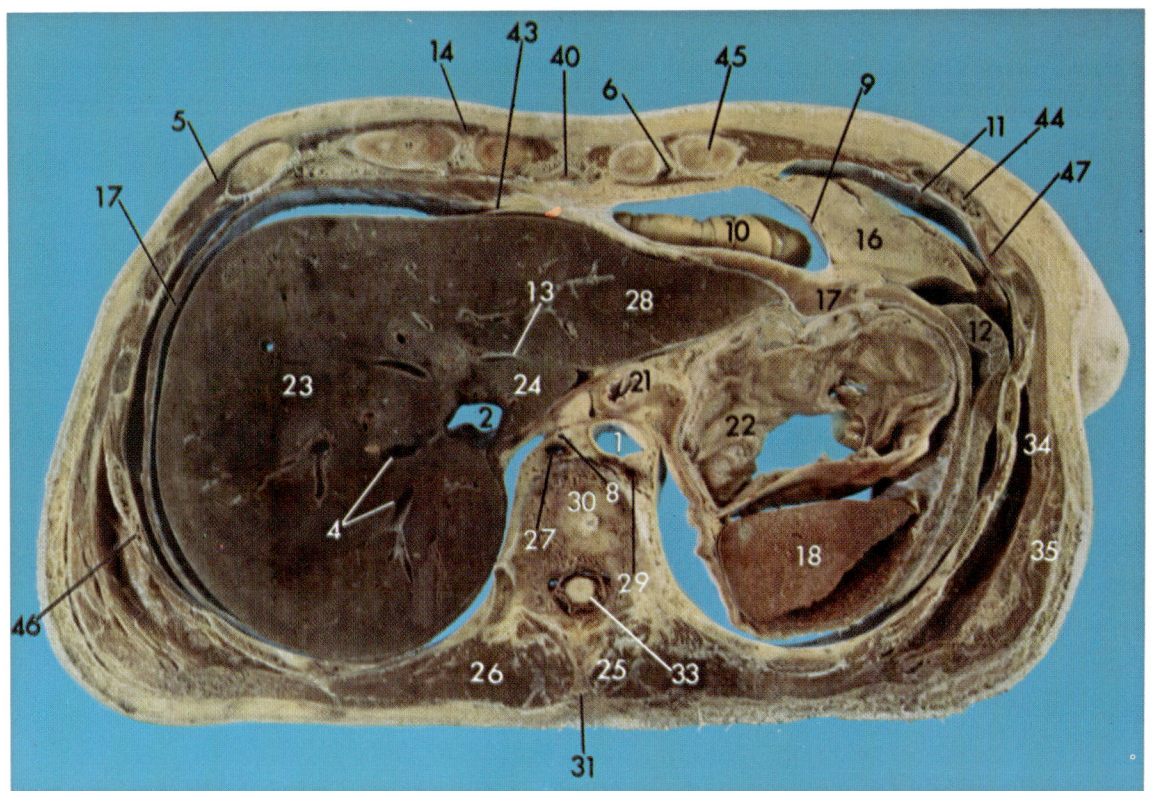

1. Aorta
2. Inferior vena cava
4. Hepatic veins
5. External oblique muscle
6. Internal mammary vessels
7. Apex of heart
8. Thoracic duct
9. Pericardium
10. Epicardial fat
11. Parietal pleura
12. Left lung
13. Lesser omentum (hepatogastric ligament)
14. Rectus abdominis muscle
16. Fat pad external to pericardium
17. Diaphragm
18. Spleen
21. Esophagus
22. Cardia of stomach
23. Right lobe of liver
24. Caudate lobe of liver
25. Multifidus muscle
26. Erector spinae muscle
27. Azygos vein
28. Left lobe of liver
29. Hemiazygos vein
30. Body of tenth thoracic vertebra
31. Spinous process of tenth thoracic vertebra
33. Spinal cord
34. Serratus anterior muscle
35. Latissimus dorsi muscle
40. Xiphoid process
42. Fluid in pleural cavity
43. Falciform ligament
44. Rib
45. Costal cartilage
46. Intercostal vessel
47. Intercostal muscle

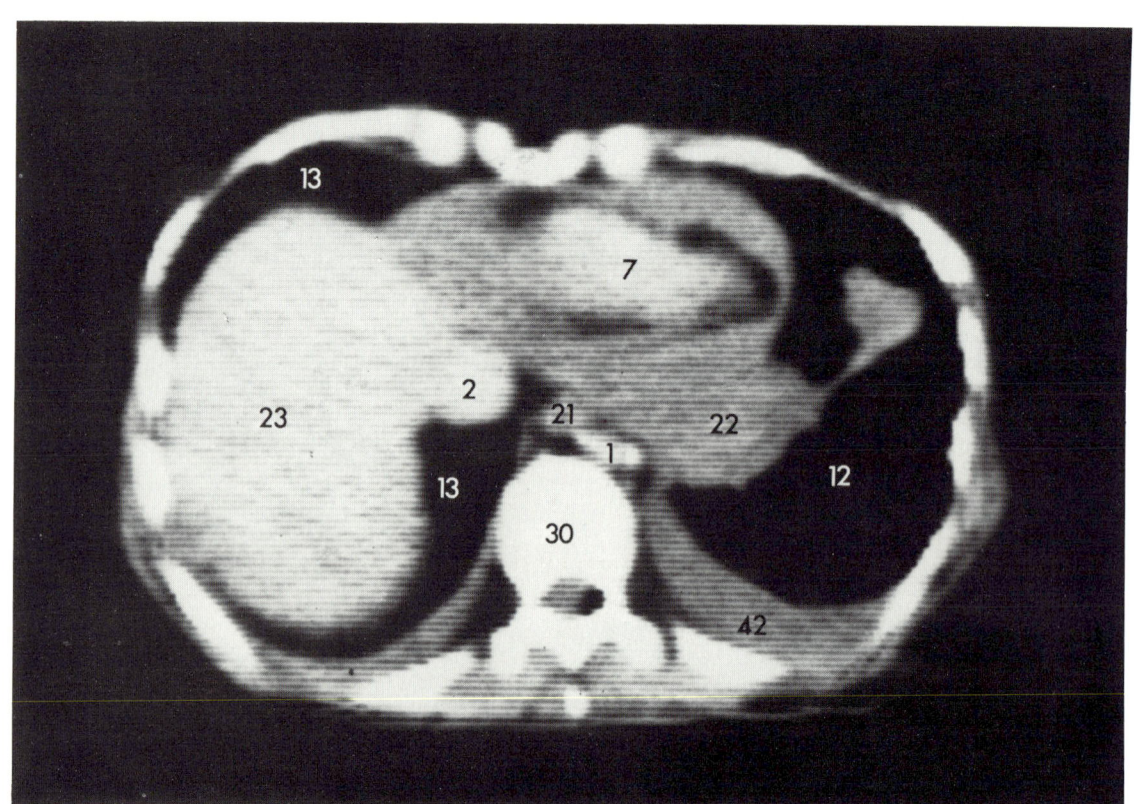

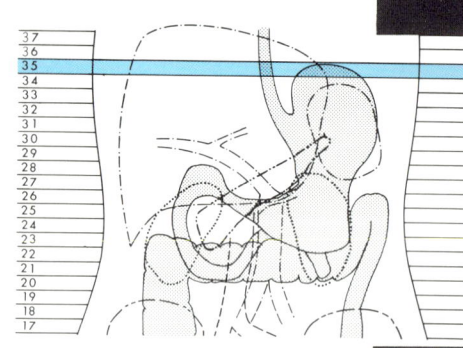

ABDOMEN AND PELVIS

Level 35

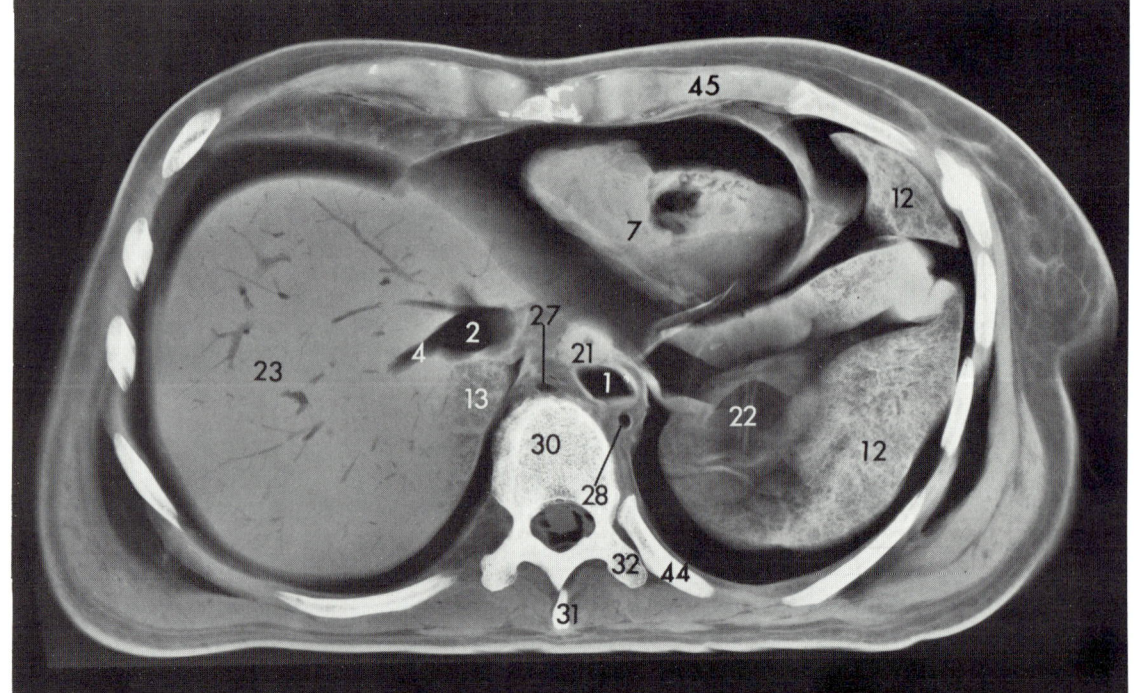

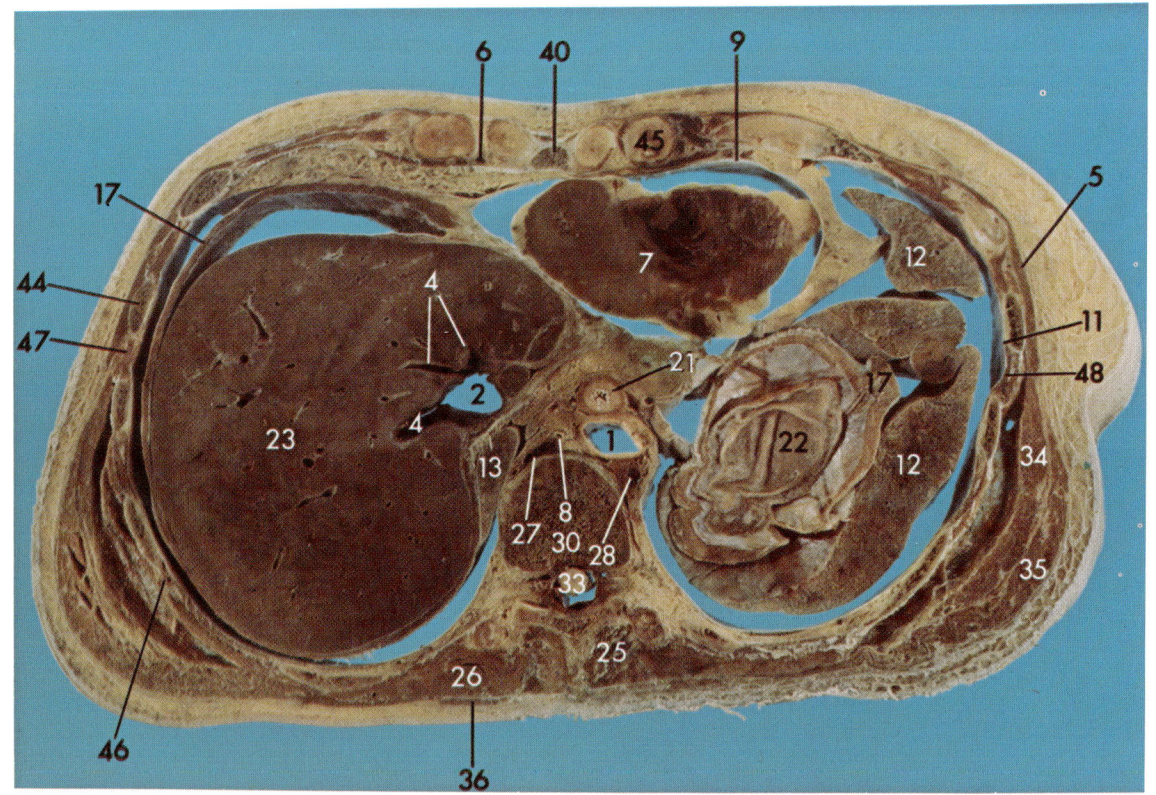

1. Aorta
2. Inferior vena cava
4. Hepatic vein
5. External oblique muscle
6. Internal mammary vessels
7. Heart
8. Thoracic duct
9. Pericardium
11. Parietal pleura
12. Left lung
13. Right lung
17. Diaphragm
21. Esophagus
22. Cardia of stomach
23. Right lobe of liver
25. Multifidus muscle
26. Erector spinae muscle
27. Azygos vein
28. Hemiazygos vein
30. Body of tenth thoracic vertebra
31. Spinous process of tenth thoracic vertebra
32. Transverse process of tenth thoracic vertebra
33. Spinal cord
34. Serratus anterior muscle
35. Latissimus dorsi muscle
36. Trapezius muscle
40. Xiphoid process
42. Fluid in pleural cavity
44. Rib
45. Costal cartilage
46. Intercostal vessels
47. External intercostal muscle
48. Internal intercostal muscle

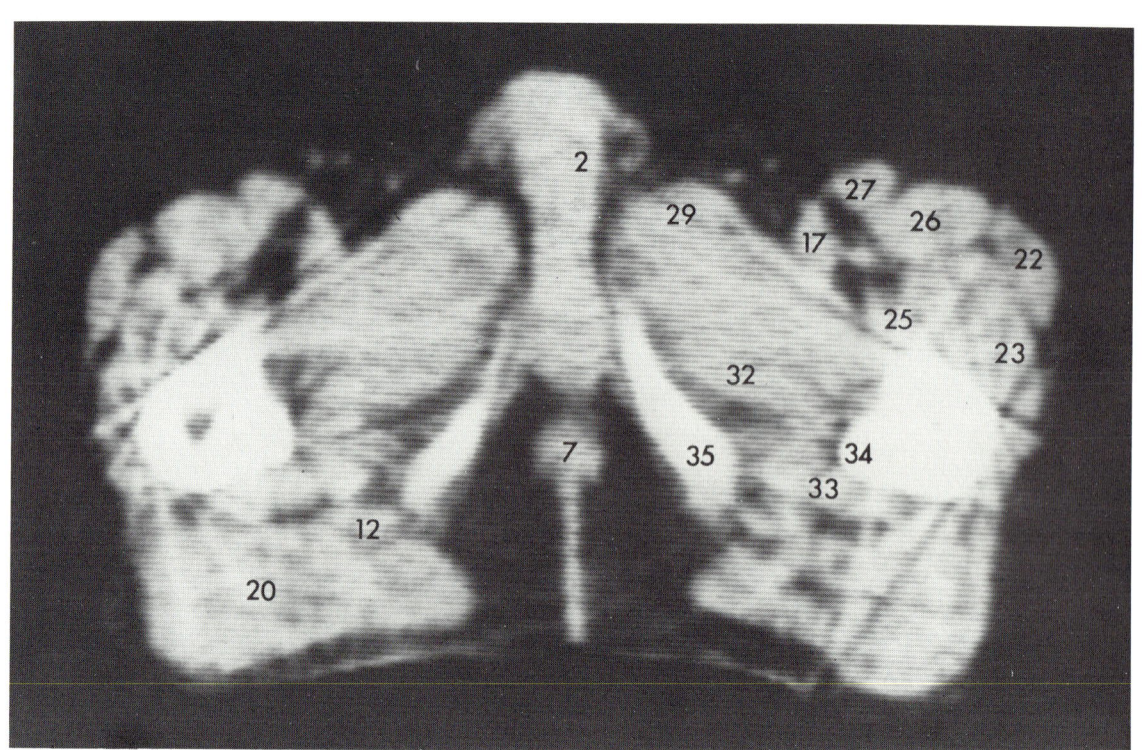

*

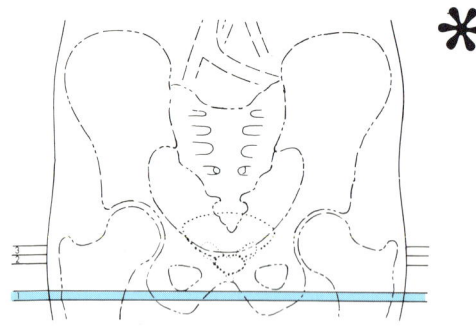

**ABDOMEN AND
PELVIS:
MALE PELVIS**

Level M1

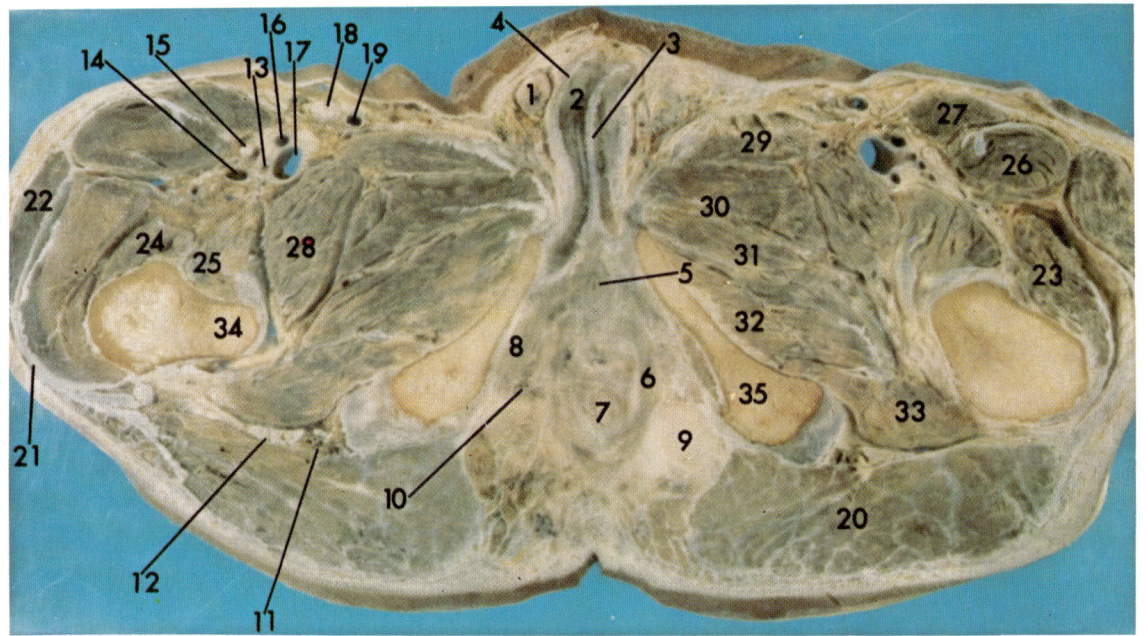

1. Spermatic cord
2. Corpus cavernosum of penis
3. Septum of penis
4. Fascia of penis
5. Cavernous urethra
6. Anal sphincter
7. Anus
8. Ischiocavernosus muscle
9. Ischiorectal fossa
10. Internal pudendal vessels
11. Inferior gluteal vessels
12. Sciatic nerve
13. Deep femoral artery
14. Deep femoral vein
15. Femoral nerve
16. Superficial femoral artery
17. Superficial femoral vein
18. Inguinal lymph node
19. Greater saphenous vein
20. Gluteus maximus muscle
21. Fascia lata
22. Tensor fasciae latae muscle
23. Vastus lateralis muscle
24. Vastus intermedius muscle
25. Iliopsoas muscle
26. Rectus femoris muscle
27. Sartorius muscle
28. Pectineus muscle
29. Adductor longus muscle
30. Adductor brevis muscle
31. Adductor minimus muscle
32. Obturator externus muscle
33. Quadratus femoris muscle
34. Lesser trochanter of femur
35. Ischium

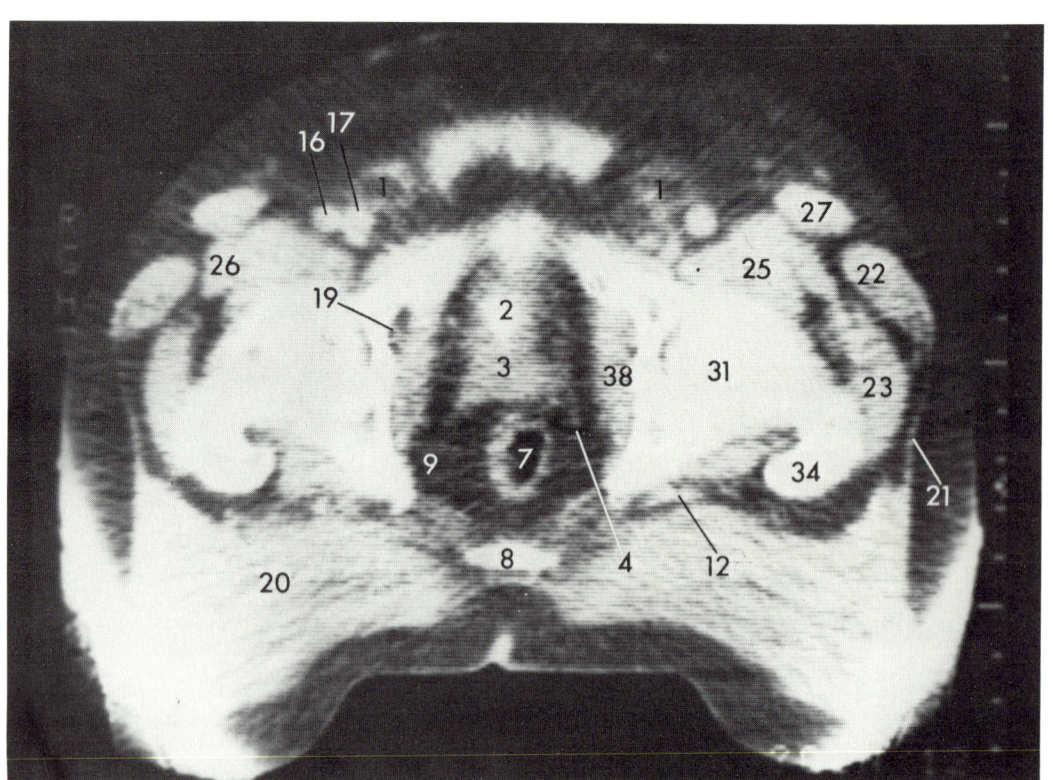

*

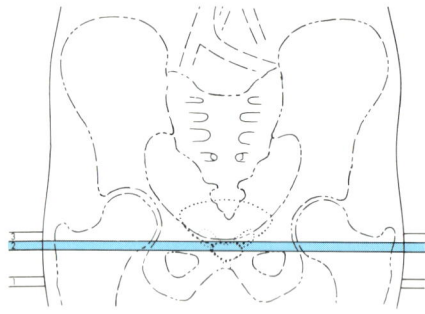

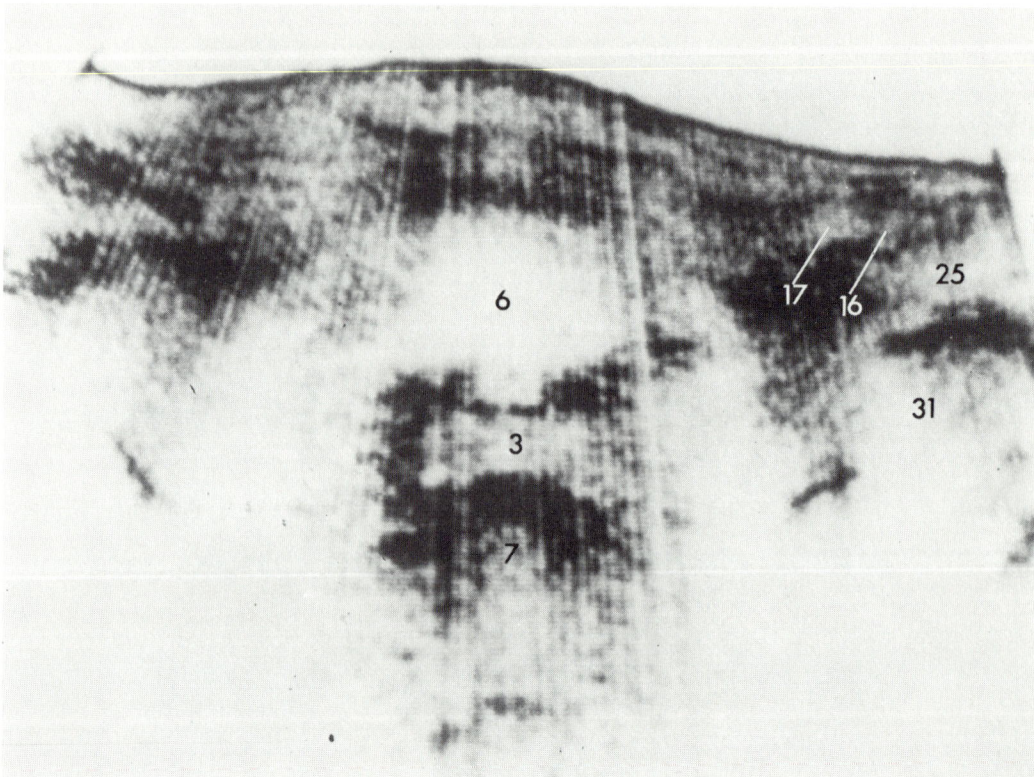

ABDOMEN AND PELVIS: MALE PELVIS

Level M2

*

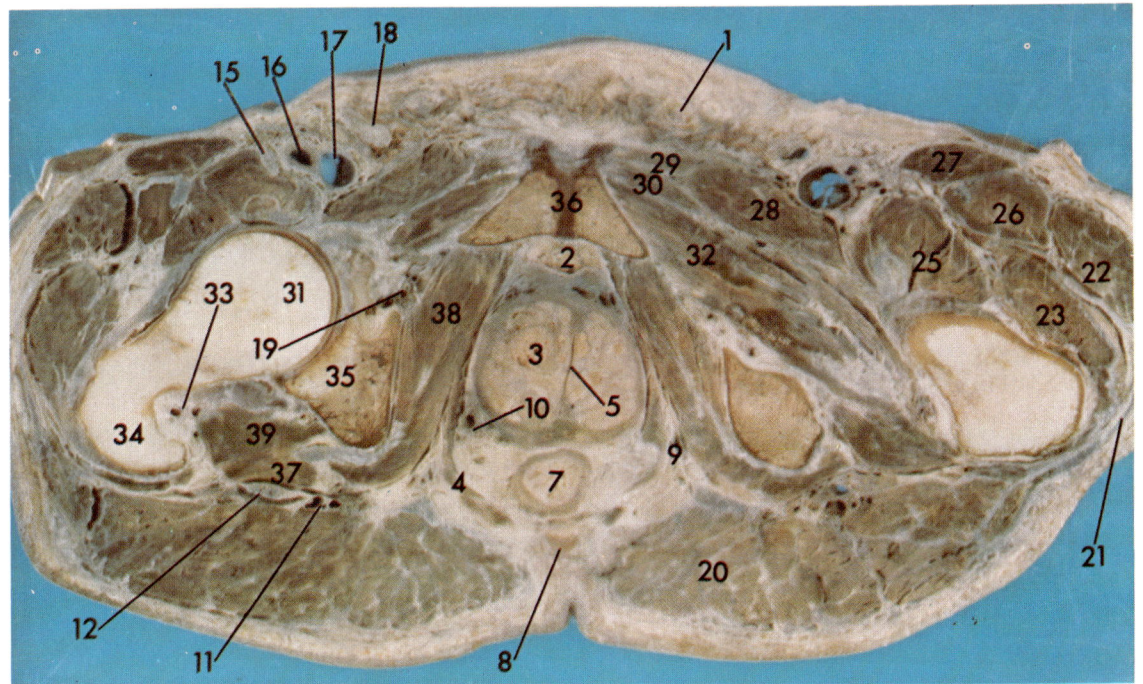

1. Spermatic cord
2. Base of bladder
3. Prostate gland
4. Levator ani muscle
5. Prostatic urethra
6. Bladder
7. Rectum
8. Coccyx
9. Ischiorectal fossa
10. Internal pudendal vessels
11. Inferior gluteal vessels
12. Sciatic nerve
15. Femoral nerve
16. Femoral artery
17. Femoral vein
18. Inguinal lymph node
19. Obturator vessels and nerves
20. Gluteus maximus muscle
21. Fascia lata
22. Tensor fasciae latae muscle
23. Vastus lateralis muscle
25. Iliopsoas muscle
26. Rectus femoris muscle
27. Sartorius muscle
28. Pectineus muscle
29. Adductor longus muscle
30. Adductor brevis muscle
31. Femoral head
32. Obturator externus muscle
33. Deep circumflex femoral vessels
34. Greater trochanter of femur
35. Ischium
36. Pubic symphysis
37. Gemellus superior muscle
38. Obturator internus muscle
39. Gemellus inferior muscle

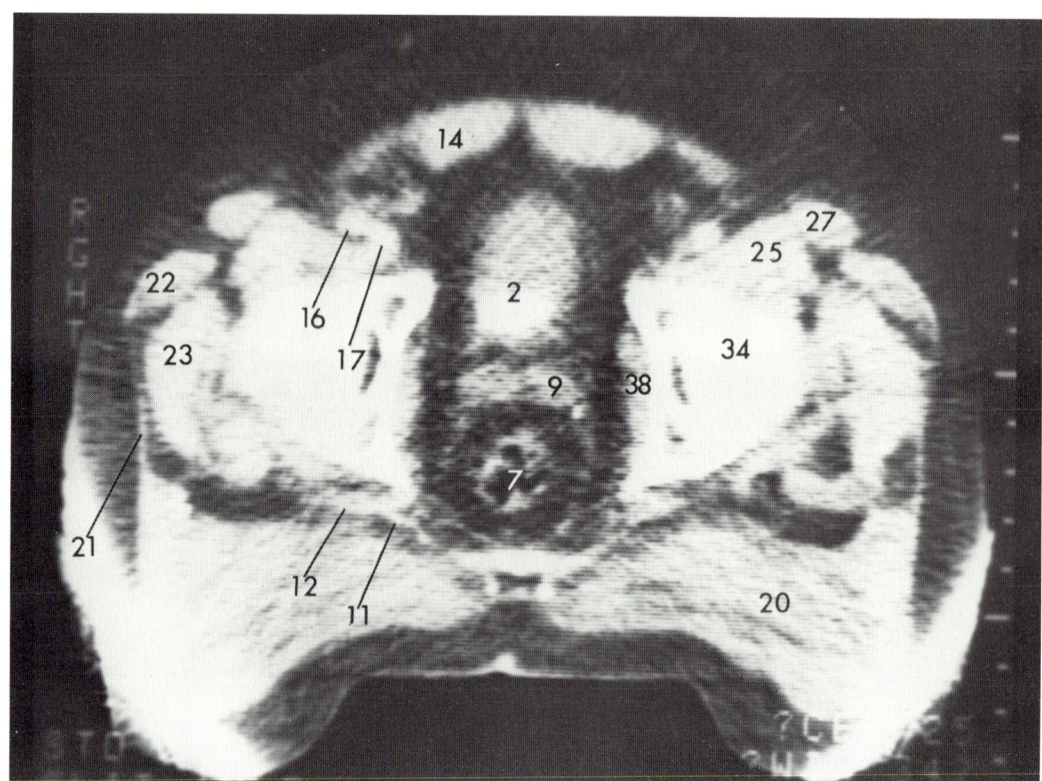

*

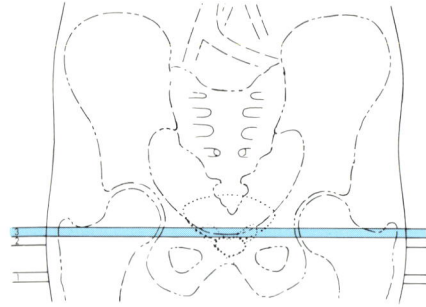

ABDOMEN AND PELVIS: MALE PELVIS

Level M3

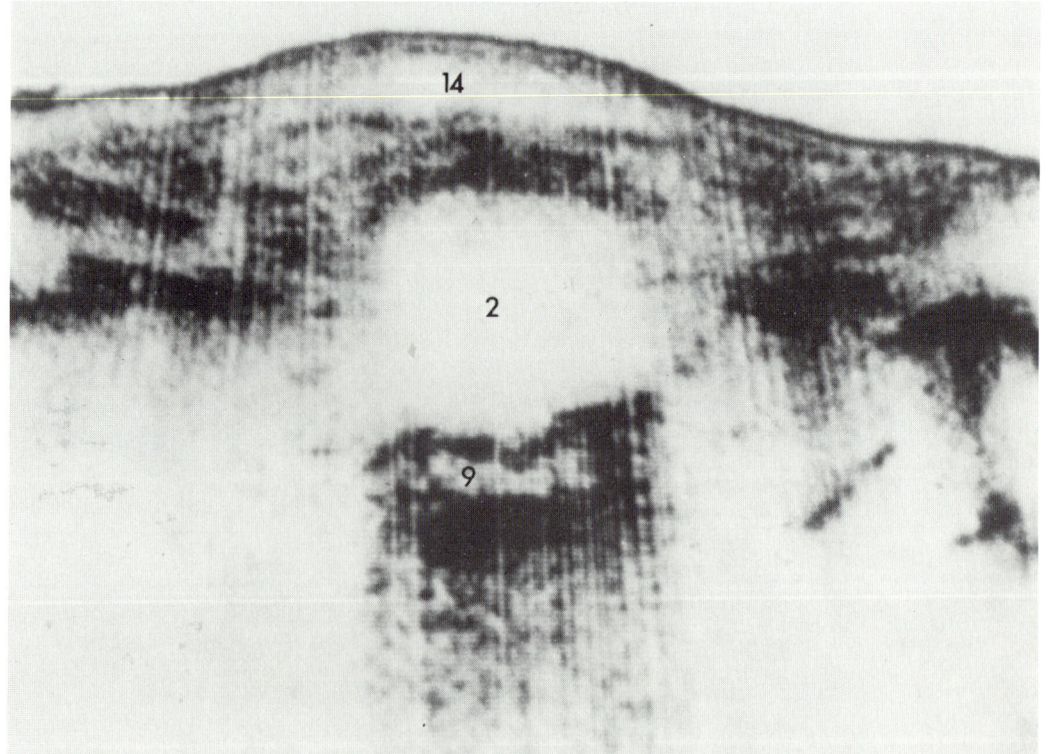

*

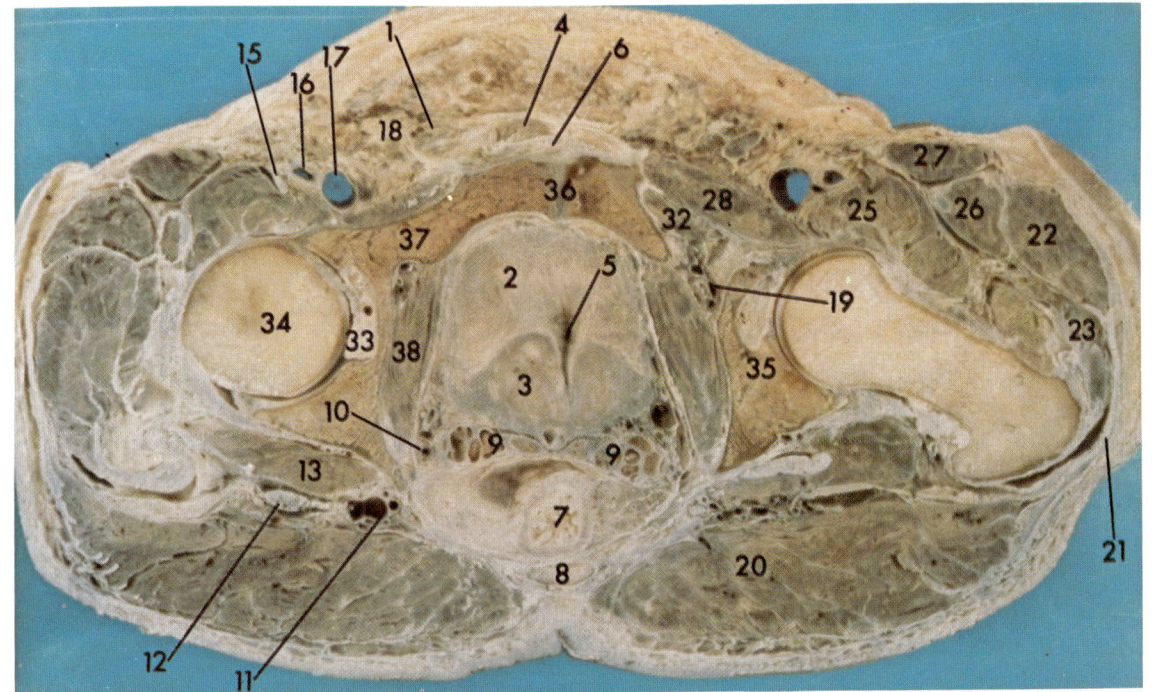

1. Spermatic cord
2. Bladder
3. Prostate gland
4. Pyramidalis muscle
5. Urethra opening into base of bladder
6. Tendon of rectus abdominis muscle
7. Rectum
8. Coccyx
9. Seminal vesicle
10. Internal pudendal vessels
11. Inferior gluteal vessels
12. Sciatic nerve
13. Piriformis muscle
14. Rectus abdominis muscle
15. Femoral nerve
16. Femoral artery
17. Femoral vein
18. Inguinal lymph node
19. Obturator vessels
20. Gluteus maximus muscle
21. Fascia lata
22. Tensor fasciae latae muscle
23. Vastus lateralis muscle
25. Iliopsoas muscle
26. Rectus femoris muscle
27. Sartorius muscle
28. Pectineus muscle
32. Obturator externus muscle
33. Acetabular fossa (fat)
34. Femoral head
35. Ischium
36. Pubic symphysis
37. Pubis
38. Obturator internus muscle

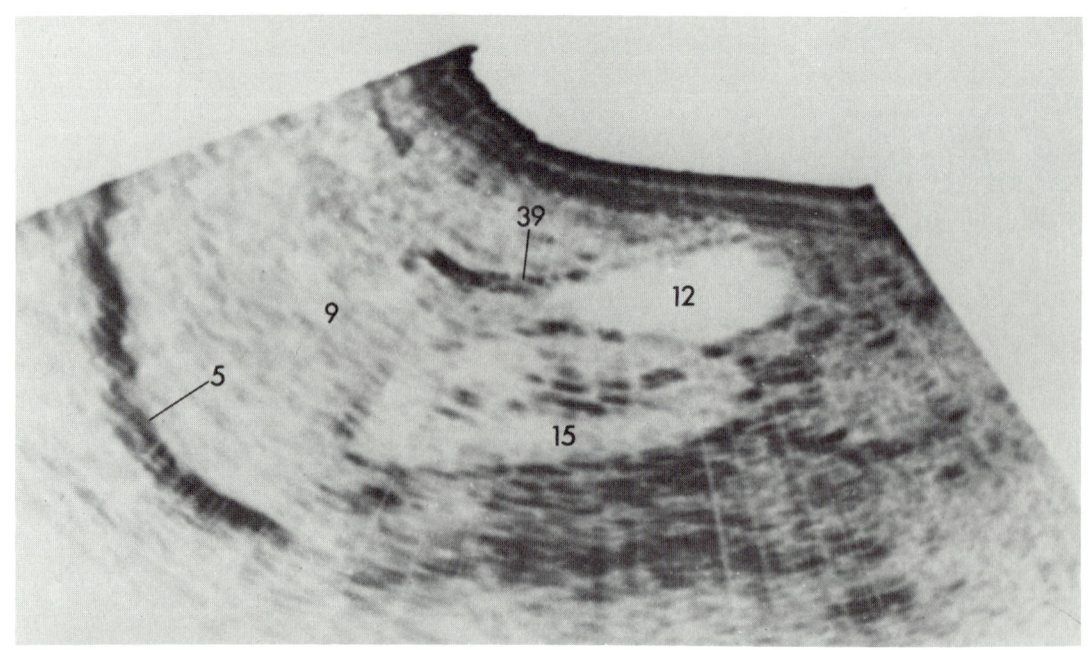

*

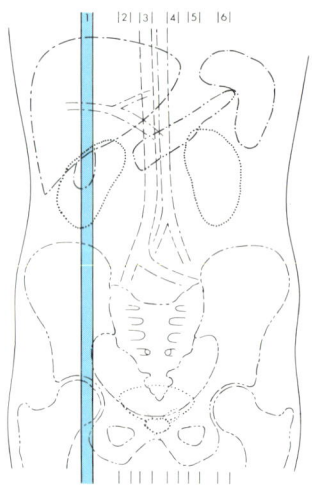

ABDOMEN AND PELVIS: LONGITUDINAL SECTION

Level L1

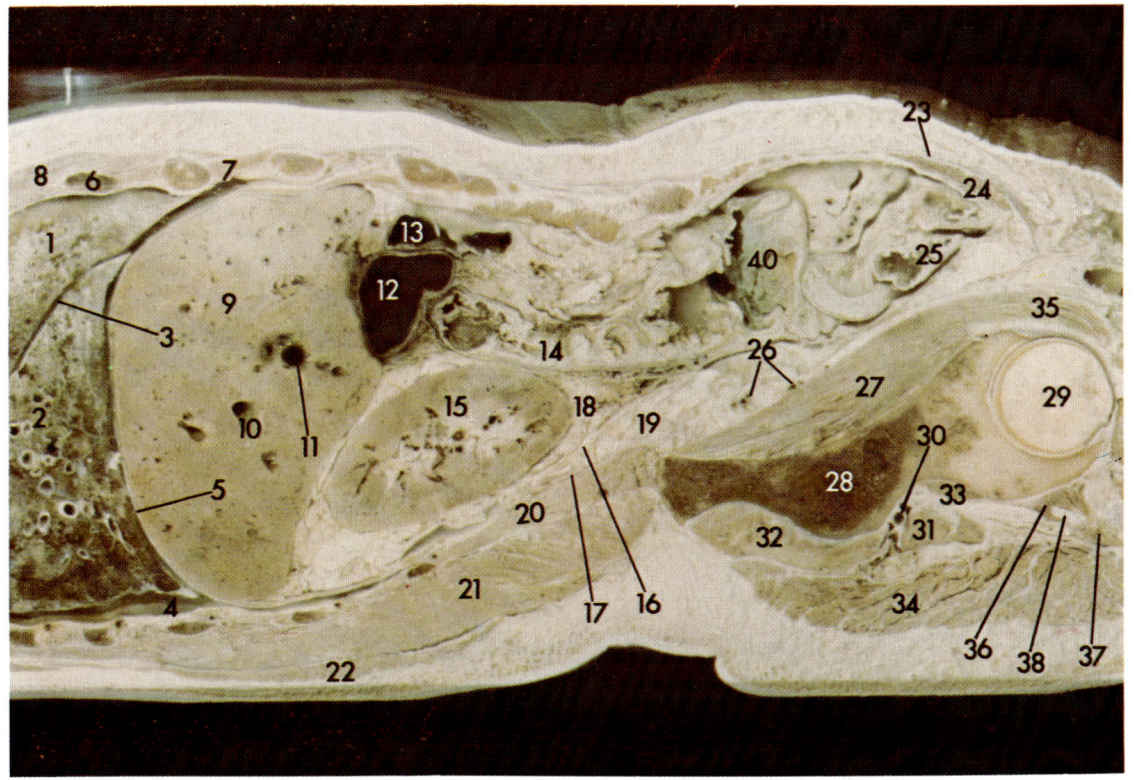

1. Middle lobe of right lung
2. Lower lobe of right lung
3. Major fissure
4. Pleural cavity
5. Right hemidiaphragm
6. Rib
7. Intercostal muscle
8. Pectoralis major muscle
9. Right lobe of liver
10. Hepatic vein
11. Portal vein
12. Gall bladder
13. Transverse colon
14. Ascending colon
15. Right kidney
16. Renal fascia (Gerota)
17. Transversalis fascia
18. Perirenal fat
19. Pararenal fat
20. Quadratus lumborum muscle
21. Erector spinae muscle
22. Latissimus dorsi muscle
23. Aponeurosis of external oblique muscle
24. Internal oblique and transversus abdominis muscles
25. Small intestine
26. Branches of iliolumbar vessels
27. Iliacus muscle
28. Ilium
29. Head of femur
30. Superior gluteal vessels
31. Piriformis muscle
32. Gluteus medius muscle
33. Gluteus minimus muscle
34. Gluteus maximus muscle
35. Iliopsoas muscle
36. Gemellus superior muscle
37. Gemellus inferior muscle
38. Obturator internus tendon
39. Cystic duct
40. Cecum

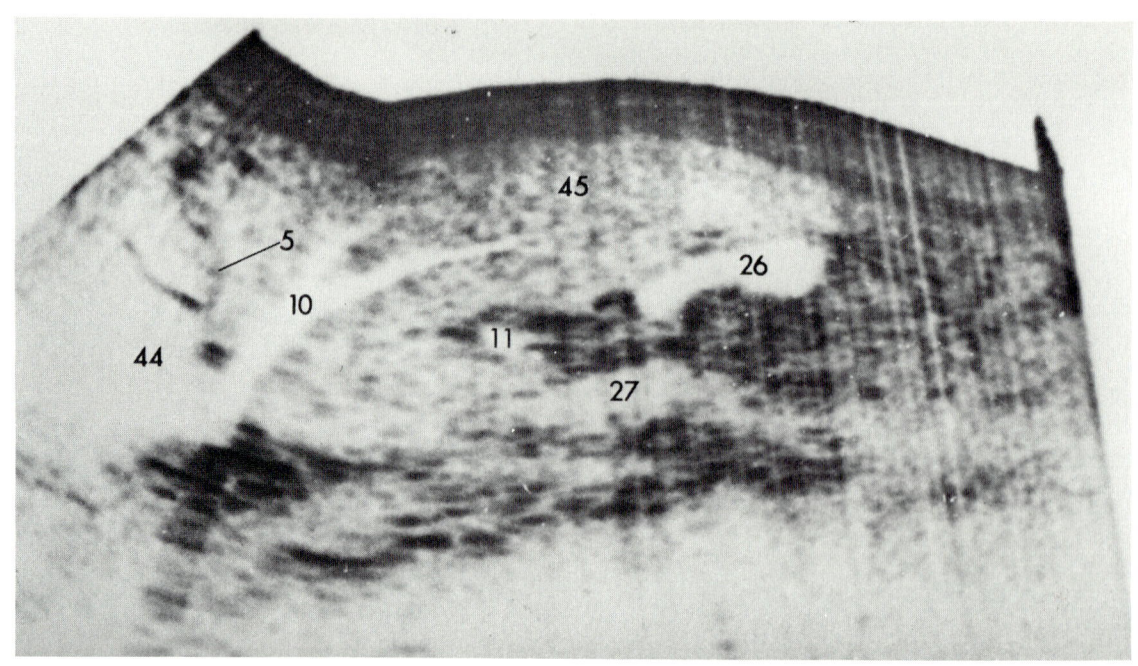

*

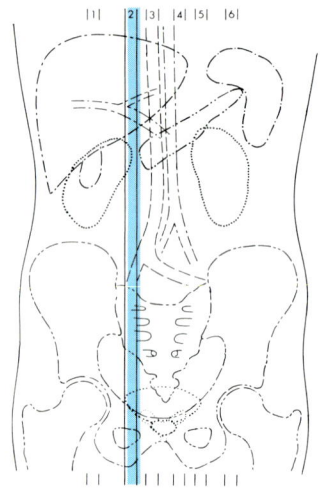

ABDOMEN AND PELVIS: LONGITUDINAL SECTION

Level L2

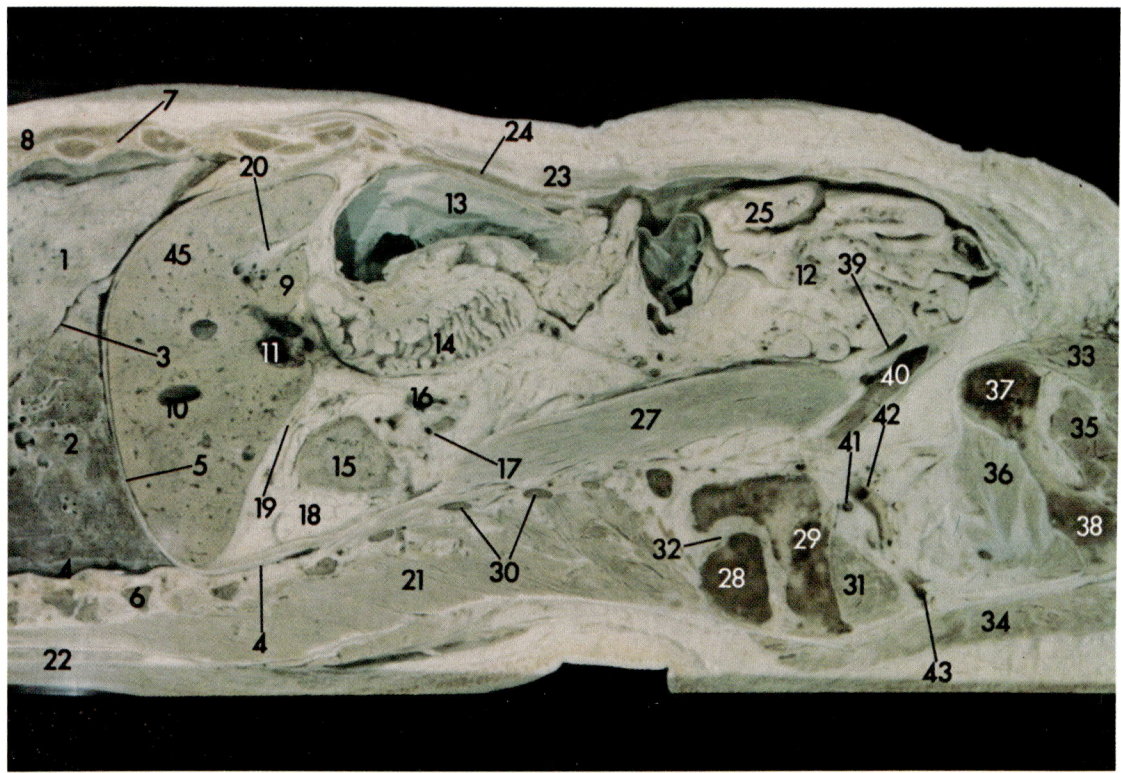

1. Middle lobe of right lung
2. Lower lobe of right lung
3. Major fissure
4. Pleural cavity
5. Right hemidiaphragm
6. Rib
7. Intercostal muscle
8. Pectoralis major muscle
9. Quadrate lobe of liver
10. Hepatic vein
11. Portal vein
12. Mesentery of small intestine
13. Transverse colon
14. Second portion of duodenum
15. Upper pole of right kidney
16. Renal vein
17. Renal artery
18. Perirenal fat
19. Right adrenal gland
20. Fat surrounding ligamentum teres
21. Erector spinae muscle
22. Latissimus dorsi muscle
23. External oblique muscle
24. Transversus abdominis muscle
25. Small intestine
26. Gall bladder
27. Psoas muscle
28. Ilium
29. Sacrum
30. Transverse process of lumbar vertebra
31. Piriformis muscle
32. Sacroiliac joint
33. Pectineus muscle
34. Gluteus maximus muscle
35. Obturator externus muscle
36. Obturator internus muscle
37. Pubis
38. Ischium
39. External iliac artery
40. External iliac vein
41. Internal iliac artery
42. Internal iliac vein
43. Superior gluteal vessels
44. Right atrium
45. Right lobe of liver

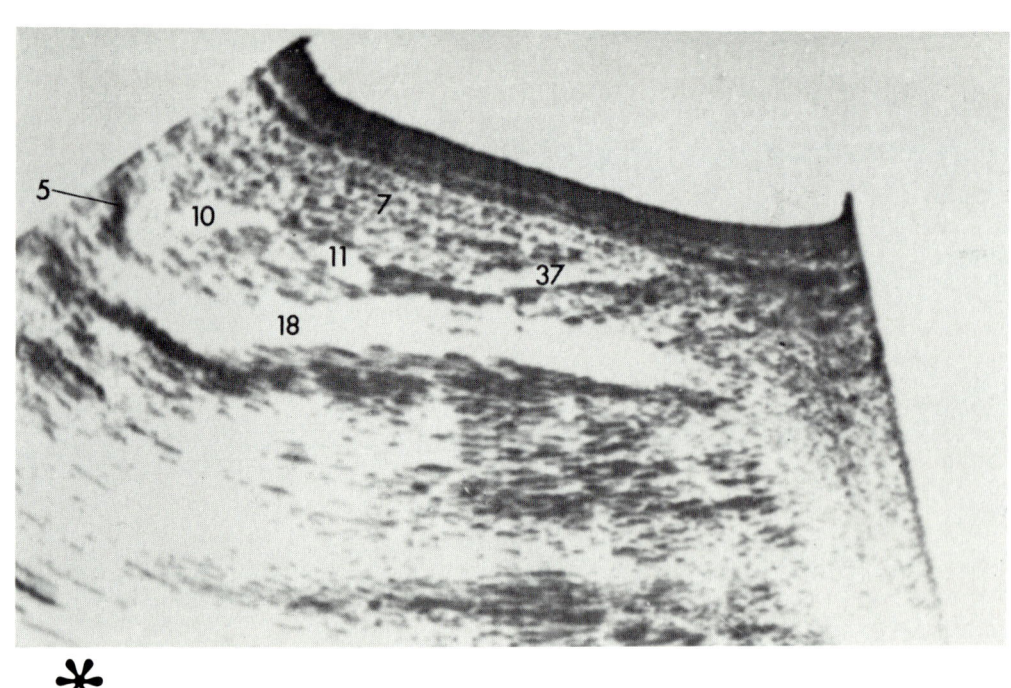

*

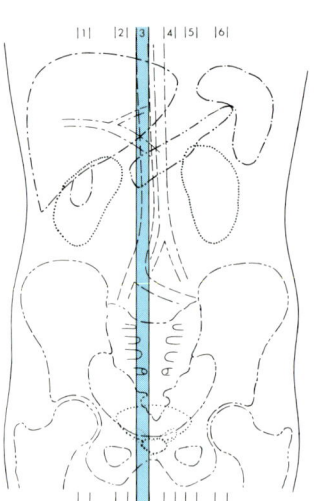

ABDOMEN AND PELVIS: LONGITUDINAL SECTION

Level L3

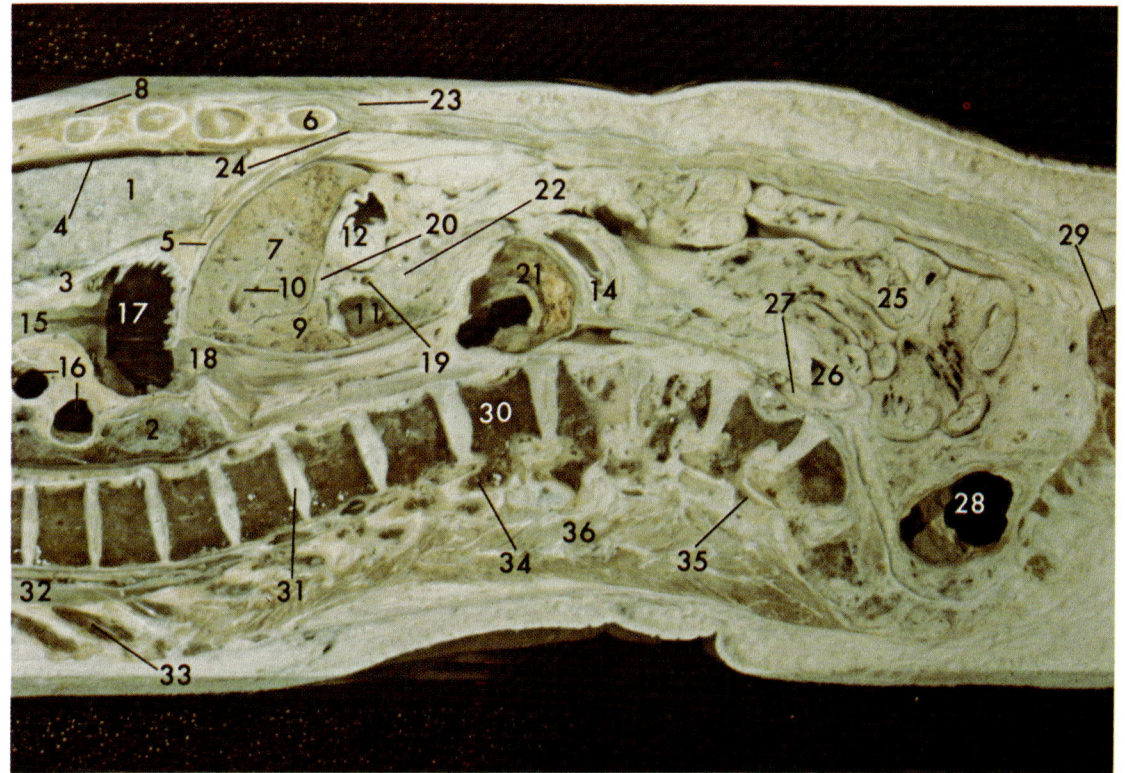

1. Middle lobe of right lung
2. Lower lobe of right lung
3. Pericardium
4. Pleural cavity
5. Right hemidiaphragm
6. Costal cartilage
7. Left lobe of liver
8. Pectoralis major muscle
9. Caudate lobe of liver
10. Hepatic vein
11. Portal vein
12. Antrum of stomach
14. Third portion of duodenum
15. Superior vena cava
16. Pulmonary veins
17. Right atrium
18. Inferior vena cava
19. Hepatic artery
20. Hepatogastric ligament (lesser omentum)
21. Abdominal aorta (aneurysm)
22. Head of pancreas
23. External oblique muscle
24. Transversus abdominis and internal oblique muscles
25. Small intestine
26. Common iliac artery
27. Common iliac vein
28. Rectum
29. Pubis
30. Body of second lumbar vertebra
31. T11–12 intervertebral disc
32. Spinal canal
33. Spinous process of eighth thoracic vertebra
34. Superior articular process of second lumbar vertebra
35. Inferior articular process of fifth lumbar vertebra
36. Erector spinae muscle
37. Superior mesenteric vein

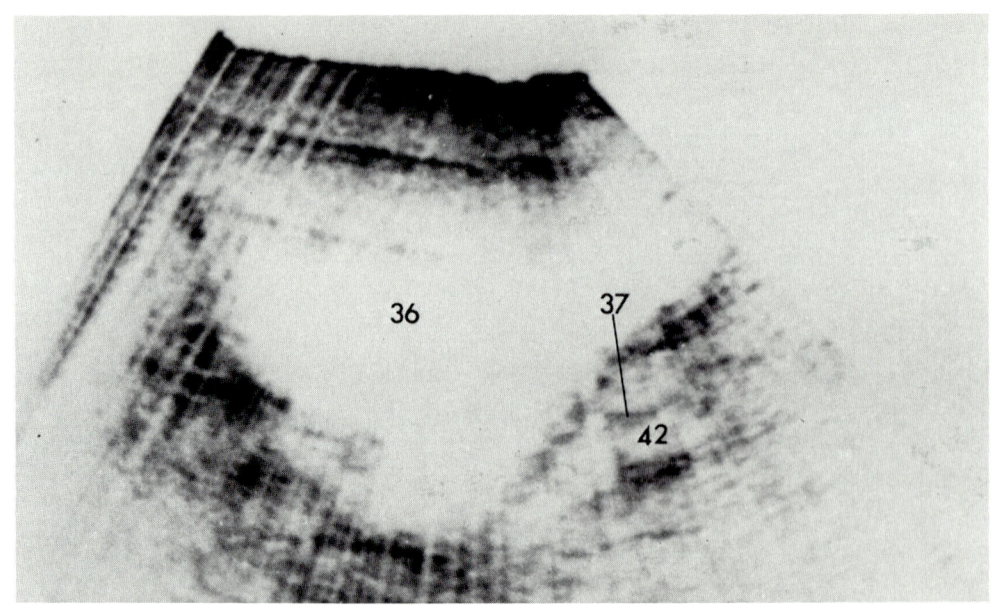

*

1. Middle lobe of right lung
2. Sternum
3. Linea alba
4. Pleural cavity
5. Left hemidiaphragm
6. Xiphoid process of sternum
7. Left lobe of liver
8. Ascending thoracic aorta
9. Esophagogastric junction
10. Left atrium
11. Descending thoracic aorta
12. Antrum of stomach

ABDOMEN AND PELVIS: LONGITUDINAL SECTION

Level L4

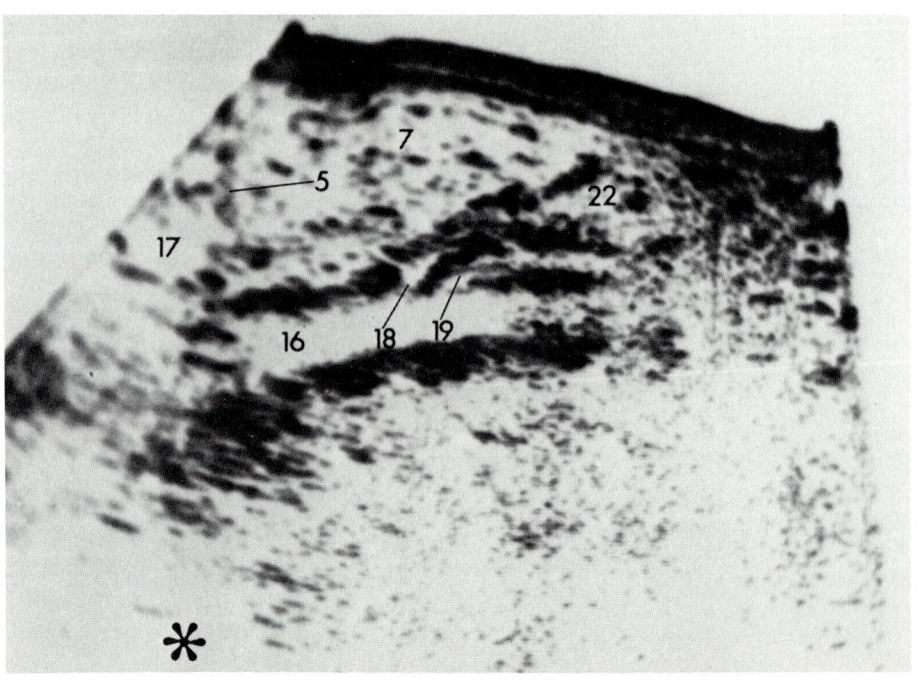

*

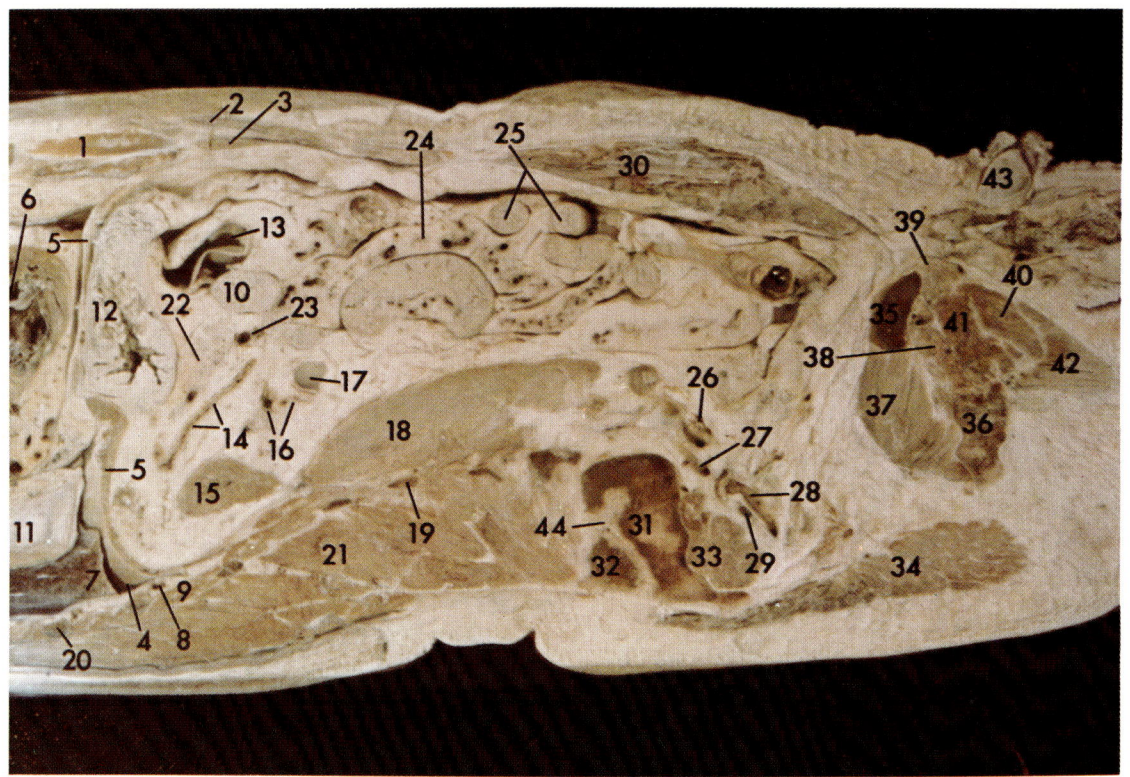

1. Costal cartilage
2. External oblique muscle
3. Transversus abdominis muscle
4. Pleural cavity
5. Left hemidiaphragm
6. Right ventricle
7. Lower lobe of left lung
8. Intercostal vessels
9. Intercostal muscle
10. Junction of duodenum and jejunum
11. Descending thoracic aorta
12. Fundus of stomach
13. Transverse colon
14. Left adrenal gland
15. Upper pole of left kidney
16. Renal vessels
17. Left renal pelvis
18. Psoas muscle
19. Transverse process of lumbar vertebra
20. Rib
21. Erector spinae muscle
22. Body of pancreas
23. Splenic vein
24. Mesentery of small intestine
25. Small intestine
26. Common iliac artery
27. Common iliac vein
28. Internal iliac artery
29. Internal iliac vein
30. Rectus abdominis muscle
31. Sacrum
32. Ilium
33. Piriformis muscle
34. Gluteus maximus muscle
35. Pubis
36. Ischium
37. Obturator internus muscle
38. Obturator externus muscle
39. Adductor longus muscle
40. Adductor brevis muscle
41. Adductor minimus muscle
42. Quadratus femoris muscle
43. Penis
44. Sacroiliac joint
45. Left lobe of liver
46. Splenic artery
47. Inferior phrenic vein
48. Antrum of stomach
49. Spleen

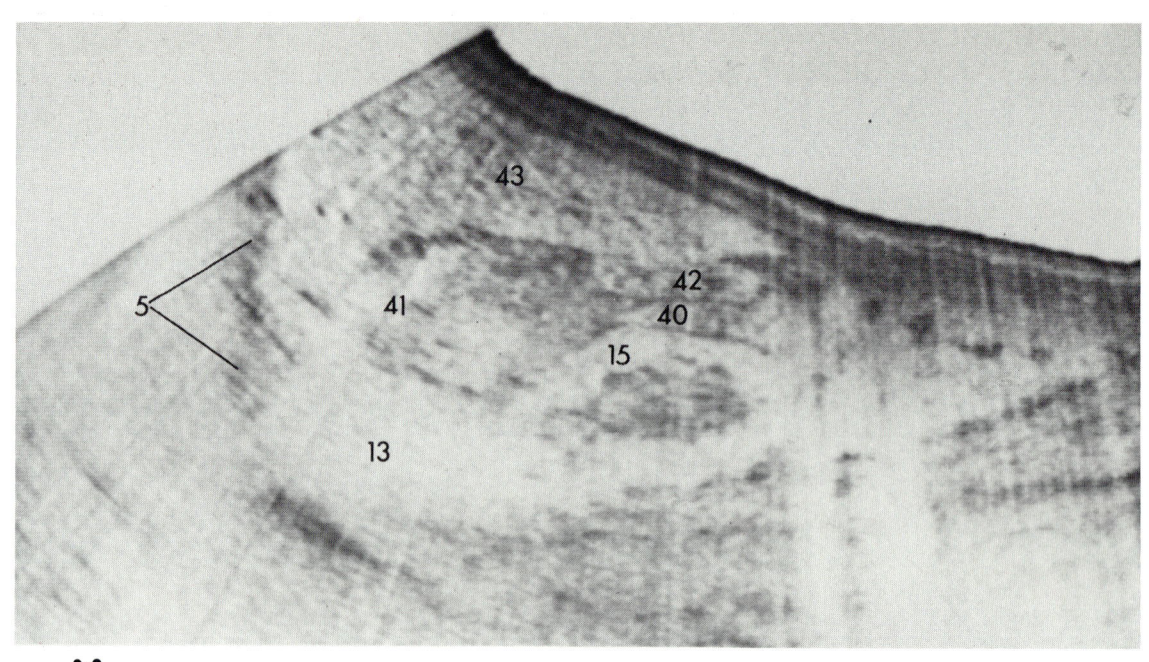

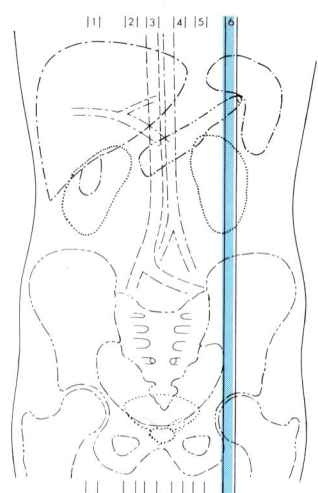

ABDOMEN AND PELVIS: LONGITUDINAL SECTION

Level L6

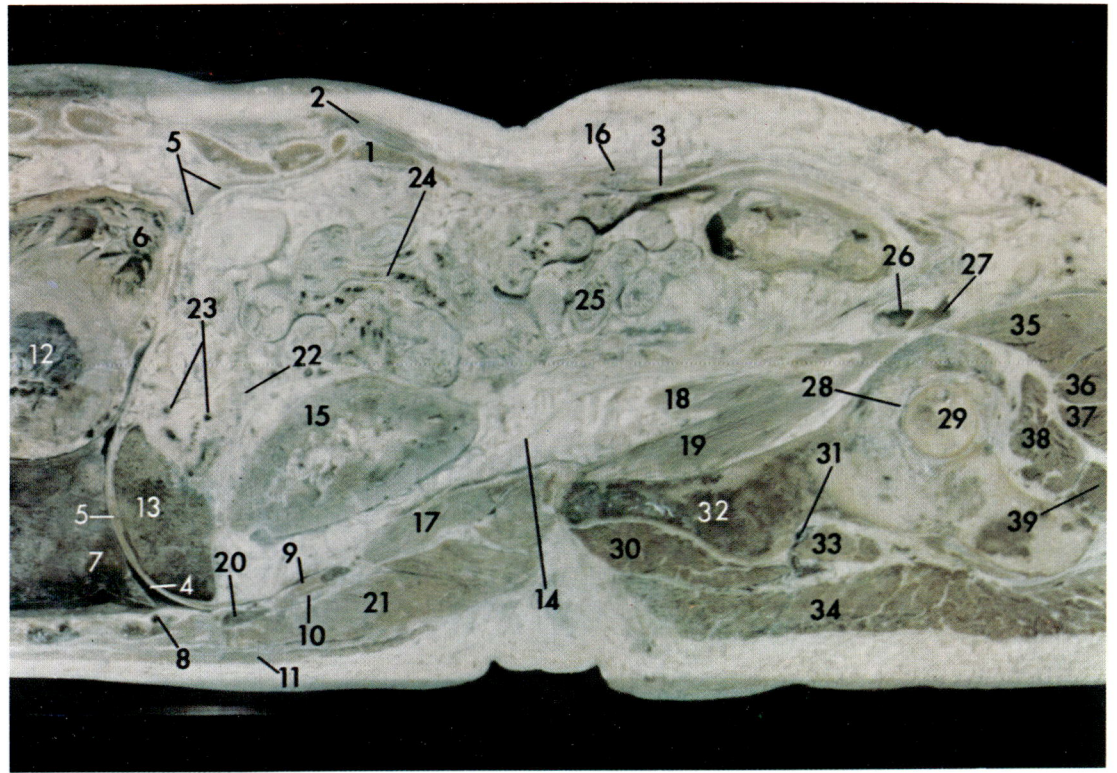

1. Costal cartilage
2. External oblique muscle
3. Transversus abdominis muscle
4. Pleural cavity
5. Left hemidiaphragm
6. Right ventricle
7. Lower lobe of left lung
8. Intercostal vessels
9. Internal intercostal muscle
10. External intercostal muscle
11. Latissimus dorsi muscle
12. Left ventricle
13. Spleen
14. Renal fascia (Gerota)
15. Left kidney
16. Internal oblique muscle
17. Quadratus lumborum muscle
18. Psoas muscle
19. Iliacus muscle
20. Rib
21. Erector spinae muscle
22. Tail of pancreas
23. Splenic vessels
24. Mesentery of small intestine
25. Small intestine
26. External iliac artery
27. External iliac vein
28. Acetabular fossa
29. Head of femur
30. Gluteus medius muscle
31. Superior gluteal vessels
32. Ilium
33. Piriformis muscle
34. Gluteus maximus muscle
35. Pectineus muscle
36. Adductor brevis muscle
37. Adductor magnus muscle
38. Obturator externus muscle
39. Quadratus femoris muscle
40. Body of pancreas
41. Fundus of stomach
42. Body of stomach
43. Left lobe of liver

219

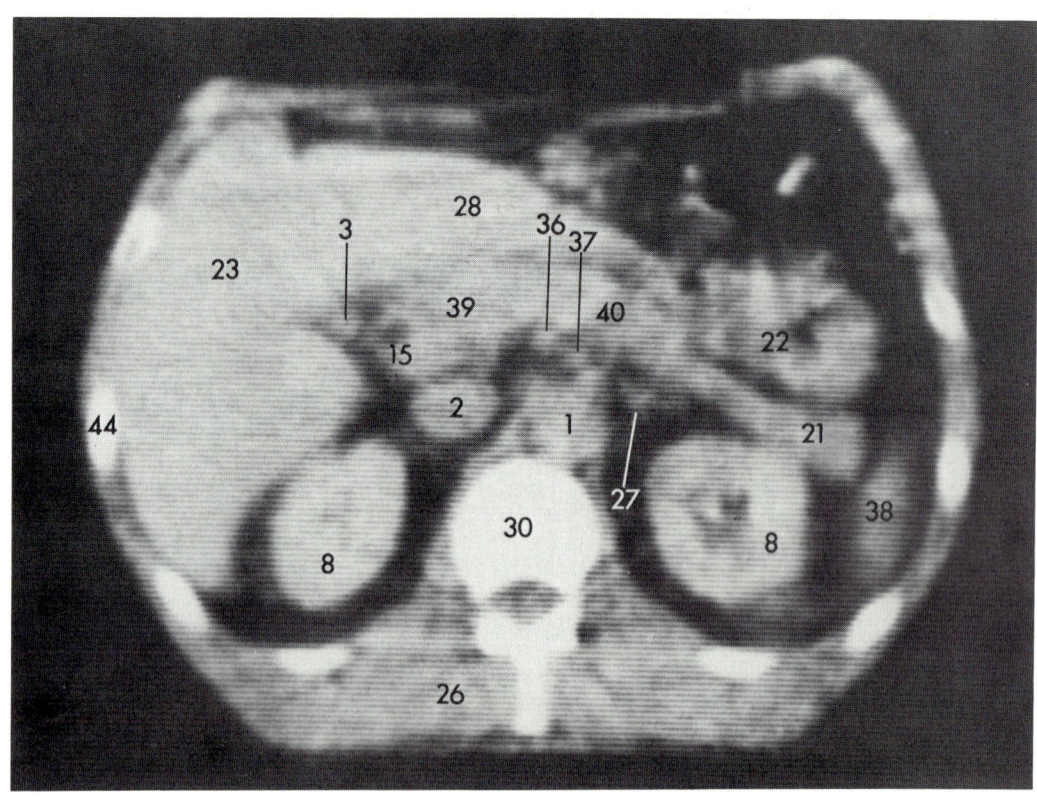

Fig. 6-1. Pancreas.

Fig. 6-2. Pancreas.

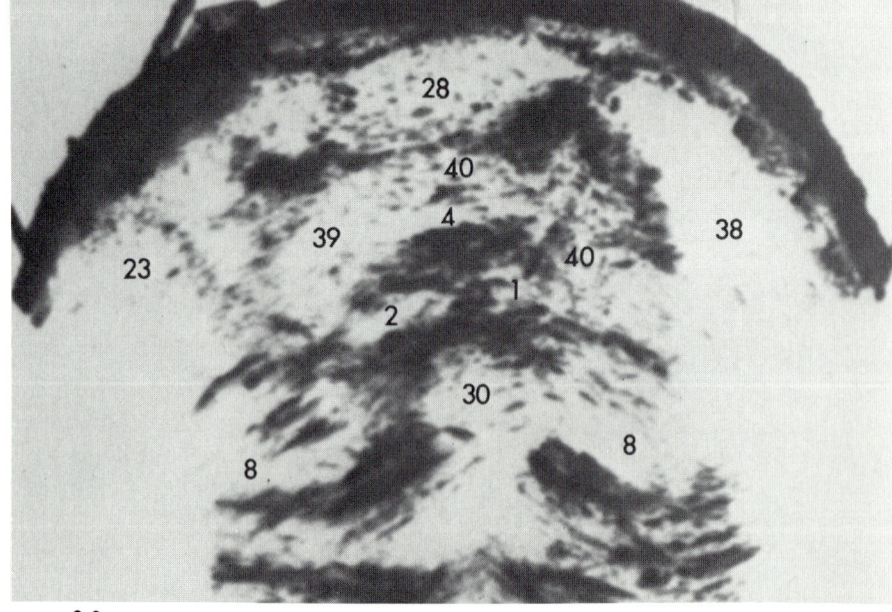

ABDOMEN AND PELVIS

Normal *In Vivo* **Studies**

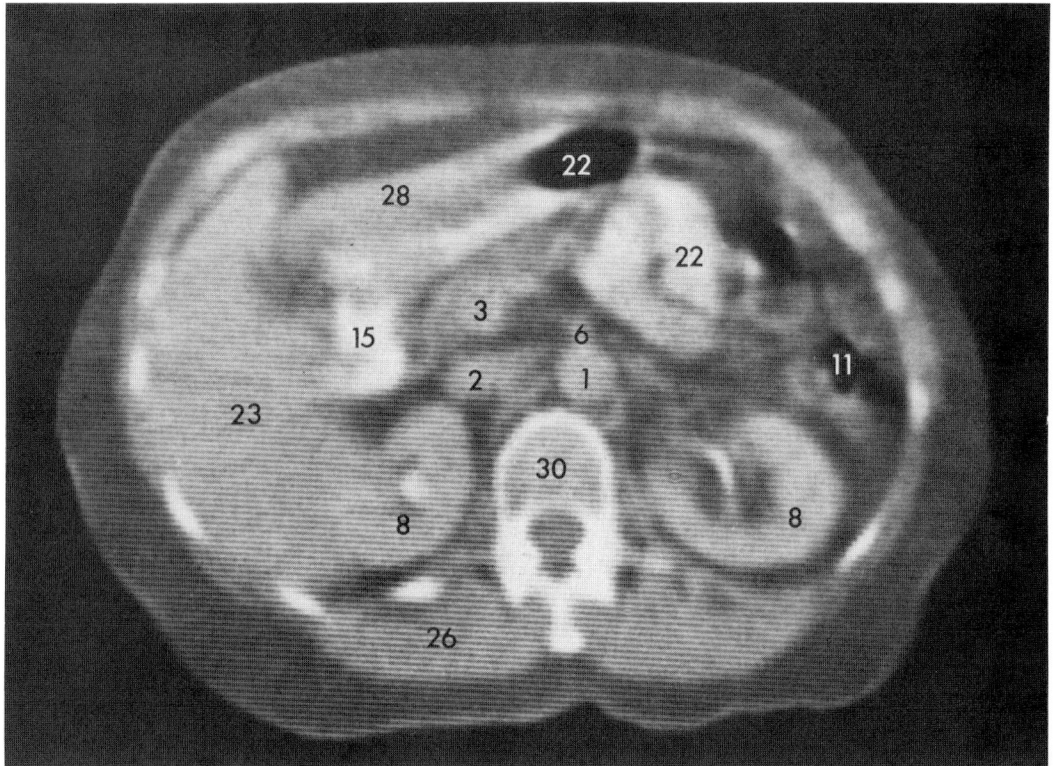

Fig. 6-3. Celiac artery and portal vein.

1. Aorta
2. Inferior vena cava
3. Portal vein
4. Splenic vein
6. Celiac artery
8. Kidney
11. Descending colon
12. Left crus of diaphragm
13. Right crus of diaphragm
15. Second portion of duodenum
17. Left renal vein
18. Right renal artery
21. Tail of pancreas
22. Stomach
23. Right lobe of liver
26. Erector spinae muscle
27. Left adrenal gland
28. Left lobe of liver
30. Body of lumbar vertebra
36. Superior mesenteric vein
37. Superior mesenteric artery
38. Spleen
39. Head of pancreas
40. Body of pancreas
44. Rib
46. Right branch of portal vein

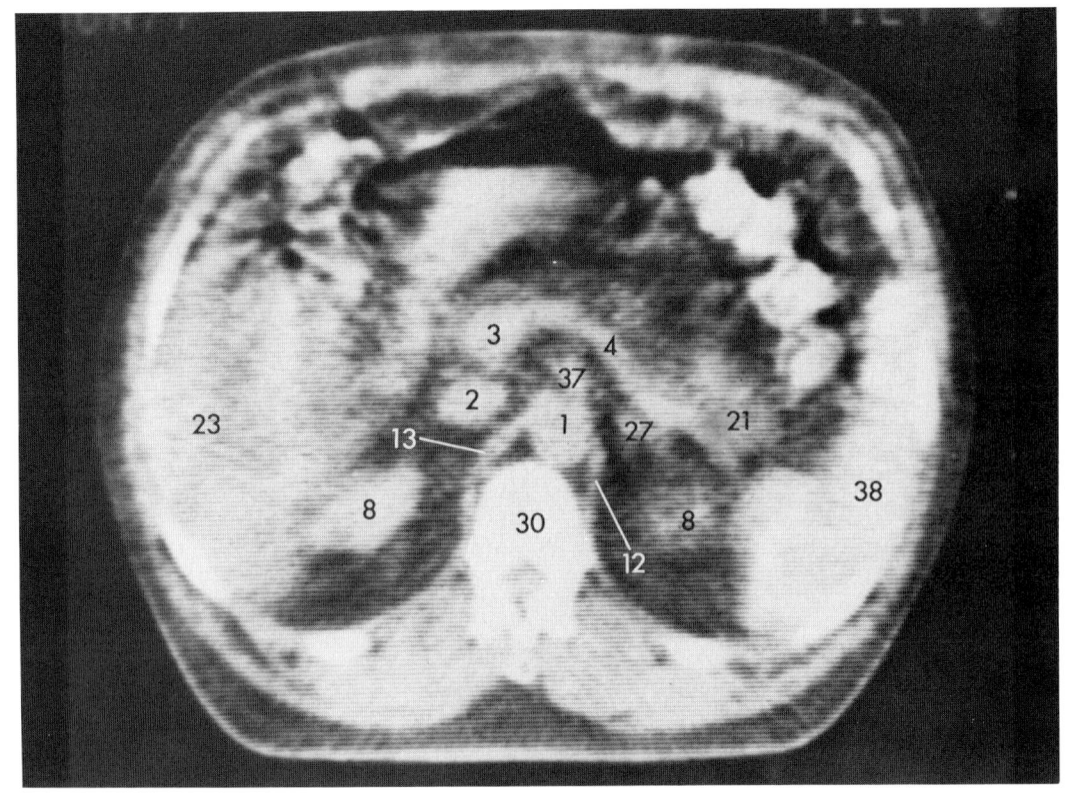

Fig. 6-4. Splenic and portal veins.

Fig. 6-5. Splenic and portal veins.

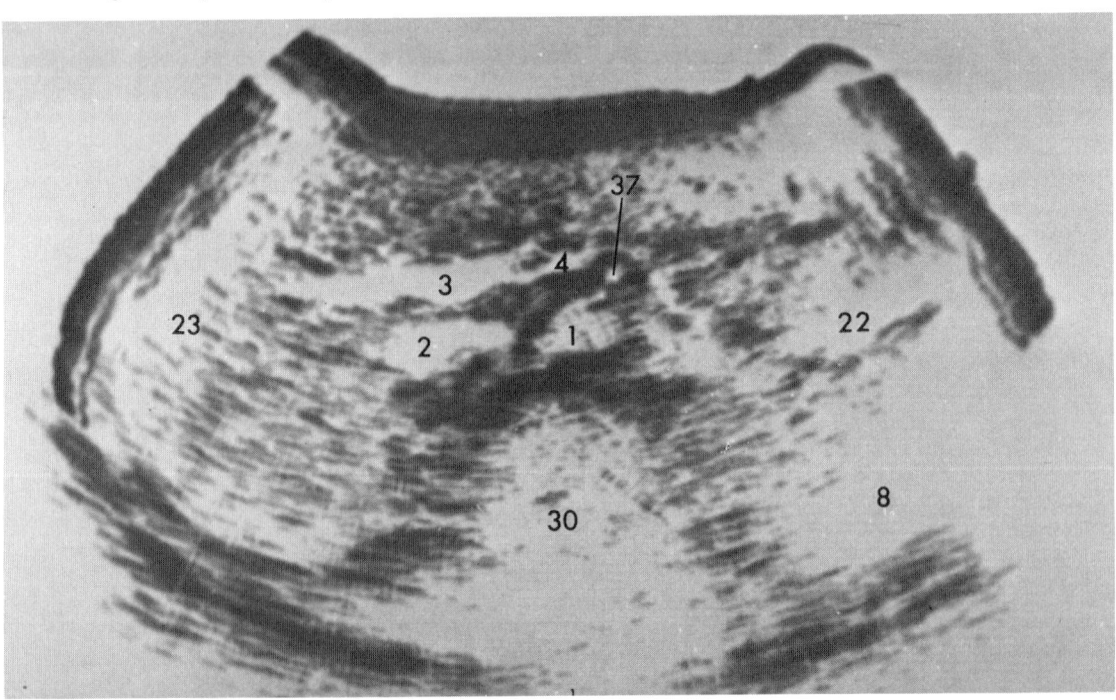

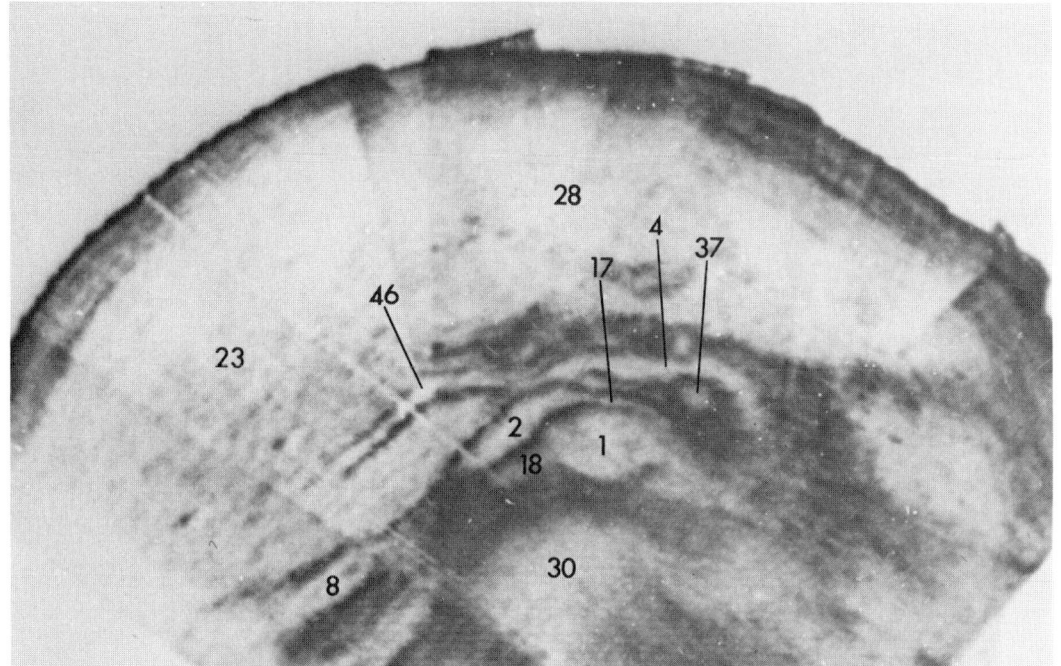

Fig. 6-6. Splenic vein and left renal vein.

1. Aorta
2. Inferior vena cava
3. Portal vein
4. Splenic vein
6. Celiac artery
8. Kidney
11. Descending colon
12. Left crus of diaphragm
13. Right crus of diaphragm
15. Second portion of duodenum
17. Left renal vein
18. Right renal artery
21. Tail of pancreas
22. Stomach
23. Right lobe of liver
26. Erector spinae muscle
27. Left adrenal gland
28. Left lobe of liver
30. Body of lumbar vertebra
36. Superior mesenteric vein
37. Superior mesenteric artery
38. Spleen
39. Head of pancreas
40. Body of pancreas
44. Rib
46. Right branch of portal vein

7
Extremities

E. MARK LEVINSOHN

An effort has been made in this chapter to limit the number of levels to those that demonstrate key areas of anatomy. Where profound changes occur over short distances, e.g., in the vicinity of joints, sequential levels have been shown. In general, the anatomic slices are viewed from below (distal aspect). However, at three levels (W3, A3, K2) the gross anatomy was best seen from above and at these levels the gross specimens are shown as visualized from above (proximal aspect).* Studies of the region of the hip joints may be found in Chapter 6, The Abdomen and Pelvis.

Some distortion of gross anatomy occurred in the preparation and fixation of the cadaver. This was most marked in the muscular regions of the midhumerus and midthigh and at the elbow joint. Sections of the elbow were obtained with the elbow flexed 115 degrees, and the reader is cautioned that these levels do not display true "transaxial" cross-sectional anatomy. Also, the computed tomographic studies in the region of the elbow were performed after the humerus had been sectioned, allowing some air into the brachial vessels.

Computed tomography of the shoulder region was obtained with a 45-cm scanning circle diameter. A 25- or 29-cm scanning circle was used for all other levels. Computed tomographic studies of the extremities were obtained with a center setting of approximately 100 Hounsfield units and a window width of approximately 500 Hounsfield units, a combination which was found to be optimal for demonstration of the combination of bone and soft-tissue structures. When bony detail was desired without particular need for soft-tissue detail, a center of 200–250 Hounsfield units with a window width of 600–700 Hounsfield units has proved to be optimal.

*In order to maintain consistency of the left and right sides, the photographs of the gross specimens at these levels have been reversed left for right in printing.

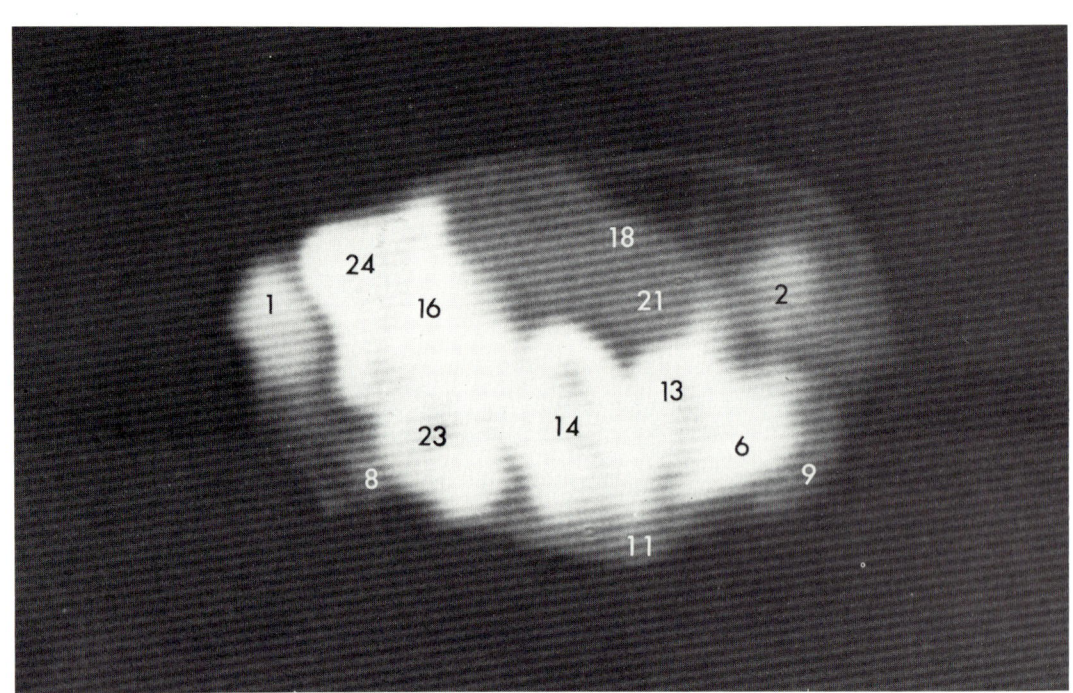

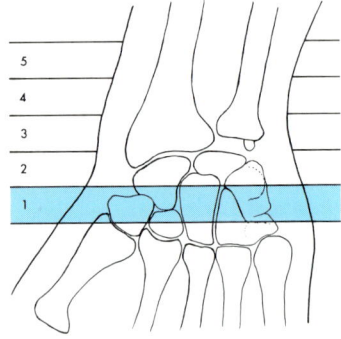

EXTREMITIES: WRIST

Level W1

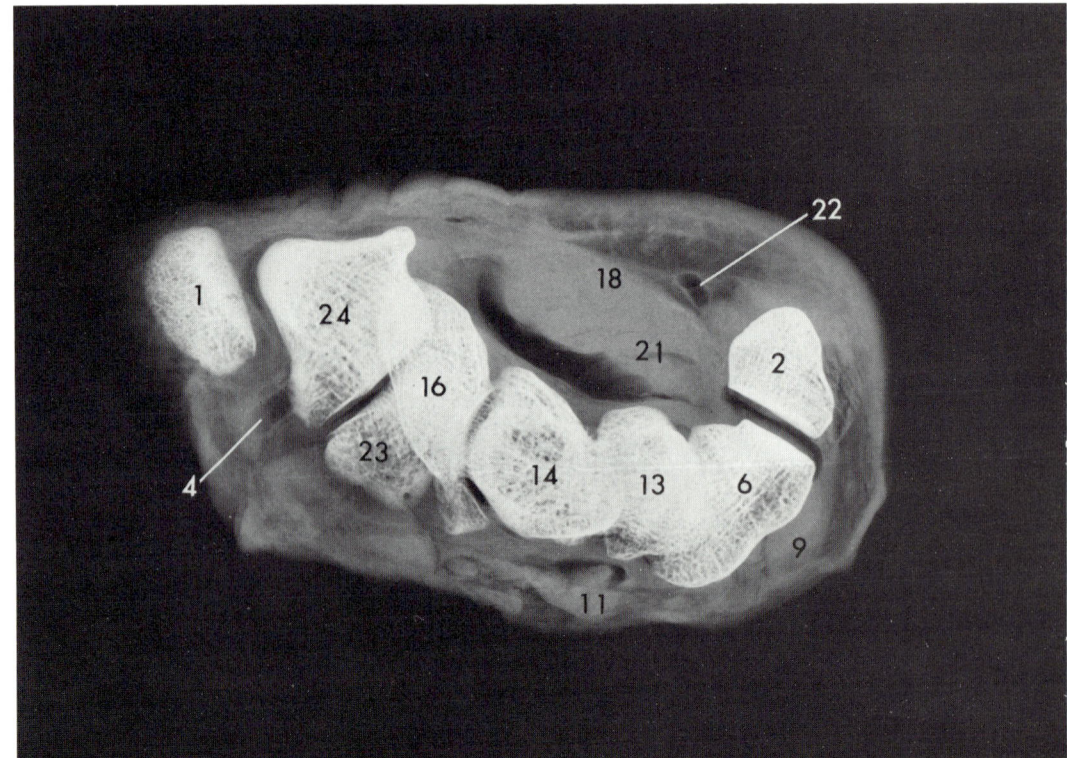

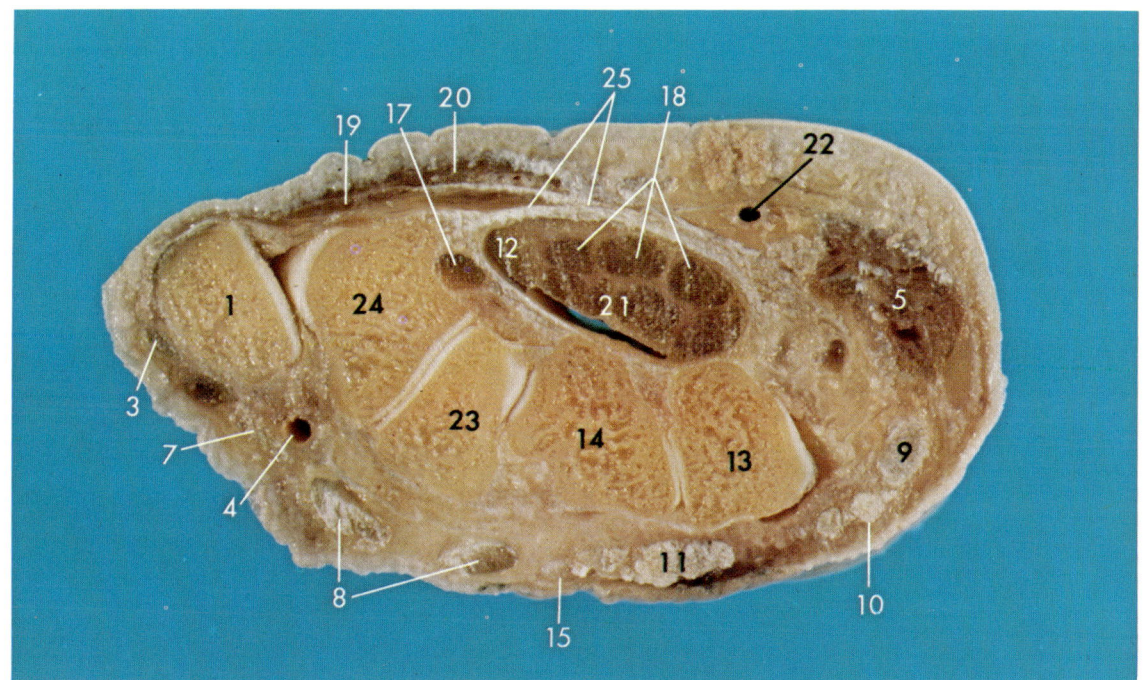

1. First metacarpal
2. Pisiform
3. Extensor pollicis brevis tendon
4. Radial artery
5. Abductor digiti minimi muscle
6. Triquetrum
7. Extensor pollicis longus tendon
8. Extensor carpi radialis longus and brevis tendons
9. Extensor carpi ulnaris tendon
10. Extensor digiti minimi tendon
11. Extensor digitorum tendons
12. Flexor pollicis longus tendon
13. Hamate
14. Capitate
15. Extensor indicis tendon
16. Navicular
17. Flexor carpi radialis tendon
18. Flexor digitorum superficialis tendons
19. Opponens pollicis muscle
20. Abductor pollicis brevis muscle
21. Flexor digitorum profundus tendons
22. Ulnar artery
23. Lesser multangular (trapezoid)
24. Greater multangular (trapezium)
25. Flexor retinaculum

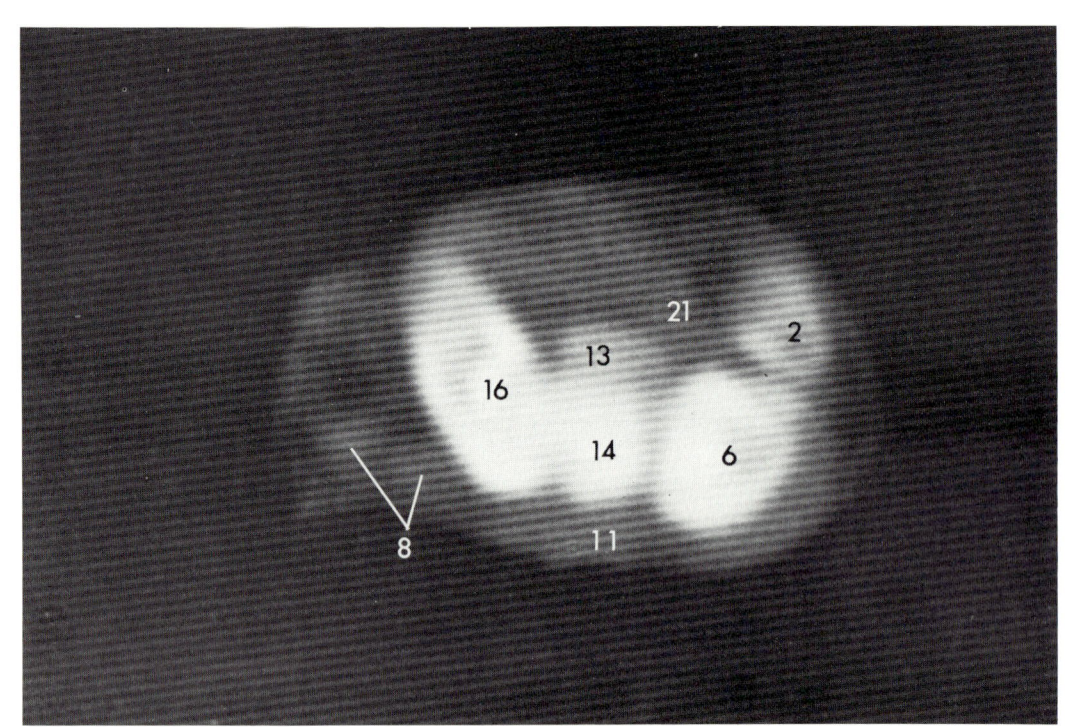

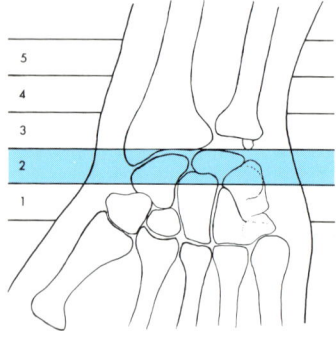

EXTREMITIES: WRIST

Level W2

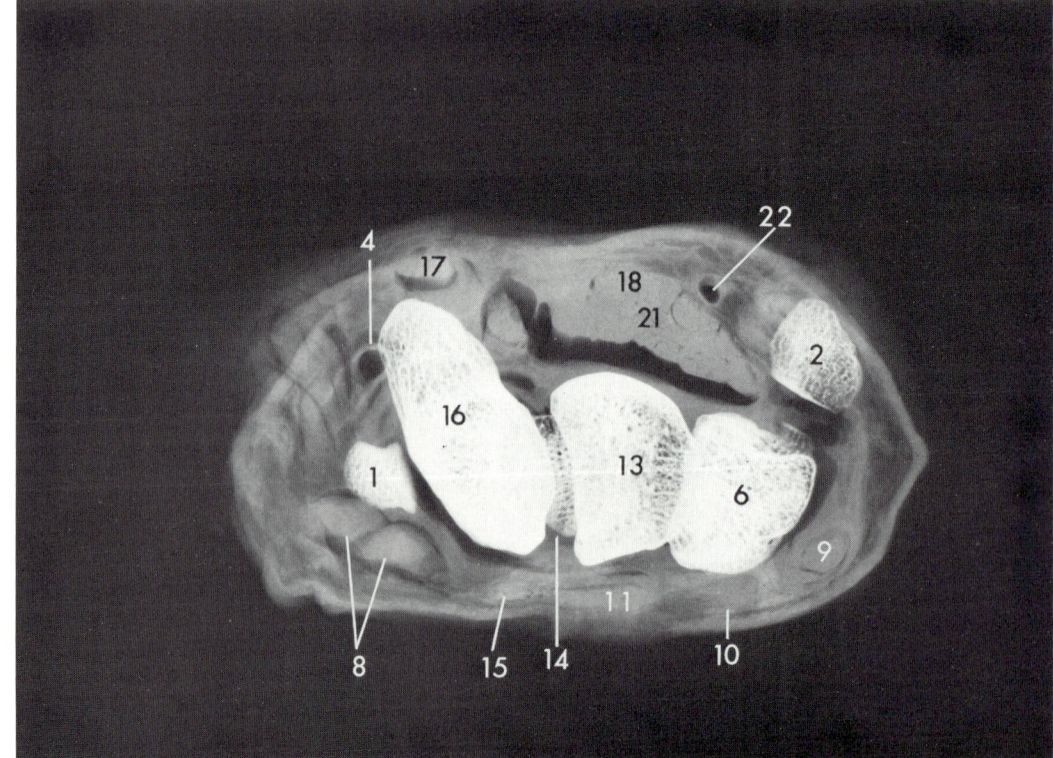

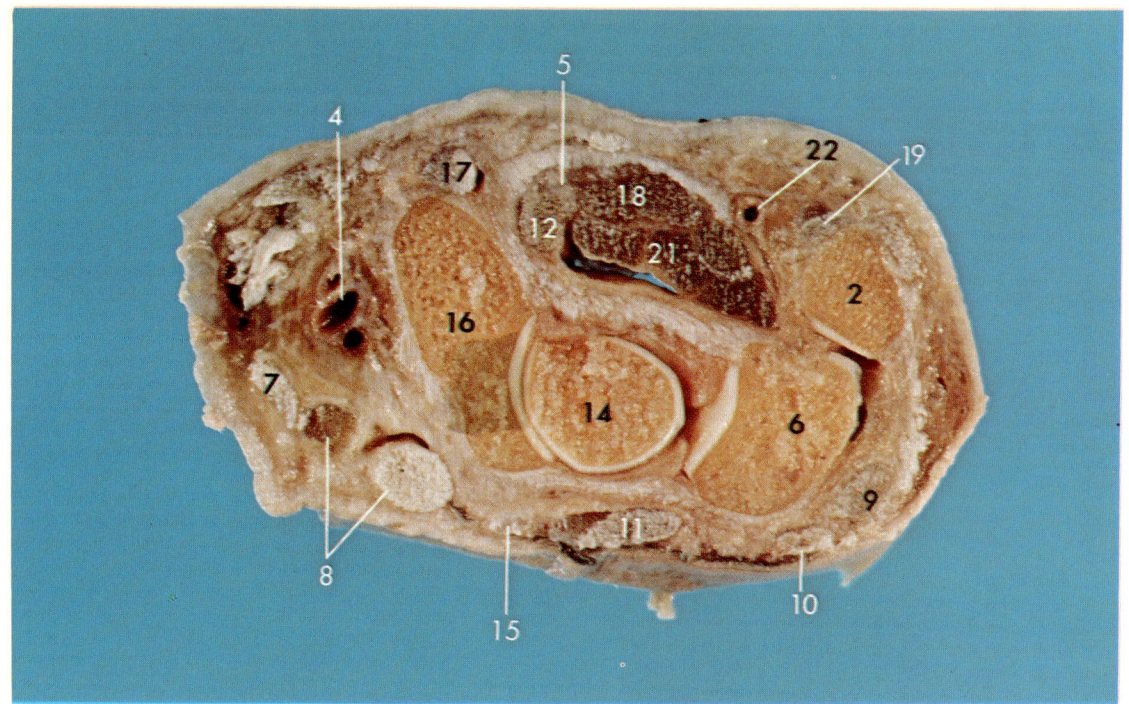

1. Styloid process of radius
2. Pisiform
4. Radial artery
5. Median nerve
6. Triquetrum
7. Extensor pollicis longus tendon
8. Extensor carpi radialis longus and brevis tendons
9. Extensor carpi ulnaris tendon
10. Extensor digiti minimi tendon
11. Extensor digitorum tendons
12. Flexor pollicis longus tendon
13. Lunate
14. Capitate
15. Extensor indicis tendon
16. Navicular
17. Flexor carpi radialis tendon
18. Flexor digitorum superficialis tendons
19. Flexor carpi ulnaris tendon
21. Flexor digitorum profundus tendons
22. Ulnar artery

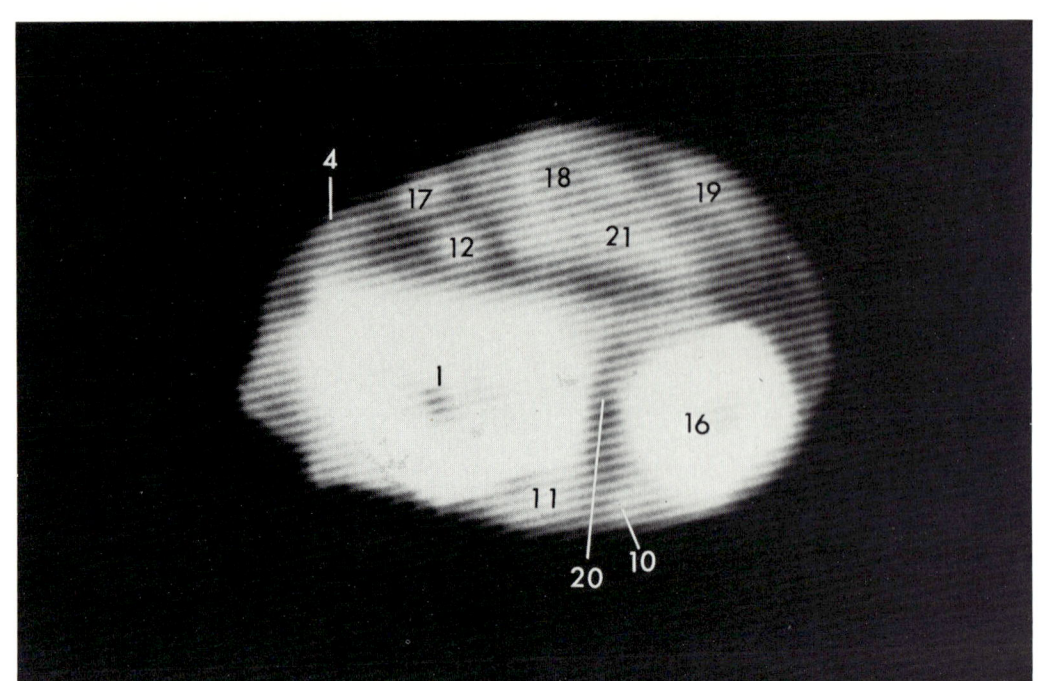

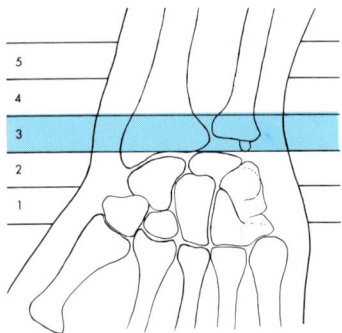

EXTREMITIES: WRIST

**Level W3
(Superior [proximal] aspect)**

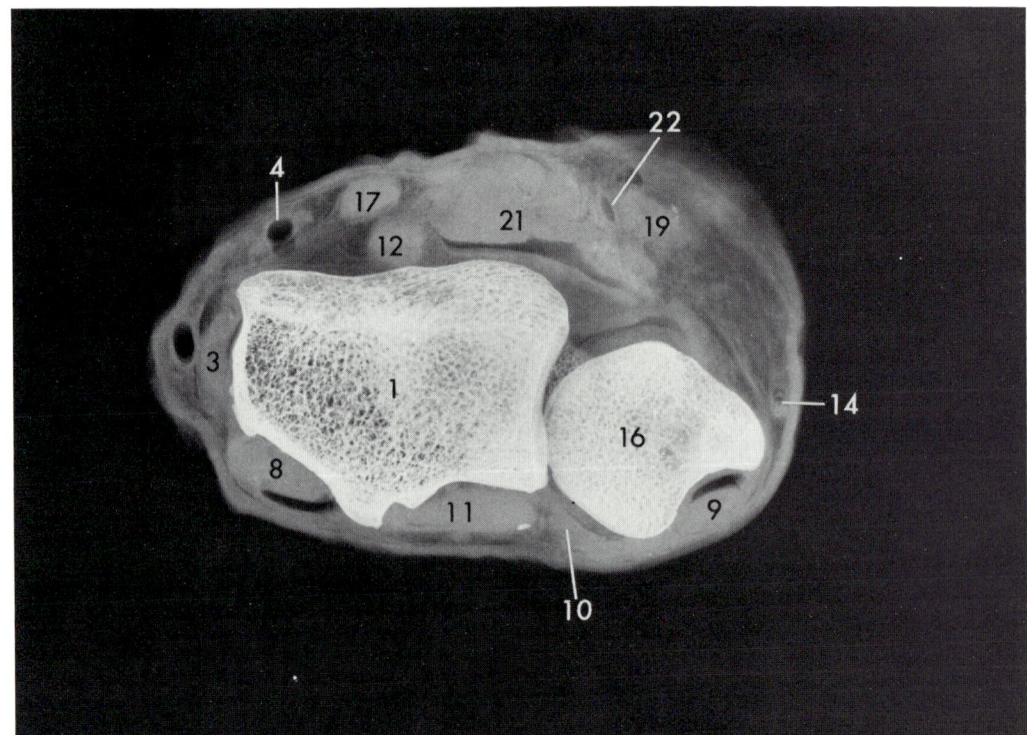

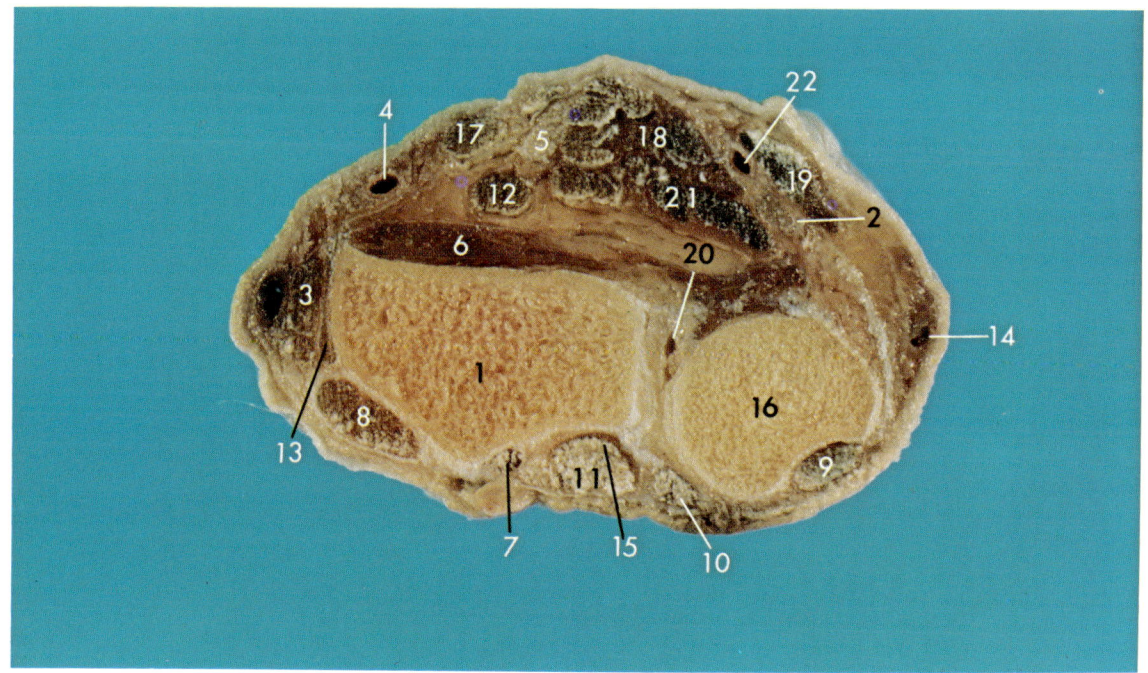

1. Radius
2. Ulnar nerve
3. Abductor pollicis longus and extensor pollicis brevis tendons
4. Radial artery
5. Median nerve
6. Pronator quadratus muscle
7. Extensor pollicis longus tendon
8. Extensor carpi radialis longus and brevis tendons
9. Extensor carpi ulnaris tendon
10. Extensor digiti minimi tendon
11. Extensor digitorum tendons
12. Flexor pollicis longus muscle
13. Brachioradialis tendon
14. Basilic vein
15. Extensor indicis tendon
16. Ulna
17. Flexor carpi radialis tendon
18. Flexor digitorum superficialis muscle and tendon
19. Flexor carpi ulnaris muscle
20. Distal radioulnar joint cavity
21. Flexor digitorum profundus muscle and tendon
22. Ulnar artery

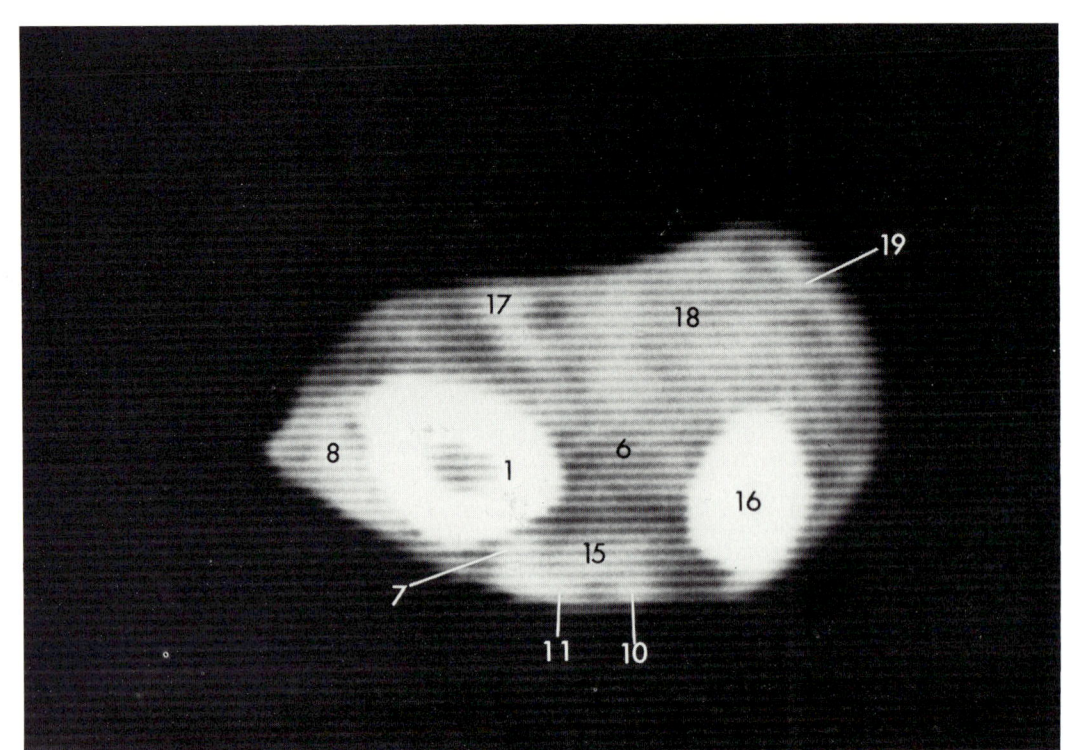

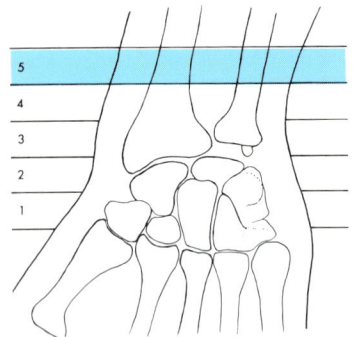

EXTREMITIES: WRIST

Level W5

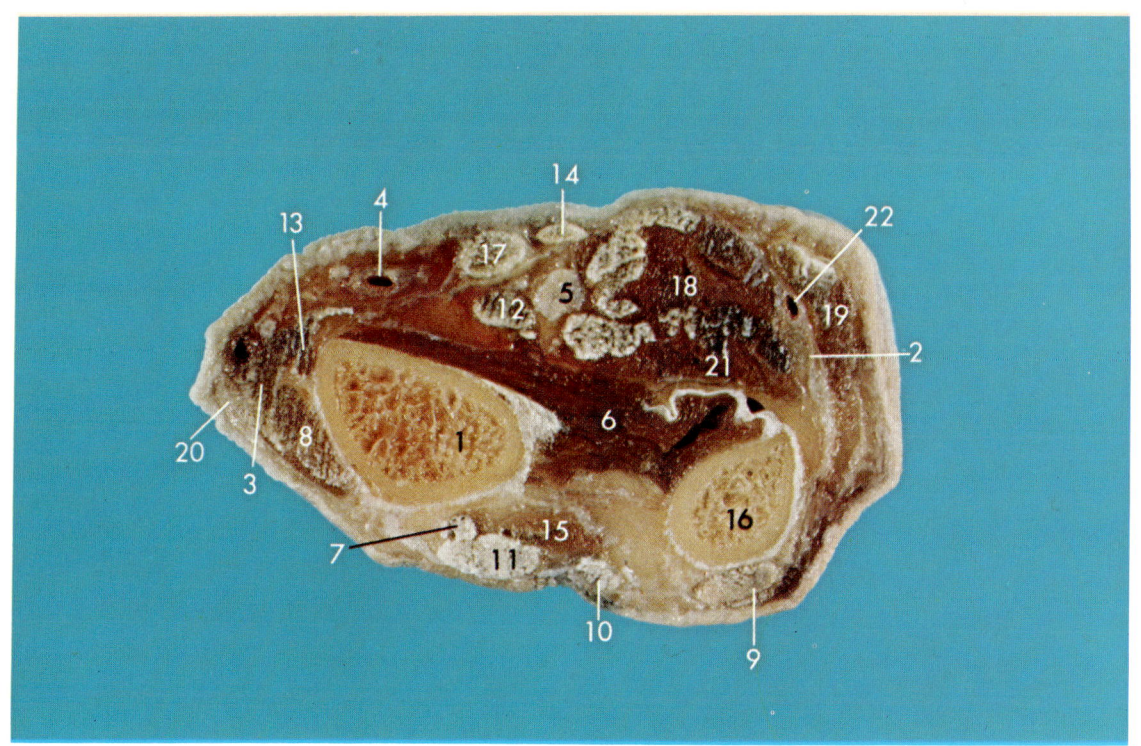

1. Radius
2. Ulnar nerve
3. Abductor pollicis longus and extensor pollicis brevis tendons
4. Radial artery
5. Median nerve
6. Pronator quadratus muscle
7. Extensor pollicis longus tendon
8. Extensor carpi radialis longus and brevis tendons
9. Extensor carpi ulnaris tendon
10. Extensor digiti minimi tendon
11. Extensor digitorum tendons
12. Flexor pollicis longus muscle
13. Brachioradialis tendon
14. Palmaris longus tendon
15. Extensor indicis muscle
16. Ulna
17. Flexor carpi radialis tendon
18. Flexor digitorum superficialis muscle
19. Flexor carpi ulnaris muscle
20. Superficial radial nerve
21. Flexor digitorum profundus muscle
22. Ulnar artery

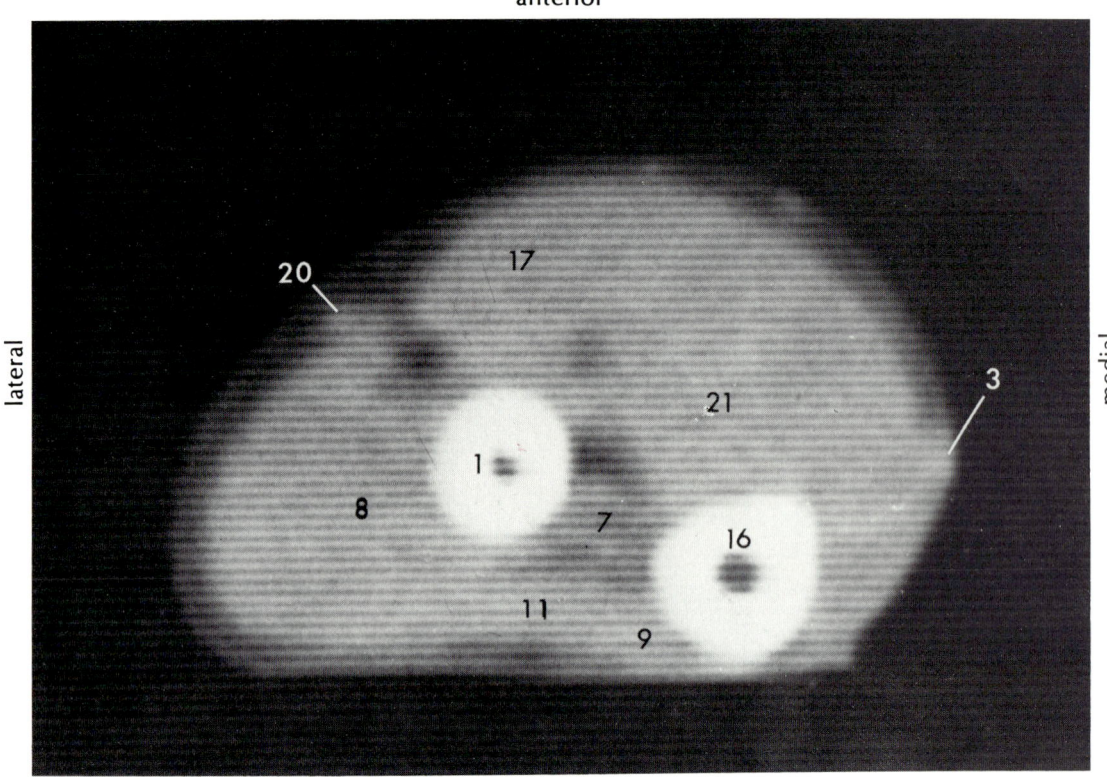

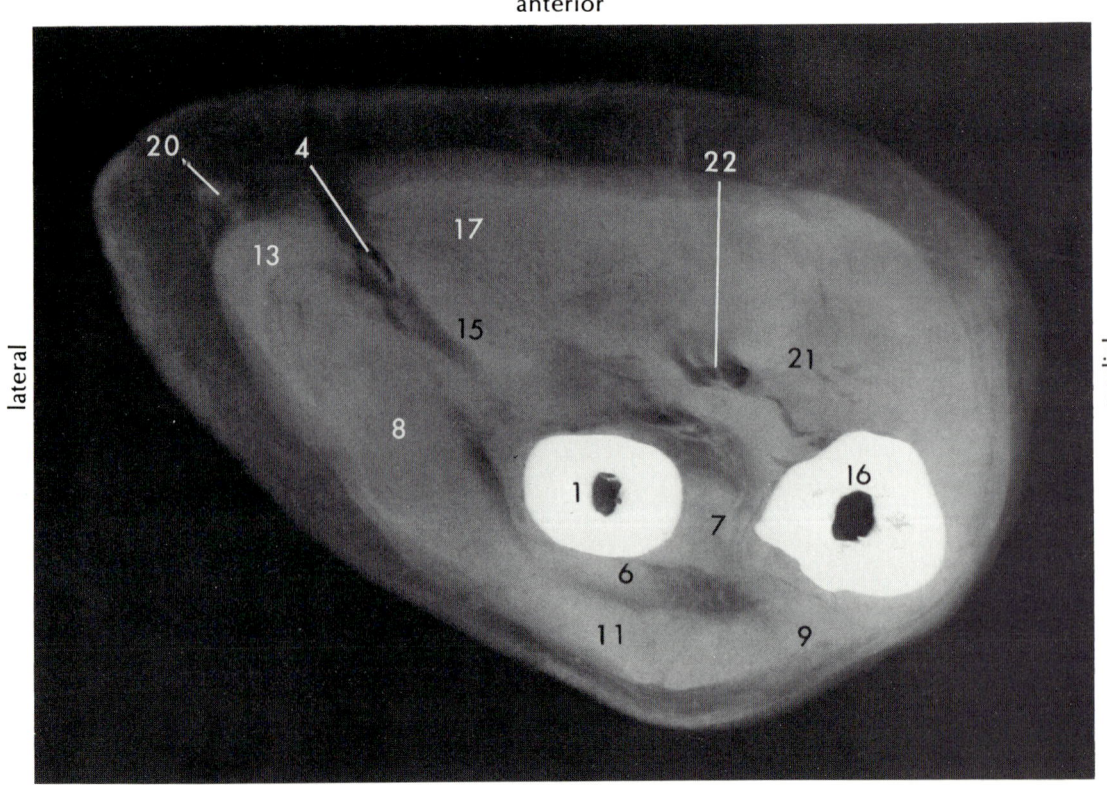

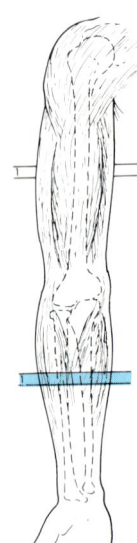

EXTREMITIES: FOREARM

Level F1

anterior

posterior

lateral — medial

1. Radius
2. Ulnar nerve
3. Basilic vein
4. Radial artery
5. Median nerve
6. Supinator muscle
7. Extensor pollicis longus muscle
8. Extensor carpi radialis longus and brevis muscles
9. Extensor carpi ulnaris muscle
10. Extensor digiti minimi muscle
11. Extensor digitorum muscle
12. Flexor pollicis longus muscle
13. Brachioradialis muscle
14. Palmaris longus muscle
15. Pronator teres muscle
16. Ulna
17. Flexor carpi radialis muscle
18. Flexor digitorum superficialis muscle
19. Flexor carpi ulnaris muscle
20. Cephalic vein
21. Flexor digitorum profundus muscle
22. Ulnar artery
23. Interosseous membrane
24. Interosseous nerve and artery

237

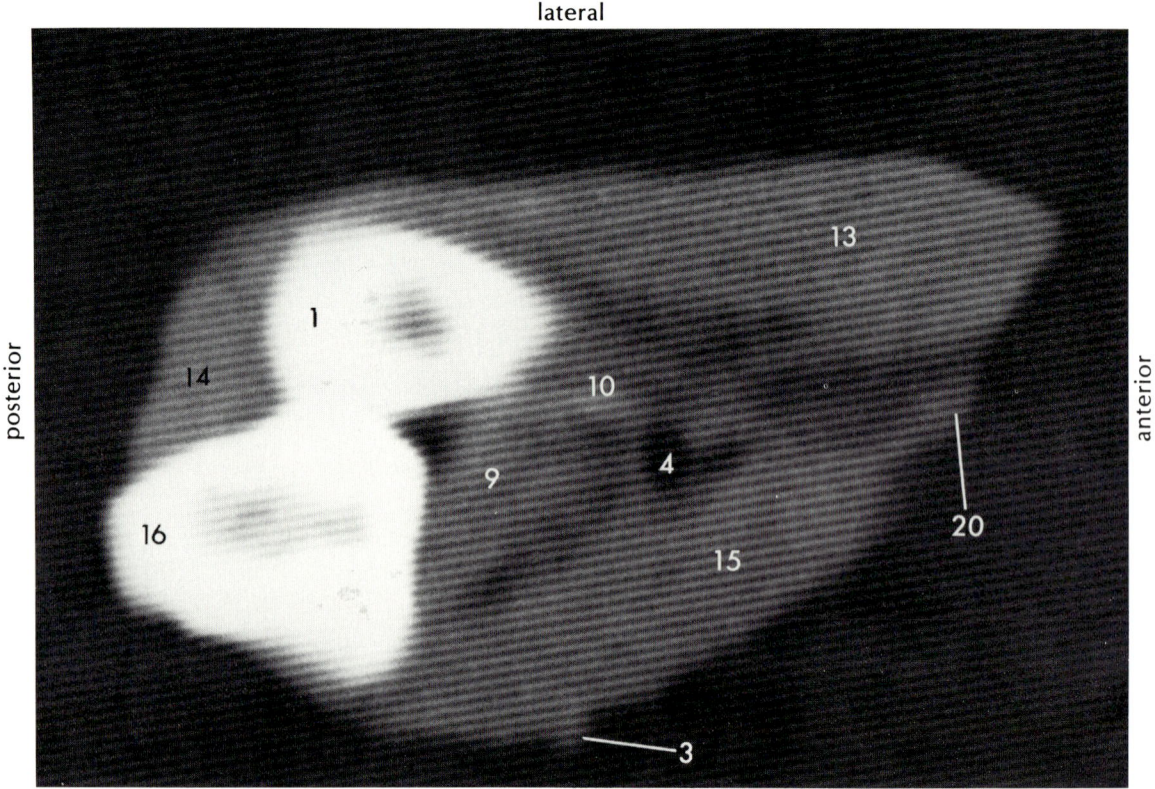

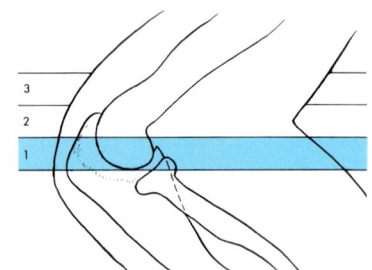

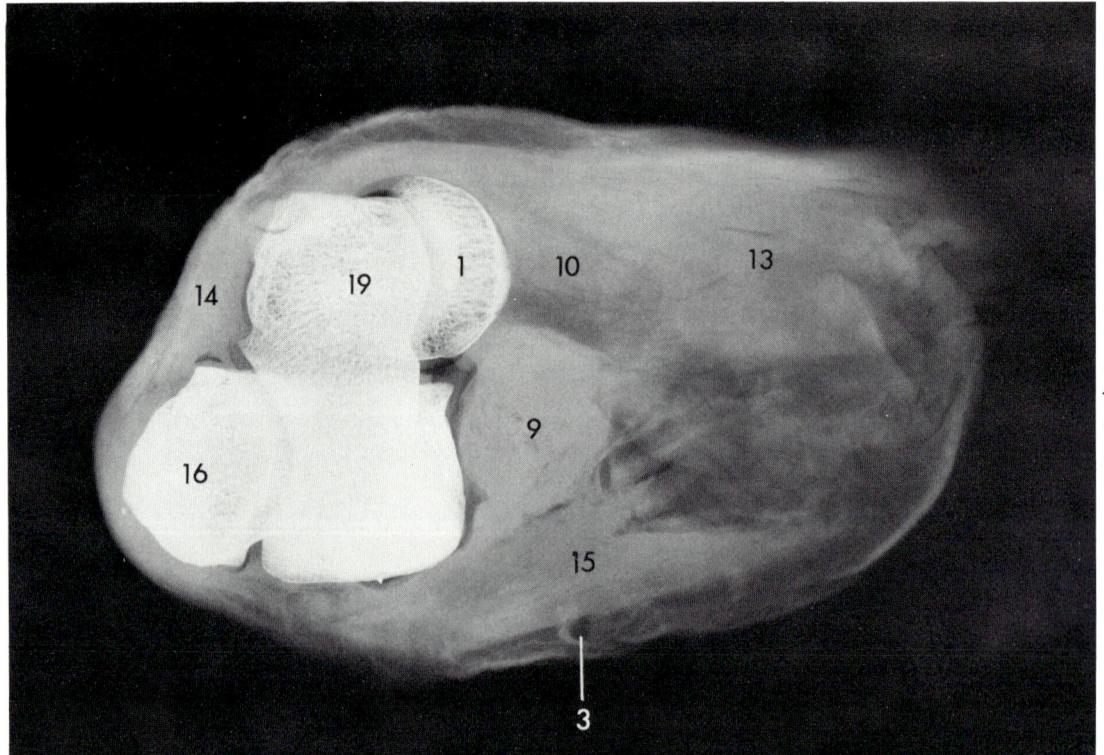

EXTREMITIES: ELBOW

Level E1

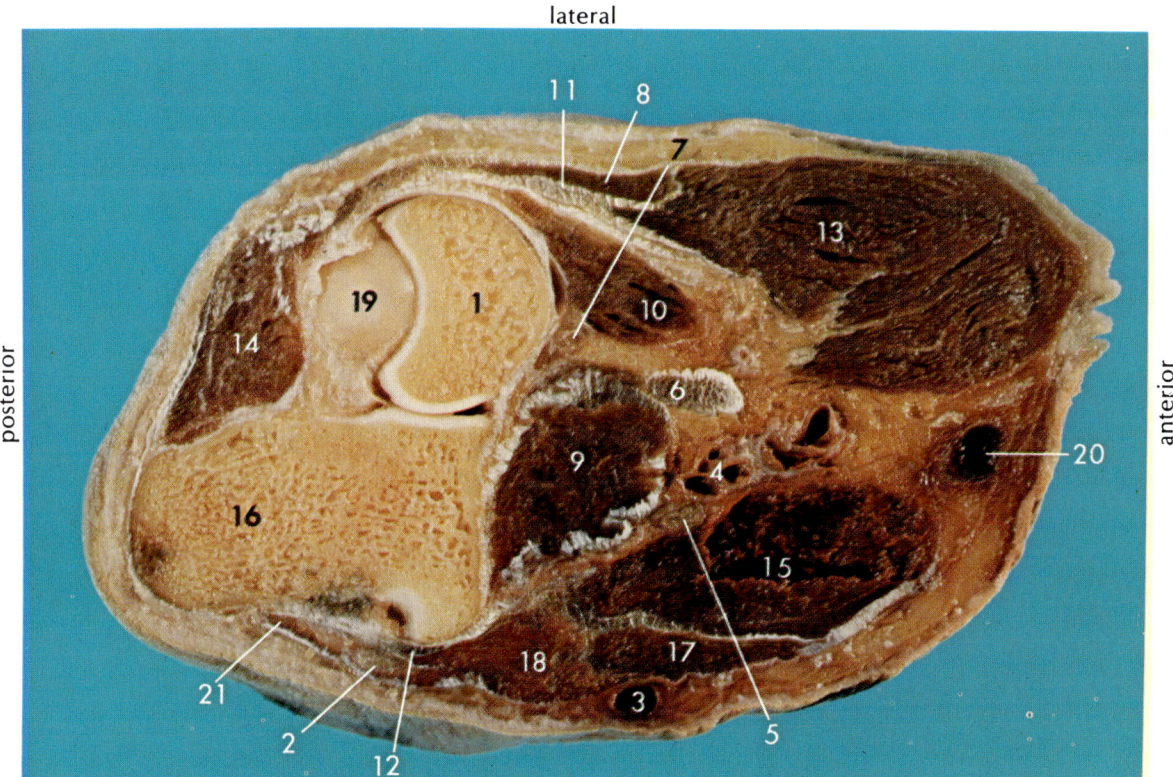

1. Head of radius
2. Ulnar nerve
3. Basilic vein
4. Brachial artery
5. Median nerve
6. Biceps brachii tendon
7. Radial nerve
8. Extensor carpi radialis longus muscle
9. Brachialis muscle
10. Extensor carpi radialis brevis muscle
11. Common extensor tendon
12. Ulnar collateral ligament
13. Brachioradialis muscle
14. Anconeus muscle
15. Pronator teres muscle
16. Olecranon process of ulna
17. Flexor carpi radialis muscle
18. Flexor digitorum superficialis muscle
19. Capitulum of humerus
20. Cephalic vein
21. Flexor digitorum profundus muscle

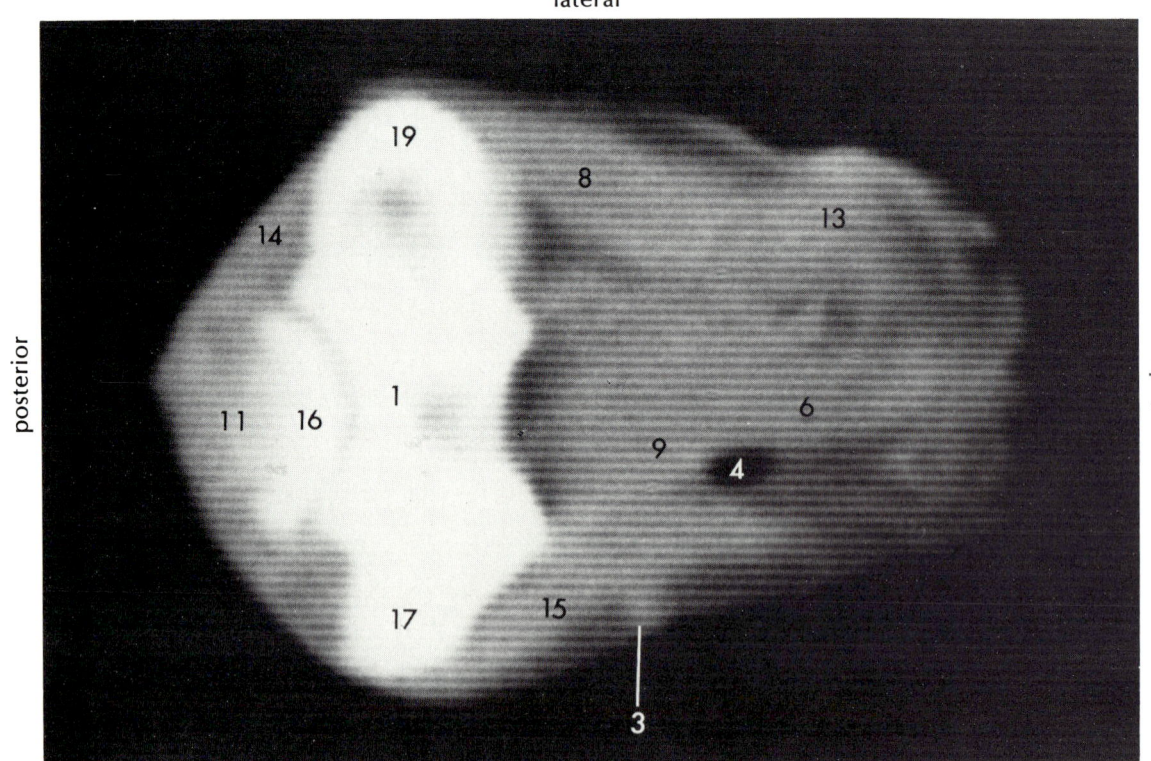

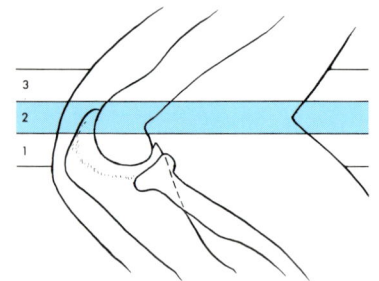

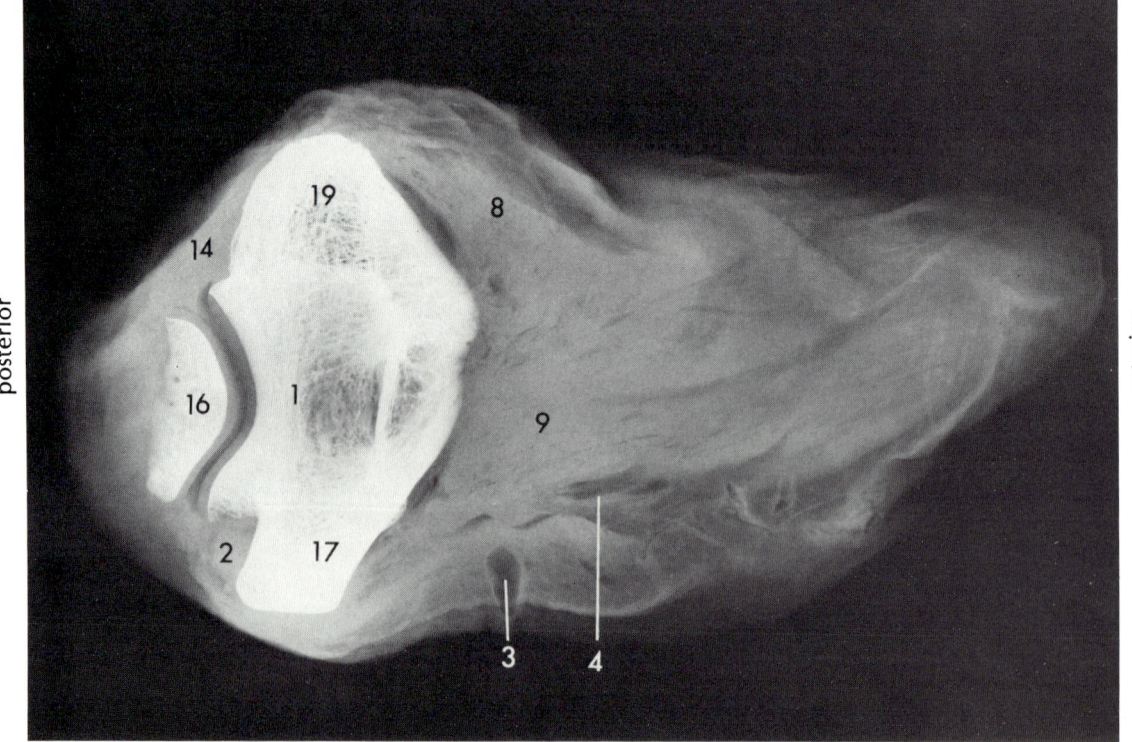

EXTREMITIES: ELBOW

Level E2

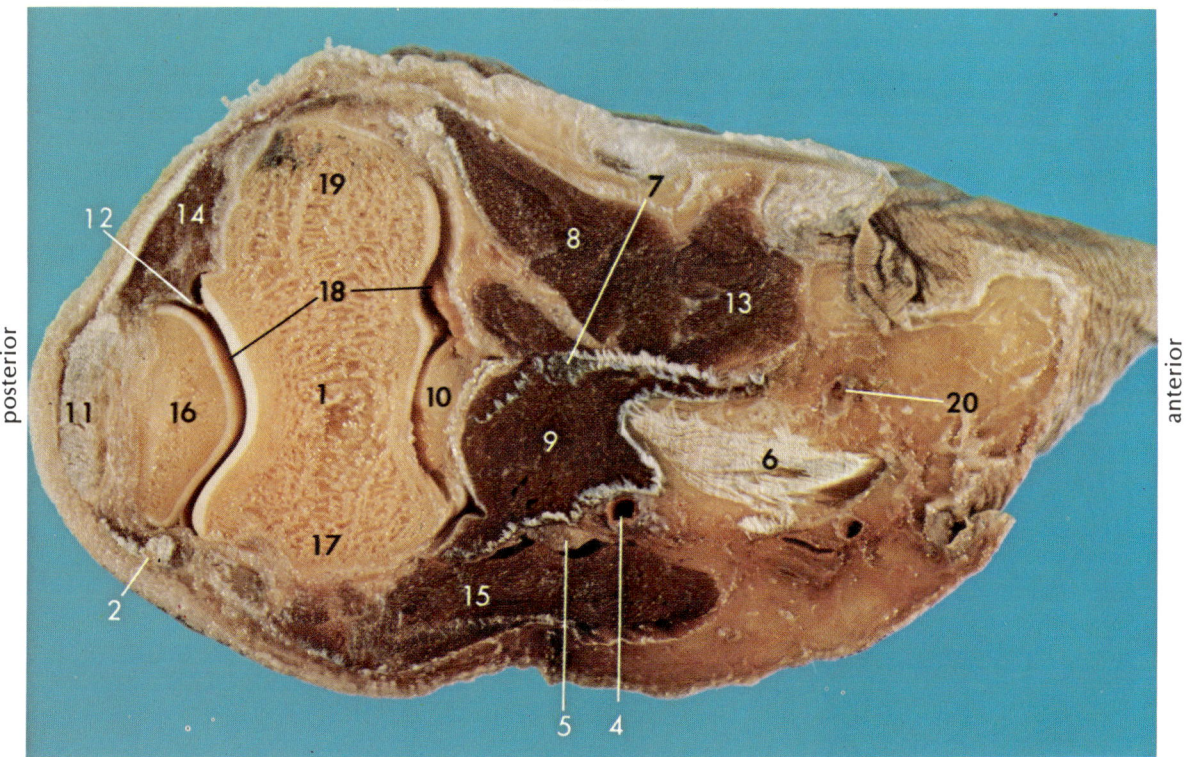

1. Humerus
2. Ulnar nerve
3. Basilic vein
4. Brachial artery
5. Median nerve
6. Biceps brachii tendon
7. Radial nerve
8. Extensor carpi radialis longus muscle
9. Brachialis muscle
10. Coronoid process of ulna
11. Triceps brachii tendon
12. Articular capsule of elbow joint
13. Brachioradialis muscle
14. Anconeus muscle
15. Pronator teres muscle
16. Olecranon process of ulna
17. Trochlea of humerus
18. Elbow joint cavity
19. Capitulum of humerus
20. Cephalic vein

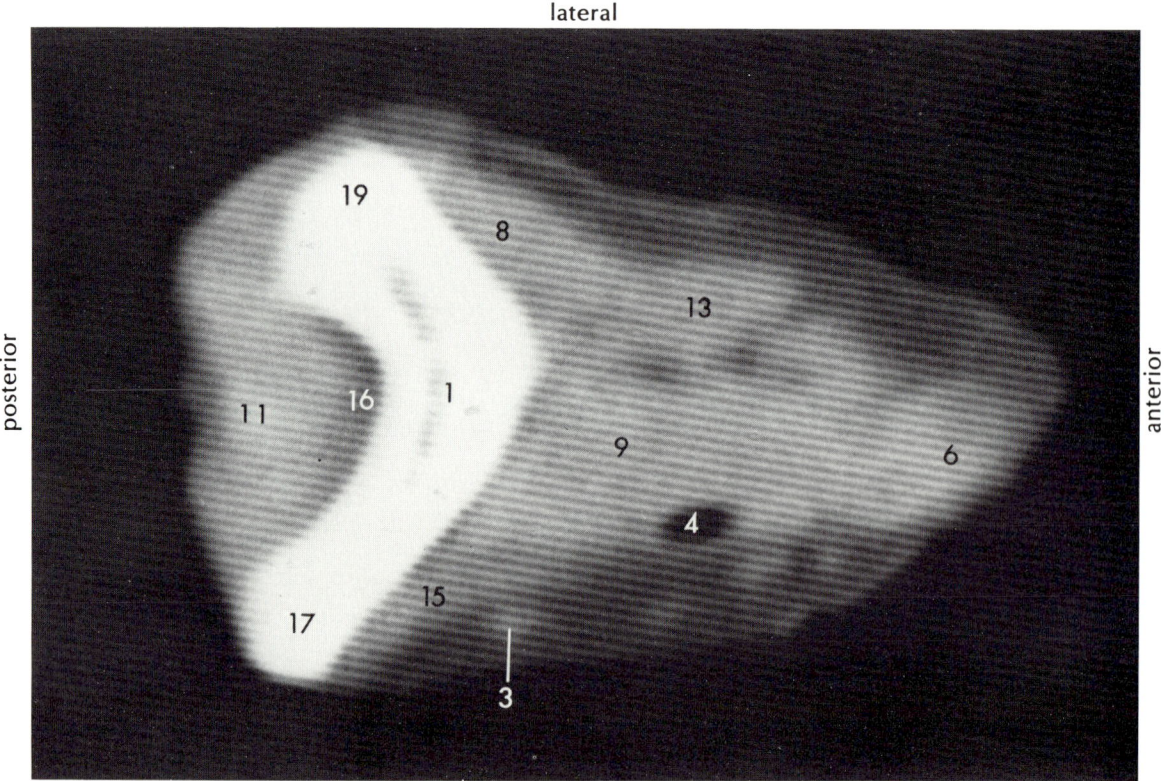

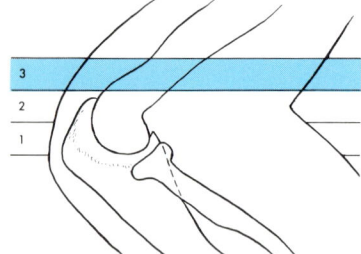

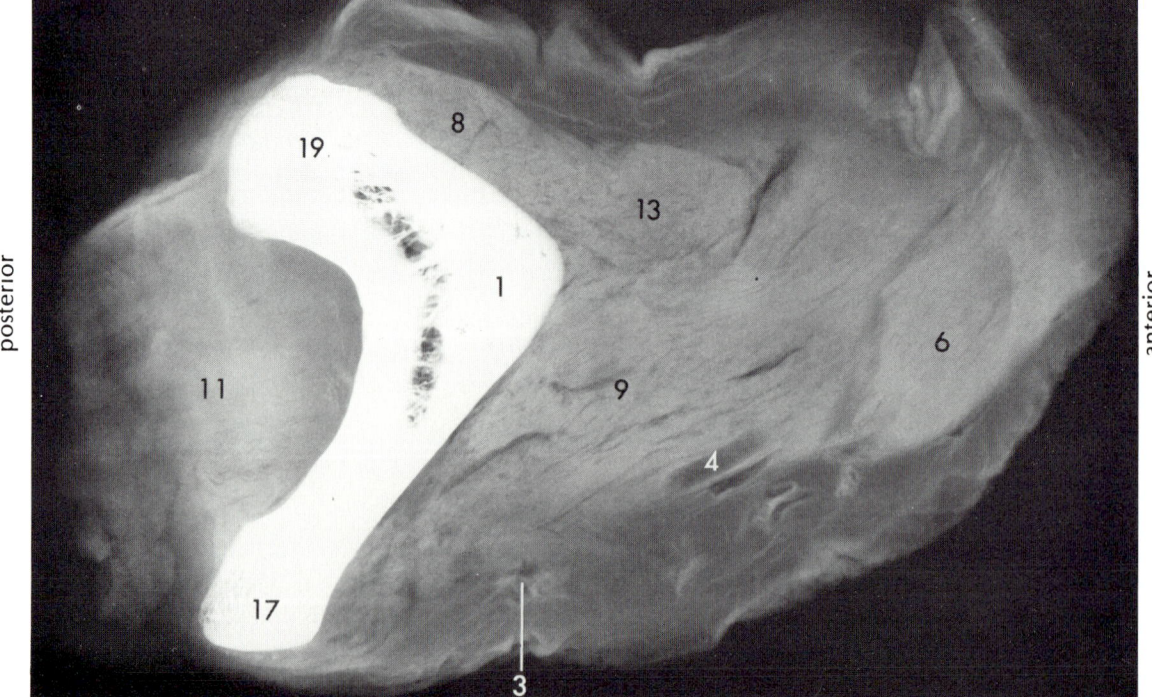

EXTREMITIES: ELBOW

Level E3

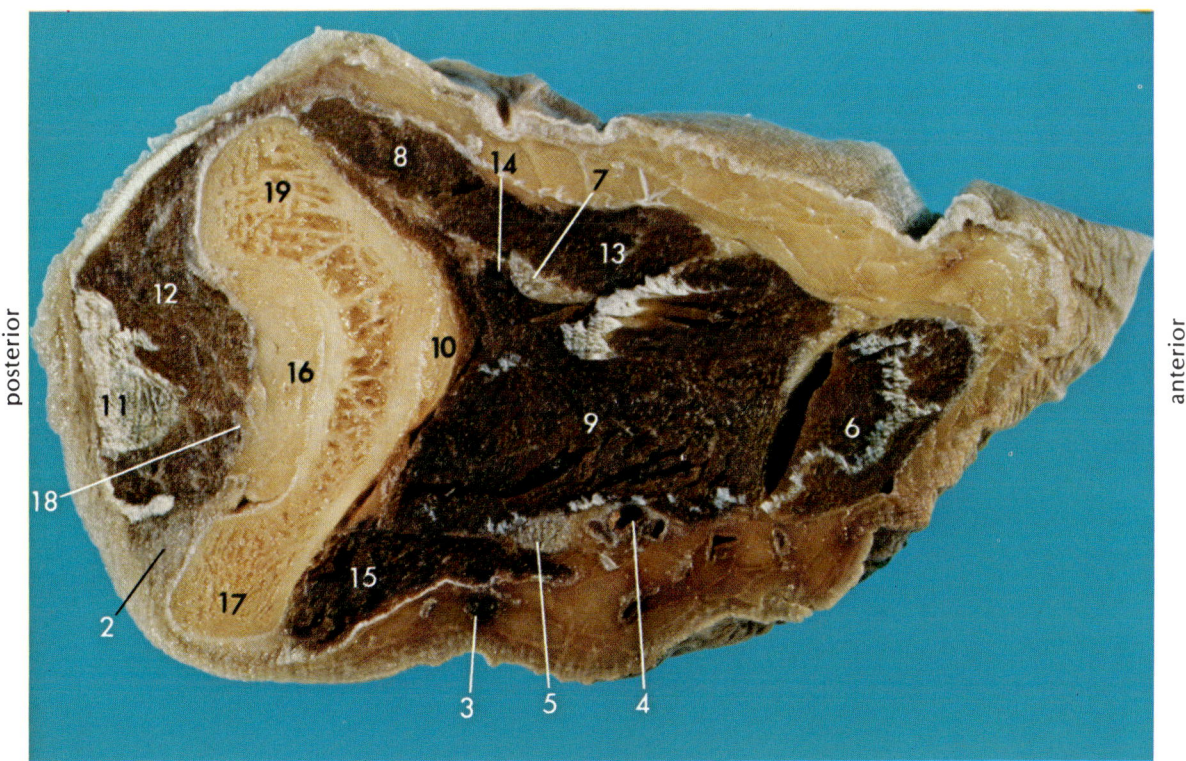

1. Humerus
2. Ulnar nerve
3. Basilic vein
4. Brachial artery
5. Median nerve
6. Biceps brachii muscle
7. Radial nerve
8. Extensor carpi radialis longus muscle
9. Brachialis muscle
10. Coronoid fossa of humerus
11. Triceps brachii tendon
12. Triceps brachii muscle
13. Brachioradialis muscle
14. Radial recurrent artery
15. Pronator teres muscle
16. Olecranon fossa of humerus
17. Medial epicondyle of humerus
18. Elbow joint capsule
19. Lateral epicondyle of humerus

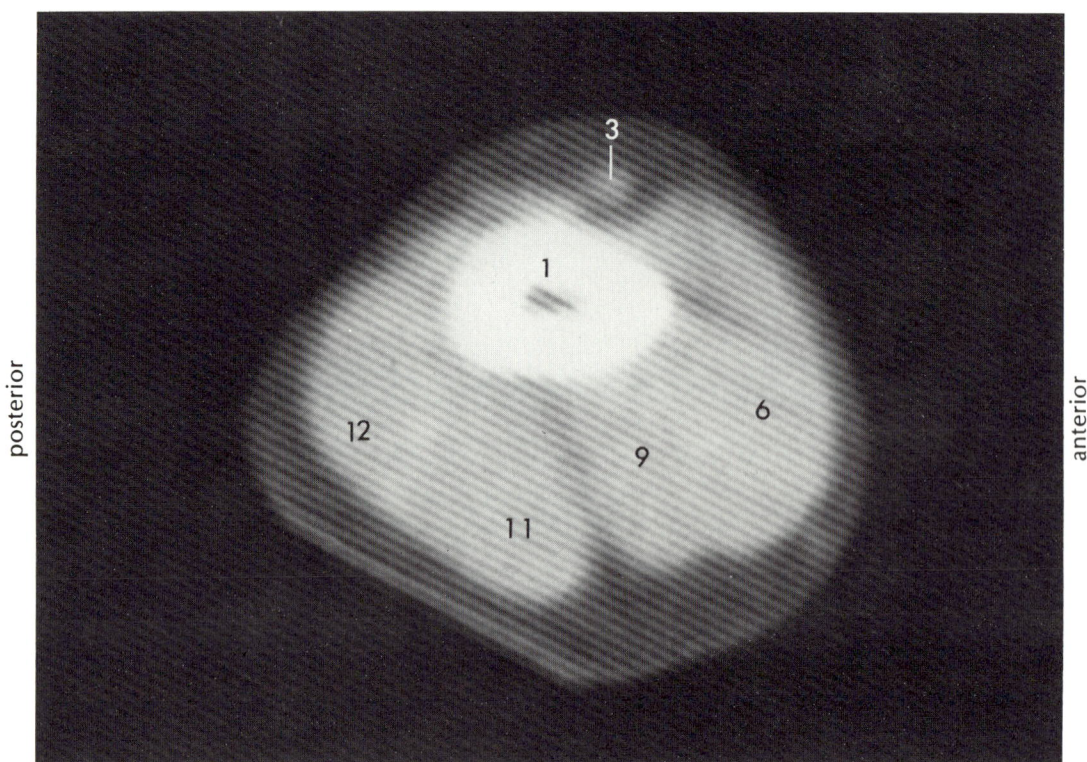

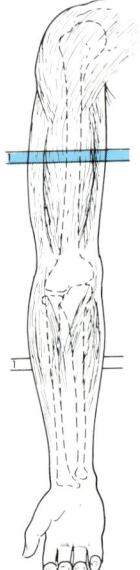

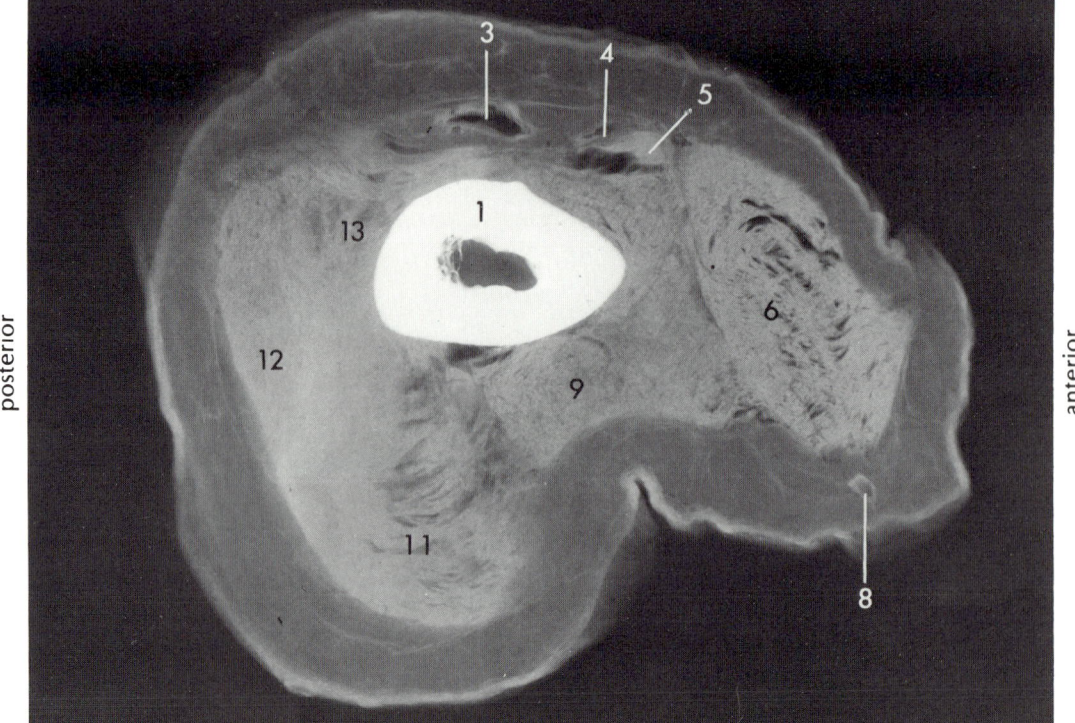

EXTREMITIES: UPPER ARM

Level U1

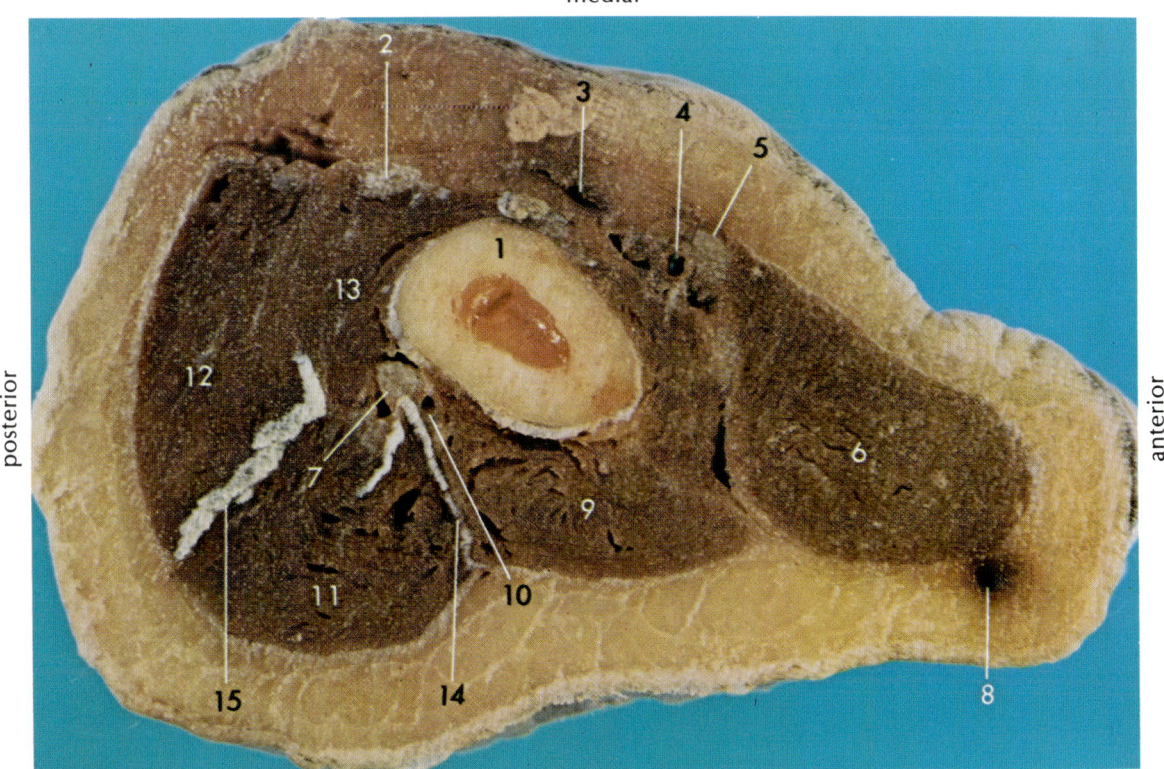

1. Humerus
2. Ulnar nerve
3. Basilic vein
4. Brachial artery
5. Median nerve
6. Biceps muscle
7. Radial nerve
8. Cephalic vein
9. Brachialis muscle
10. Radial recurrent artery
11. Triceps brachii muscle (lateral head)
12. Triceps brachii muscle (long head)
13. Triceps brachii muscle (medial head)
14. Lateral intermuscular septum
15. Triceps brachii muscle and tendon

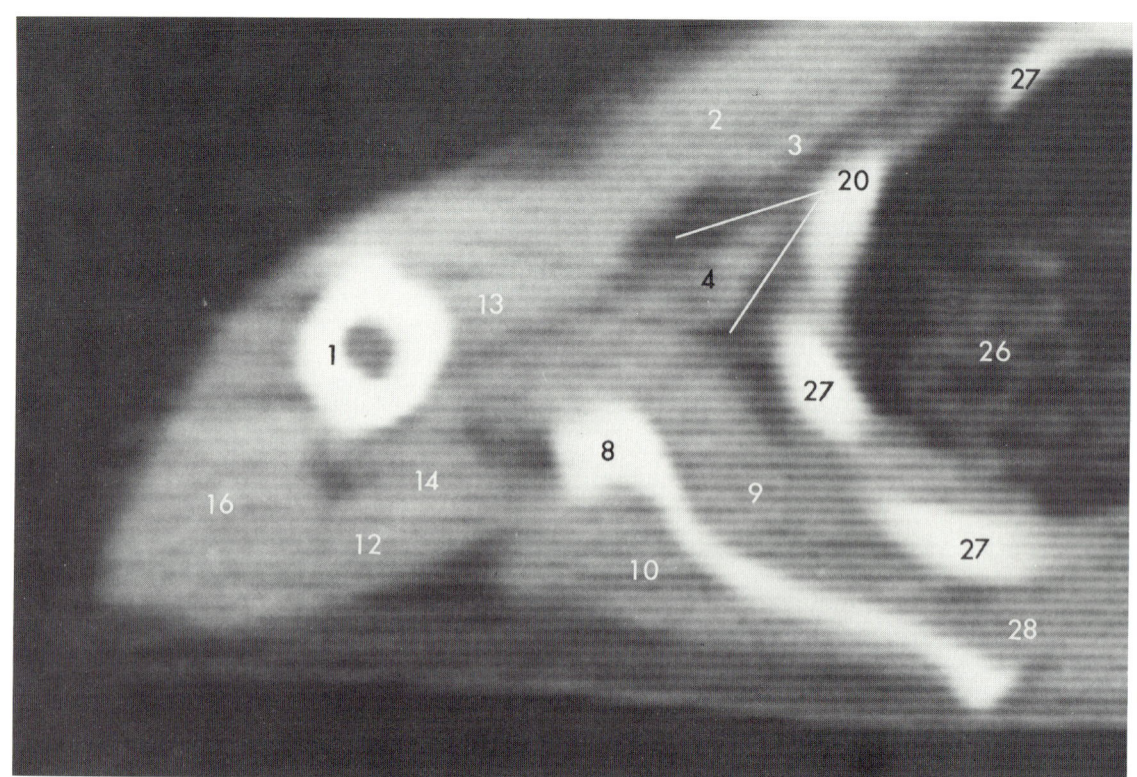

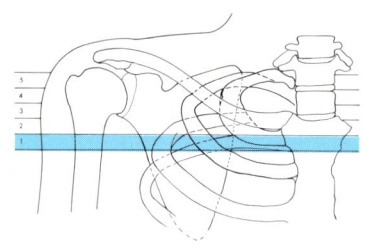

EXTREMITIES: SHOULDER

Level S1

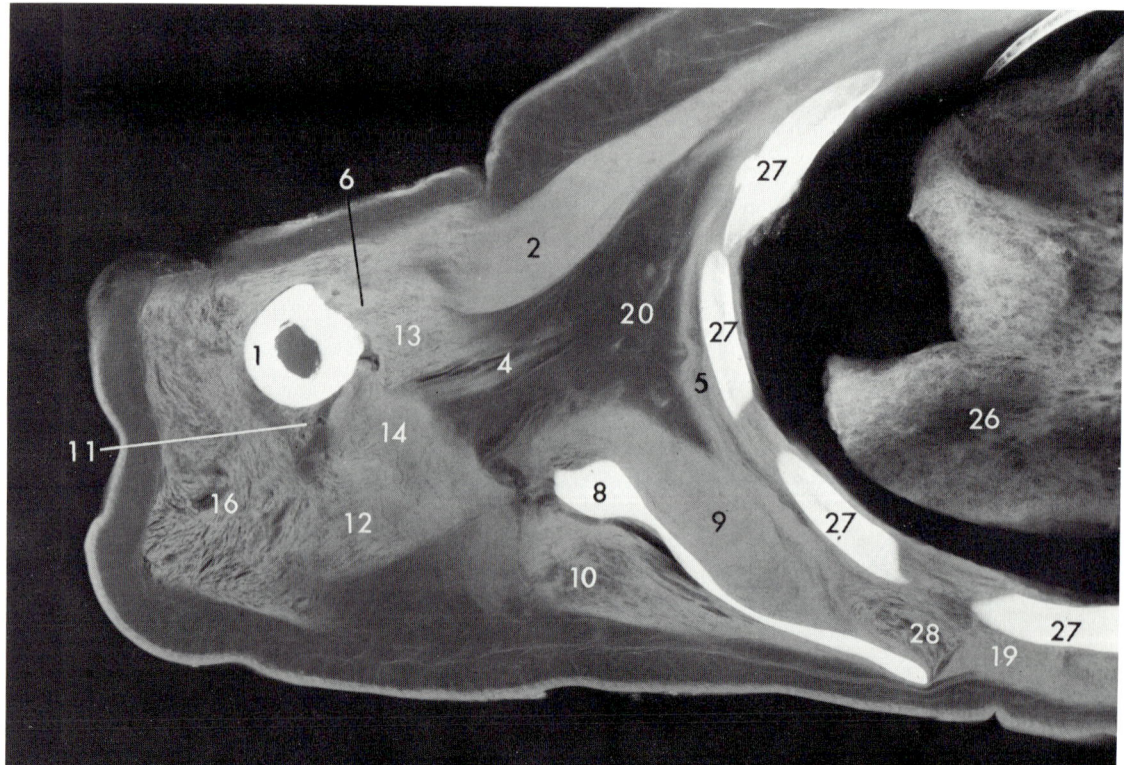

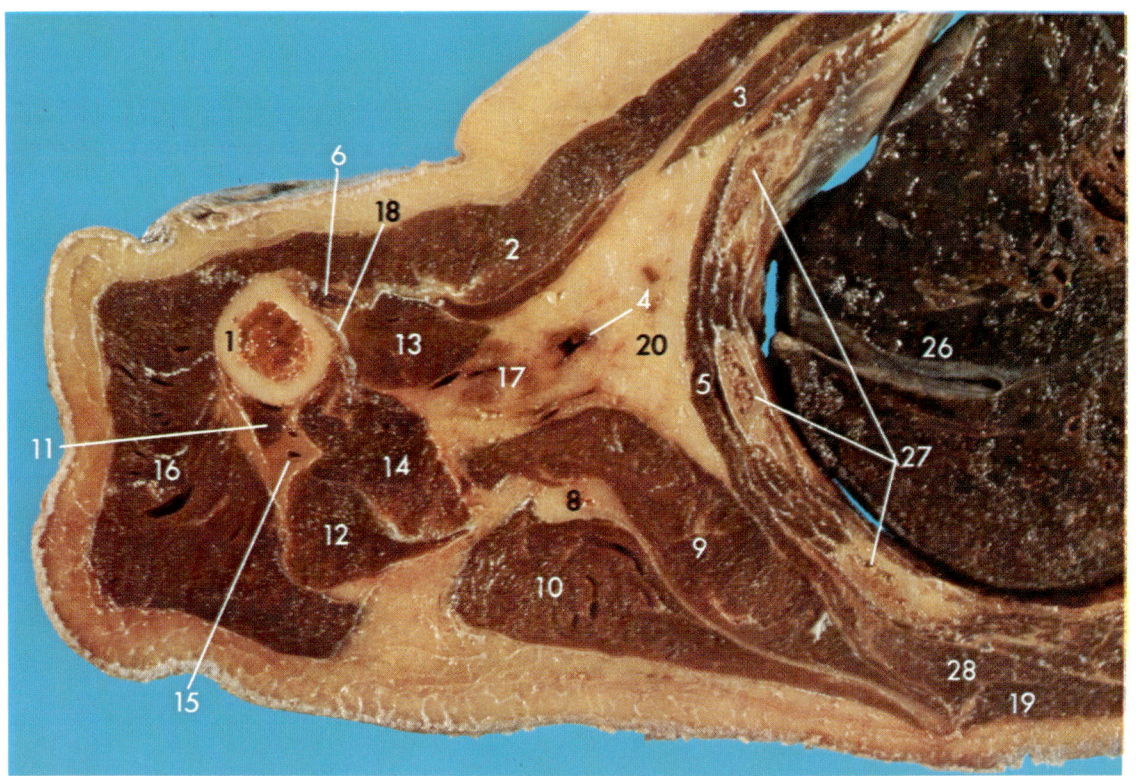

1. Humerus
2. Pectoralis major muscle
3. Pectoralis minor muscle
4. Axillary artery and vein
5. Serratus anterior muscle
6. Biceps brachii tendon (long head)
8. Scapula
9. Subscapularis muscle
10. Infraspinatus muscle
11. Triceps brachii muscle (lateral head)
12. Triceps brachii muscle (long head)
13. Biceps brachii muscle (short head)
14. Teres major muscle
15. Posterior circumflex humeral artery and vein
16. Deltoid muscle
17. Brachial plexus
18. Latissimus dorsi tendon
19. Trapezius muscle
20. Axillary space (fat)
26. Lung
27. Thoracic ribs
28. Rhomboideus major muscle

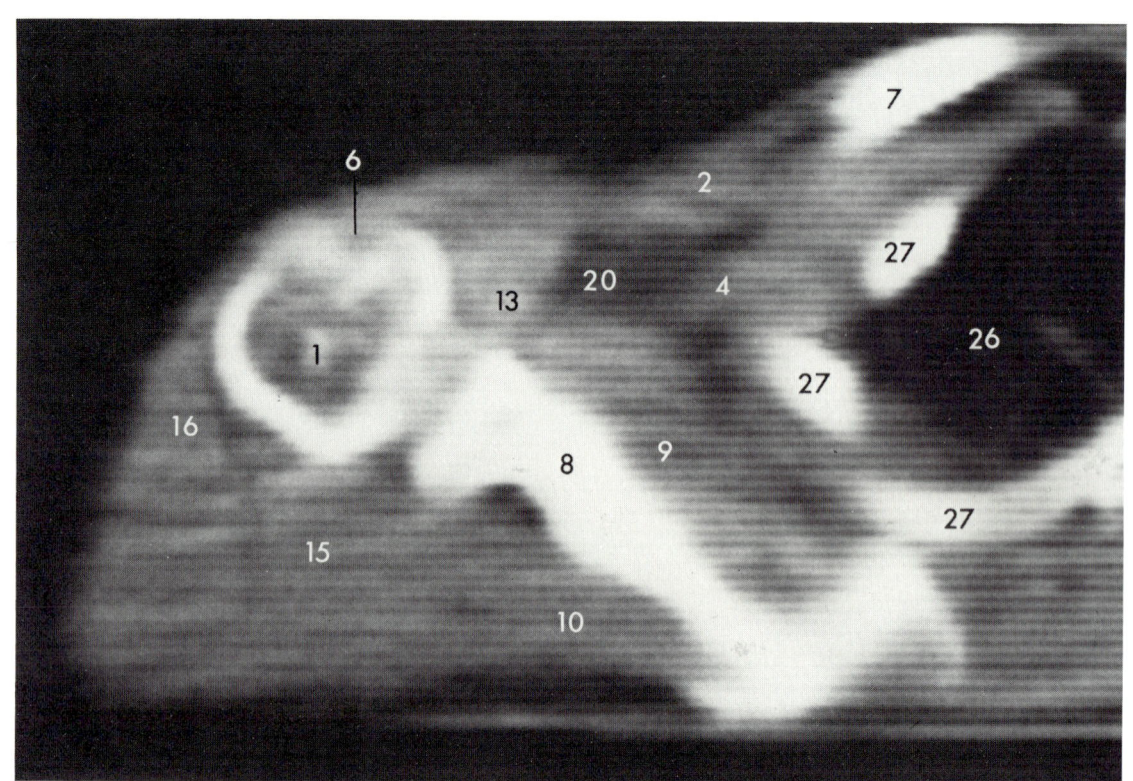

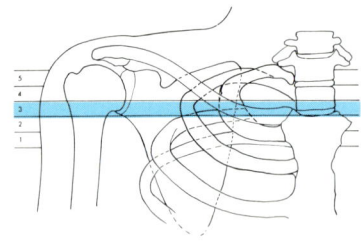

EXTREMITIES: SHOULDER

Level S3

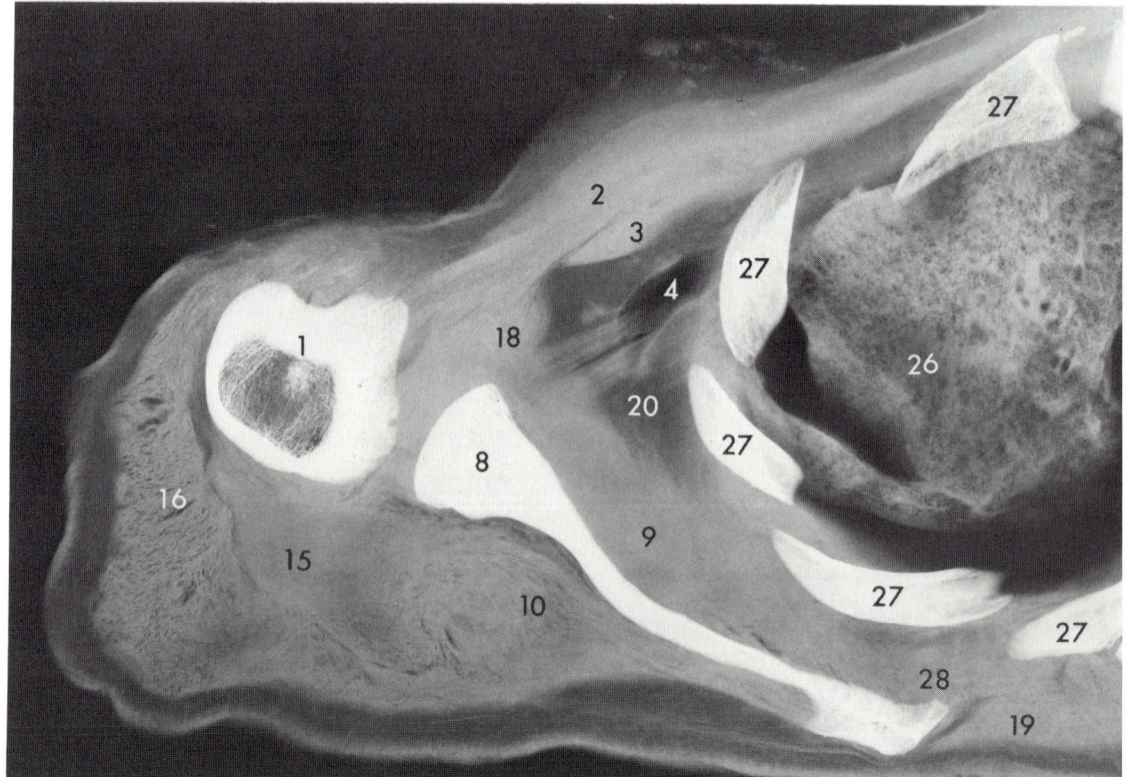

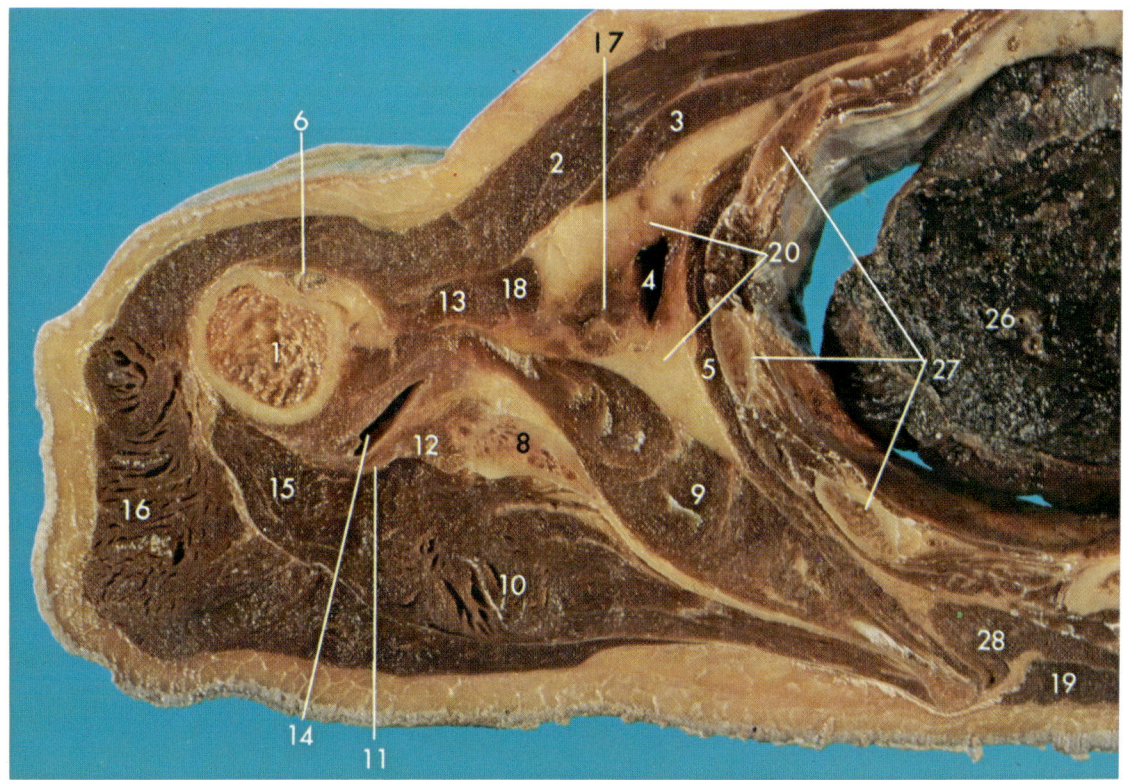

1. Humerus
2. Pectoralis major muscle
3. Pectoralis minor muscle
4. Axillary artery and vein
5. Serratus anterior muscle
6. Biceps brachii tendon (long head)
7. Clavicle
8. Scapula
9. Subscapularis muscle
10. Infraspinatus muscle
11. Inferior glenohumeral ligament
12. Triceps brachii muscle (long head)
13. Biceps brachii muscle (short head)
14. Subscapularis bursa
15. Teres minor muscle
16. Deltoid muscle
17. Axillary lymph nodes
18. Coracobrachialis muscle
19. Trapezius muscle
20. Axillary space (fat)
26. Lung
27. Thoracic ribs
28. Romboideus major muscle

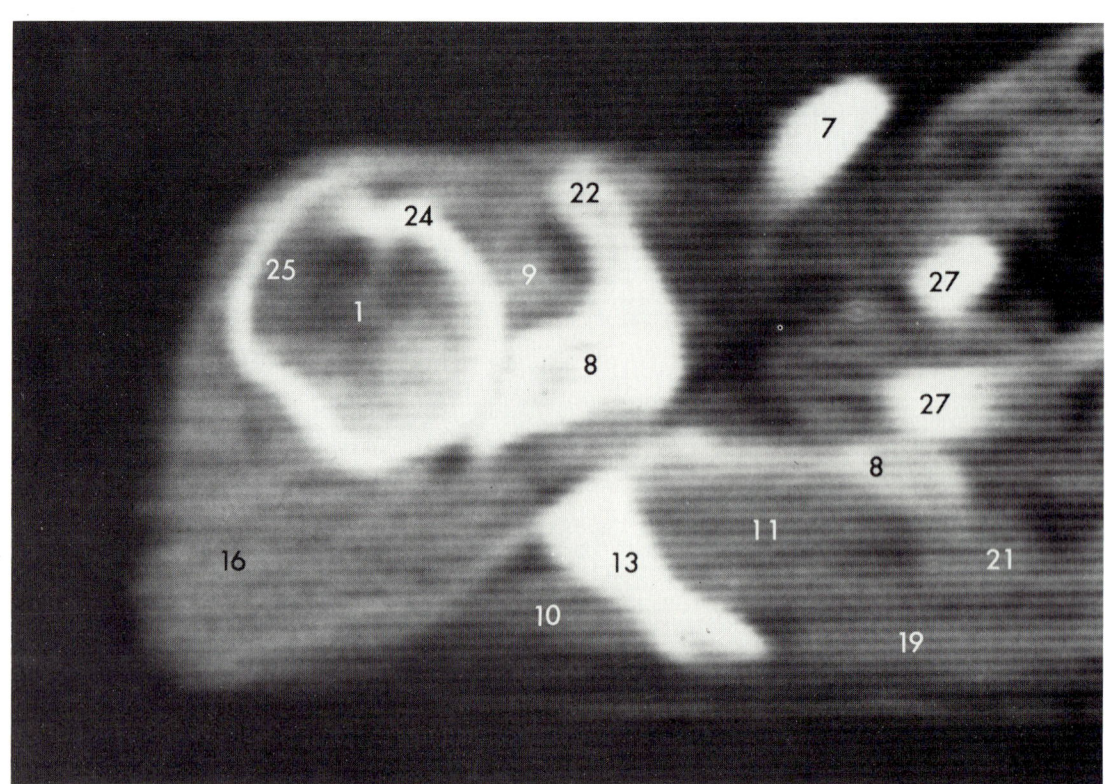

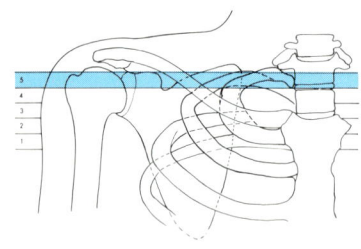

EXTREMITIES: SHOULDER

Level S5

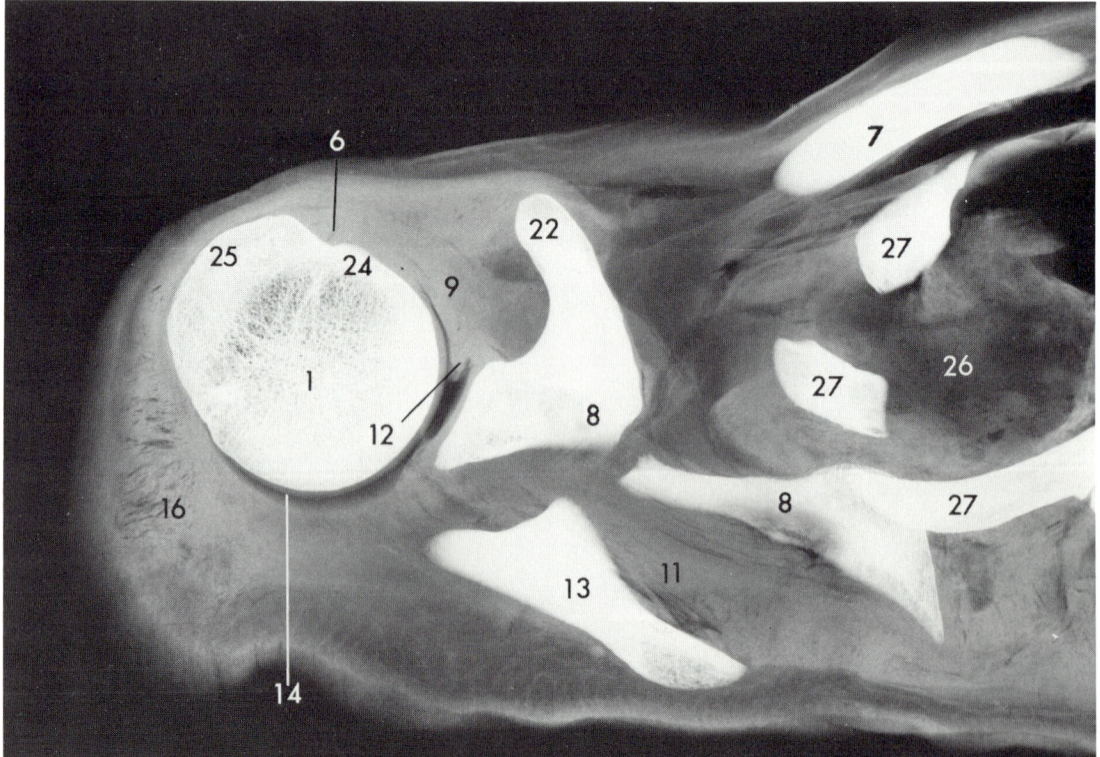

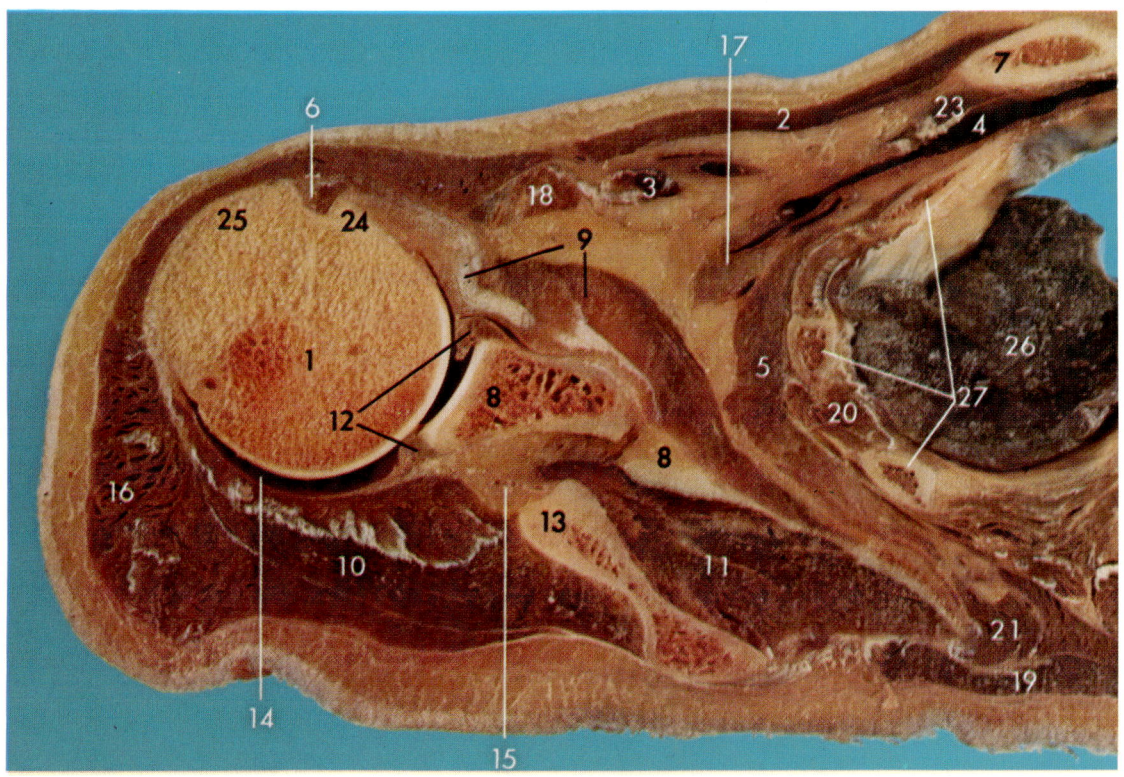

1. Head of humerus
2. Pectoralis major muscle
3. Pectoralis minor muscle
4. Subclavian vein
5. Serratus anterior muscle
6. Biceps brachii tendon (long head)
7. Clavicle
8. Scapula
9. Subscapularis muscle and tendon
10. Infraspinatus muscle
11. Supraspinatus muscle
12. Glenoid labrum of scapula
13. Spine of scapula
14. Shoulder joint cavity
15. Suprascapular artery and vein
16. Deltoid muscle
17. Brachial plexus
18. Coracobrachialis muscle and biceps brachii tendon (short head)
19. Trapezius muscle
20. Intercostal muscle
21. Rhomboideus minor muscle
22. Coracoid process of scapula
23. Subclavius muscle
24. Lesser tubercle of humerus
25. Greater tubercle of humerus
26. Lung
27. Thoracic ribs

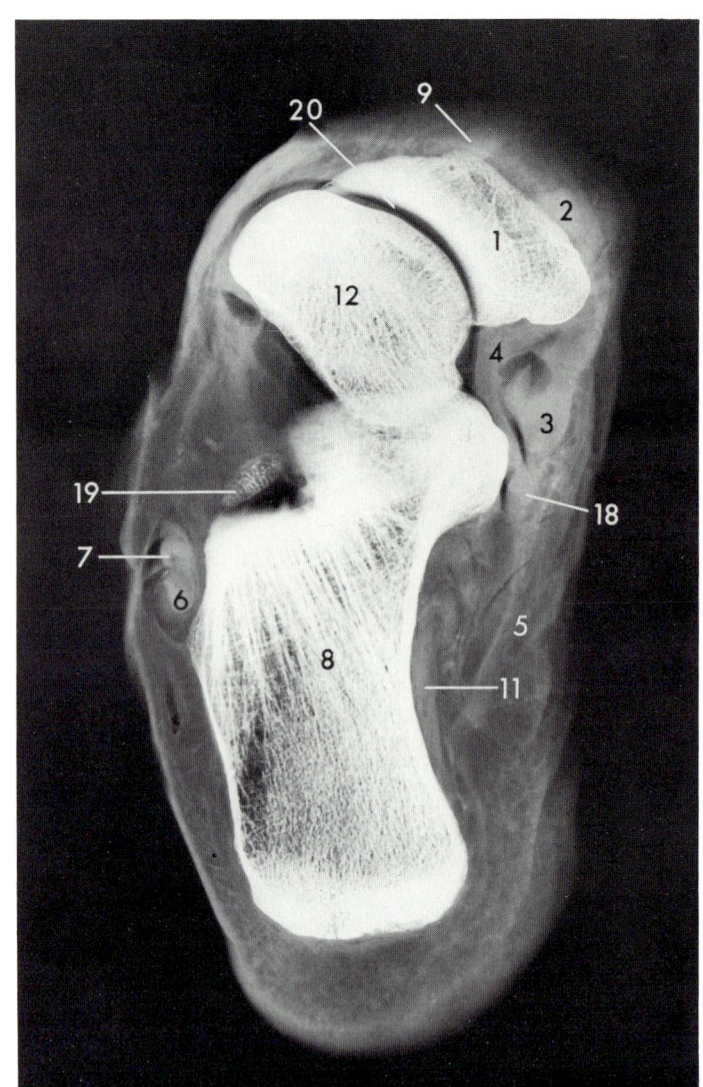
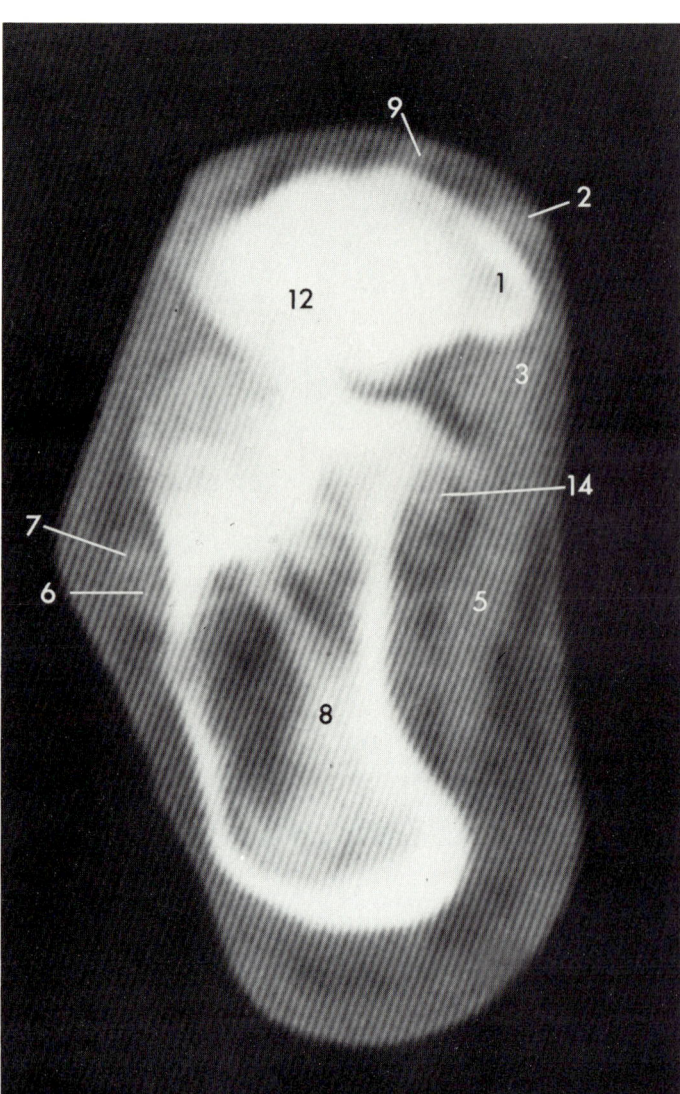
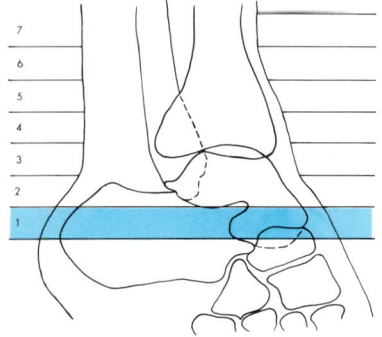

EXTREMITIES: ANKLE

Level A1

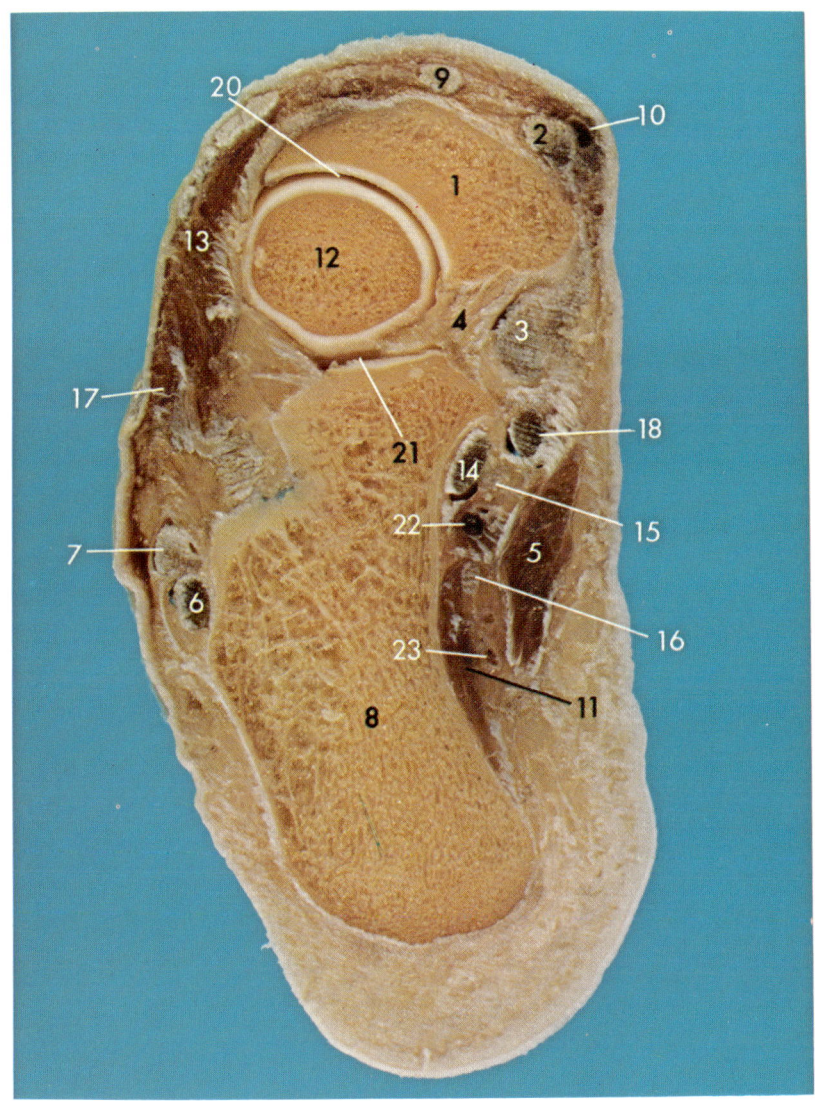

1. Navicular
2. Tibialis anterior tendon
3. Tibialis posterior tendon
4. Plantar calcaneonavicular (spring) ligament
5. Abductor hallucis muscle
6. Peroneus longus tendon
7. Peroneus brevis tendon
8. Calcaneus
9. Extensor hallucis longus tendon
10. Great saphenous vein
11. Quadratus plantae muscle
12. Head of talus
13. Extensor hallucis brevis muscle
14. Flexor hallucis longus tendon
15. Medial plantar nerve
16. Lateral plantar nerve
17. Extensor digitorum brevis muscle
18. Flexor digitorum longus tendon
19. Lateral process of talus
20. Talonavicular joint cavity
21. Talocalcaneal joint cavity
22. Medial plantar artery and vein
23. Lateral plantar artery and vein

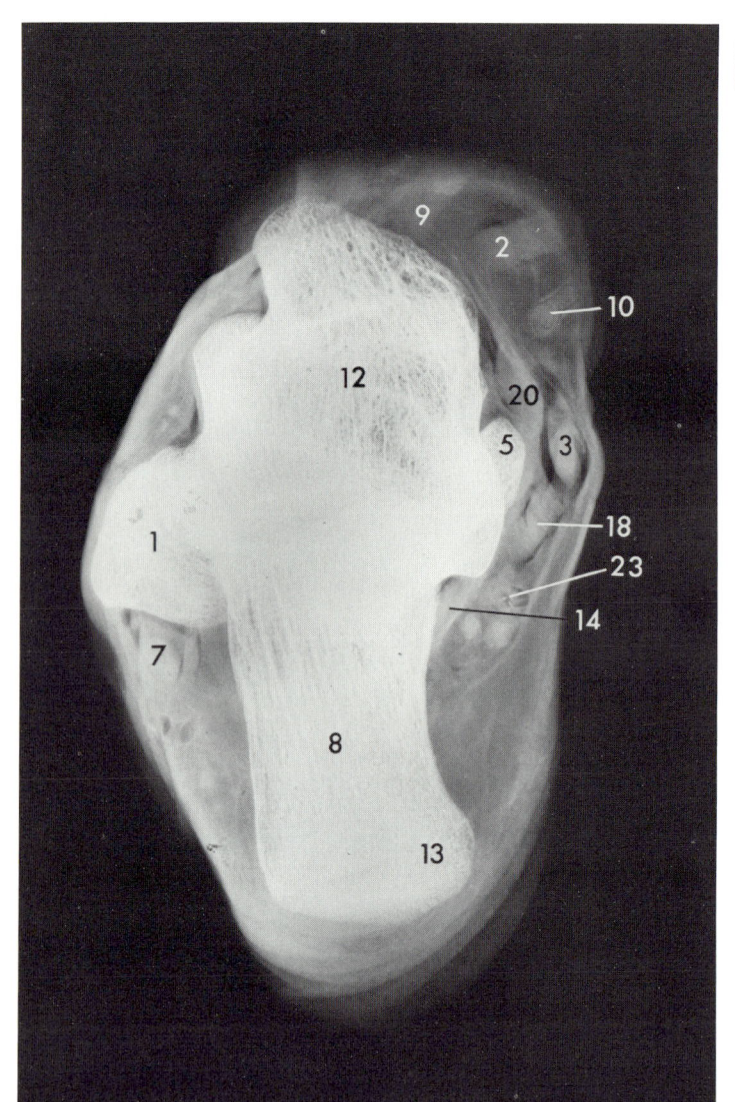
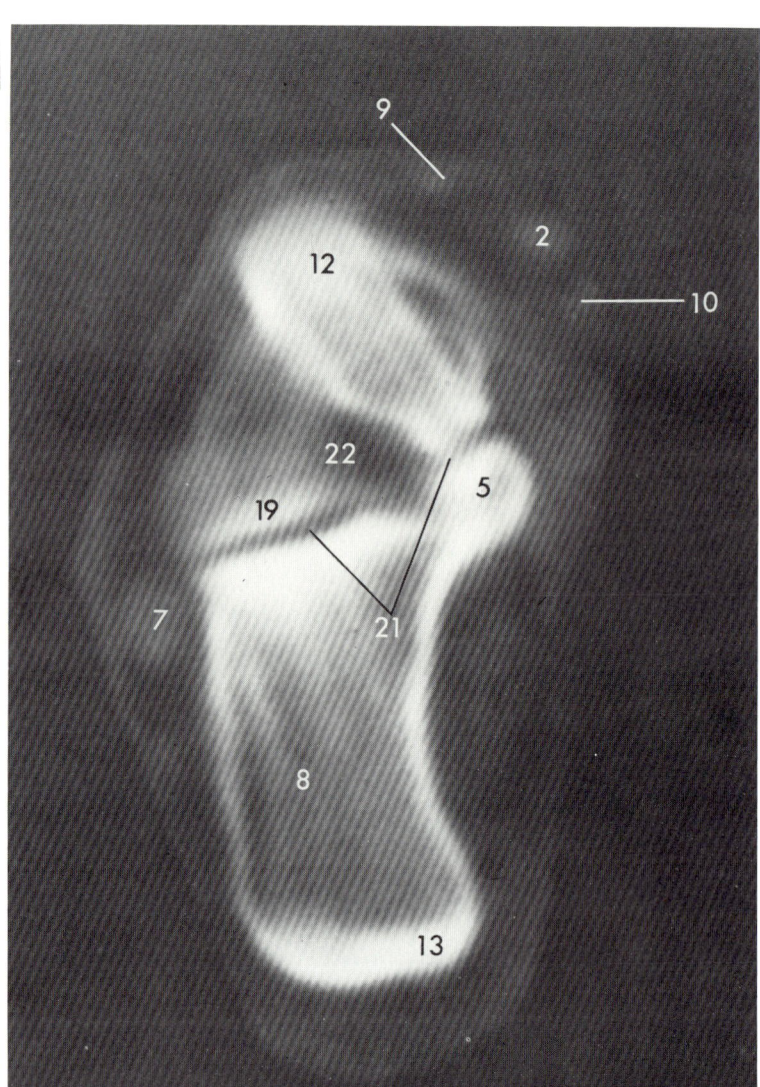
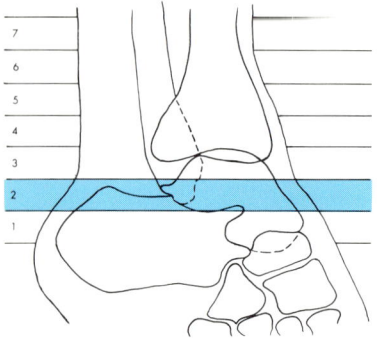

**EXTREMITIES:
ANKLE**

Level A2

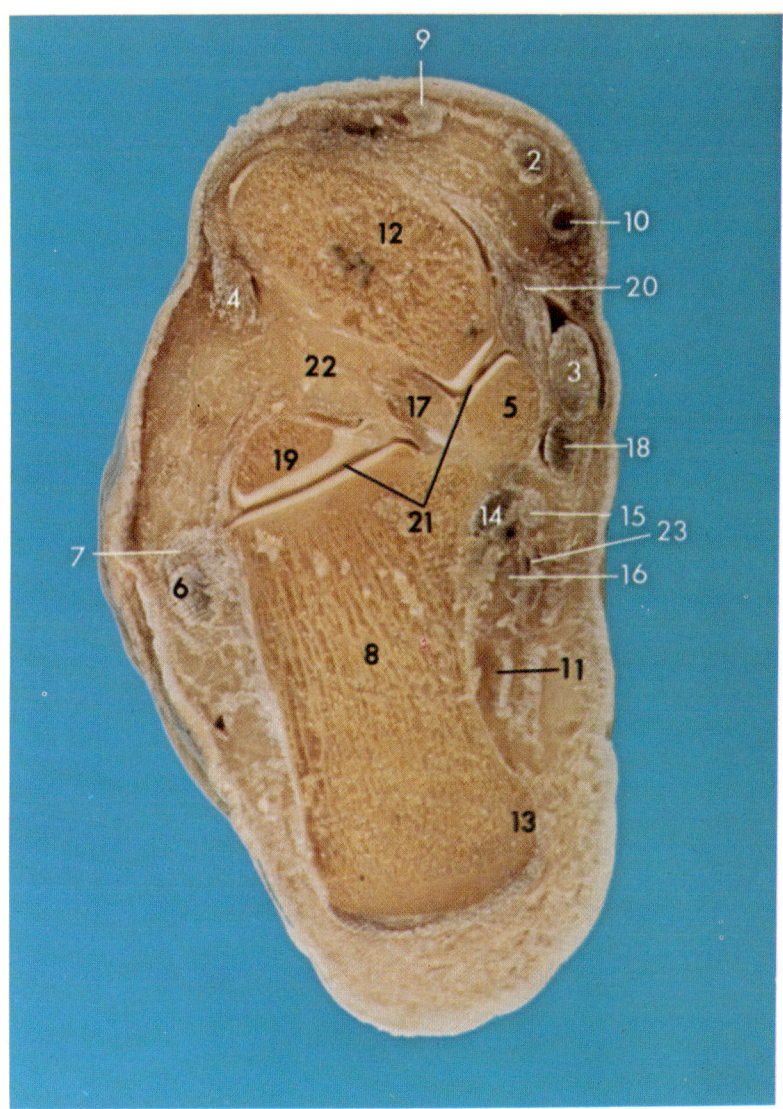

1. Lateral malleolus (fibula)
2. Tibialis anterior tendon
3. Tibialis posterior tendon
4. Lateral talocalcaneal ligament
5. Sustentaculum tali
6. Peroneus longus tendon
7. Peroneus brevis tendon
8. Calcaneus
9. Extensor hallucis longus tendon
10. Great saphenous vein
11. Quadratus plantae muscle
12. Body of talus
13. Tuberosity of calcaneus
14. Flexor hallucis longus tendon
15. Medial plantar nerve
16. Lateral plantar nerve
17. Interosseous talocalcaneal ligament
18. Flexor digitorum longus tendon
19. Posterior process of talus
20. Deltoid ligament
21. Talocalcaneal joint cavity
22. Sulcus tali
23. Lateral plantar artery and vein

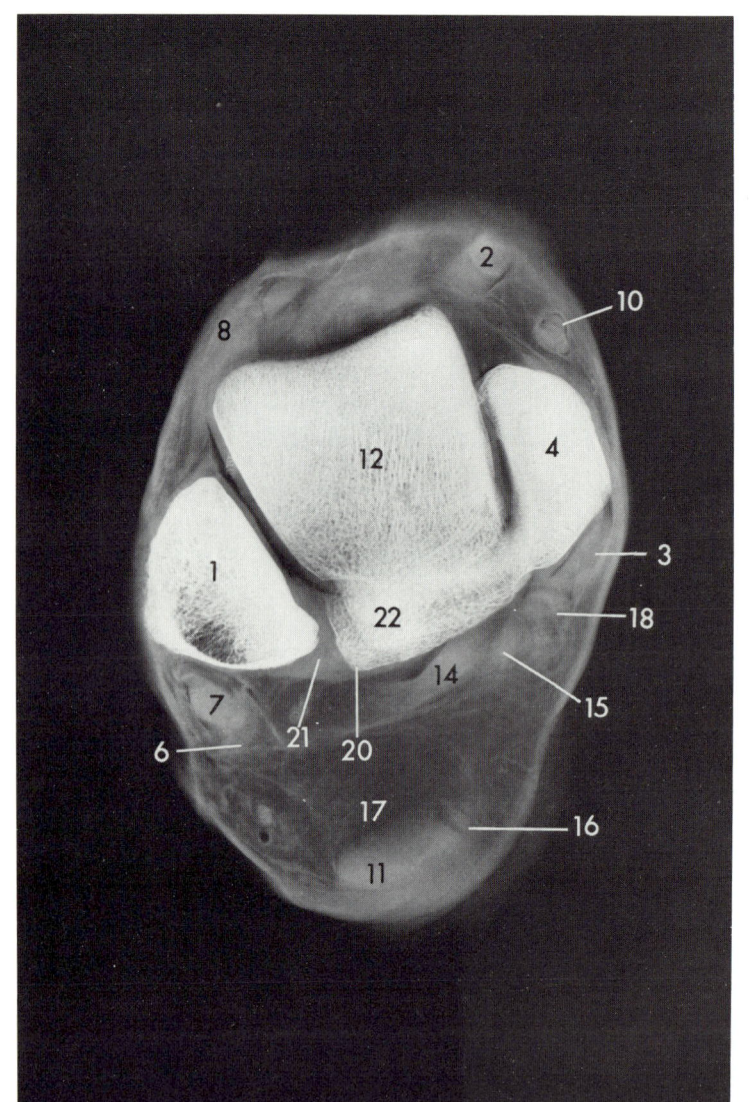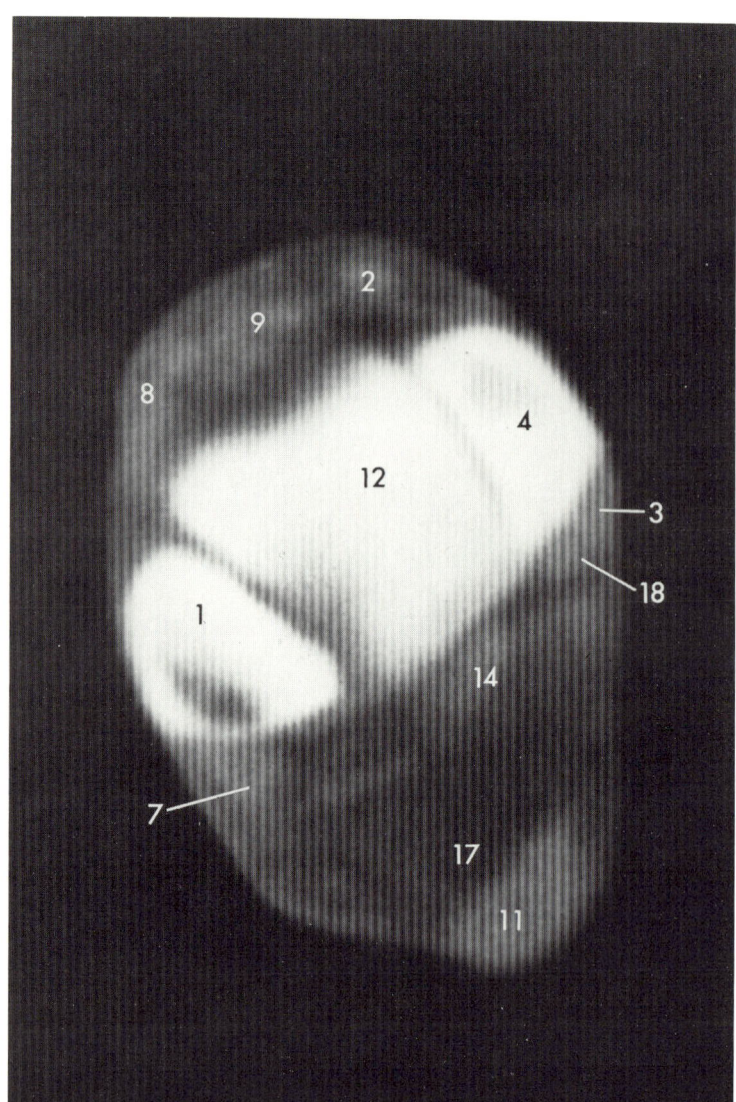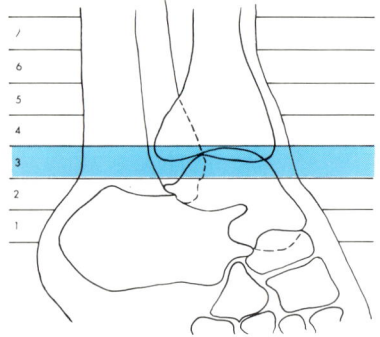

EXTREMITIES: ANKLE

Level A3 (Superior [proximal] aspect)

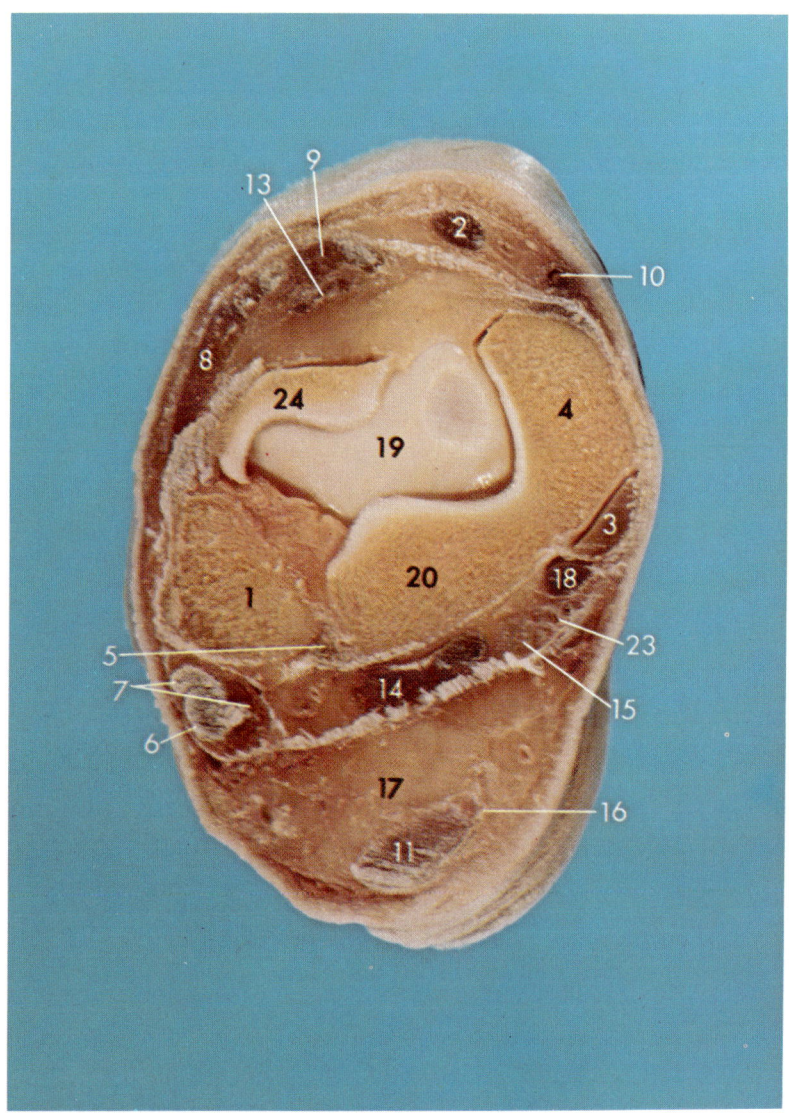

1. Lateral malleolus (fibula)
2. Tibialis anterior tendon
3. Tibialis posterior tendon
4. Medial malleolus (tibia)
5. Posterior tibiofibular ligament
6. Peroneus longus tendon
7. Peroneus brevis muscle and tendon
8. Extensor digitorum longus muscle
9. Extensor hallucis longus tendon
10. Great saphenous vein
11. Achilles tendon
12. Body of talus
13. Anterior tibial artery and vein
14. Flexor hallucis longus muscle and tendon
15. Tibial nerve
16. Plantaris tendon
17. Pre-Achilles space (fat)
18. Flexor digitorum longus tendon
19. Trochlea of talus
20. Posterior malleolus (tibia)
21. Posterior talofibular ligament
22. Posterior process of talus
23. Posterior tibial artery and vein
24. Tibia (distal aspect of anterior surface)

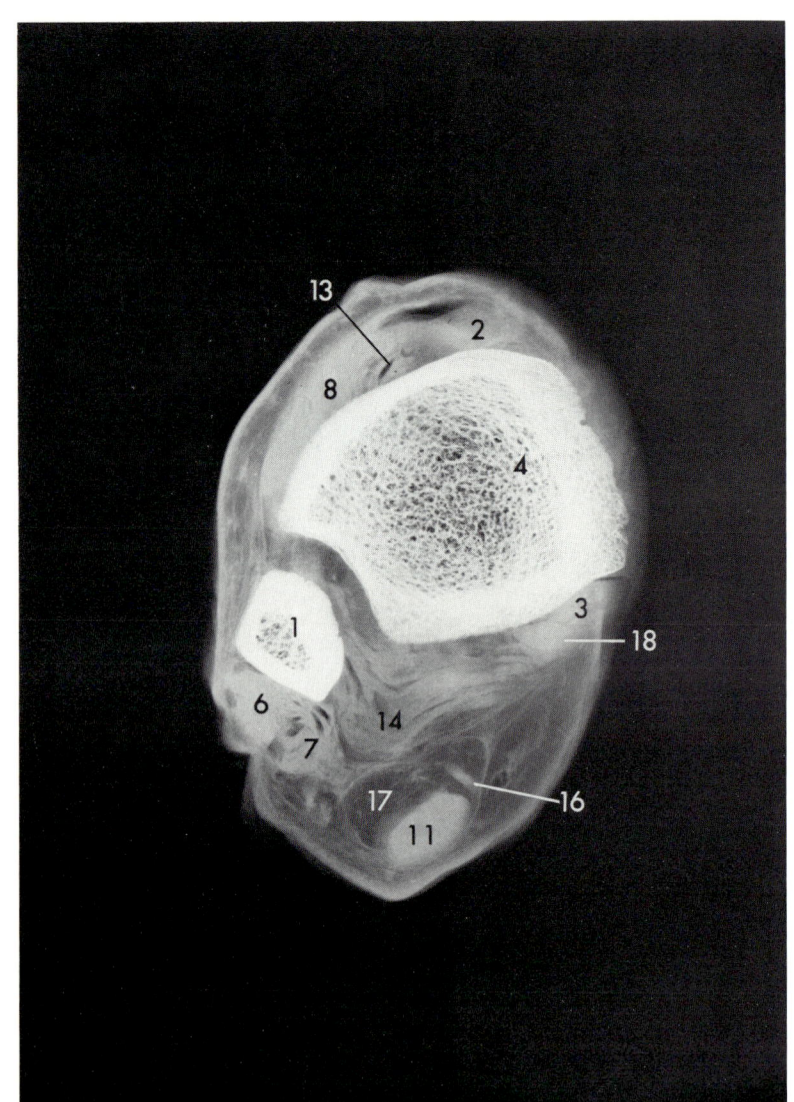
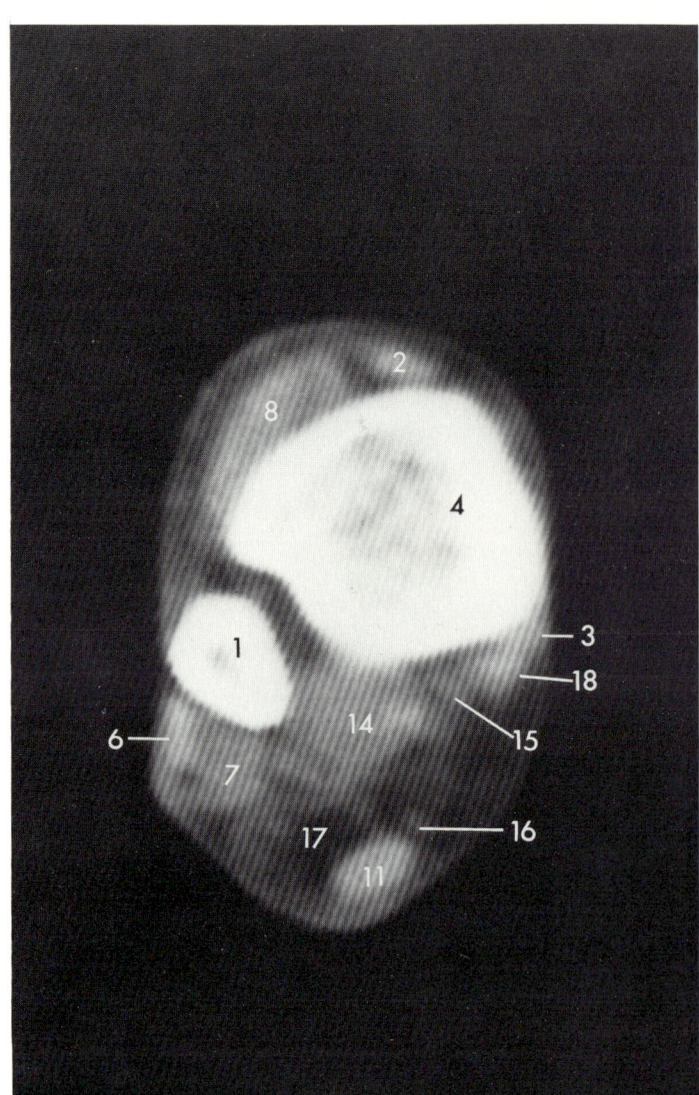
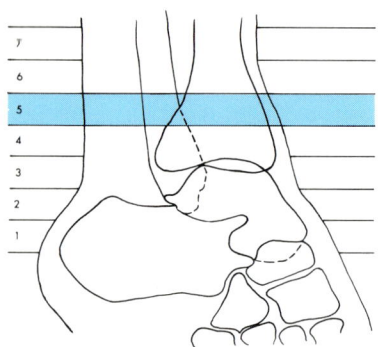

EXTREMITIES: ANKLE

Level A5

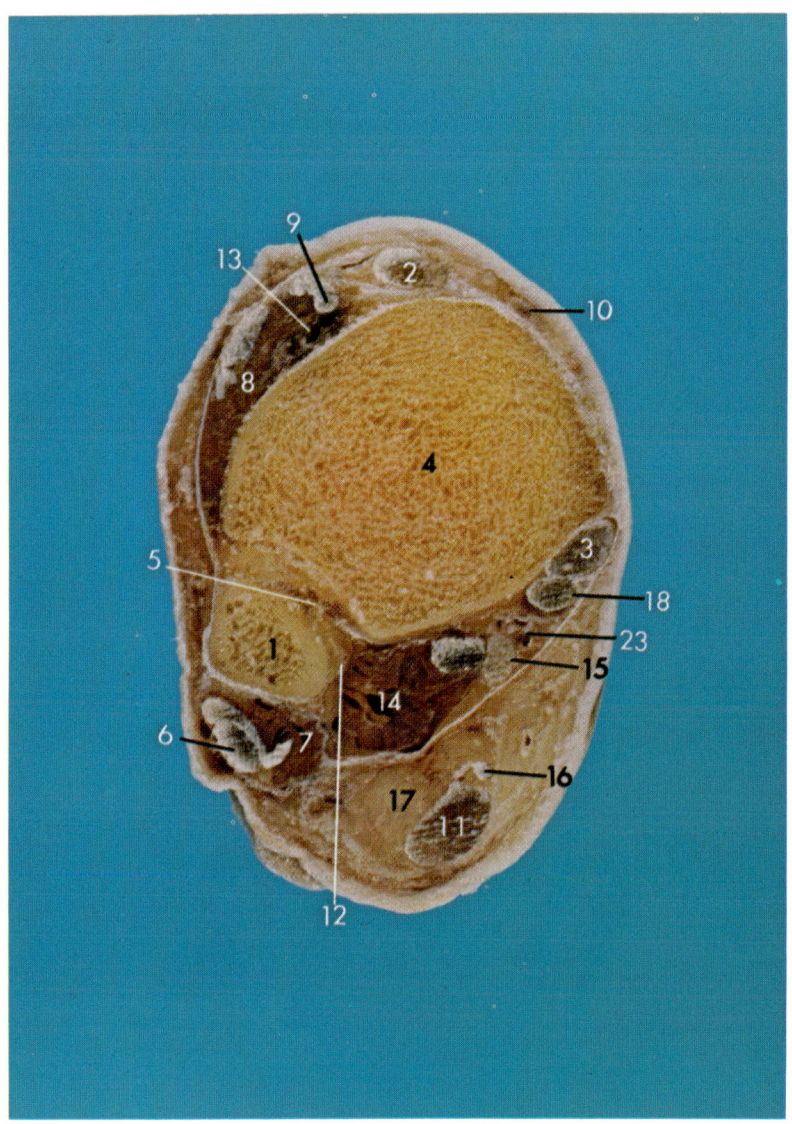

1. Fibula
2. Tibialis anterior tendon
3. Tibialis posterior tendon
4. Tibia
5. Posterior tibiofibular ligament
6. Peroneus longus tendon
7. Peroneus brevis muscle
8. Extensor digitorum longus muscle
9. Extensor hallucis longus tendon
10. Great saphenous vein
11. Achilles tendon
12. Peroneal artery and vein
13. Anterior tibial artery and vein
14. Flexor hallucis longus muscle
15. Tibial nerve
16. Plantaris tendon
17. Pre-Achilles space (fat)
18. Flexor digitorum longus tendon
23. Posterior tibial artery and vein

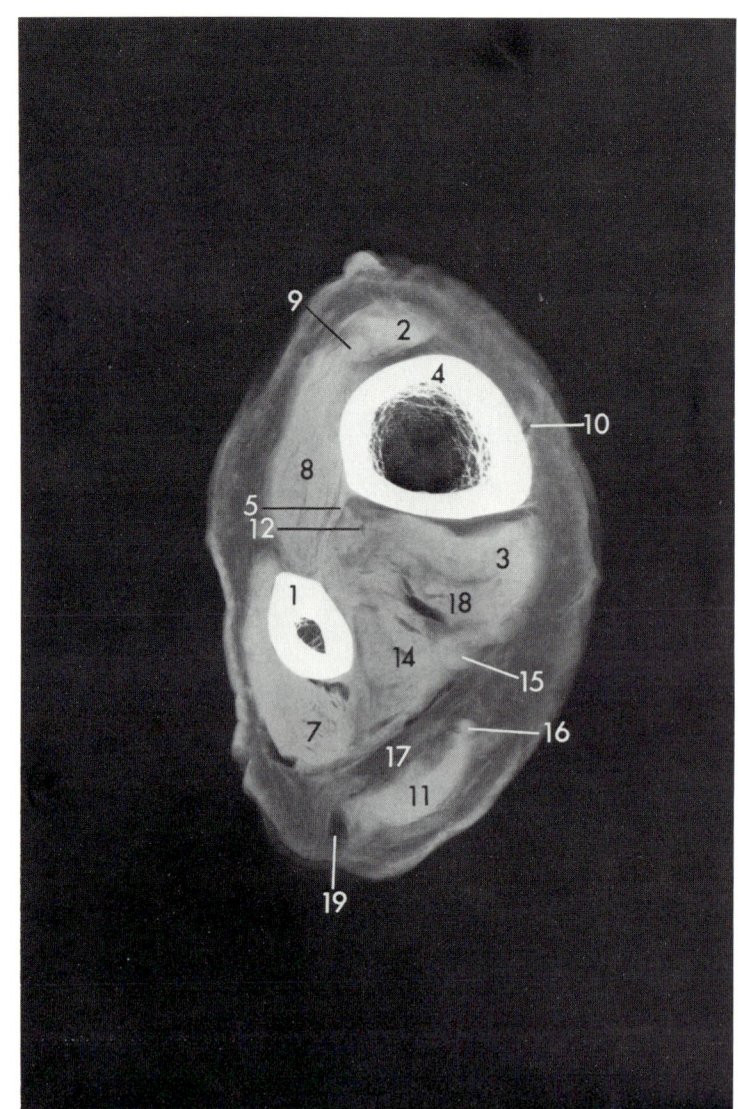
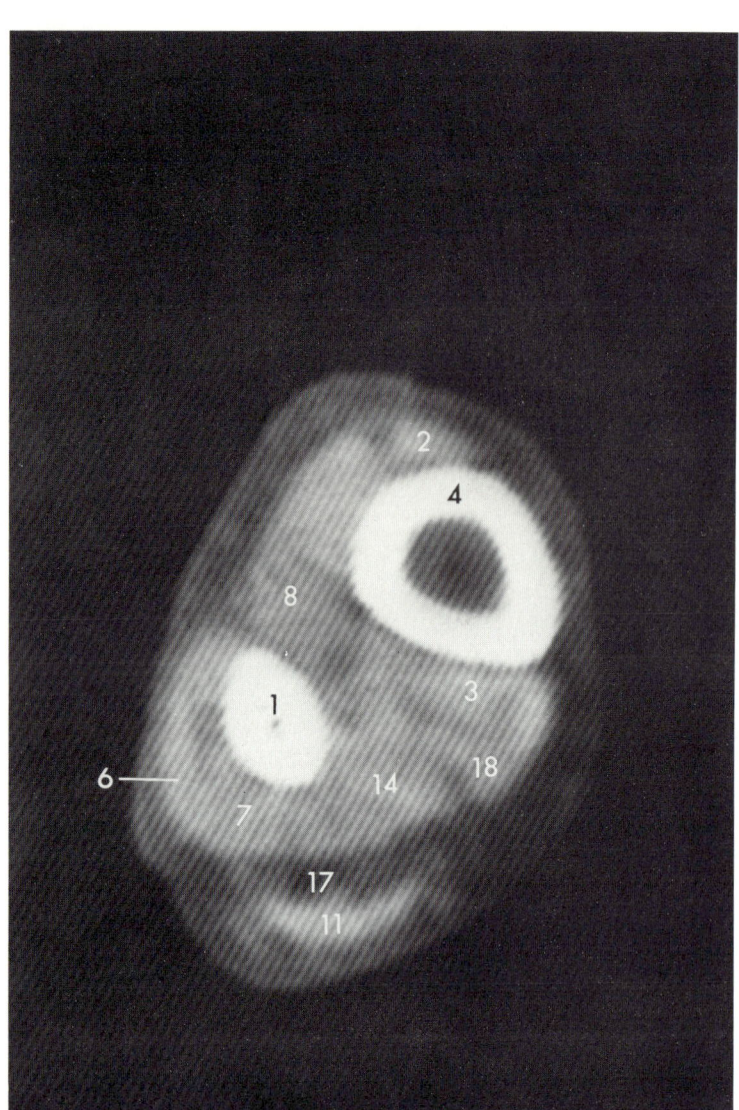
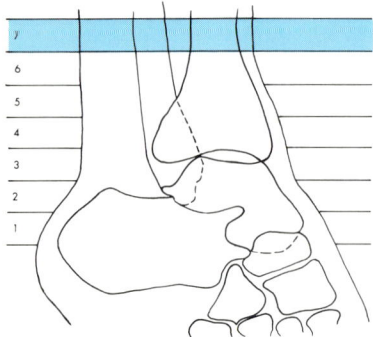

EXTREMITIES: ANKLE

Level A7

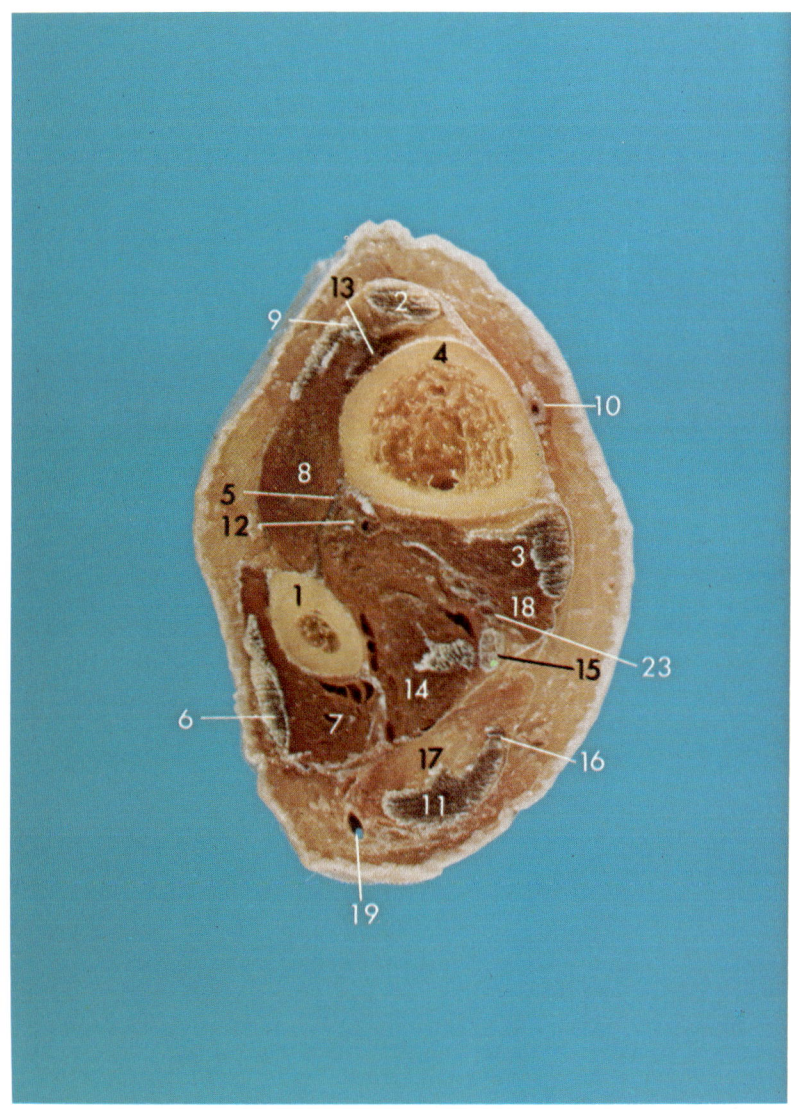

1. Fibula
2. Tibialis anterior tendon
3. Tibialis posterior muscle and tendon
4. Tibia
5. Interosseous membrane
6. Peroneus longus muscle and tendon
7. Peroneus brevis muscle
8. Extensor digitorum longus muscle
9. Extensor hallucis longus muscle and tendon
10. Great saphenous vein
11. Achilles tendon
12. Peroneal artery and vein
13. Anterior tibial artery
14. Flexor hallucis longus muscle
15. Tibial nerve
16. Plantaris tendon
17. Pre-Achilles space (fat)
18. Flexor digitorum longus muscle
19. Small saphenous vein
23. Posterior tibial artery and vein

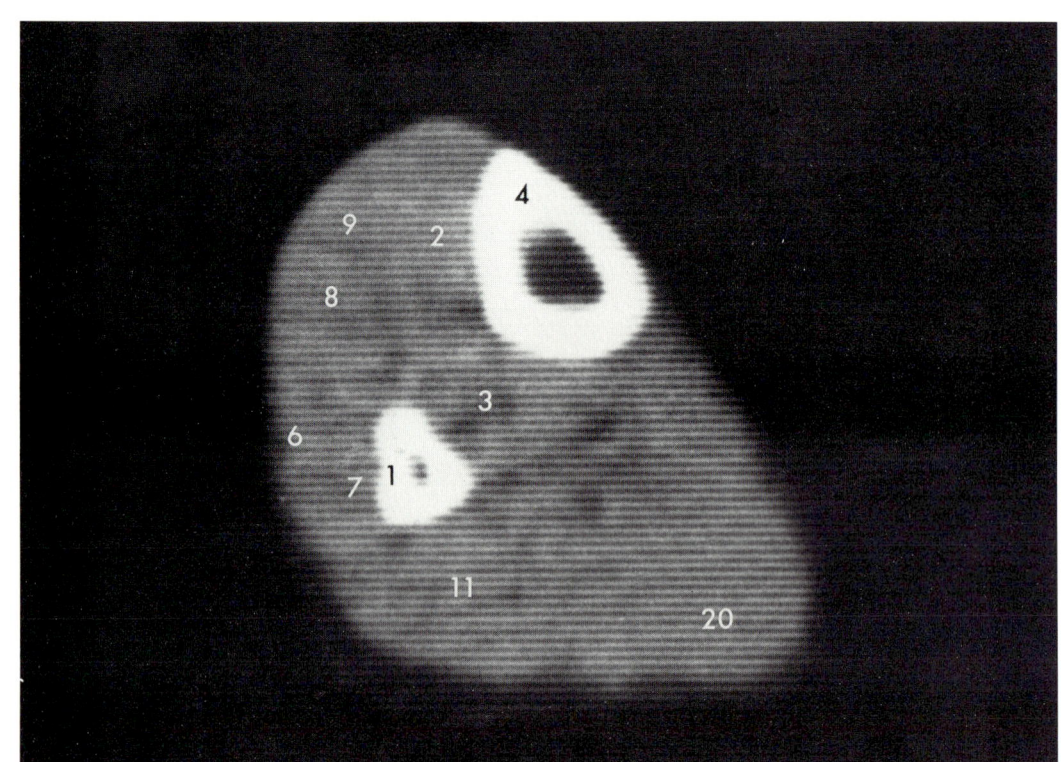

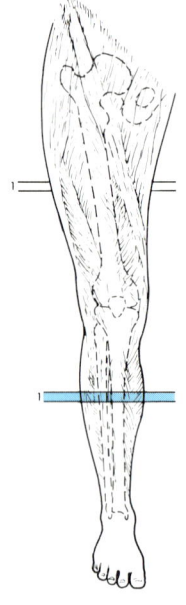

EXTREMITIES: LOWER LEG

Level L1

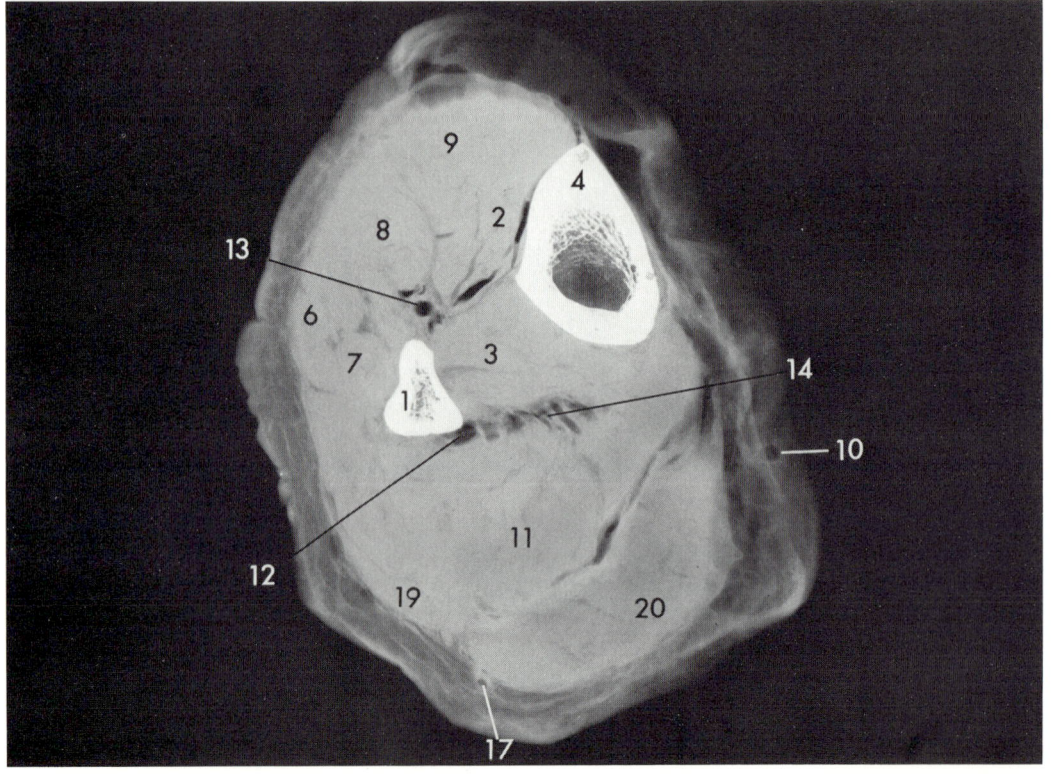

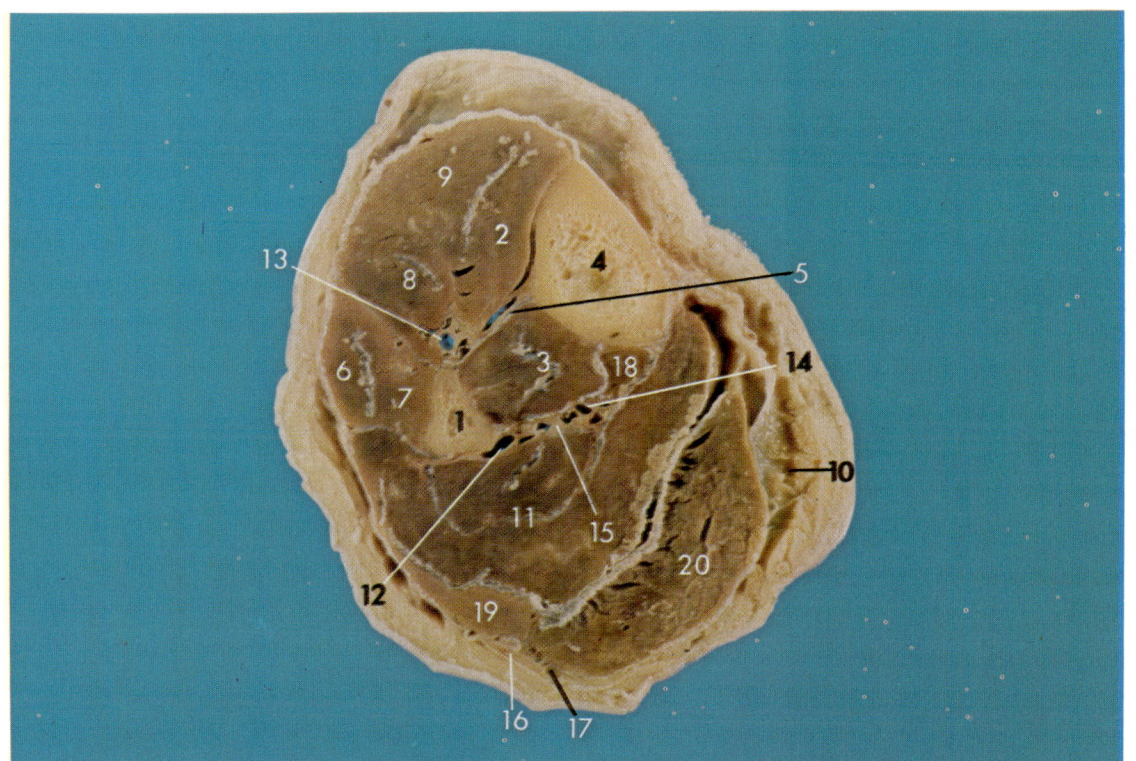

1. Fibula
2. Tibialis anterior muscle
3. Tibialis posterior muscle
4. Tibia
5. Interosseous membrane
6. Peroneus longus muscle
7. Peroneus brevis muscle
8. Extensor digitorum longus muscle
9. Extensor hallucis longus muscle
10. Great saphenous vein
11. Soleus muscle
12. Peroneal artery and vein
13. Anterior tibial artery and vein
14. Posterior tibial artery and vein
15. Tibial nerve
16. Sural nerve
17. Small saphenous vein
18. Flexor digitorum longus muscle
19. Gastrocnemius muscle (lateral head)
20. Gastrocnemius muscle (medial head)

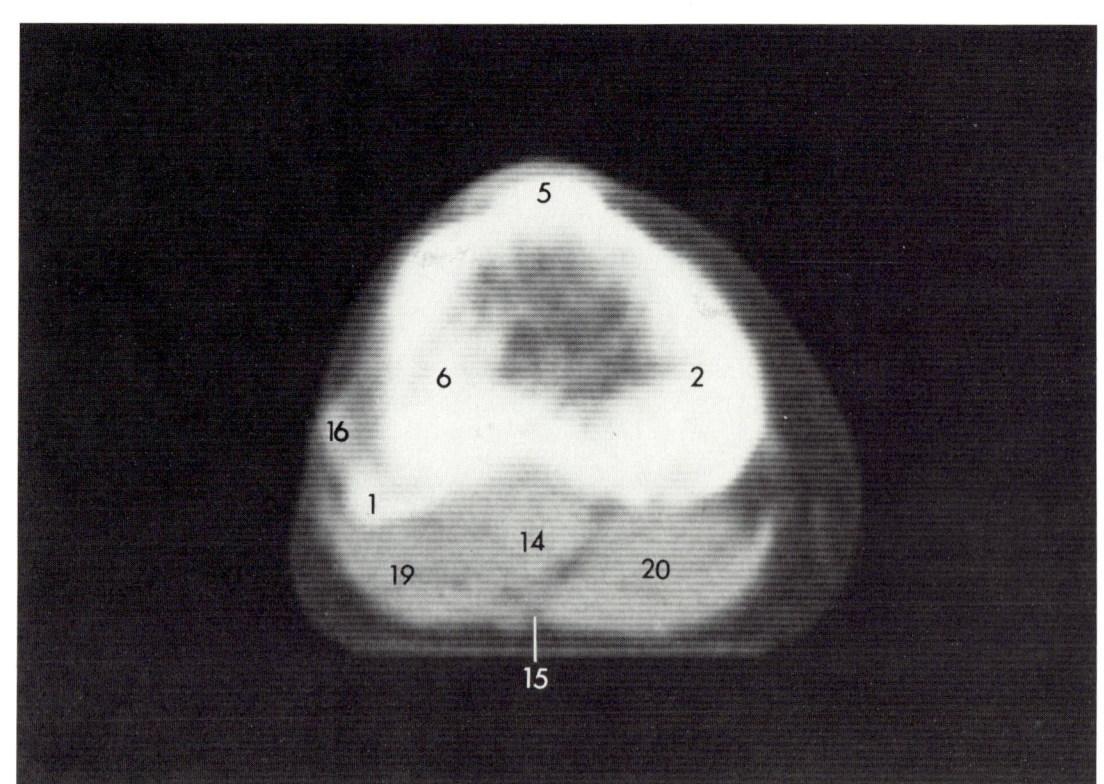

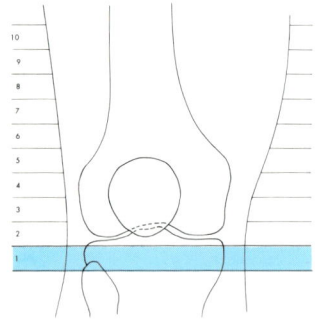

EXTREMITIES: KNEE

Level K1

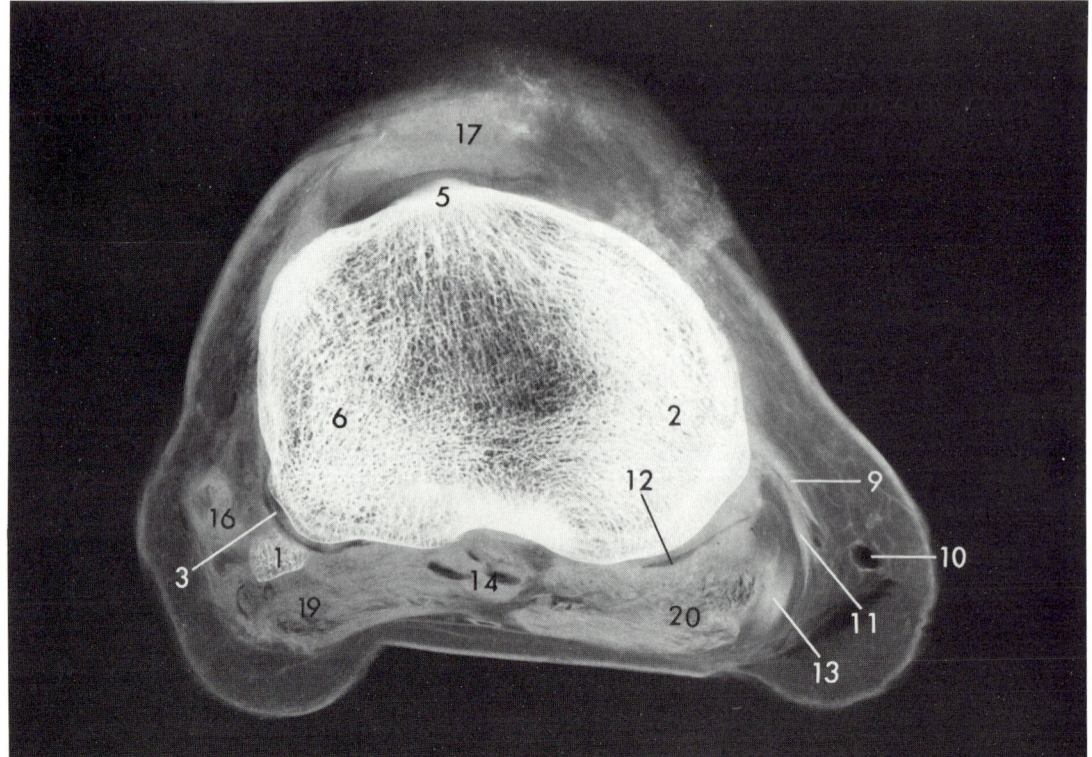

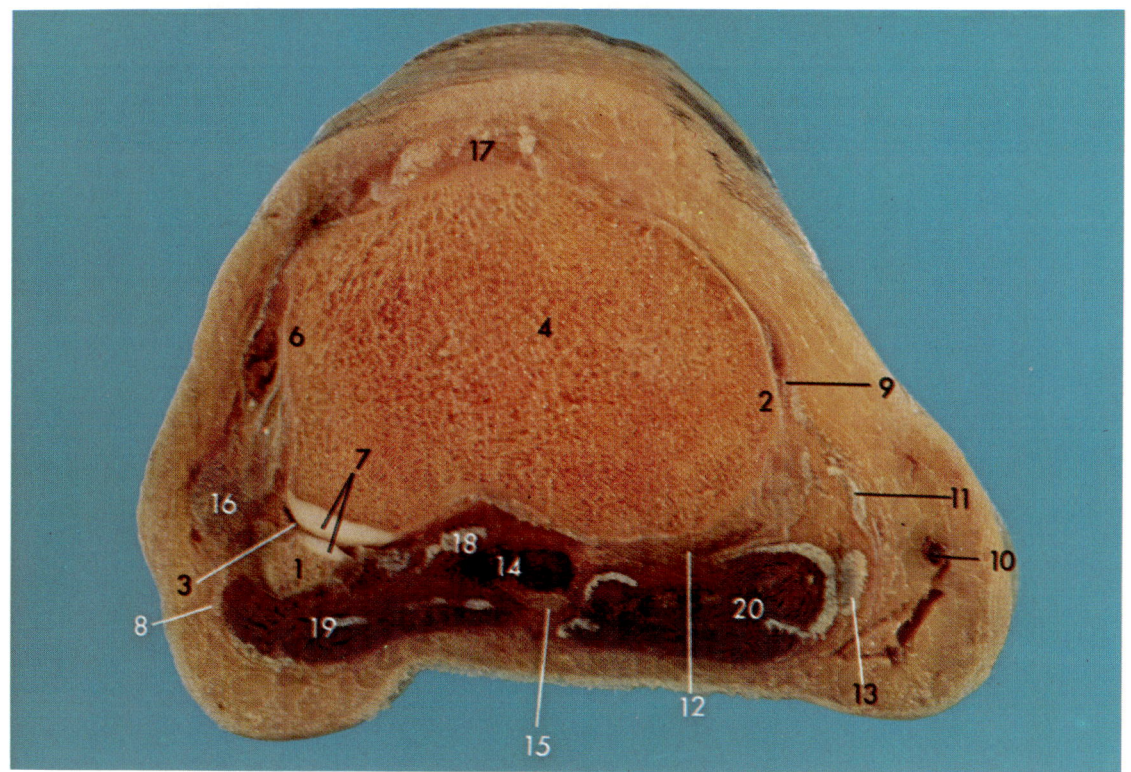

1. Fibula
2. Medial condyle of tibia
3. Tibiofibular joint cavity
4. Tibia
5. Tuberosity of tibia
6. Lateral condyle of tibia
7. Articular cartilage
8. Common peroneal nerve
9. Sartorius tendon
10. Great saphenous vein
11. Gracilis tendon
12. Semimembranosus tendon
13. Semitendinosus tendon
14. Popliteal artery and vein
15. Tibial nerve
16. Biceps femoris tendon
17. Patellar ligament
18. Popliteus muscle
19. Gastrocnemius (lateral head) and soleus muscles
20. Gastrocnemius muscle (medial head)

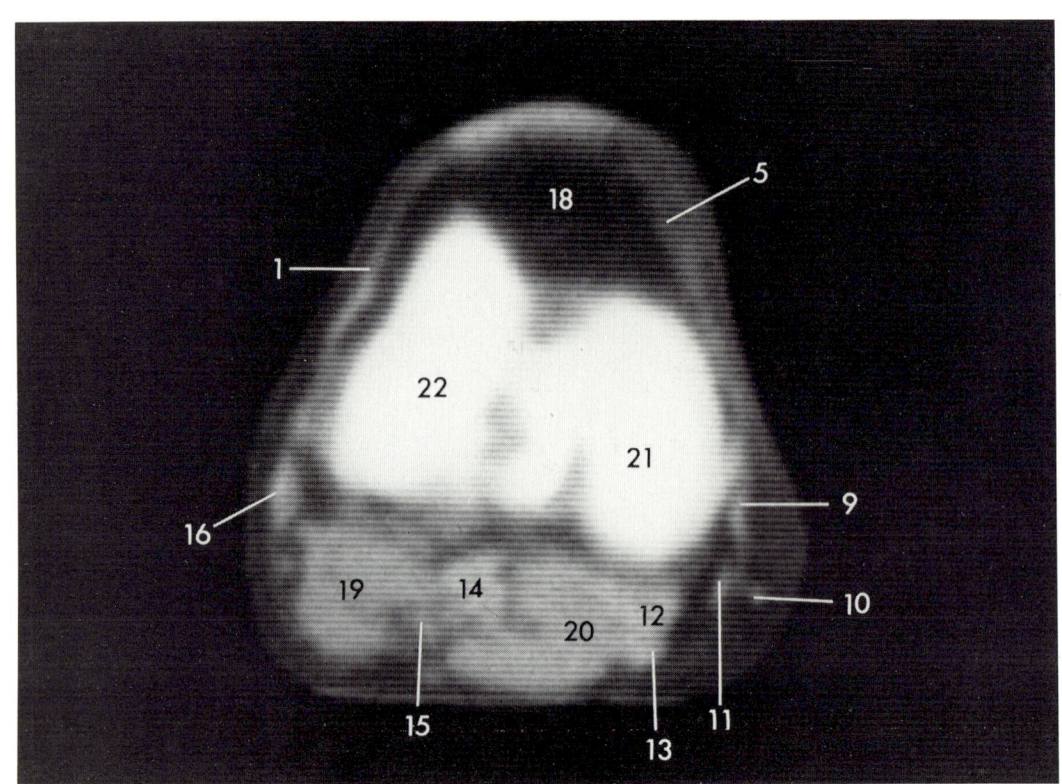

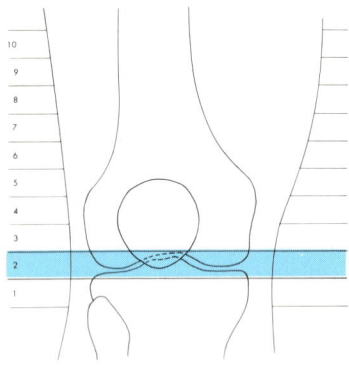

EXTREMITIES: KNEE

Level K2 (Superior [proximal] aspect)

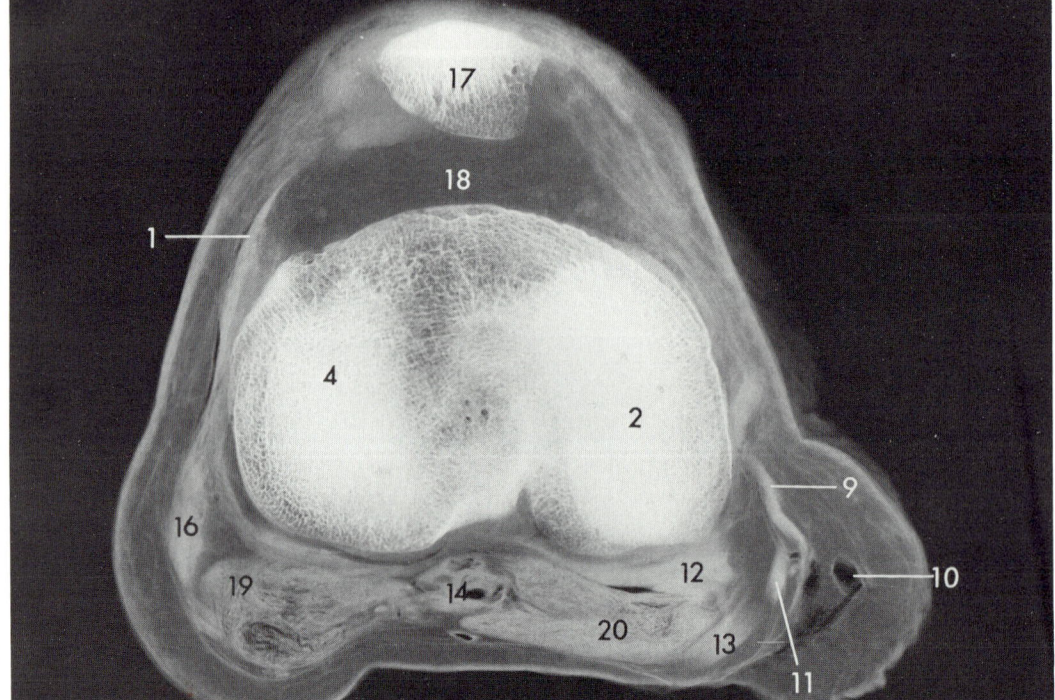

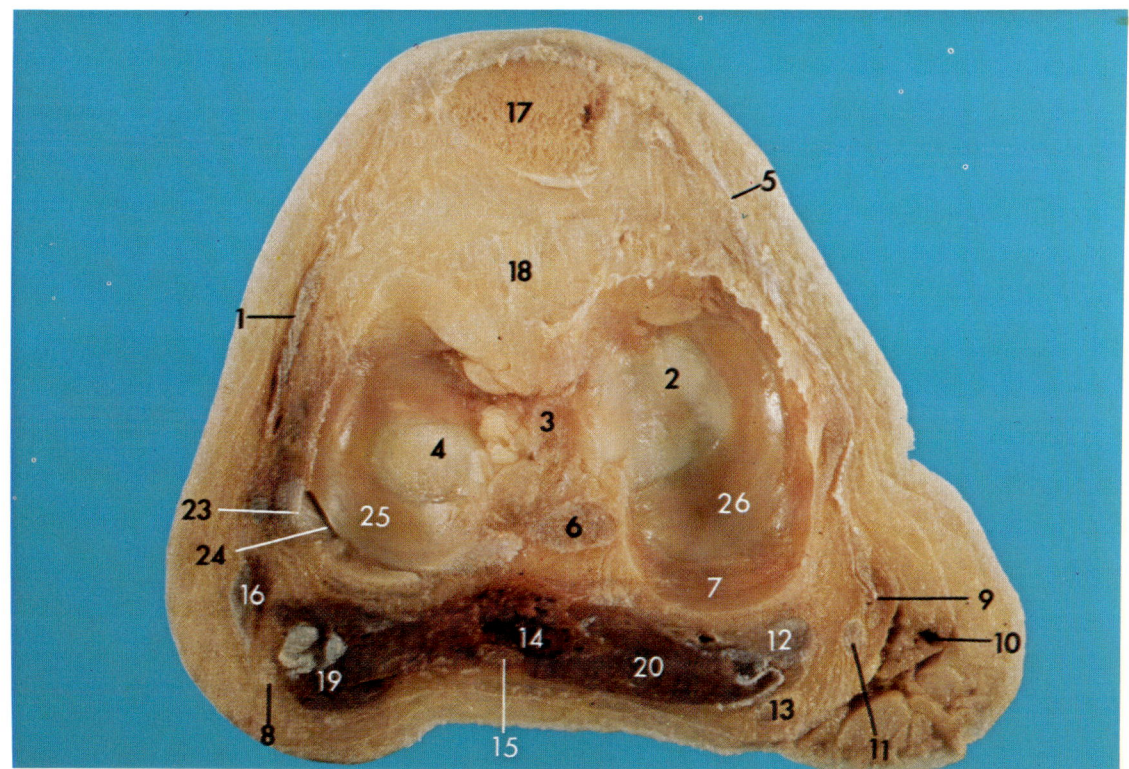

1. Iliotibial tract
2. Medial condyle of tibia (articular surface)
3. Anterior cruciate ligament
4. Lateral condyle of tibia (articular surface)
5. Medial patellar retinaculum
6. Posterior cruciate ligament
7. Capsule of knee joint
8. Common peroneal nerve
9. Sartorius muscle
10. Great saphenous vein
11. Gracilis tendon
12. Semimembranosus tendon
13. Semitendinosus tendon
14. Popliteal artery and vein
15. Tibial nerve
16. Biceps femoris tendon
17. Patella
18. Infrapatellar fat pad
19. Gastrocnemius muscle (lateral head)
20. Gastrocnemius muscle (medial head)
21. Medial condyle of femur
22. Lateral condyle of femur
23. Popliteus tendon
24. Popliteus bursa
25. Lateral meniscus
26. Medial meniscus

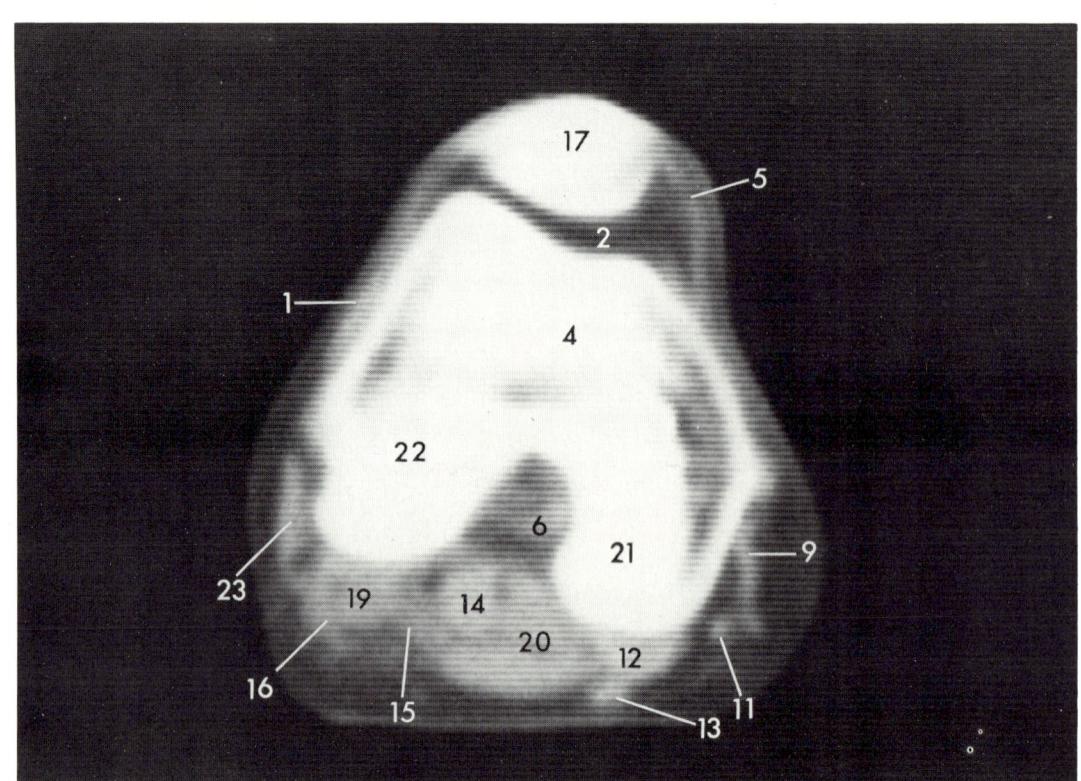

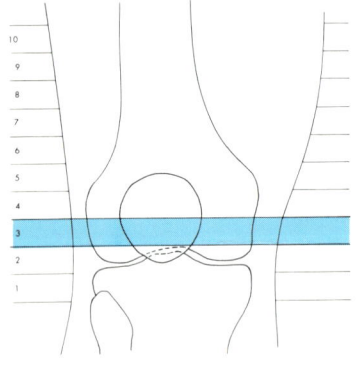

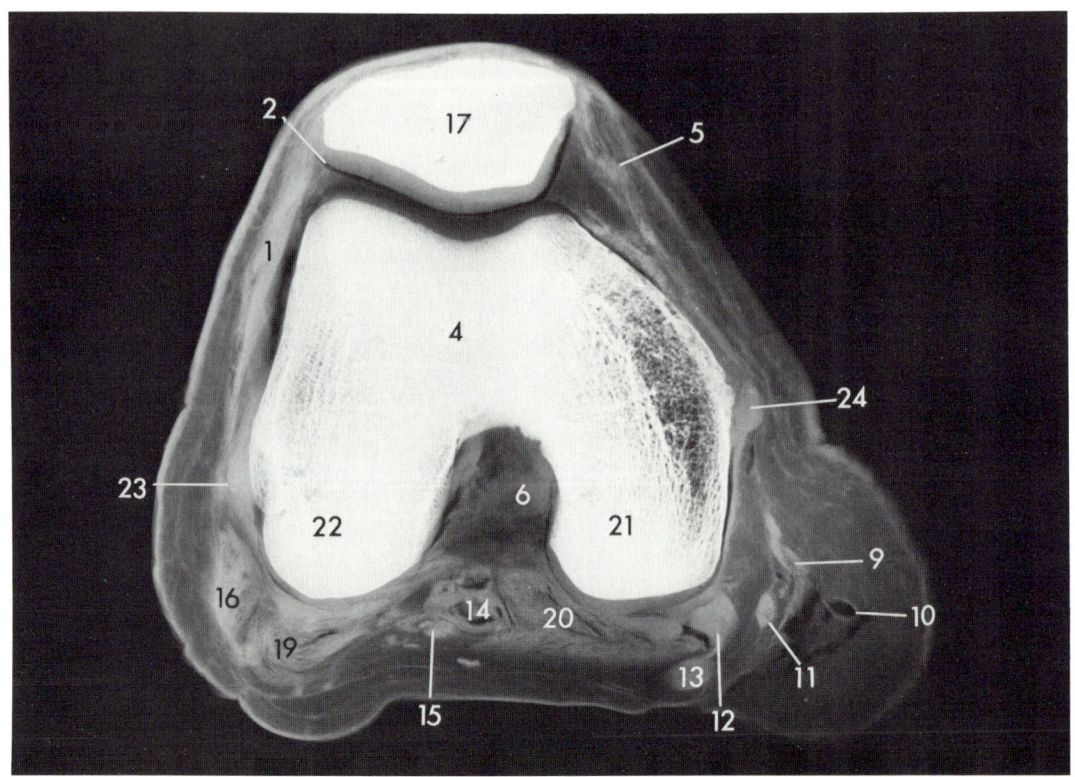

EXTREMITIES: KNEE

Level K3

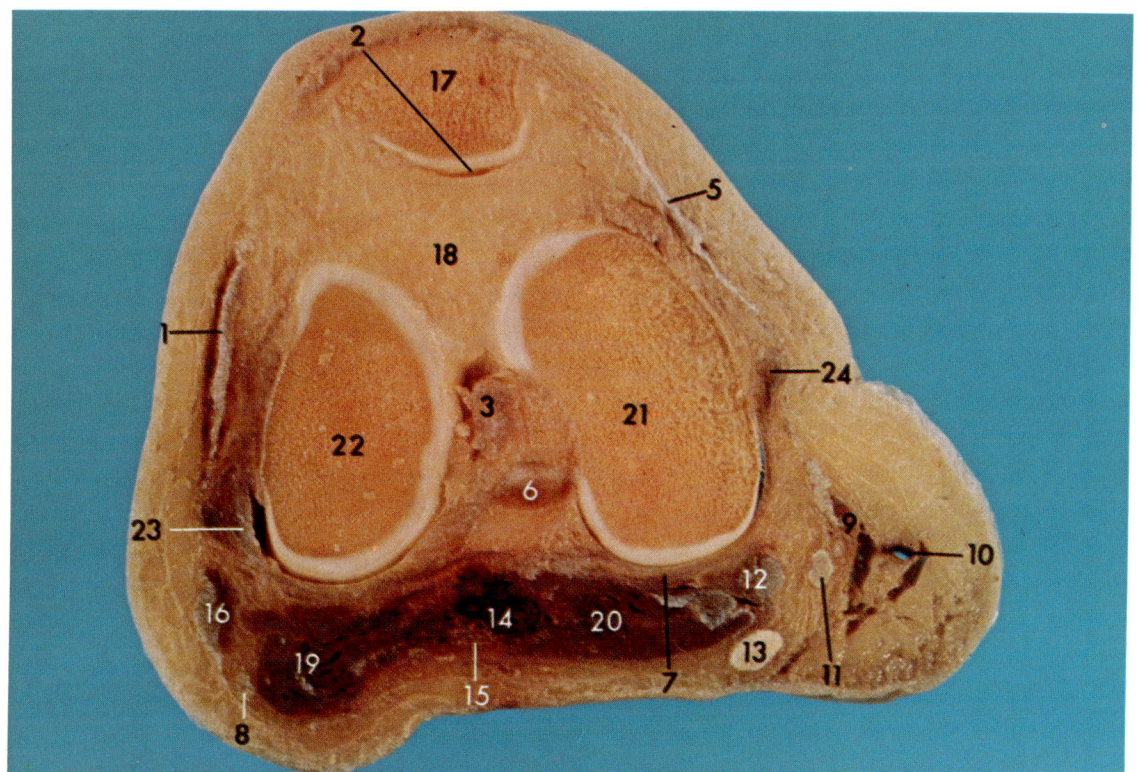

1. Iliotibial tract
2. Knee joint cavity
3. Anterior cruciate ligament
4. Femur
5. Medial patellar retinaculum
6. Posterior cruciate ligament
7. Capsule of knee joint
8. Common peroneal nerve
9. Sartorius muscle
10. Great saphenous vein
11. Gracilis tendon
12. Semimembranosus tendon
13. Semitendinosus tendon
14. Popliteal artery and vein
15. Tibial nerve
16. Biceps femoris muscle and tendon
17. Patella
18. Infrapatellar fat pad
19. Gastrocnemius muscle (lateral head)
20. Gastrocnemius muscle (medial head)
21. Medial condyle of femur
22. Lateral condyle of femur
23. Fibular collateral ligament
24. Tibial collateral ligament

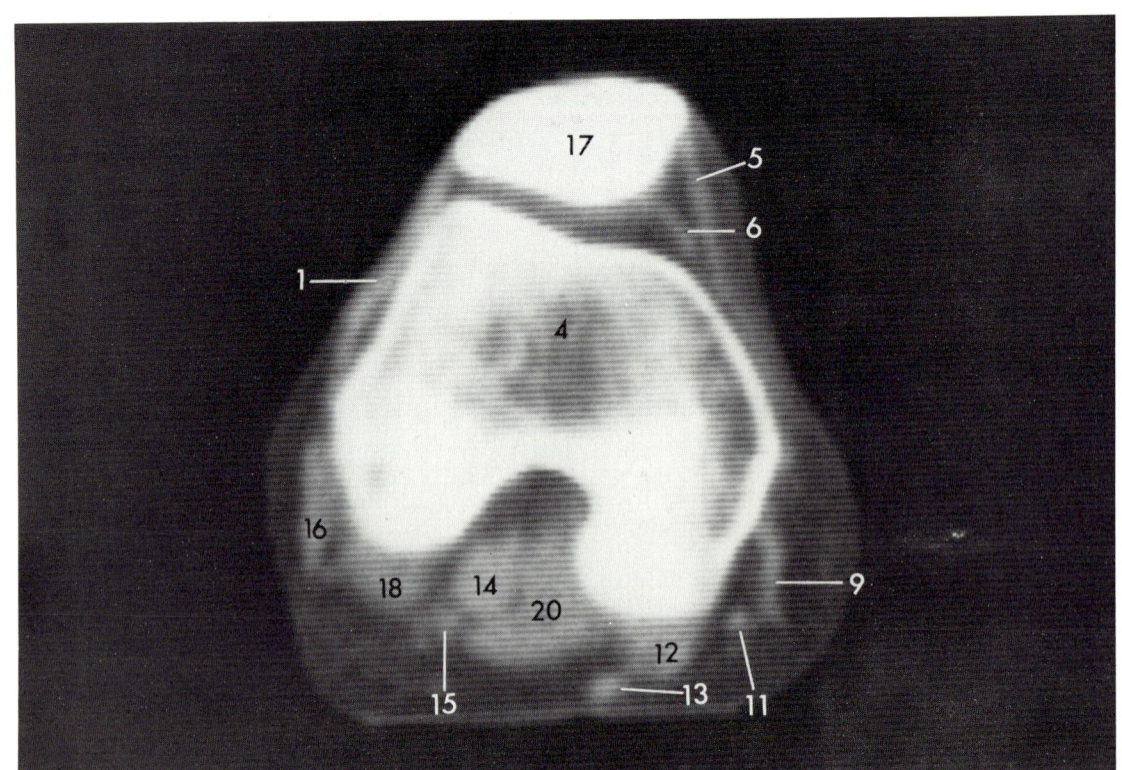

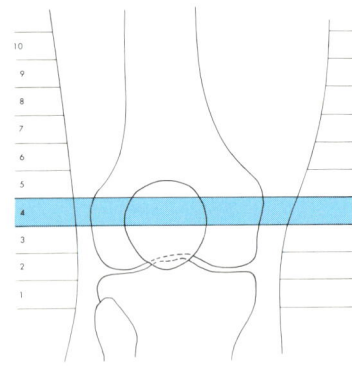

EXTREMITIES: KNEE

Level K4

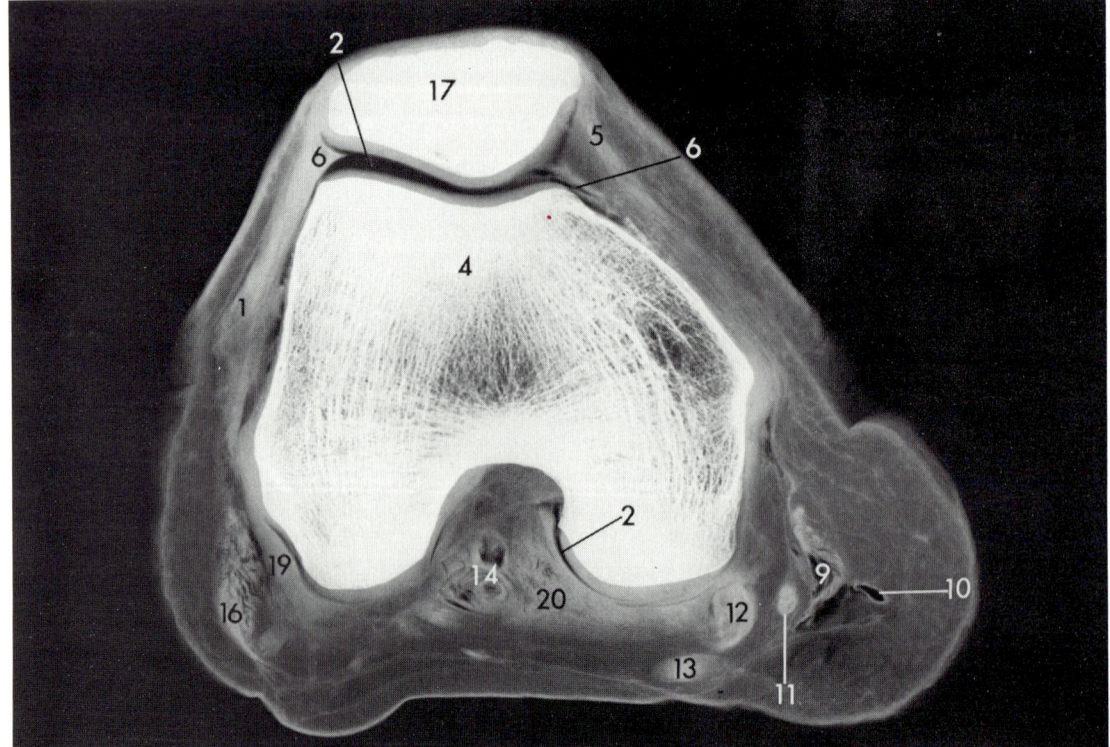

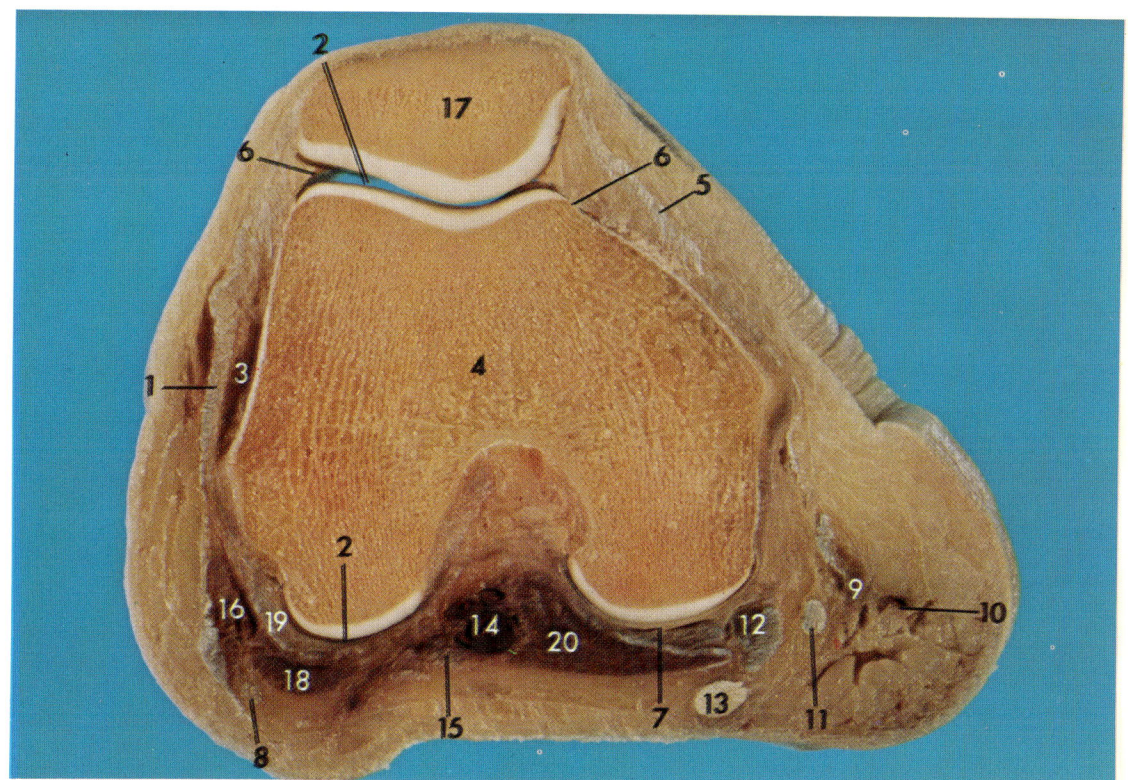

1. Iliotibial tract
2. Knee joint cavity
3. Vastus lateralis muscle
4. Femur
5. Medial patellar retinaculum
6. Alar fold (synovial)
7. Capsule of knee joint
8. Common peroneal nerve
9. Sartorius muscle
10. Great saphenous vein
11. Gracilis tendon
12. Semimembranosus tendon
13. Semitendinosus tendon
14. Popliteal artery and vein
15. Tibial nerve
16. Biceps femoris muscle
17. Patella
18. Plantaris muscle
19. Gastrocnemius tendon (lateral head)
20. Gastrocnemius muscle (medial head)

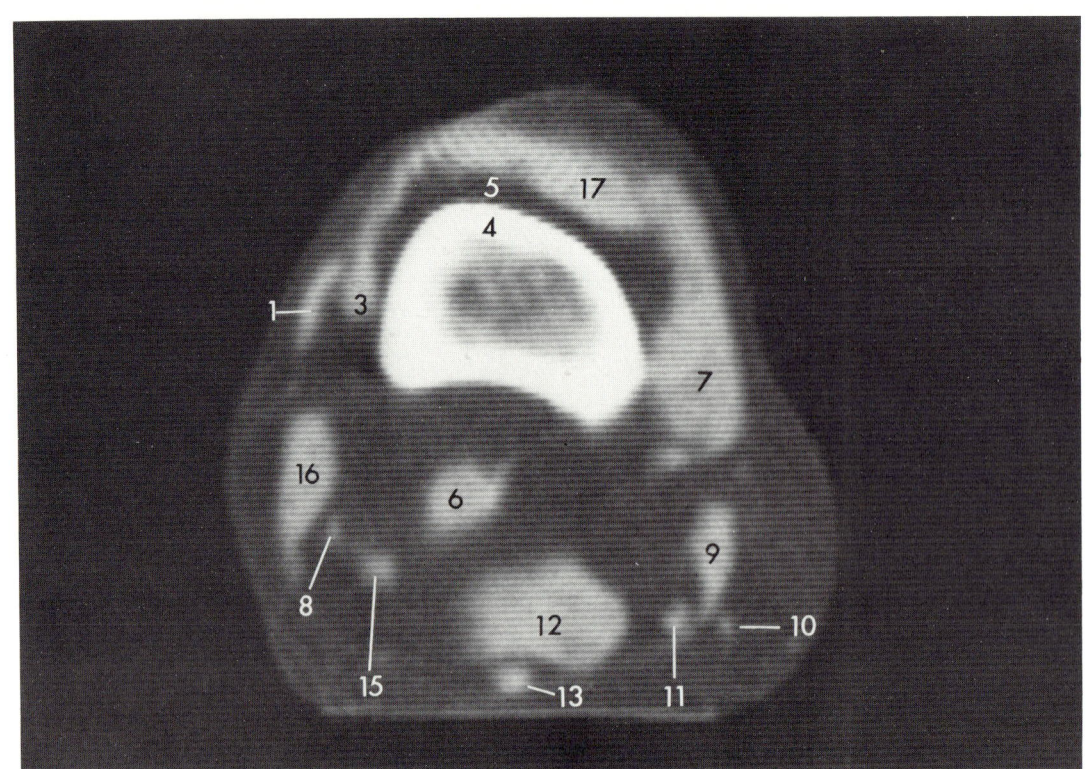

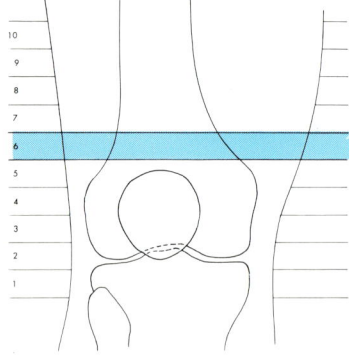

EXTREMITIES: KNEE

Level K6

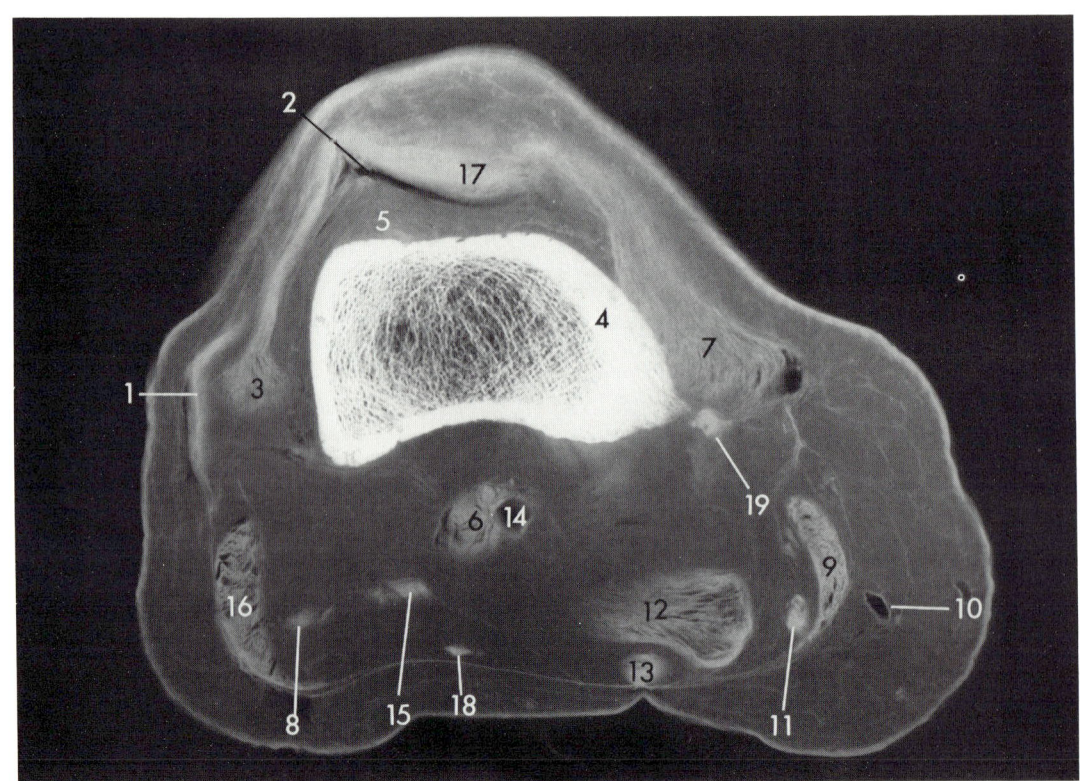

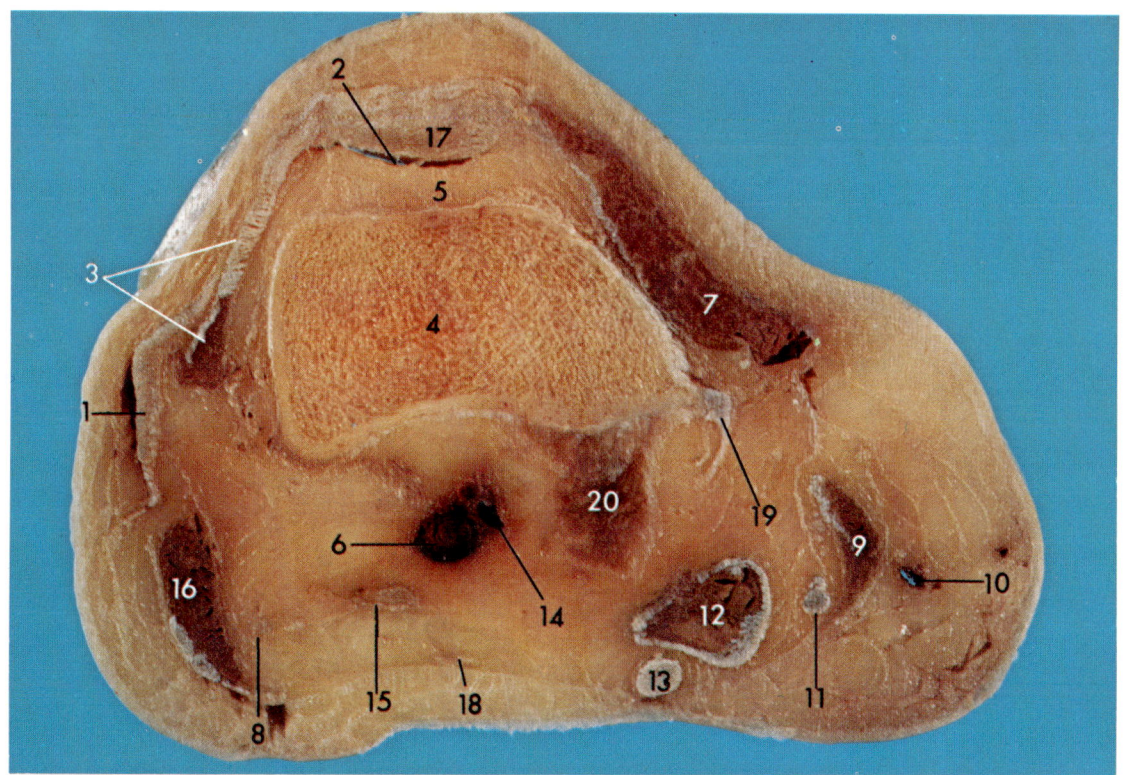

1. Iliotibial tract
2. Suprapatellar bursa
3. Vastus lateralis muscle and tendon
4. Femur
5. Prefemoral fat
6. Popliteal vein
7. Vastus medialis muscle
8. Common peroneal nerve
9. Sartorius muscle
10. Great saphenous vein
11. Gracilis tendon
12. Semimembranosus muscle
13. Semitendinosus tendon
14. Popliteal artery
15. Tibial nerve
16. Biceps femoris muscle (short head)
17. Quadriceps tendon
18. Small saphenous vein
19. Adductor magnus tendon
20. Gastrocnemius muscle (medial head)

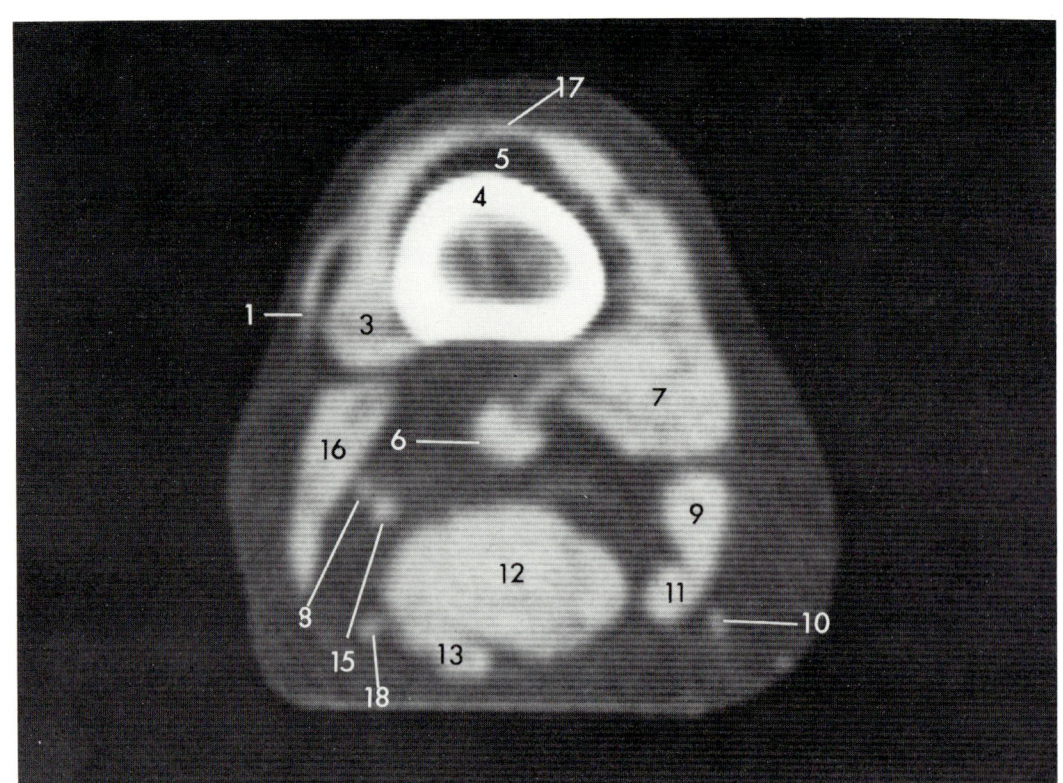

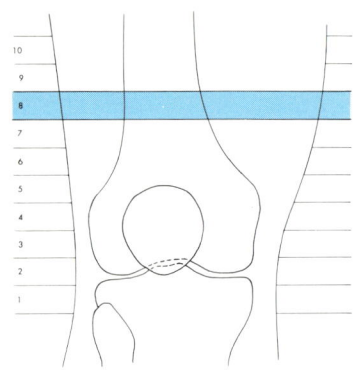

EXTREMITIES: KNEE

Level K8

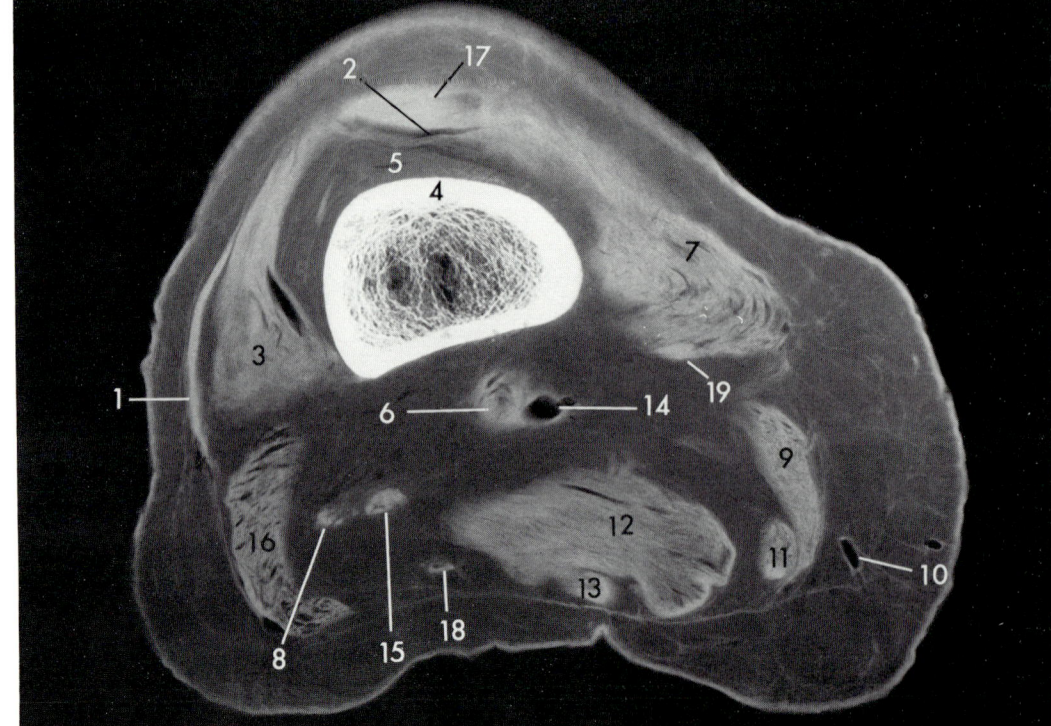

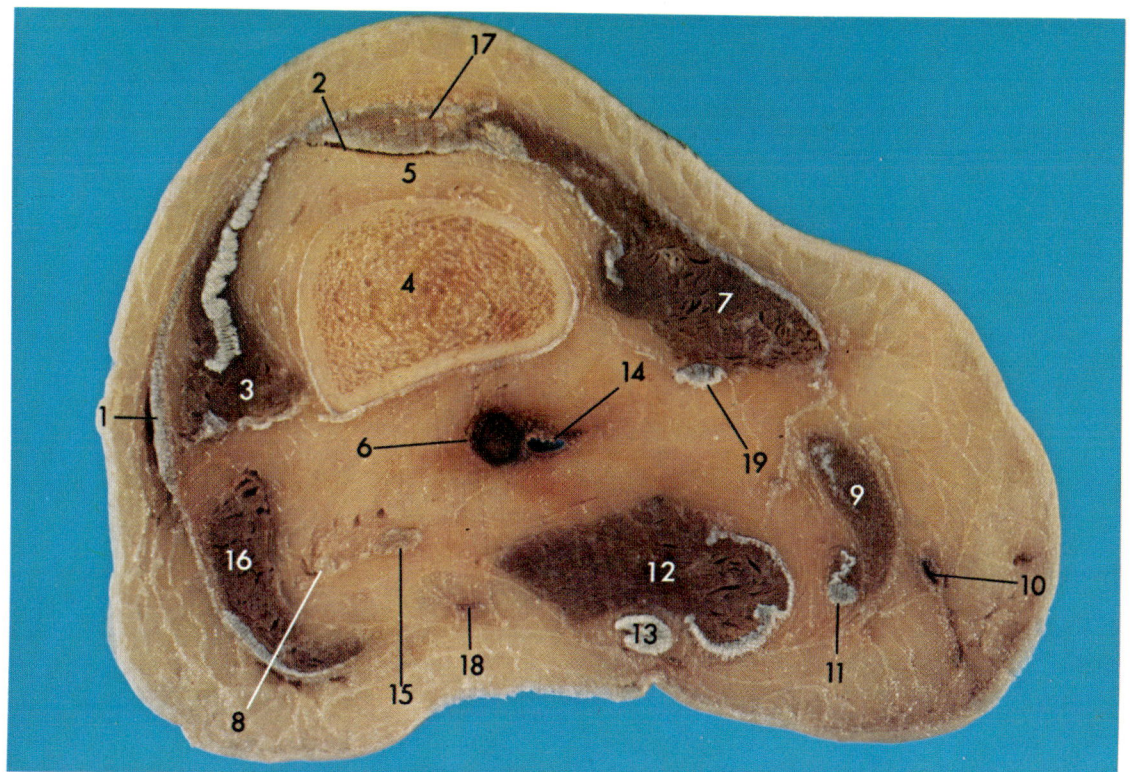

1. Iliotibial tract
2. Suprapatellar bursa
3. Vastus lateralis muscle
4. Femur
5. Prefemoral fat
6. Popliteal vein
7. Vastus medialis muscle
8. Common peroneal nerve
9. Sartorius muscle
10. Great saphenous vein
11. Gracilis muscle and tendon
12. Semimembranosus muscle
13. Semitendinosus tendon
14. Popliteal artery
15. Tibial nerve
16. Biceps femoris muscle (short head)
17. Quadriceps tendon
18. Small saphenous vein
19. Adductor magnus tendon

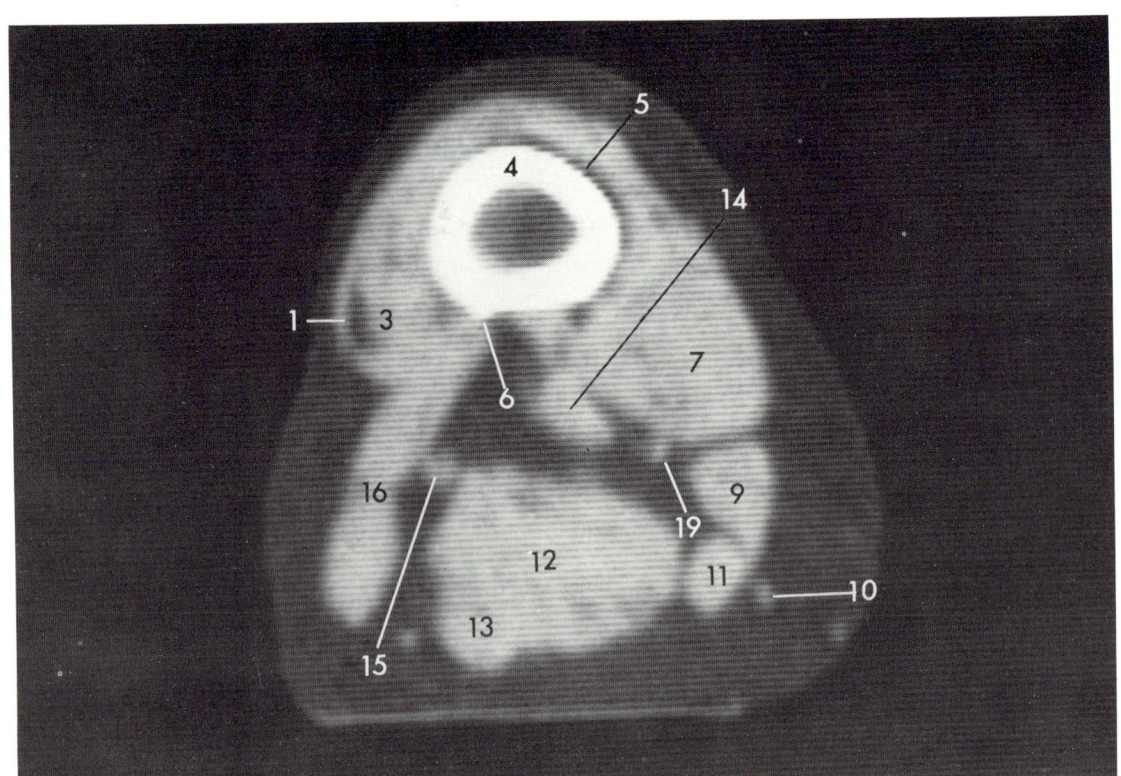

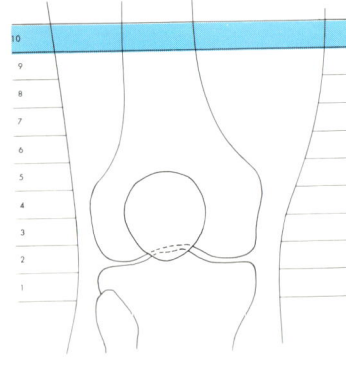

EXTREMITIES:
KNEE

Level K10

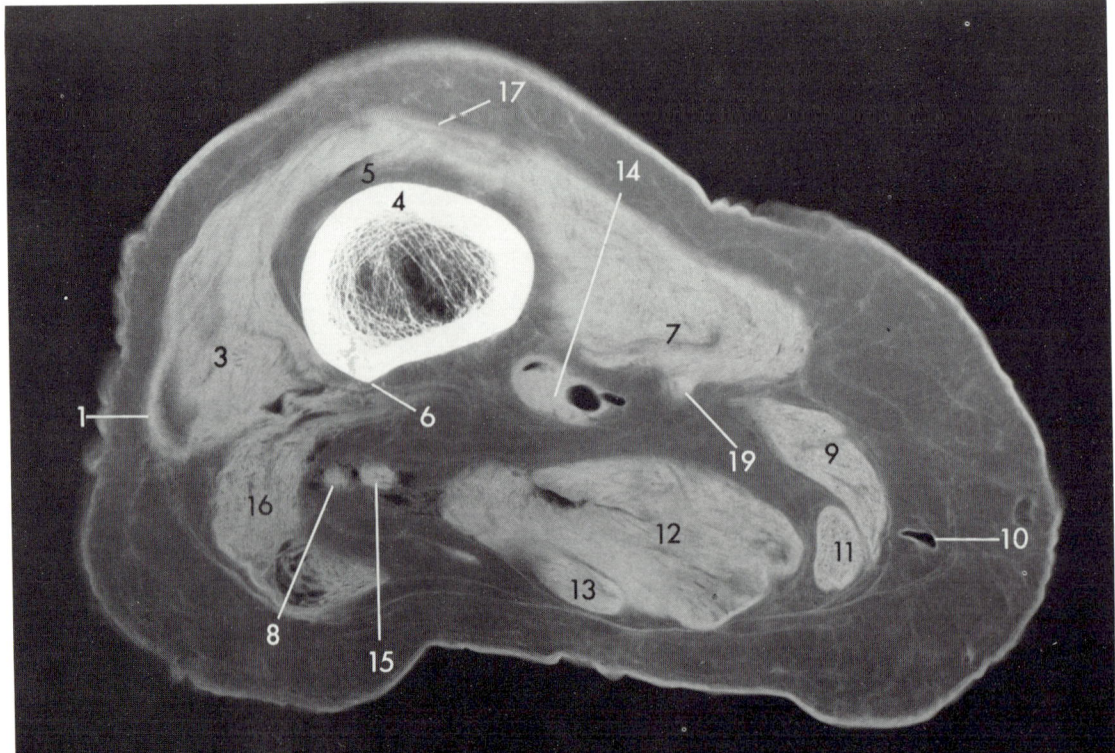

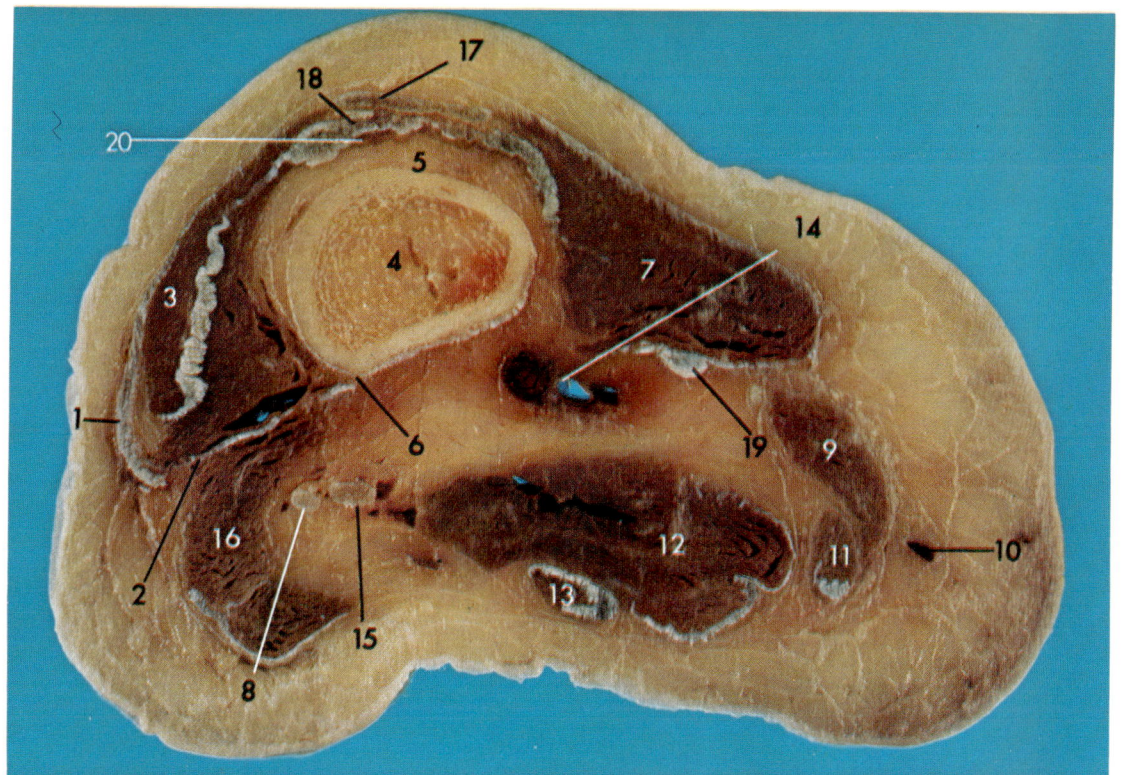

1. Iliotibial tract
2. Lateral intermuscular septum
3. Vastus lateralis muscle
4. Femur
5. Prefemoral fat
6. Linea aspera of femur
7. Vastus medialis muscle
8. Common peroneal nerve
9. Sartorius muscle
10. Great saphenous vein
11. Gracilis muscle
12. Semimembranosus muscle
13. Semitendinosus muscle
14. Femoral artery and vein
15. Tibial nerve
16. Biceps femoris muscle (short head)
17. Rectus femoris tendon
18. Vastus intermedius tendon
19. Adductor magnus tendon
20. Articularis genus muscle

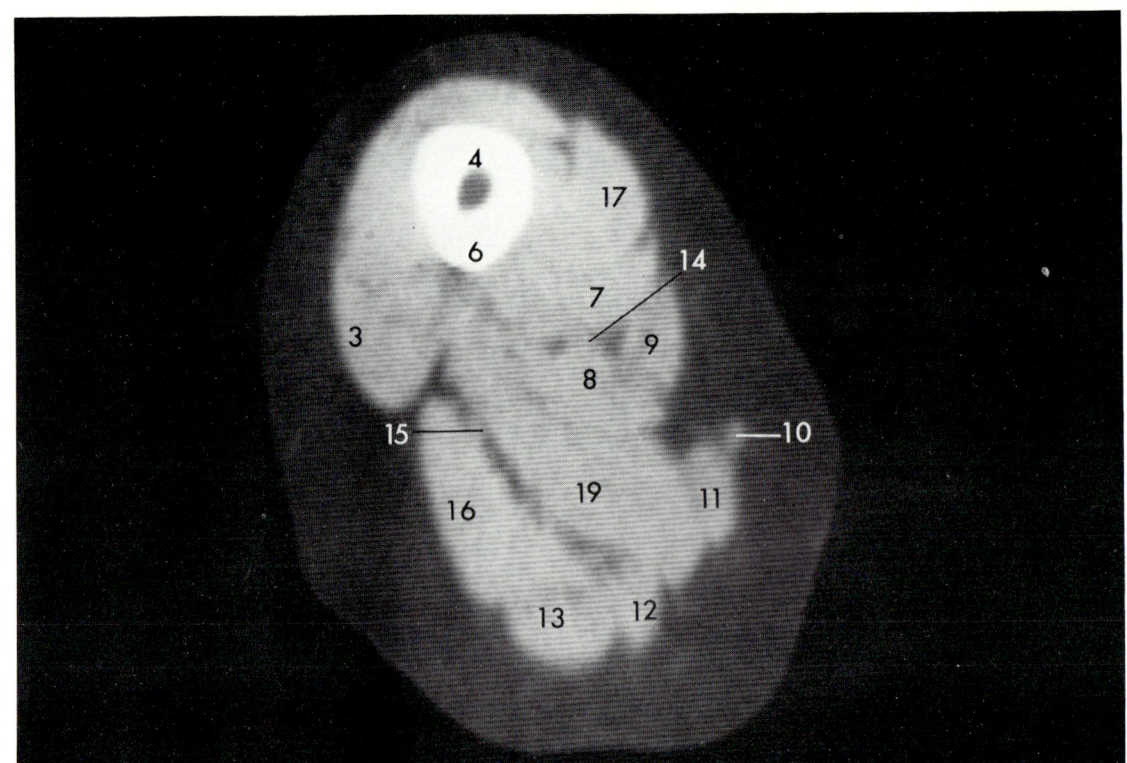

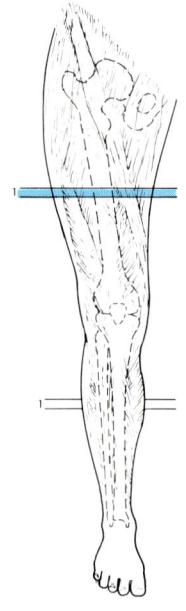

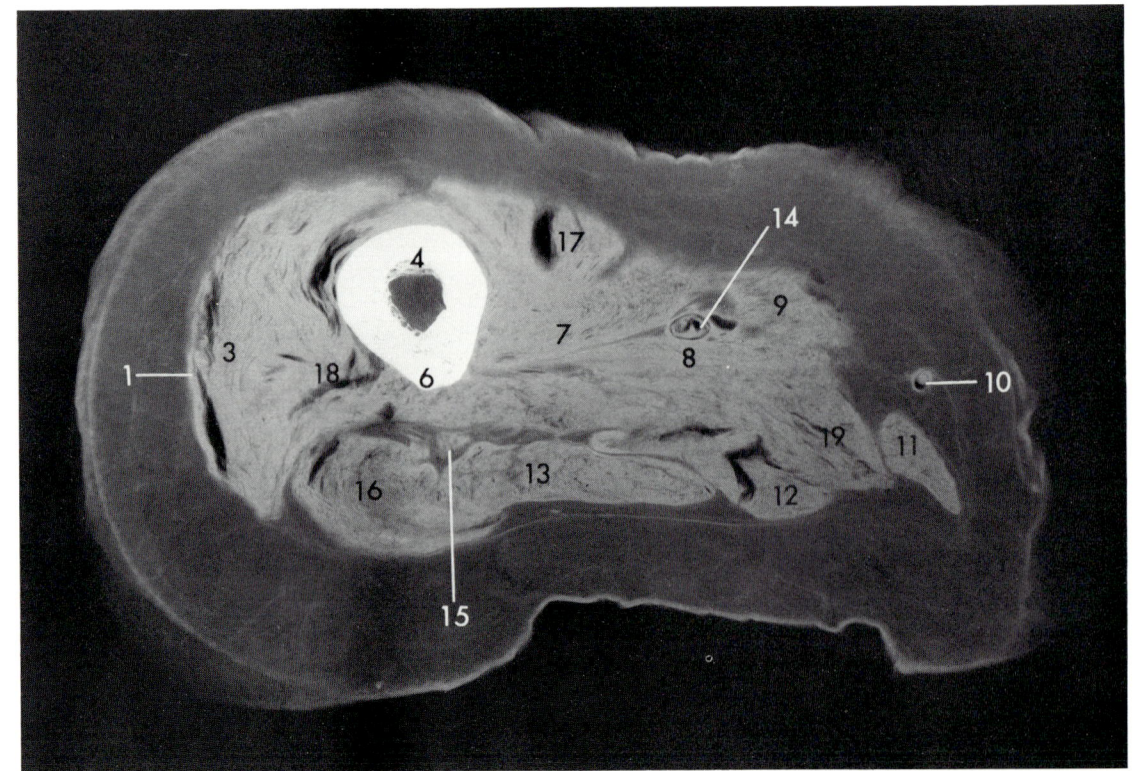

EXTREMITIES: THIGH

Level T1

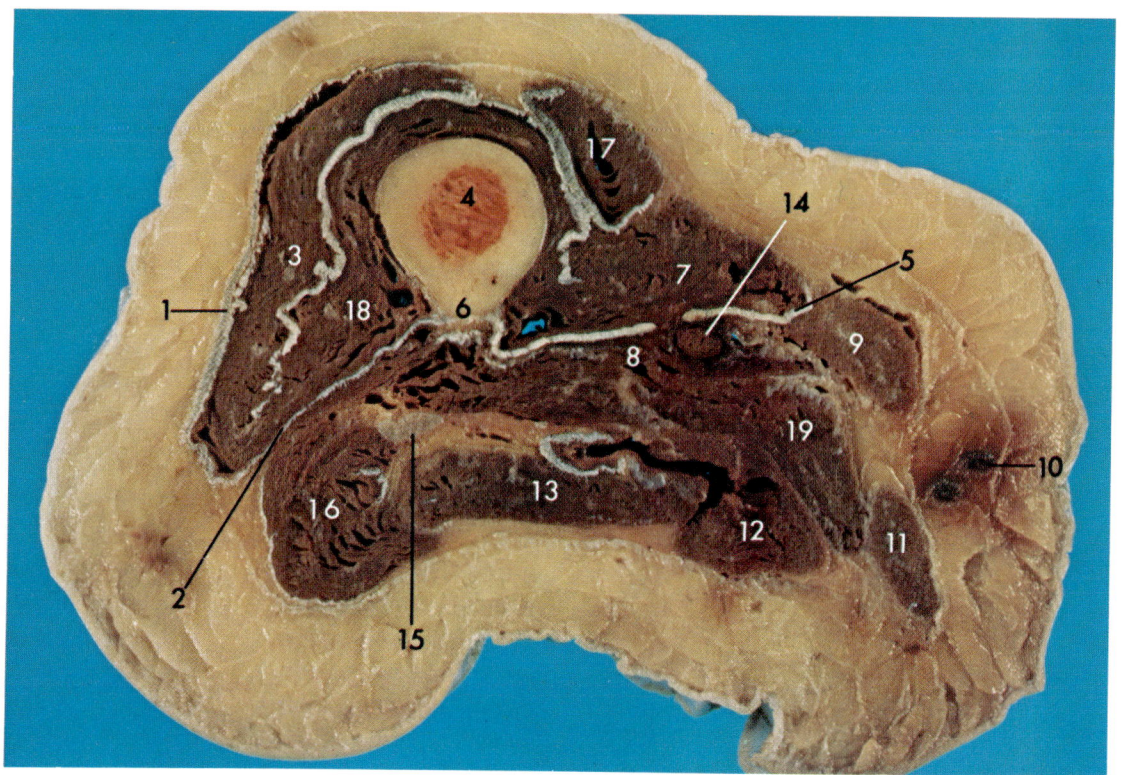

1. Iliotibial tract
2. Lateral intermuscular septum
3. Vastus lateralis muscle
4. Femur
5. Medial intermuscular septum
6. Linea aspera of femur
7. Vastus medialis muscle
8. Adductor longus muscle
9. Sartorius muscle
10. Great saphenous vein
11. Gracilis muscle
12. Semimembranosus muscle
13. Semitendinosus muscle
14. Femoral artery and vein
15. Sciatic nerve
16. Biceps femoris muscle (long head)
17. Rectus femoris muscle
18. Vastus intermedius muscle
19. Adductor magnus muscle

Index

Abdomen, computed tomography of, 144–223
   in female, 144–201
   in male, 202–207
Abdominal aorta, 84–87, 174–201, 212–215
   in *in vivo* studies, 220–223
Abductor digiti minimi muscle, hand, 228–229
Abductor hallucis muscle, 252–253
Abductor pollicis brevis muscle, 228–229
Abductor pollicis longus tendon, 232–235
Accessory hemiazygos vein, 110–113
Acetabular fossa, 206–207, 218–219
Acetabulum, 154–157
Achilles tendon, 256–261
Adductor brevis muscle, 146–153, 202–205, 216–219
Adductor longus muscle, 146–153, 202–205, 216–217, 278–279
Adductor magnus muscle, 146–147, 218–219
Adductor magnus tendon
   in knee, 272–277
   in thigh, 278–279
Adductor minimus muscle, 146–151, 202–203, 216–217
Adrenal gland, 192–197
   left, 86–87, 188–191, 216–217
      in *in vivo* studies, 220–223
   right, 86–87, 210–211
Alar fold, synovial, 270–271
Alveolar ridge of maxilla, superior, 66–67
Ambient (circummesencephalic) cistern, 46–47
   in *in vivo* studies using metrizamide, 30, 35
Amipaque (metrizamide), intrathecal injection of
   in computed tomography of skull and brain, 3, 30–35
   in *in vivo* studies of spine, 98–100
Amygdaloid nucleus, 10–11, 46–47
Anconeus muscle, 238–241
Angular gyrus, 18–19
Ankle, computed tomography of, 252–261
Anterior commissure, 10–11
Anterior junction line
   area of, 124–127
   definition of, 102
   in *in vivo* studies, 139–140
Antrum of stomach, 212–217
Anus, 146–147, 202–203
   sphincter of, 146–147, 202–203, 214–215
Aorta
   abdominal, 84–87, 174–201, 212–215
      in *in vivo* studies, 220–223
   root of, in *in vivo* studies, 138
   thoracic, 88–89
      ascending, 118–125
         in *in vivo* studies, 138–139
      descending, 104–125
         in *in vivo* studies, 138–139
Aortic arch, 128–129
   anterior portion of, 126–127
      in *in vivo* studies, 139–140
   posterior portion of, 126–127
      in *in vivo* studies, 139–140

Aortic-pulmonic window, 126–127
   definition of, 102
   lateral aspect of, lymph nodes at, 126–127
   medial aspect of, lymph nodes at, 124–127
   posterior aspect of, left lower lobe of lung in, in *in vivo* studies, 139
Aortic valve, 114–117
Aponeurosis of external oblique muscle, 162–167, 208–209
Apophyseal joint, C4–5, 62–63
Apophyseal joint, L2–3, 84–85
Appendices epiploicae of sigmoid colon, 160–163
Aqueduct of Sylvius, 10–13, 46–47
Arachnoid granulation, 22–23
Arch
   anterior of first cervical vertebra, 66–71, 92–93
      in *in vivo* studies using metrizamide, 98–100
   aortic. See Aortic arch
   pharyngopalatine, 66–67
Arm, upper, computed tomography of, 244–245
Artery(ies)
   axillary, 246–249
      left, 130–135
      right, 132–135
   basilar, 8–9, 42–45
      in *in vivo* studies using metrizamide, 33
   brachial
      in elbow, 238–243
      in upper arm, 244–245
   carotid
      common
         left, in chest, 128–137
            in *in vivo* studies, 141
         in neck and face, 54–61
         right, in chest, 134–137
            in *in vivo* studies, 141
      external
         in neck and face, 62–63, 66–67
         in spine, 92–97
      internal
         in *in vivo* studies using metrizamide, 33
         in neck and face, 62–73, 90–97
         in skull, 4–7, 40–45
         supraclinoid portion of, 8–9
   celiac, 190–193, 214–215
      in *in vivo* studies, 221
   cerebellar, posterior inferior, 4–5
   cerebral
      anterior, 10–11
         in *in vivo* studies, 26
      middle, 8–9
         in *in vivo* studies, 26
      posterior, in *in vivo* studies, 26
   cervical, deep, 94–97
   coronary, descending
      left anterior, 108–109, 114–115
      right posterior, 106–109
   epigastric, inferior, 162–173
   femoral

Artery(ies), femoral (*continued*)
      in abdomen and pelvis, 152–161, 202–207
      deep, in abdomen and pelvis, 146–151, 202–203
      in knee, 276–277
      superficial, in abdomen and pelvis, 146–151, 202–207
      in thigh, 278–279
   gastroduodenal, 186–189
   hepatic, 190–197, 212–213
   humeral, posterior circumflex, 246–247
   iliac
      common, 80–83, 170–173, 212–217
      external, 78–79, 162–169, 210–211, 218–219
      internal, 166–169, 210–211, 216–217
   innominate, 128–133
   interosseous, 236–237
   mammary, internal, 126–127
   maxillary, internal, 70–71
   mesenteric
      inferior, 174–177
      superior, 178–189, 214–215
         in *in vivo* studies, 220–223
   peroneal
      in ankle, 258–261
      in lower leg, 262–263
   phrenic, inferior, 196–197
   plantar
      lateral, 252–255
      medial, 252–253
   popliteal, 264–275
   pulmonary
      anterior segmental left upper lobe, 124–125
      interlobar
         definition of, 102
         left, 120–123
            in *in vivo* studies, 138
         right, 118–121
      left, 122–125
         in *in vivo* studies, 139
      main, 120–123
         in *in vivo* studies, 138
      right, 120–123
         in *in vivo* studies, 138–139
      truncus anterior of, 124–125
      right lower lobe, 116–117
   radial
      in forearm, 236–237
      in wrist, 228–235
   radial recurrent
      in elbow, 242–243
      in upper arm, 244–245
   renal, 182–185, 210–211, 216–217
      left, 188–189
      right, in *in vivo* studies, 220–223
   splenic, 190–195, 216–219
   subclavian
      left, 128–137
         in *in vivo* studies, 141
      right, 134–137
         in *in vivo* studies, 141
   suprascapular, 250–251

INDEX 283

Artery(ies) (continued)
  tibial
    anterior
      in ankle, 256-261
      in lower leg, 262-263
    posterior
      in ankle, 256-261
      in lower leg, 262-263
  ulnar
    in forearm, 236-237
    in wrist, 228-235
  umbilical, 172-173
  vertebral
    left, in chest, 136-137
    in neck and face, 54-57, 60-61, 64-67
    right, in chest, 136-137
    in skull and brain, 4-5
    in spine, 96-97
      in *in vivo* studies using metrizamide, 100
Articular capsule of elbow joint, 240-241
Articular cartilage of knee, 264-265
Articular facet, L3-4, in *in vivo* studies using metrizamide, 98-99
Articularis genus muscle, 276-277
Aryepiglottic fold(s)
  in neck and face, 60-61
  in spinal level, 90-91
Arytenoid cartilage, 58-59
Atrial appendage
  left, 120-121
  right, 116-119
Atrium
  of lateral ventricle, 12-15
    in *in vivo* studies, 25
  left, 112-121, 214-215
    in *in vivo* studies, 138
  right, 108-115, 210-215
    in *in vivo* studies, 138
Auditory canal, external, 4-5, 40-41, 72-73
Auditory meatus, internal, 72-73
Auditory tube, 68-69
  orifice of, 70-71
Axillary artery, 246-249
  left, 130-135
  right, 132-135
Axillary lymph nodes, 248-249
Axillary space, 126-127, 246-249
Axillary vein, 246-249
  left, 132-133
  right, 132-135
Azygoesophageal recess
  definition of, 102
  right lower lobe of lung in, 114-121
  in *in vivo* studies, 138
Azygos fissure in *in vivo* studies, 140
Azygos vein
  in abdomen and pelvis, 194-201
  arch of
    anterior portion of, 124-125
    in *in vivo* studies, 139-140
    posterior portion of, 124-125
  in chest, 106-123
  in spine, 86-89

Basilar artery, 8-9, 42-45
  in *in vivo* studies using metrizamide, 33

Basilic vein
  in elbow, 238-243
  in forearm, 236-237
  in upper arm, 244-245
  in wrist, 232-233
Basiocciput, clivus, 4-5
Basisphenoid, clivus, 4-7, 40-41, 70-71
Biceps brachii muscle, 242-249
Biceps brachii tendon
  in elbow, 238-241
  in shoulder, 246-251
Biceps femoris muscle
  in abdomen and pelvis, 146-149
  in ankle, 268-277
  in thigh, 278-279
Biceps femoris tendon, 264-269
Bifurcation of trachea, 124-125
Bile duct, common, 182-191
Bladder, 150-163, 166-167, 204-207, 214-215
  base of, 204-205
  dome of, 164-165
Blood vessels. *See* Artery(ies); Vein(s); Vessels
Bone(s)
  basiocciput (clivus), 4-5
  basisphenoid (clivus), 4-7, 40-41, 70-71
  calcaneus, 252-255
    tuberosity of, 254-255
  capitate, 228-231
  capitulum of humerus, 238-241
  clavicle, 132-137, 248-251
  ethmoid, perpendicular plate of, 40-43
  femur, 146-153, 268-279
    greater trochanter of, 156-161, 204-205
    head of, 154-163, 204-209, 218-219
    lateral condyle of, 266-269
    lesser trochanter of, 146-149, 202-203
    linea aspera of
      in knee, 276-277
      in thigh, 278-279
    medial condyle of, 266-269
    neck of, 154-159
  fibula, 254-265
  frontal, 46-47
    in *in vivo* studies, 48-49
    zygomatic process of, 46-47
  greater multangular (trapezium), 228-229
  hamate, 228-229
  humerus, 228-249
    capitulum of, 238-241
    coronoid fossa of, 242-243
    head of, 136-137, 250-251
    lateral epicondyle of, 242-243
    medial epicondyle of, 242-243
    olecranon fossa of, 242-243
    trochlea, 240-241
    tubercles of, 250-251
  hyoid bone
    body of, 60-61, 90-91
    greater cornu of, 60-61, 90-91
  ilium, 162-173, 208-211, 216-219
    wing of, 78-81
  ischium, 158-161, 202-207, 210-211, 216-217
  lesser multangular (trapezoid), 228-229
  lunate, 230-231
  mandible, 58-63, 94-95
    condyle of, 4-7, 68-73
    coronoid process of, 68-71
    ramus of, 64-69
  maxilla, 40-41
    anterior nasal spine of, 68-69
    palatine process of, 68-69

Bones, maxilla (continued)
    superior alveolar ridge of, 66-67
  metacarpal, first, 228-229
  nasal, 40-45
    in *in vivo* studies, 48-49
  navicular
    in ankle, 252-253
    in wrist, 228-231
  occipital, 66-69
    basiocciput (clivus), 4-5
    condyle of, 68-69
    jugular process of, 4-7
  parietal, 22-23
  patella, 266-271
  pisiform, 228-231
  pubis, 158-161, 206-207, 210-217
    ramus of, superior, 156-157
  sacrum, 164-167, 210-211, 214-217
    wing of, 78-83
  scapula, 116-137, 246-251
    coracoid process, 136-137, 250-251
    glenoid labrum of, 250-251
    spine of, 130-137, 250-251
  sphenoid
    basisphenoid (clivus), 4-7, 40-41, 70-71
    body of
      in neck and face, 72-73
      in skull, 4-7
    greater wing of
      in *in vivo* studies, 48-49
      in neck and face, 72-73
      in skull, 4-9, 40-47
    lesser wing of, 44-45
    pterygoid process of, 70-73
  sternum, 114-129, 214-215
    manubrium of, 130-133
  talus
    body of, 254-257
    head of, 252-253
    lateral process of, 252-253
    posterior process of, 254-257
    trochlea of, 256-257
  temporal
    mastoid portion of, 4-9, 40-45, 66-73
    petrous portion of, 4-9, 40-45, 72-73
      in *in vivo* studies, 24
        using metrizamide, 32, 35
    squamous portion of, 42-45
    styloid process of, 66-69
  tibia, 256-265
    lateral condyle of, 264-267
    medial condyle of, 264-267
    tuberosity of, 264-265
  triquetrum, 228-231
  ulna, 232-237
    coronoid process of, 240-241
    olecranon process of, 238-241
  vomer, 68-73
  zygoma, 40-43, 68-73
    frontal process of, 44-45
    in *in vivo* studies, 48-49
Bony nasal septum, 68-73
Bowel, small, 78-79
Brachial artery
  in elbow, 238-243
  in upper arm, 244-245
Brachial plexus
  in chest, 134-135
  inferior trunk of, 132-133
  in shoulder, 246-247, 250-251
Brachialis muscle

Brachialis muscle (*continued*)
  in elbow, 238–243
  in upper arm, 244–245
Brachiocephalic vein, 130–135
  left, 132–135
    in *in vivo* studies, 141
  right, in *in vivo* studies, 141
Brachioradialis muscle
  in elbow, 238–243
  in forearm, 236–237
Brachioradialis tendon, 232–235
Brachium pontis, 8–9
Brain, computed tomography of, 2–35
Breast, 112–119
Bronchus(i)
  left lower lobe, 118–121
  left main, 122–123
    in *in vivo* studies, 139
  left upper lobe, 122–123
    in *in vivo* studies, 138
  lingular, 120–123
  right lower lobe, 118–119
  right main, 122–123
    in *in vivo* studies, 139
  right middle lobe, 118–119
  right upper lobe
    in *in vivo* studies, 138
  segmental
    anterior
      left upper lobe, 124–125
      right upper lobe, 122–123
    apical, right upper lobe, 124–125
    left lower lobe, 116–117
    right lower lobe, 116–117
    superior
      left lower lobe, 120–121
      right lower lobe, 118–119
Bronchus intermedius, 120–121
Buccinator muscle, 64–67
Bursa
  popliteus, 266–267
  subscapularis, 248–249
  suprapatellar, 272–275
  trochanteric, 156–159

Calcaneus, 252–255
  tuberosity of, 254–255
Calcarine fissure, 16–17
Callosal sulcus, 16–17
Canal
  auditory, external, 4–5, 40–41, 72–73
  carotid, 4–7, 40–41, 70–73
  hypoglossal, 4–5
    in *in vivo* studies using metrizamide, 100
  infraorbital, 40–41
  nasolacrimal, 72–73
  optic, 8–9
    cranial opening of, 44–45
    orbital opening of, 44–45
  sacral, 168–171
  semicircular
    lateral, 40–41
    superior, 72–73
  spinal, 78–85, 212–213
Capitate, 228–231

Capitulum of humerus, 238–241
Capsule
  elbow joint, 242–243
  external, 12–13
  extreme, 12–13
  internal
    anterior limb of, 10–13
    posterior limb of, 12–13
  of knee joint, 266–271
Cardia of stomach, 198–201
Cardiac apex, 104–105, 198–199
Cardiac vein
  great, 108–109, 114–115
  middle, 106–109
Cardiophrenic angle
  definition of, 102
  left, 104–105
Carina of trachea in *in vivo* studies, 139
Carotid artery
  common
    left, in chest, 128–137
      in *in vivo* studies, 141
    in neck and face, 54–61
    right, in chest, 134–137
      in *in vivo* studies, 141
  external
    in neck and face, 62–63, 66–67
    in spine, 92–97
  internal
    in *in vivo* studies using metrizamide, 33
    in neck and face, 62–73
    in skull, 4–7, 40–45
    in spine, 90–97
    supraclinoid portion of, 8–9
Carotid canal, 4–7, 40–41, 70–73
Cartilage
  articular, of knee, 264–265
  arytenoid, 58–59
  costal, 184–185, 198–201, 212–213, 216–219
  of first rib, 130–131
  cricoid, lamina of, 56–57
  epiglottic, 60–61
  thyroid
    lamina of, 56–59
    superior cornu of, 60–61, 90–91
Cauda equina, 180–181
Caudate lobe of liver, 192–199, 212–213
Caudate nucleus, head of, 10–13
Cavity
  elbow joint, 240–241
  knee joint, 268–271
  middle ear, 40–41
  oral, 66–67
  pericardial, 110–111, 124–125
  peritoneal, 104–105, 192–193
    rectouterine pouch of, 158–163
  pleural, 128–129, 192–193, 208–218
    fluid in, 120–121, 198–201
  radioulnar joint, distal, 232–233
  shoulder joint, 250–251
  talocalcaneal joint, 252–255
  talonavicular joint, 252–253
  tibiofibular joint, 264–265
  tympanic, 40–41, 72–73
Cavum septum pellucidum in *in vivo* studies, 28
Cecum, 168–169, 208–209
Celiac artery, 190–193, 214–215
  in *in vivo* studies, 221
Center settings for computed tomography
  of abdomen and pelvis, 145

Center settings for computed tomography (*continued*)
  of chest, 102–141
  of extremities, 227
  of neck and face, 53
  of orbit, 39
  of skull and brain, 3
  of spine, 77
Central (Rolandic) fissure, 14–23
Centrum semiovale, 14–19
  in *in vivo* studies, 27
Cephalic vein
  in elbow, 238–241
  in forearm, 236–237
  in upper arm, 244–245
Cerebellar artery, posterior inferior, 4–5
Cerebellar cistern, superior, in *in vivo* studies using metrizamide, 34–35
Cerebellar flocculus, 40–41
Cerebellar hemisphere, 8–11, 42–45
  in *in vivo* studies, 29
Cerebellar peduncle
  inferior, in *in vivo* studies using metrizamide, 32
  middle, 8–9
Cerebellar tonsil
  in skull and brain, 6–7
  in *in vivo* studies using metrizamide, 32, 34
  in spine, 92–93
  in *in vivo* studies using metrizamide, 100
Cerebellar vermis, 8–13
Cerebellopontine angle cistern, 44–45
  in *in vivo* studies using metrizamide, 33, 35
Cerebellum
  superior aspect of, sulci on, in *in vivo* studies using metrizamide, 30
Cerebral artery
  anterior, 10–11
    in *in vivo* studies, 26
  middle, 8–9
    in *in vivo* studies, 26
  posterior, in *in vivo* studies, 26
Cerebral cortex in *in vivo* studies, 27
Cerebral hemispheres in *in vivo* studies using metrizamide, 31
Cerebral peduncle, 10–11, 46–47
Cervical artery, deep, 94–97
Cervical nerve, fourth, 90–91
  dorsal root ganglion of, 90–91
Cervical spinal cord, 92–93, 96–97
Cervical vertebra
  fifth, body of, 60–61
  first
    anterior arch of, 66–71, 92–93
      in *in vivo* studies using metrizamide, 100
    inferior articular facet of, in *in vivo* studies using metrizamide, 100
    posterior arch of, 66–67, 92–93
      in *in vivo* studies using metrizamide, 100
    superior articular facet of, 92–93
    transverse process of, 92–93
  fourth
    body of, 62–63, 90–91
    lamina of, 90–91
    lateral mass of, 90–91
    pedicle of, 90–91
    spinous process of, 90–91
    superior articular facet of, 96–97

INDEX   285

Cervical vertebra (continued)
  second
    body of, 64-67
    lamina of, 64-65
    odontoid process of, 66-69, 92-93
      in in vivo studies using metrizamide, 100
    spinous process of, 64-65
  seventh
    body of, 56-57
    lamina of, 56-57
    spinous process of, 56-57
  sixth
    body of, 58-59
      in in vivo studies using metrizamide, 98-99
    spinous process of, 58-59
  third
    body of, 94-95, 96-97
      in in vivo studies using metrizamide, 98-99
    inferior articular facet of, 96-97
    lamina of, 94-95, 96-97
    lateral mass of, 94-95
    pedicle of, 94-95
    spinous process of, 94-95, 96-97
    transverse process of, 94-95
Cervix, 158-159, 214-215
  anterior lip of, 156-157
Chest, computed tomography of, 102-141
Chiasm, optic, 46-47
Choroid plexus of lateral ventricle, glomus of, 14-15
  in in vivo studies, 28
Choroidal fissure, 10-11, 46-47
  in in vivo studies using metrizamide, 30
Cingulate gyrus, 10-17
Circumflex femoral vessels, 146-153, 204-205
Circumflex humeral artery, posterior, 246-247
Circumflex humeral vein, posterior, 246-247
Circumflex iliac vessels, deep, 166-171
Circummesencephalic cistern, 10-11, 46-47
  in in vivo studies using metrizamide, 30, 35
Cistern
  ambient (circummesencephalic), 46-47
    in in vivo studies using metrizamide, 30, 35
  cerebellar, superior, in in vivo studies using metrizamide, 34-35
  cerebellopontine angle, 44-45
    in in vivo studies using metrizamide, 33, 35
  circummesencephalic, 10-11, 46-47
    in in vivo studies using metrizamide, 30, 35
  crural, 10-11, 46-47
    in in vivo studies using metrizamide, 30
  interpeduncular, 10-11, 46-47
    in in vivo studies, 26
      using metrizamide, 30
  medullary, in in vivo studies using metrizamide, 32, 100
  pontine, in in vivo studies, 24, 29
    using metrizamide, 33
  quadrigeminal, 10-13, 46-47
    in in vivo studies, 24, 25, 26
      using metrizamide, 30, 35
  retropulvinar, 12-13
    in in vivo studies, 28
      using metrizamide, 30
  suprasellar
    in vivo studies of, 24, 26

Cistern, suprasellar (continued)
    using metrizamide, 33
  of velum interpositum in in vivo studies, 25, 28
    using metrizamide, 31
Cisterna magna
  in in vivo studies, 29
    using metrizamide, 32
  vallecula of, in in vivo studies using metrizamide, 34
Claustrum, 12-13
Clavicle, 132-137, 248-251
Clinoid process, anterior, 8-9, 44-45
Clivus
  basiocciput, 4-5
  basisphenoid, 4-7, 40-41, 70-71
    in in vivo studies using metrizamide, 32
Coccygeus muscle, 156-163
Coccyx, 154-163, 204-207, 214-216
Collateral ligament
  fibular, 268-269
  tibial, 268-269
  ulnar, 238-239
Colliculus
  inferior, 10-11, 46-47
    in in vivo studies using metrizamide, 35
  superior, 12-13
Colon
  ascending, 170-177, 208-209
  descending, 168-189
    in in vivo studies, 220-223
  hepatic flexure of, 178-181
  sigmoid, 164-167, 214-215
    appendices epiploicae of, 160-163
    loop of, in rectouterine pouch of peritoneal cavity, 162-163
    mesentery of, 166-167
  splenic flexure of, 190-191
  transverse, 174-185, 208-211, 216
    distal, 186-189
Commissure, anterior, 10-11
Computed tomography
  of abdomen and pelvis, 144-223
  of ankle, 252-261
  of chest, 102-141
  of elbow, 238-243
  of extremities, 227-279
  of forearm, 236-237
  of knee, 264-277
  of lower leg, 262-263
  of orbit, 39-49
  of shoulder, 246-251
  of skull and brain, 2-35
  of spine, 77-100
  of thigh, 278-279
  of upper arm, 244-245
  of wrist, 227-235
Concha, nasal
  inferior, 70-71
  middle, 72-73
Condylar vein, 4-7
Condyle
  lateral
    of femur, 266-269
    of tibia, 264-267
  mandibular, 4-7, 68-73
  medial
    of femur, 266-269
    of tibia, 264-267
  occipital, 68-69

Contrast medium, intravenous injection of, in computed tomography of skull and brain, 3
Conus medullaris of spinal cord, 86-87 182-183
Coracobrachialis muscle, 248-251
Coracoid process of scapula, 136-137, 250-251
Cornea, 44-45
Cornu
  greater, of hyoid bone, 90-91
  superior, of thyroid cartilage, 90-91
Corona radiata, 14-19
Coronary artery, descending
  left anterior, 108-109, 114-115
  right posterior, 106-109
Coronary sinus, 108-117
Coronoid fossa of humerus, 242-243
Coronoid process
  of mandible, 68-71
  of ulna, 240-241
Corpus callosum
  body of, 14-17
  genu of, 10-13
  splenium of, in in vivo studies using metrizamide, 31
Corpus cavernosum of penis, 202-203
Cortex, cerebral, in in vivo studies, 27
Costal cartilage, 184-185, 198-201, 212-213, 216-219
  of first rib, 130-131
Cranial fossa
  middle, 72-73
  posterior, 68-73
Cranial opening of optic canal, 44-45
Crest, occipital, internal, 8-9
Cricoid cartilage, lamina of, 56-57
Crista galli, 46-47
Cruciate ligaments, 266-269
Crural cistern, 10-11, 46-47
  in in vivo studies in metrizamide, 30
Cuneus, 14-19
Cystic duct, 192-193, 208-209

Deltoid ligament, 254-255
Deltoid muscle, 246-251
Demifacet for head of eighth rib, 88-89
Dentate ligament, 86-89
Dentate nucleus, 10-11
Diaphragm, 192-201
  left crus of, 188-197, 214-215
    in in vivo studies, 220-223
  right crus of, 86-87, 182-197
    in in vivo studies, 220-223
Diaphragma sellae, foramen of, 44-45
Diploe, 22-23
Diploic vein, 22-23
Disc, intervertebral
  C2-3, 64-65
  C3-4, 90-91
  C5-6, 60-61
  C6-7, 58-59
  L1-2, 180-181
  L3-4, 214-215
  L5-S1, 80-83, 170-171
  S1-2, 78-79
  T7-8, 88-89

Disc, intervertebral (continued)
  T11-12, 192-193, 212-213
  T12-L1, 188-189
Dorsal root ganglion of fourth cervical nerve, 90-91
Dorsum sellae, 8-9, 44-45
Douglas, pouch of, 158-163
Duct(s)
  bile, common, 182-191
  cystic, 192-193, 208-209
  hepatic, 196-197
  hepatic, common, 194-195
  lymphatic, right, in chest, 136-137
  thoracic, 112-123, 126-127, 134-137, 198-201
Ductus node, 126-127
Duodenal bulb, 184-185, 188-191
Duodenum
  fourth portion of, 180-185
  and jejunum, junction of, 216-217
  second portion of, 180-187, 210-211
    in in vivo studies, 220-223
  third portion of, 174-177, 212-215
    and second portion of, junction of, 178-179
Dura mater, 4-5
  spinal, 78-83, 86-97

Elbow, computed tomography of, 238-243
Emissary vein, 4-7
Epicardial fat, 198-199
Epicondyle
  lateral, of humerus, 242-243
  medial, of humerus, 242-243
Epidural venous plexus, spinal, 94-95
Epigastric artery, inferior, 162-173
Epiglottic cartilage, 60-61
Epipericardial fat pad
  left, 104-107
  right, 108-109
Erector spinae muscle, 80-81, 84-89, 168-201, 208-219
  in in vivo studies, 220-223
Esophagogastric junction, 214-215
Esophagus, 54-57, 88-89, 104-137, 198-201
  in in vivo studies, 140-141
Ethmoid, perpendicular plate of, 40-43
Ethmoid sinus, 4-5, 40-45
  in in vivo studies, 48-49
Eustachian tube, 68-69
  orifice of, 70-71
Extensor carpi radialis brevis muscle
  in elbow, 238-239
  in forearm, 236-237
Extensor carpi radialis brevis tendon, 228-235
Extensor carpi radialis longus muscle
  in elbow, 238-243
  in forearm, 236-237
Extensor carpi radialis longus tendon, 228-235
Extensor carpi ulnaris muscle, 236-237
Extensor carpi ulnaris tendon, 228-235
Extensor digiti minimi muscle, hand, 236-237
Extensor digiti minimi tendon, hand, 228-235
Extensor digitorum brevis muscle, 252-253
Extensor digitorum longus muscle
  in ankle, 256-261
  in lower leg, 262-263
Extensor digitorum muscle, hand, 236-237
Extensor digitorum tendons, hand, 228-235
Extensor hallucis brevis tendon, 252-253
Extensor hallucis longus muscle
  in ankle, 260-261
  in lower leg, 262-263
Extensor hallucis longus tendon, 252-261
Extensor indicis muscle, 234-235
Extensor indicis tendon, 228-233
Extensor pollicis brevis tendon, 228-229, 232-235
Extensor pollicis longus muscle, 236-237
Extensor pollicis longus tendon, 228-235
Extensor tendon, common, hand, 238-239
Extreme capsule, 12-13
Extremities, computed tomography of, 227-279
Eyelid
  lower, 40-41
  upper, 42-47

Falciform ligament, 104-105, 174-175, 182-183, 186-199
Falx cerebri, 8-23
  in in vivo studies, 27, 29
Fascia
  lateroconal, 174-181
  penile, 202-203
  prevertebral, 90-91
  renal, 174-183, 208-209, 218-219
  transversalis, 174-183, 186-187, 208-209
Fascia lata, 146-167, 202-207
Fat
  in axillary space, 246-249
  epicardial, 198-199
  epipericardial pad of
    left, 104-107
    right, 108-109
  external to pericardium, 198-199
  infrapatellar pad of, 266-269
  mediastinal
    anterior, 124-127
    in in vivo studies, 139
  orbital, 40-41, 46-47, 72-73
  pararenal, 208-209
  perirenal, 208-211
  in pre-Achilles space, 256-261
  in prefemoral, 272-277
  in renal sinus, 182-183, 186-187
  retrobulbar, 42-45
    in in vivo studies, 48-49
  retropancreatic, 186-189
  subcutaneous, 170-175
  surrounding ligamentum teres, 210-211
Femoral artery
  in abdomen and pelvis, 152-161, 202-207
  deep, in abdomen and pelvis, 146-151, 202-203
  in knee, 276-277
  superficial, in abdomen and pelvis, 146-151, 202-207
  in thigh, 278-279
Femoral nerve, 146-161, 162-173, 202-207
Femoral vein
  in abdomen and pelvis, 146-161, 202-207
  in knee, 276-277
  in thigh, 278-279

Femoral vessels, circumflex, 146-153, 204-205
Femur, 146-153, 268-279
  greater trochanter of, 156-161, 204-205
  head of, 154-163, 204-209, 218-219
  lateral condyle of, 266-269
  lesser trochanter of, 146-149, 202-203
  linea aspera of
    in knee, 276-277
    in thigh, 278-279
  medial condyle of, 266-269
  neck of, 154-159
Fibula, 254-265
Fibular collateral ligament, 268-269
Fissure
  azygos, in in vivo studies, 140
  calcarine, 16-17
  central (Rolandic), 14-23
  choroidal, 10-11, 46-47
    in in vivo studies using metrizamide, 30
  interhemispheric, in in vivo studies, 28
    using metrizamide, 30-33
  major, of lung, 208-211
    left, 114-115, 124-129
    right, 110-115, 122-125
  orbital
    inferior, 40-41
    superior, 6-7, 42-45
  parieto-occipital, 14-19
  Rolandic, 14-23
  Sylvian, 10-17, 46-47
    in in vivo studies, 24
    using metrizamide, 30, 33
Flexor carpi radialis muscle
  in elbow, 238-239
  in forearm, 236-237
Flexor carpi radialis tendon, 228-235
Flexor carpi ulnaris muscle
  in forearm, 236-237
  in wrist, 232-235
Flexor carpi ulnaris tendon, 230-231
Flexor digitorum longus muscle
  in ankle, 260-261
  in lower leg, 262-263
Flexor digitorum longus tendon, 252-259
Flexor digitorum profundus muscle
  in elbow, 238-239
  in forearm, 236-237
  in wrist, 232-235
Flexor digitorum profundus tendons, 228-233
Flexor digitorum superficialis muscle
  in elbow, 238-239
  in forearm, 236-237
  in wrist, 232-235
Flexor digitorum superficialis tendon, 228-233
Flexor hallucis longus muscle, 256-261
Flexor hallucis longus tendon, 252-257
Flexor pollicis longus muscle
  in forearm, 236-237
  in wrist, 232-235
Flexor pollicis longus tendon, 228-231
Flexor retinaculum, 228-229
Flocculus of cerebellum, 40-41
Foramen
  of diaphragma sellae, 44-45
  intervertebral
    C3-4, 96-97
    L2-3, 84-85
    L5-S1, 82-83
  jugular, 4-7, 70-71
  of Monro, 12-13
  sacral

Foramen, sacral (*continued*)
   anterior, 78–81, 168–169
   posterior, 78–81
Foramen magnum, 68–71
   anterior margin of, in *in vivo* studies using metrizamide, 100
   posterior margin of, 6–7
      in *in vivo* studies using metrizamide, 100
Foramen ovale, 4–7, 40–41, 70–73
Foramen spinosum, 40–41, 70–73
Foramen transversarium, of cervical vertebrae, 90–97
   in *in vivo* studies using metrizamide, 98–99
Forearm, computed tomography of, 236–237
Fornix
   columns of, 10–13
      in *in vivo* studies, 24
   posterior, of vagina, 158–159
Fossa
   acetabular, 206–207, 218–219
   coronoid, of humerus, 242–243
   cranial
      middle, 72–73
      posterior, 68–73
   hypophyseal, 44–45
   ischiorectal, 152–157, 202–205
   nasal, 40–43, 70–73
   olecranon, of humerus, 242–243
   pterygopalatine, 72–73
   of Rosenmüller, 68–71
Frontal bone, 46–47
   in *in vivo* studies, 48–49
   zygomatic process of, 46–47
Frontal gyrus
   inferior, 8–13
   middle, 8–19
   superior, 8–21
Frontal horn of lateral ventricle, 10–13
   in *in vivo* studies, 24, 25, 26, 28
      using metrizamide, 30
Frontal lobe, 6–21, 22–23, 46–47
   sulci on surface of, in *in vivo* studies, 25
Frontal process of zygoma, 44–45
Frontal sinus, 4–7, 46–47
Fundus of stomach, 104–105, 216–219
Fusiform gyrus, 10–13, 46–47

Gall bladder, 180–191, 208–211
   neck of, 192–193
Ganglion
   dorsal root, of fourth cervical nerve, 90–91
   gasserian, 40–43
   sphenopalatine, 40–41
Gasserian ganglion, 40–43
Gastric vein
   left, 192–197
   short, 196–197
Gastrocnemius muscle
   in knee, 264–273
   in lower leg, 262–263
Gastrocnemius tendon, 270–271
Gastroduodenal artery, 186–189
Gemellus inferior muscle, 156–159, 204–205, 208–209
Gemellus superior muscle, 158–159, 204–205, 208–209

Genioglossus muscle, 62–63
Genu of corpus callosum, 10–13
Gerota's fascia, 174–183, 208–209, 218–219
Gland
   adrenal, 192–197
      left, 86–87, 188–191, 216–217
         in *in vivo* studies, 220–223
      right, 86–87, 210–211
   lacrimal, 46–47
   parotid, 64–67
   pineal, calcified, 12–13
      in *in vivo* studies, 25
   pituitary, infundibulum of, 8–9
      in *in vivo* studies, 26
         using metrizamide, 33
   prostate, 204–207, 214–215
   submaxillary, 60–65, 90–91, 96–97
   thyroid, lateral lobe of, 54–59
Glenohumeral joint, right, in *in vivo* studies, 141
Glenoid labrum of scapula, 250–251
Globe, 4–7, 40–47
   in *in vivo* studies, 48–49
Globus pallidus, 12–13
Glomus of choroid plexus of lateral ventricle, 14–15
   in *in vivo* studies, 25
Glottis, rima of, 58–59
Gluteal vessels
   inferior, 164–165, 202–207
   superior, 166–169, 208–211, 218–219
Gluteus maximus muscle, 146–171, 202–211, 216–219
Gluteus medius muscle, 154–173, 208–209, 218–219
Gluteus minimus muscle, 156–171, 208–209
Gracilis muscle
   in abdomen and pelvis, 146–149
   in knee, 274–277
   in thigh, 278–279
Gracilis tendon, 266–275
Granulation
   arachnoid (pacchionian), 22–23
Greater cornu of hyoid bone, 60–61, 90–91
Greater multangular (trapezium), 228–229
Greater wing of sphenoid, 4–9, 72–73
   in *in vivo* studies, 48–49
Gyrus(i)
   angular, 18–19
   cingulate, 10–17
   frontal
      inferior, 8–13
      middle, 8–19
      superior, 8–21
   fusiform, 10–13, 46–47
   occipital
      lateral, 14–17
      superior, 18–19
   orbital
      medial, 46–47
      posterior, 46–47
   parahippocampal, 10–13, 46–47
   postcentral, 14–21
   precentral, 10–21, 22–23
   supramarginal, 18–19
   temporal
      inferior, 10–17, 46–47
      middle, 10–17, 46–47
      superior, 10–17, 46–47
Gyrus rectus, 6–9, 46–47

Hamate, 228–229
Hamulus, pterygoid, 66–67
Heart, 104–141, 200–201
   apex of, 104–105, 198–199
Hemiazygos vein, 106–109, 196–201
   accessory, 110–113, 124–127
Hemidiaphragm
   left, 104–105, 214–219
      dome of, 106–107
   right, 104–105, 208–213
      dome of, 110–111
Hemispheres
   cerebellar, 8–11, 42–45
      in *in vivo* studies, 29
   cerebral, in *in vivo* studies using metrizamide, 31
Hemorrhoidal vessels
   inferior, 214–215
   superior, 154–161, 166–167
Hepatic artery, 190–197, 212–213
Hepatic duct(s), 196–197
   common, 194–195
Hepatic flexure of colon, 178–181
Hepatic veins, 198–201, 208–213
   in chest entering inferior vena cava, 104–105
Hepatogastric ligament, 198–199, 212–213
Hilar lymph nodes, right, 122–123
Hip joint, capsule of, 156–157
Hippocampus, 10–13, 46–47
Horn(s) of lateral ventricle
   frontal, in *in vivo* studies, 24, 25, 26
      using metrizamide, 30
   occipital, 14–15
      in *in vivo* studies, 28
   temporal, 10–13, 46–47
      in *in vivo* studies, 24
Humeral artery, posterior circumflex, 246–247
Humeral vein, posterior circumflex, 246–247
Humerus, 240–249
   capitulum of, 238–241
   coronoid fossa of, 242–243
   head of, 136–137, 250–251
   lateral epicondyle of, 242–243
   medial epicondyle of, 242–243
   olecranon fossa of, 242–243
   trochlea of, 240–241
   tubercles of, 250–251
Hyoid bone
   body of, 60–61, 90–91
   greater cornu of, 60–61, 90–91
Hypoglossal canal, 4–5
   in *in vivo* studies using metrizamide, 100
Hypoglossal nerve (XII), 4–5
Hypopharynx, 58–61, 90–91
Hypophyseal fossa, 44–45

Ileum, 162–167, 172–173
Iliac artery
   common, 80–83, 170–173, 212–217
   external, 78–79, 162–169, 210–211, 218–219
   internal, 166–169, 210–211, 216–217
Iliac vein
   common, 80–83, 170–171, 212–217
   external, 78–79, 162–169, 210–211, 218–219
   internal, 166–169, 210–211, 216–217

Iliac vessels, circumflex, deep, 166-171
Iliacus muscle, 168-173, 208-209, 218-219
Iliocecal valve, 168-169
Iliofemoral ligament, 156-159
Iliolumbar vessels, branches of, 208-209
Iliopsoas muscle, 148-167, 202-209
Iliotibial tract
   in knee, 266-271
   in thigh, 278-279
Ilium, 162-173, 208-211, 216-219
   wing of, 78-81
Inferior articular facet
   of fifth lumbar vertebra, 82-83
   of first cervical vertebra in *in vivo* studies using metrizamide, 98-100
   of second lumbar vertebra, 84-85
   of third cervical vertebra, 96-97
   of twelfth thoracic vertebra, 86-87
Inferior articular process of seventh thoracic vertebra, 88-89
Inferior cerebellar artery, posterior, 4-5
Inferior cerebellar peduncle in *in vivo* studies using metrizamide, 32
Inferior colliculus, 10-11, 46-47
   in *in vivo* studies using metrizamide, 35
Inferior frontal gyrus, 8-13
Inferior nasal concha, 70-71
Inferior oblique muscle, 40-43
Inferior orbital fissure, 40-41
Inferior parietal lobule, 18-19
Inferior pubic ramus, 146-151
Inferior rectus muscle, 40-43
   in *in vivo* studies, 48-49
Inferior temporal gyrus, 10-17, 46-47
Inferior vena cava
   in abdomen and pelvis, 84-85, 172-201, 212-213
   in chest, 104-109
   entering right atrium, 110-113
Infraorbital canal, 40-41
Infrapatellar fat pad, 266-269
Infraspinatus muscle
   in chest, 122-137
   in shoulder, 246-251
Infundibulum of pituitary gland, 8-9, 44-45
   in *in vivo* studies, 26
      using metrizamide, 33
Inguinal ligament, 158-159
Inguinal lymph node, 202-207
Innominate artery, 128-133
Innominate vein, 130-135
   left, 132-135
      in *in vivo* studies, 141
   right, in *in vivo* studies, 141
Insula, 10-13
Intercostal muscle
   in abdomen and pelvis, 188-199, 208-211, 216-217
   external, 200-201, 218-219
   internal, 200-201, 218-219
   in shoulder, 250-251
Intercostal vein
   entering azygos vein, 106-107
   left superior, 134-135
Intercostal vessels, 198-201, 216-219
Interhemispheric fissure in *in vivo* studies, 28
   using metrizamide, 30-33
Interlobar pulmonary artery
   definition of, 102
   left, 120, 122-123
      in *in vivo* studies, 138

Interlobar pulmonary artery (*continued*)
   right, 118-121
Intermuscular septum
   lateral
      in knee, 276-277
      in thigh, 278-279
      in upper arm, 244-245
   medial, 278-279
Internal auditory meatus, 72-73
Internal capsule
   anterior limb of, 10-13
   posterior limb of, 12-13
Internal carotid artery
   in neck and face, 62-73
   in skull and brain, 4-7, 40-45
      in *in vivo* studies using metrizamide, 33
   in spine, 90-97
   supraclinoid portion of, 8-9
Interosseous artery, 236-237
Interosseous membrane
   in forearm, 236-237
   in lower leg, 262-263
Interosseous nerve, 236-237
Interosseous talocalcaneal ligament, 254-255
Interpeduncular cistern, 10-11, 46-47
   in *in vivo* studies, 26
      using metrizamide, 30
Interventricular septum, 106-115
Intervertebral disc
   C2-3, 64-65
   C3-4, 90-91
   C5-6, 60-61
   C6-7, 58-59
   L1-2, 180-181
   L3-4, 214-215
   L5-S1, 80-83, 170-171
   S1-2, 78-79
   T7-8, 88-89
   T11-12, 192-193, 212-213
   T12-L1, 188-189
Intervertebral foramen
   C3-4, 96-97
   L2-3, 84-85
   L5-S1, 82-83
Intestine, small, 168-171, 174-177, 208-219
   mesentery of, 168-177, 210-211, 216-219
Introitus, vaginal, 146-147
Ischial tuberosity, 148-153
Ischiocavernosus muscle, 148-149, 202-203
Ischiorectal fossa, 152-157, 202-205
Ischium, 158-161, 202-207, 210-211, 216-217

Jejunum, 172-173, 178-187
   and duodenum, junction of, 216-217
Joint(s)
   ankle, computed tomography of, 252-261
   apophyseal
      C4-5, 62-63
      L2-3, 84-85
   elbow, computed tomography of, 238-243
   glenohumeral, right, in *in vivo* studies, 141
   hip, capsule of, 156-157
   knee, computed tomography of, 264-277
   sacroiliac, 78-83, 166-171, 210-211, 216-217
   sternoclavicular, 132-133

Joint(s) (*continued*)
   tibiofibular, cavity of, 264-265
   wrist, computed tomography of, 227-235
Jugular foramen, 4-7, 70-71
Jugular process of occipital bone, 4-7
Jugular vein
   external, branches of, 60-61
   internal, 4-7
      left, in chest, 136-137
      in neck and face, 54-69
      right, in chest, 136-137
      in spine, 90-97
Junction line area, anterior, 124-127
   in *in vivo* studies, 139-140

Knee, computed tomography of, 264-277
Kidney, 176-191
   in *in vivo* studies, 220-223
   left, 84-87, 218-219
      upper pole of, 216-217
   lower pole of, 174-175
   right, 208-209
      upper pole of, 210-211
   upper pole of, 192-193

Lacrimal gland, 46-47
Lamina
   of cricoid cartilage, 56-57
   of fifth lumbar vertebra, 82-83
   of first sacral vertebra, 80-81
   of first thoracic vertebra, 54-55
   of fourth cervical vertebra, 90-91
   of second cervical vertebra, 64-65
   of second lumbar vertebra, 84-85
   of second sacral vertebra, 78-79
   of seventh cervical vertebra, 56-57
   of seventh thoracic vertebra, 88-89
   of third cervical vertebra, 94-95, 96-97
   of third lumbar vertebra, 214-215
   of thyroid cartilage, 56-59
   of twelfth thoracic vertebra, 86-87
      in *in vivo* studies using metrizamide, 98-99
Larynx
   anterior commissure of, 56-57
   vallecula of, 60-61
Lateral lobe of thyroid gland, 54-59
Lateral mass of second cervical vertebra, 94-95
Lateral occipital gyrus, 14-17
Lateral pterygoid plate, 66-69, 92-93
Lateral rectus muscle, 4-7, 42-45
   in *in vivo* studies, 48-49
Lateral semicircular canal, 40-41
Lateral sinus, 12-13
Lateral ventricle
   atrium of, 12-15
      in *in vivo* studies, 25
   body of, 14-17
      in *in vivo* studies, 25
      posterior portion of, in *in vivo* studies using metrizamide, 31
   choroid plexus of, glomus of, 14-15

Lateral ventricle (continued)
  horns of
    frontal, 10–13
      in in vivo studies, 24, 25, 26, 28
        using metrizamide, 30
    occipital, 14–15
      in in vivo studies, 28
    temporal, 10–13, 46–47
      in in vivo studies, 24
Lateroconal fascia, 174–181
Latissimus dorsi muscle, 104–107, 112–123, 182–201, 208–211, 218–219
Latissimus dorsi tendon, 246–247
Leg, lower, computed tomography of, 262–263
Lens, 42–45
Lesser multangular (trapezoid), 228–229
Lesser wing of sphenoid, 44–45
Levator ani muscle, 148–155, 204–205
Levator palpebrae superioris muscle, 46–47
  in in vivo studies, 48–49
Levator scapulae muscle, 54–63
Levator veli palatini muscle, 70–71
Ligament(s)
  broad, of uterus, 162–165
  collateral
    fibular, 268–269
    tibial, 268–269
    ulnar, 238–239
  cruciate, 266–269
  deltoid, 254–255
  dentate, 86–89
  falciform
    in abdomen and pelvis, 174–175, 182–183, 186–199
    in chest, 104–105
  hepatogastric, 198–199, 212–213
  iliofemoral, 156–159
  inguinal, 158–159
  odontoid, transverse, 92–93
  patellar, 264–265
  petroclinoid, 8–13, 44–45
  plantar calcaneonavicular, 252–253
  round, 158–159
  talocalcaneal
    interosseous, 254–255
    lateral, 254–255
  talofibular, posterior, 256–257
  tibiofibular, posterior, 256–259
  umbilical
    medial, 172–173
    median, 172–173
Ligamentum nuchae, 4–7
Ligamentum teres, 188–193
  fat surrounding, 210–211
Ligamentum teres femoris, 158–159
Linea alba, 178–179, 182–183, 188–192, 214–215
Linea aspera of femur
  in knee, 276–277
  in thigh, 278–279
Lingula of left lung, 112–121
Lingular bronchus, 120–123
Lip
  lower, 62–65
  upper, 64–65
Liver, 86–87
  caudate lobe of, 192–199, 212–213
  left lobe of, 104–105, 182–183, 186–199, 212–219
    in in vivo studies, 220–223
  quadrate lobe of, 186, 188–195, 210–211

Liver (continued)
  right lobe of, 104–109, 176–201, 208–211
    in in vivo studies, 220–223
Lobe(s)
  frontal, 6–21, 22–23, 46–47
    sulci on surface of, in in vivo studies, 25
  of liver. See Liver.
  of lung. See Lung
  occipital, 14–19
  parietal, 14–23
  temporal, 6–17, 40–47
    uncus of, in in vivo studies using metrizamide, 30
  of thyroid gland, lateral, 54–59
Lobule
  paracentral, 18–23
  parietal
    inferior, 18–19
    superior, 20–23
Longissimus capitis muscle, 64–65
Longissimus cervicis muscle, 56–57
Longus capitis muscle
  in neck and face, 68–71
  in spine, 92–95
Longus colli muscle
  in neck and face, 54–55, 62–65
  in spine, 92–95
Lumbar nerve, 170–171, 174–177
  second, 84–85
Lumbar subarachnoid space in in vivo studies using metrizamide, 98–99
Lumbar vertebra
  body of, in in vivo studies, 220–223
  fifth
    body of, 80–83, 172–173
    inferior articular facet of, 82–83
    inferior articular process of, 212–213
    lamina of, 82–83
    spinous process of, 82–83
  first
    body of, 86–87, 180–187
    pedicle of, 86–87, 182–183
    spinous process of, 178–181
    superior articular facet of, 86–87
    transverse process of, 86–87, 180–183
  fourth
    body of, in in vivo studies using metrizamide, 98–99
    spinous process of, 172–173
  second
    body of, 176–179, 212–213
    inferior articular facet of, 84–85
    lamina of, 84–85
    pedicle of, 214–215
    spinous process of, 84–85, 174–177
    superior articular facet of, 178–179
    superior articular process of, 212–213
    transverse process of, 176–179
  third
    body of, 84–85, 174–175, 214
    lamina of, 214–215
    superior articular facet of, 84–85, 174–175
  transverse process of, 210–211, 216–217
Lunate, 230–231
Lung, 246–251
  apex of, 134–135
  left, 198–201
    lingula of, 112–121
    lower lobe of, 104–129, 216–219
    upper lobe of, 122–131

Lung (continued)
  in in vivo studies, 140
  left lower, in posterior aspect of aortic-pulmonic window, in in vivo studies, 139
  right, 88–89, 200–201
    lower lobe of, 104–125, 208–213
      in azygoesophageal recess, 114–121
      in in vivo studies, 138
    middle lobe of, 110–121, 208–215
    upper lobe of, 122–133
      in in vivo studies, 140
Lymph nodes, 190–191
  axillary, 248–249
  hilar, right, 122–123
  inguinal, 202–207
  at lateral aspect of aortic-pulmonic window, 126–127
  at medial aspect of aortic-pulmonic window, 124–127
  precaval, 126–127
  pretracheal, 126–131
  subcarinal, 120–123
Lymphatic duct, right, in chest, 136–137

Malleolus
  lateral, 254–257
  medial, 256–257
  posterior, 256–257
Mamillary body, 46–47
Mamillary process, 84–85
Mammary artery, internal, 126–127
Mammary vein, internal, 126–127
Mammary vessels, internal, 198–201
Mandible, 58–63, 94–95
  condyle of, 4–7, 68–73
  coronoid process of, 68–71
  ramus of, 64–69
Mandibular nerve (V), 4–7
Manubrium of sternum, 130–134
Masseter muscle, 64–71
Masseter tendon, 64–71
Mastoid portion of temporal bone, 4–9, 40–45
Mastoid process of temporal bone, 66–73
Maxilla, 40–41
  anterior nasal spine of, 68–69
  palatine process of, 68–69
  superior alveolar ridge of, 66–67
Maxillary artery, internal, 70–71
Maxillary sinus, 40–43, 68–73
  in in vivo studies, 48–49
Meatus, auditory, internal, 72–73
Meckel's cave, 40–43
Medial orbital gyrus, 46–47
Medial pterygoid plate, 68–69
Medial rectus muscle, 4–7, 42–45
  in in vivo studies, 48–49
Median nerve
  in elbow, 238–243
  in forearm, 236–237
  in upper arm, 244–245
  in wrist, 230–235
Mediastinal fat
  anterior, 124–127
  in in vivo studies, 139

Medulla oblongata, 4-7
  in *in vivo* studies using metrizamide, 32, 35, 100
  pyramids of, 4-5
Medullary cistern in *in vivo* studies using metrizamide, 32, 100
Membrane
  interosseous
    in forearm, 236-237
    in lower leg, 262-263
  tympanic, 40-41
Meniscus
  lateral, 266-267
  medial, 266-267
Mesenteric artery
  inferior, 174-177
  superior, 178-189, 214-215
    in *in vivo* studies, 220-223
Mesenteric vein
  inferior, 174-187
  superior, 178-185, 188-189, 212-215
    in *in vivo* studies, 220-223
    and superior splenic vein, confluence of, 186-187
Metacarpal, first, 228-229
Metrizamide
  in *in vivo* computed tomographic studies of skull and brain using, 30-35
  in *in vivo* studies of spine, 98-100
  intrathecal injection of, in computed tomography of skull and brain, 3
Midbrain, 10-11, 46-47
  in *in vivo* studies, 24, 26
    using metrizamide, 30
Mitral valve, 110-113
Monro, foramen of, 12-13
Multangular, greater (trapezium), 228-229
Multangular, lesser (trapezoid), 228-229
Multifidus muscle
  in abdomen and pelvis, 168-201
  in neck and face, 54-63
  in spine, 78-91, 96-97
Muscle(s)
  abductor digiti minimi, 228-229
  abductor hallucis, 252-253
  abductor pollicis brevis, 228-229
  adductor brevis, 146-153, 202-205, 216-219
  adductor longus
    in abdomen and pelvis, 146-153, 202-205, 216-217
    in thigh, 278-279
  adductor magnus, 146-147, 218-219
  adductor minimus, 146-151, 202-203, 216-217
  anconeus, 238-241
  articularis genus, 276-277
  biceps brachii, 244-245
    in elbow, 242-243
    in shoulder, 246-249
  biceps femoris
    in abdomen and pelvis, 146-149
    in ankle, 268-277
    in thigh, 278-279
  brachialis
    in elbow, 238-243
    in upper arm, 244-245
  brachioradialis
    in elbow, 238-243
    in forearm, 236-237
  buccinator, 64-67
  coccygeus, 156-163

Muscle(s) (*continued*)
  coracobrachialis, 248-251
  deltoid, 246-251
  erector spinae, 80-81, 84-89, 168-201, 208-219
    in *in vivo* studies, 220-223
  extensor carpi radialis brevis
    in elbow, 238-239
    in forearm, 236-237
  extensor carpi radialis longus
    in elbow, 238-243
    in forearm, 236-237
  extensor carpi ulnaris, 236-237
  extensor digiti minimi, 236-237
  extensor digitorum, 236-237
  extensor digitorum brevis, 252-253
  extensor digitorum longus
    in ankle, 256-261
    in lower leg, 262-263
  extensor hallucis longus
    in ankle, 260-261
    in lower leg, 262-263
  extensor indicis, 234-235
  flexor carpi radialis
    in elbow, 238-239
    in forearm, 236-237
  flexor carpi ulnaris
    in forearm, 236-237
    in wrist, 232-235
  flexor digitorum longus
    in ankle, 260-261
    in lower leg, 262-263
  flexor digitorum profundus
    in elbow, 238-239
    in forearm, 236-237
    in wrist, 232-235
  flexor digitorum superficialis
    in elbow, 238-239
    in forearm, 236-237
    in wrist, 232-235
  flexor hallucis longus, 256-261
  flexor pollicis longus
    in forearm, 236-237
    in wrist, 232-235
  gastrocnemius
    in knee, 264-273
    in lower leg, 262-263
  gemellus inferior, 156-159, 204-205, 208-209
  gemellus superior, 158-159, 204-205, 208-209
  genioglossus, 62-63
  gluteus maximus, 146-171, 202-211, 216-219
  gluteus medius, 154-173, 208-209, 218-219
  gluteus minimus, 156-171, 208-209
  gracilis
    in abdomen and pelvis, 146-149
    in knee, 274-277
    in thigh, 278-279
  iliacus, 168-173, 208-209, 218-219
  iliopsoas, 148-167, 202-209
  infraspinatus
    in chest, 122-137
    in shoulder, 246-251
  intercostal
    in abdomen and pelvis, 188-199, 208-211, 216-217
    external, 200-201, 218-219
    internal, 200-201, 218-219
    in shoulder, 250-251
  ischiocavernosus, 148-149, 202-203
  latissimus dorsi

Muscle(s), latissimus dorsi (*continued*)
    in abdomen and pelvis, 182-201, 208-211, 218-219
    in chest, 104-107, 112-123
  levator ani, 148-155, 204-205
  levator palpebrae superioris, 46-47
    in *in vivo* studies, 48-49
  levator scapulae, 54-63
  levator veli palatini, 70-71
  longissimus capitis, 64-65
  longissimus cervicus, 56-57
  longus capitis
    in neck and face, 68-71
    in spine, 92-95
  longus colli
    in neck and face, 54-55, 62-65
    in spine, 92-95
  lumbospinalis, 186-187
    description of, 145
  masseter, 64-71
  multifidus
    in abdomen and pelvis, 168-201
    in neck and face, 54-63
    spinal, 78-91, 96-97
  oblique
    external
      in abdomen and pelvis, 172-201, 210-213, 216-219
      aponeurosis of, 162-167, 208-209
    inferior, 40-43
    internal, 162-183, 208-209, 212-213, 218-219
    superior, 46-47
  obliquus capitis inferior, 66-67
  obturator externus, 150-157, 202-207, 210-211, 216-219
  obturator internus, 150-156, 204-207, 210-211, 216-217
  occipitalis, 72-73
  omohyoid, 58-61
  opponens pollicis, 228-229
  orbicularis oculi, 46-47
  orbicularis oris, 64-65
  palmaris longus, 236-237
  pectineus, 148-157, 202-207, 210-211, 218-219
  pectoralis major
    in abdomen and pelvis, 208-213
    in chest, 118-135
      in *in vivo* studies, 141
    in shoulder, 246-251
  pectoralis minor
    in chest, 122-133
      in *in vivo* studies, 141
    in shoulder, 246-251
  peroneus brevis
    in ankle, 256-261
    in lower leg, 262-263
  peroneus longus
    in ankle, 260-261
    in lower leg, 262-263
  pharyngopalatine, 66-67
  piriformis, 162-167, 206-211, 216-219
  plantaris, 270-271
  popliteus, 264-265
  pronator teres
    in elbow, 238-243
    in forearm, 236-237
  psoas, 80-87, 168-171, 210-211, 216-217
  pterygoid
    external

Muscle(s), pterygoid, external (continued)
    in neck, 68–71
    in spine, 92–93
  internal
    in neck, 66–69
    in spine, 92–93
  pyramidalis, 206–207
  quadratus femoris, 148–157, 202–203, 216–219
  quadratus lumborum, 174–191, 208–209, 218–219
  quadratus plantae, 252–255
  rectus
    inferior, 40–43
      in in vivo studies, 48–49
    lateral, 4–7, 42–45
      in in vivo studies, 48–49
    medial, 4–7, 42–45
      in in vivo studies, 48–49
    superior, 46–47
      in in vivo studies, 48–49
  rectus abdominis, 154–199, 206–207, 216–217
    tendon of, 206–207
  rectus capitis posterior
    in neck and face, 66–69
    in skull and brain, 4–7
    in spine, 92–95
  rectus femoris
    in abdomen and pelvis, 146–161, 202–207
    in thigh, 278–279
  rhomboideus major
    in chest, 122–133, 136–137
    in shoulder, 246–249
  rhomboideus minor
    in chest, 136–137
    in neck and face, 54–57
    in shoulder, 250–251
  sartorius
    in abdomen and pelvis, 146–165, 202–207
    in knee, 266–267
    in thigh, 278–279
  scalenus anterior
    in chest, 134–137
    in neck and face, 54–55
  scalenus medius
    in chest, 136–137
    in neck and face, 54–59
  scalenus posterior
    in chest, 136–137
    in neck and face, 54–59
  semimembranosus
    in knee, 272–277
    in thigh, 278–279
  semispinalis capitis
    in neck and face, 54–71
    in skull and brain, 4–7
    in spine, 90–95
  semispinalis cervicis
    in neck and face, 54–59, 62–65
    in spine, 90–91, 96–97
  semitendinosus
    in knee, 276–277
    in thigh, 278–279
  serratus anterior
    in abdomen and pelvis, 194–201
    in chest, 106–107, 112–123, 126–127, 132–133, 136–137
    in shoulder, 246–251
  serratus posterior inferior
    in abdomen and pelvis, 186–195
    in chest, 104–105

Muscle(s) (continued)
  soleus
    in knee, 264–265
    in lower leg, 262–263
  splenius capitis
    in neck and face, 54–67
    in skull, 4–7
    in spine, 90–93
  splenius cervicis, 54–55
  sternocleidomastoid
    in chest, 136–137
    in neck and face, 54–71
  sternohyoid, 54–61
  sternothyroid, 54–55
  subclavius
    in chest, 134–137
    in shoulder, 250–251
  subscapularis
    in chest, 120–135
    in shoulder, 246–251
  supinator, 236–237
  supraspinatus
    in chest, 130–137
    in shoulder, 250–251
  temporalis, 4–7, 40–45, 70–73
  tensor fasciae latae, 146–167, 202–207
  teres major
    in chest, 120–127
    in shoulder, 246–247
  teres minor, 248–249
  thyrohyoid, 58–59
  tibialis anterior, 262–263
  tibialis posterior
    in ankle, 260–261
    in lower leg, 262–263
  transversus abdominis, 166–183, 186–193, 208–213, 216–219
  trapezius, 200–201
    in abdomen and pelvis, 200–201
    in chest, 122–137
    in neck and face, 54–61
    in shoulder, 246–251
  triceps brachii
    in elbow, 242–243
    in shoulder, 246–249
    in upper arm, 244–245
  vastus intermedius
    in abdomen and pelvis, 146–155, 202–203
    in thigh, 278–279
  vastus lateralis
    in abdomen and pelvis, 146–153, 202–207
    in knee, 270–277
    in thigh, 278–279
  vastus medialis
    of abdomen and pelvis, 146–147
    of knee, 272–277
    of thigh, 278–279

Nasal bone, 40–45
  in in vivo studies, 48–49
Nasal concha
  inferior, 70–71
  middle, 72–73
Nasal fossa, 40–43, 70–73
Nasal septum, bony, 68–73
Nasal spine of maxilla, anterior, 68–69

Nasolacrimal canal, 72–73
Nasopharynx, 68–71, 92–93
Navicular
  in ankle, 252–253
  in wrist, 228–231
Nerve(s)
  cervical, fourth, 90–91
    dorsal root ganglion of, 90–91
  femoral, 146–161, 162–173, 202–207
  hypoglossal (XII), 4–5
  interosseous, 236–237
  lumbar, 170–171, 174–177
    second, 84–85
  mandibular (V_1), 4–7
  median
    in elbow, 238–243
    in forearm, 236–237
    in upper arm, 244–245
    in wrist, 230–235
  obturator, 204–205
  oculomotor (III), 8–9, 44–45
  optic (II), 4–9, 44–45
    in in vivo studies, 48–49
  peroneal, common, 264–277
  plantar
    lateral, 252–255
    medial, 252–255
  pudendal, 162–165
  radial
    in elbow, 238–243
    superficial, 234–235
    in upper arm, 244–245
  sacral, 166–169
    first, 78–79
  sciatic
    in abdomen and pelvis, 146–165, 202–207
    in thigh, 278–279
  sural, 262–263
  tibial
    in ankle, 256–261
    in knee, 264–277
    in lower leg, 262–263
  trigeminal (V), 8–9
  ulnar
    in elbow, 238–243
    in forearm, 236–237
    in upper arm, 244–245
    in wrist, 232–235
Nucleus
  amygdaloid, 10–11, 46–47
  caudate, head of, 10–13
  dentate, 10–11
  red, 10–11

Oblique muscle
  external
    in abdomen and pelvis, 172–201, 210–213, 216–219
    aponeurosis of, 162–167, 208–209
  inferior, 40–43
  internal, 162–183, 208–209, 212–213, 218–219
  superior, 46–47
    in in vivo studies, 48–49
Oblique pericardial sinus, 114–115
Obliquus capitis inferior muscle, 66–67
Obturator externus muscle, 150–157, 202–207, 210–211, 216–219

Obturator internus muscle, 150–165, 204–207, 210–211, 216–217
Obturator internus tendon, 208–209
Obturator nerve, 204–205
Obturator vessels, 154–165, 204–207
Occipital bone, 66–69
  jugular process of, 4–7
Occipital condyle, 68–69
Occipital crest, internal, 8–9, 70–73
Occipital gryus
  lateral, 14–17
  superior, 18–19
Occipital horn of lateral ventricle, 14–15
  in in vivo studies, 28
Occipital lobe, 14–19
Occipital sinus, 10–11
Occipitalis muscle, 72–73
Oculomotor nerve (III), 8–9, 44–45
Odontoid ligament, transverse, 92–93
Odontoid process of second cervical vertebra, 66–69, 92–93
  in in vivo studies using metrizamide, 98–100
Olecranon fossa of humerus, 242–243
Olecranon process of ulna, 238–241
Omentum
  greater, 214–215
  lesser, 196–199, 212–213
Omohyoid muscle, 58–61
Opponens pollicis muscle, 228–229
Optic canal, 8–9
  cranial opening of, 44–45
  orbital opening of, 44–45
Optic chiasm, 46–47
  in in vivo studies using metrizamide, 30, 33
Optic nerve (II), 4–9, 44–45
  in in vivo studies, 48–49
Optic radiations, 12–13, 16–17
Optic tract, 10–11
Oral cavity, 66–67
Orbicularis oculi muscle, 46–47
Orbicularis oris muscle, 64–65
Orbit
  computed tomographic studies of, 39–49
  floor of, 72–73
Orbital fat, 40–41, 46–47, 72–73
Orbital fissure
  inferior, 40–41
  superior, 6–7, 42–45
Orbital gyrus
  medial, 46–47
  posterior, 46–47
Orbital opening of optic canal, 44–45
Orbital roof, 46–47
  in in vivo studies, 48–49
Oropharynx, 62–67, 94–97
Ovarian vessels, 170–173
Ovary, 162–165

Pacchionian granulation, 22–23
Palate
  hard, 68–69
  soft, 66–69
Palatine process of maxilla, 68–69
Palatine tonsil, 66–67
Palmaris longus muscle, 236–237
Palmaris longus tendon, 234–235

Pancreas
  body of, 182–183, 186–193, 214–219
    in in vivo studies, 220–223
  head of, 180–189, 212–213
    in in vivo studies, 220–223
  in vivo studies of, 220
  tail of, 194–195, 218–219
    in in vivo studies, 220–223
  uncinate process of, 180–181
Pancreaticoduodenal vessels, posterior superior, 186–187
Paracentral lobule, 18–23
Parahippocampal gyrus, 10–13, 46–47
Pararenal fat, 208–209
Paraspinal area, left, 116–117
Paratracheal stripe, right, 126–127, 130–135
  definition of, 102
  in in vivo studies, 140
Parietal bone, 22–23
Parietal lobe, 14–23
Parietal lobule
  inferior, 18–19
  superior, 20–23
Parietal peritoneum, 174–179, 188–189
Parietal pleura, 128–129, 198–201
Parietal trigone
  definition of, 102
  in in vivo studies, 140
Parieto-occipital fissure, 14–19
Parotid gland, 64–67
Partial volume effect in computed tomography of skull and brain, 3
Patella, 266–271
Patellar ligament, 264–265
Patellar retinaculum, medial, 266–271
Pectineus muscle, 148–157, 202–207, 210–211, 218–219
Pectoralis major muscle
  in abdomen and pelvis, 208–213
  in chest, 118–135
    in in vivo studies, 141
  in shoulder, 246–251
Pectoralis minor muscle
  in chest, 122–133
    in in vivo studies, 141
  in shoulder, 246–247
Pedicle
  of eighth thoracic vertebra, 88–89
  of first lumbar vertebra, 86–87, 182–183
  of fourth cervical vertebra, 90–91
  of third cervical vertebra, 94–95
Peduncle
  cerebellar
    inferior, in in vivo studies using metrizamide, 32
    middle, 8–9
  cerebral, 10–11, 46–47
Pelvis
  computed tomography of, 144–173
  female, computed tomography of, 144–173
  male, computed tomography of, 202–207
  renal, 178–185, 216–217
Penis, 214–217
  corpus cavernosum of, 202–203, 214–215
  fascia of, 202–203
  septum of, 202–203
Pericardial cavity, 110–111, 124–125
Pericardial sinus
  oblique, 114–115
  transverse, 120–121
Pericardium, 108–109, 198–201, 212–213

Perirenal fat, 208–211
Peritoneal cavity, 104–105, 192–193
  rectouterine pouch of, 158–163
Peritoneal sac, lesser, 182–183
Peritoneum, parietal, 174–179, 188–189
Peroneal artery
  in ankle, 258–261
  in lower leg, 262–263
Peroneal nerve, common, 264–277
Peroneal vein
  in ankle, 258–261
  in lower leg, 262–263
Peroneus brevis muscle
  in ankle, 256–261
  in lower leg, 262–263
Peroneus brevis tendon, 252–257
Peroneus longus muscle
  in ankle, 260–261
  in lower leg, 262–263
Peroneus longus tendon, 252–261
Perpendicular plate of ethmoid, 40–43
Petroclinoid ligament, 8–13, 44–45
Petrous portion of temporal bone, 4–9, 40–45, 72–73
  in in vivo studies using metrizamide, 32, 35
Petrous pyramid in in vivo studies, 24
Pharyngeal recess, 68–71
Pharyngopalatine arch, 66–67
Pharyngopalatine muscle, 66–67
Phrenic artery, inferior, 196–197
Phrenic vein, inferior, 190–191, 216–217
Pineal gland, calcified, 12–13
  in in vivo studies, 25
Pinna, 66–67
Piriformis muscle, 162–167, 206–211, 216–219
Pisiform, 228–231
Pituitary gland, infundibulum of, 8–9
  in in vivo studies, 26
  using metrizamide, 33
Plane of computed tomography sections
  of neck and face, 53
  of orbit, 39
  of skull and brain, 2
Plantar artery
  lateral, 252–255
  medial, 252–253
Plantar calcaneonavicular ligament, 252–253
Plantar nerve
  lateral, 252–255
  medial, 252–255
Plantar vein
  lateral, 252–255
  medial, 252–253
Plantaris muscle, 270–271
Plantaris tendon, 256–261
Pleura
  parietal, 128–129, 198–201
  visceral, 128–129
Pleural cavity, 128–129, 192–193, 208–218
  fluid in, 120–121, 198–201
Pleural space, 104–105
Plexus
  brachial
    in chest, 134–135
    inferior trunk of, 132–133
    in shoulder, 246–247, 250–251
  choroid, of lateral ventricle, glomus of, 14–15
    in in vivo studies, 25
  vascular, uterovaginal, 156–163
Pons, 8–9, 40–45
  in in vivo studies, 24, 29

Pons, in *in vivo* studies (*continued*)
  using metrizamide, 33, 35
Pontine cistern in *in vivo* studies, 24, 29
  using metrizamide, 33
Popliteal artery, 264–275
Popliteal vein, 264–275
Popliteus bursa, 266–267
Popliteus muscle, 264–265
Popliteus tendon, 266–267
Portal vein
  in abdomen and pelvis, 184–185, 188–197, 208–213
  in *in vivo* studies of, 221–222
  right branch of, in *in vivo* studies, 220–223
Postcentral gyrus, 14–21
Pouch, rectouterine, 158–163
Pre-Achilles space, 256–261
Precaval lymph nodes, 126–127
Precentral gyrus, 10–21, 22–23
Precuneus, 18–21
Prefemoral fat, 272–277
Pretracheal lymph nodes, 126–131
Prevertebral fascia, 90–91
Pronator quadratus muscle, 232–235
Pronator teres muscle
  in elbow, 238–243
  in forearm, 236–237
Prostate gland, 204–207, 214–215
Prostatic urethra, 204–205
Psoas muscle, 80–87, 168–191, 210–211, 216–219
Pterygoid hamulus, 66–67
Pterygoid muscle
  external
    in neck, 68–71
    in spine, 92–93
  internal
    in neck, 66–69
    in spine, 92–93
Pterygoid plates of sphenoid bone
  lateral, 66–69, 92–93
  medial, 68–69, 92–93
Pterygoid process of sphenoid bone, 70–73
Pterygopalatine fossa, 72–73
Pubic ramus
  inferior, 146–151
  superior, 156–157
Pubic symphysis, 150–155, 204–207
Pubis, 158–161, 206–207, 210–217
Pudendal nerve, 162–165
Pudendal vessels, internal, 152–153, 202–207
Pulmonary artery
  anterior segmental, left upper lobe, 124–125
  interlobar
    definition of, 102
    left, 120–123
      in *in vivo* studies, 138
    right, 118–121
  left, 122–125
    in *in vivo* studies, 139
  main, 120–123
    in *in vivo* studies, 138
  right, 120–123
    in *in vivo* studies, 138–139
      truncus anterior of, 124–125
    right lower lobe, 116–117
Pulmonary valve, 118–119
Pulmonary vein(s), 212–213
  left inferior, 116–119
    in *in vivo* studies, 138
  left superior, 122–123

Pulmonary vein(s) (*continued*)
  right inferior, 114–117
    in *in vivo* studies, 138
  right superior, 116–121
Pulvinar of thalamus, 12–13
Putamen, 10–13
Pyramidalis muscle, 206–207
Pyramids
  of medulla, 4–5
  petrous, in *in vivo* studies, 24

Quadrate lobe of liver, 186, 188–195, 210–211
Quadratus femoris muscle, 148–151, 202–203, 216–219
Quadratus lumborum muscle, 174–191, 208–209, 218–219
Quadratus plantae muscle, 252–255
Quadriceps tendon, 272–275
Quadrigeminal cistern, 10–13, 46–47
  in *in vivo* studies, 24, 25, 26
    using metrizamide, 30, 35

Radial artery
  in forearm, 236–237
  in wrist, 228–235
Radial nerve
  in elbow, 238–243
  superficial, 234–235
  in upper arm, 244–245
Radial recurrent artery
  in elbow, 242–243
  in upper arm, 244–245
Radiations, optic, 12–13, 16–17
Radioulnar joint cavity, distal, 232–233
Radius, 232–237
  head of, 238–239
  styloid process of, 230–231
Ramus
  inferior pubic, 146–151
  of mandible, 64–69
  superior pubic, 156–157
Rectouterine pouch, 158–163
Rectum, 148–165, 204–207, 212–216
Rectus abdominis muscle, 154–199, 206–207, 216–217
  tendon of, 206–207
Rectus capitis posterior muscle
  in neck and face, 66–69
  in skull and brain, 4–7
  in spine, 92–95
Rectus femoris muscle
  in abdomen and pelvis, 146–161, 202–207
  in thigh, 278–279
Rectus femoris tendon
  in abdomen and pelvis, 162–163
  in knee, 276–277
Rectus muscle
  inferior, 40–43
    in *in vivo* studies, 48–49

Rectus muscle (*continued*)
  lateral, 4–7, 42–45
    in *in vivo* studies, 48–49
  medial, 4–7, 42–45
    in *in vivo* studies, 48–49
  superior, 46–47
    in *in vivo* studies, 48–49
Red nucleus, 10–11
Renal artery, 182–185, 210–211, 216–217
  left, 188–189
  right, in *in vivo* studies, 220–223
Renal fascia, 174–183, 208–209, 218–219
Renal pelvis, 178–185, 216–217
Renal sinus, fat in, 182–183, 186–187
Renal vein, 180–181, 186–187, 210–211, 216–217
  left, 178–179, 182–185
    in *in vivo* studies, 223
  right, 176–179
Restiform body in *in vivo* studies using metrizamide, 32
Retina, 40–42, 46–47
Retinaculum
  flexor, 228–229
  patellar, medial, 266–271
Retrobulbar fat, 42–45
  in *in vivo* studies, 48–49
Retropancreatic fat, 186–189
Retropulvinar cistern, 12–13
  in *in vivo* studies, 28
    using metrizamide, 30
Rhomboideus major muscle
  in chest, 122–133, 136–137
  in shoulder, 246–249
Rhomboideus minor muscle
  in chest, 136–137
  in neck and face, 54–57
  in shoulder, 250–251
Rib(s), 182–193, 196–201, 208–211, 216–219
  eighth, 88–89
    head of, demifacet for, 88–89
  eleventh, 194–195
  first, 54–55
    costal cartilage of, 130–131
    in *in vivo* studies, 220–223
  second, 54–55
  thoracic, 246–251
Rima of glottis, 58–59
Rolandic fissure, 14–23
Rosenmüller, fossa of, 68–71

Sacral canal, 168–171
Sacral foramen
  anterior, 78–81, 168–169
  posterior, 78–81
Sacral nerves, 166–169
  first, 78–79
Sacral vertebra
  first
    body of, 78–81, 170–171
    lamina of, 80–81
    spinous process of, 80–81
    superior articular facet of, 82–83
  second, 168–169
    body of, 78–79

Sacral vertebra, second (continued)
  lamina of, 78–79
  spinous process of, 78–79
Sacroiliac joint, 78–83, 166–171, 210–211, 216–217
Sacrum, 164–167, 210–211, 214–217
  wing of, 78–83
Sagittal sinus, superior, 14–23
Saphenous vein
  in abdomen and pelvis, 146–153
  greater
    in ankle, 252–261
    in knee, 264–277
    in lower leg, 262–263
    in pelvis, 202–203
    in thigh, 278–279
  small
    in ankle, 260–261
    in knee, 272–275
    in lower leg, 262–263
Sartorius muscle
  in abdomen and pelvis, 146–165, 202–207
  in knee, 266–277
  in thigh, 278–279
Sartorius tendon, 264–265
Scalenus anterior muscle
  in chest, 134–137
  in neck and face, 54–55
Scalenus medius muscle
  in chest, 136–137
  in neck and face, 54–59
Scalenus posterior muscle
  in chest, 136–137
  in neck and face, 54–59
Scapula, 116–137, 246–251
  coracoid process, 136–137, 250–251
  glenoid labrum of, 250–251
  spine of, 130–137, 250–251
Sciatic nerve
  in abdomen and pelvis, 146–165, 202–207
  in thigh, 278–279
Sclera, 40–47
Segmental bronchus(i)
  anterior
    left upper lobe, 124–125
    right upper lobe, 122–123
  apical, right upper lobe, 124–125
  left lower lobe, 116–117
  right lower lobe, 116–117
  superior
    left lower lobe, 120–121
    right lower lobe, 118–119
Semicircular canal
  lateral, 40–41
  superior, 72–73
Semimembranosus muscle
  in knee, 272–277
  in thigh, 278–279
Semimembranosus tendon
  in abdomen and pelvis, 148–149
  in knee, 264–271
Seminal vesicle, 206–207, 214–215
Semispinalis capitis muscle
  in neck and face, 54–71
  in skull and brain, 4–7
  in spine, 90–95
Semispinalis cervicis muscle
  in neck and face, 54–59, 62–65
  in spine, 90–91, 96–97
Semitendinosus muscle

Semitendinosus muscle (continued)
  in knee, 276–277
  in thigh, 278–279
Semitendinosus tendon
  in abdomen and pelvis, 146–149
  in knee, 264–275
Septum
  intermuscular
    lateral
      in knee, 276–277
      in thigh, 278–279
      in upper arm, 244–245
    medial, 278–279
  interventricular, 106–115
  nasal, bony, 68–73
  penile, 202–203
Septum pellucidum
  cavum, in in vivo studies, 28
  in in vivo studies, 24, 25, 26
Serratus anterior muscle
  in abdomen and pelvis, 194–201
  in chest, 106–107, 112–113, 126–127, 136–137
  in shoulder, 246–251
Serratus posterior inferior muscle
  in abdomen and pelvis, 186–195
  in chest, 104–105
Shoulder, computed tomography of, 246–251
Sigmoid colon, 164–167, 214–215
  appendices epiploicae of, 160–163
  loop of, in rectouterine pouch of peritoneal cavity, 162–163
  mesentery of, 166–167
Sigmoid sinus, 8–11, 68–69
Sinus(es)
  coronary, 108–117
  ethmoid, 4–5, 40–45
    in in vivo studies, 48–49
  frontal, 4–7, 46–47
  lateral, 12–13
  maxillary, 40–43, 68–73
    in in vivo studies, 48–49
  occipital, 10–11
  pericardial
    oblique, 114–115
    transverse, 120–121
  sagittal, superior, 14–23
  renal, fat in, 182–183, 186–187
  sigmoid, 8–11, 68–69
  sphenoid, 6–7, 40–45
  transverse, 70–73
Skull, computed transaxial tomography of, 2–35
Soleus muscle
  in knee, 264–265
  in lower leg, 262–263
Spermatic cord, 202–207
Sphenoid
  body of
    in neck and face, 72–73
    in skull, 4–7
  greater wing of
    in in vivo studies, 48–49
    in neck and face, 72–73
    in skull, 4–9, 40–47
  lesser wing of, 44–45
  pterygoid plates of
    lateral, 66–69, 92–93
    medial, 68–69, 92–93
  pterygoid process of, 70–73
Sphenoid sinus, 6–7, 40–45

Sphenoid sinus, (continued)
  in in vivo studies using metrizamide, 32
Sphenopalatine ganglion, 40–41
Sphenozygomatic suture, 42–43
Sphincter, anal, 146–147, 202–203, 214–215
Spinal canal, 78–85, 212–213
Spinal cord, 90–91, 94–95, 134–135, 192–201
  cervical, 92–93, 96–97
  conus medullaris of, 86–87, 182–183
  in neck, 54–57, 64–65
  thoracic, in in vivo studies using metrizamide, 98–99
Spinal dura mater, 78–83, 86–95, 96–97
Spine
  computed tomography of, 77–100
  nasal, of maxilla, anterior, 68–69
Spine of scapula, 130–137, 250–251
Spinous process, 184–185
  of eighth thoracic vertebra, 212–213
  of eleventh thoracic vertebra, 192–197
  of fifth lumbar vertebra, 82–83
  of first lumbar vertebra, 178–181
  of first sacral vertebra, 80–81
  of first thoracic vertebra, 54–55
  of fourth cervical vertebra, 90–91
  of fourth lumbar vertebra, 172–173
  of second cervical vertebra, 64–65
  of second lumbar vertebra, 84–85, 174–177
  of second sacral vertebra, 78–79
  of seventh cervical vertebra, 56–57
  of seventh thoracic vertebra, 88–89
  of sixth cervical vertebra, 58–59
  of tenth thoracic vertebra, 198–201
  of third cervical vertebra, 94–95, 96–97
  of twelfth thoracic vertebra, 86–87, 186–191
Spleen, 104–105, 184–185, 190–199, 216–219
  in in vivo studies, 220–223
Splenic artery, 190–195, 216–219
Splenic flexure of colon, 190–191
Splenic vein
  in abdomen and pelvis, 184–197, 214–219
  in in vivo studies, 222–223
  superior, and superior mesenteric vein, confluence of, 186–187
Splenium of corpus callosum in in vivo studies using metrizamide, 31
Splenius capitis muscle
  in neck and face, 54–67
  in skull, 4–7
  in spine, 90–93
Splenius cervicis muscle, 54–55
Spring ligament, 252–253
Squamous portion of temporal bone, 42–45
Sternoclavicular joint, 132–133
Sternocleidomastoid muscle
  in chest, 136–137
  in neck and face, 54–71
Sternohyoid muscle, 54–61
Sternothyroid muscle, 54–55
Sternum, 114–129, 214–215
  manubrium of, 130–133
  xiphoid process of, 198–201, 214–215
Stomach, 180–197
  antrum of, 212–217
  body of, 218–219
  cardia of, 198–201
  fundus of, 104–105, 216–219
  in in vivo studies, 220–223
Styloid process
  of radius, 230–231

Styloid process (*continued*)
   of temporal bone, 66-69
Subarachnoid space
   lumbar, in *in vivo* studies using
      metrizamide, 98-99
   thoracic, in *in vivo* studies using
      metrizamide, 98-99
Subcarinal lymph nodes, 120-123
Subclavian artery
   left, 128-137
      in *in vivo* studies, 141
   right, 134-137
      in *in vivo* studies, 141
Subclavian vein
   left, 134-137
   right, 136-137
Subclavius muscle
   in chest, 134-137
   in shoulder, 250-251
Subcutaneous fat, 170-175
Submaxillary gland, 60-65, 90-94, 96-97
Subscapularis bursa, 248-249
Subscapularis muscle
   in chest, 120-135
   in shoulder, 246-251
Subscapularis tendon, 250-251
Substantia nigra, 46-47
Sulcus(i)
   callosal, 16-19
   on superior aspect of cerebellum, *in vivo*
      studies using metrizamide, 30
   on surface of frontal lobe in *in vivo*
      studies, 25
Sulcus tali, 254-255
Superior alveolar ridge of maxilla, 66-67
Superior articular facet
   of first cervical vertebra, 92-93
   of first lumbar vertebra, 86-87
   of first sacral vertebra, 82-83
   of fourth cervical vertebra, 96-97
   of third lumbar vertebra, 84-85
Superior articular process of eighth thoracic
   vertebra, 88-89
Superior cerebellar cistern in *in vivo* studies
   using metrizamide, 34
Superior colliculus, 12-13
Superior cornu of thyroid cartilage, 60-61,
   90-91
Superior frontal gyrus, 8-21
Superior oblique muscle, 46-47
Superior occipital gyri, 18-19
Superior orbital fissure, 6-7, 42-45
Superior parietal lobule, 20-23
Superior rectus muscle, 46-47
   in *in vivo* studies, 48-49
Superior sagittal sinus, 14-23
Superior semicircular canal, 72-73
Superior temporal gyrus, 10-17, 46-47
Superior vena cava
   in abdomen and pelvis, 212-213
   in chest, 116-129
   in *in vivo* studies, 138-140
Supinator muscle, 236-237
Supraclinoid portion of internal carotid
   artery, 8-9
Supramarginal gyrus, 18-19
Suprapatellar bursa, 272-275
Suprascapular artery, 250-251
Suprascapular vein, 250-251
S015ellar cistern in *in vivo* studies, 24, 26
   using metrizamide, 33

Supraspinatus muscle
   in chest, 130-137
   in shoulder, 250-251
Sural nerve, 262-263
Sustentaculum tali, 254-255
Suture, sphenozygomatic, 42-43
Sylvian fissure, 10-17, 46-47
   in *in vivo* studies, 24
      using metrizamide, 30, 33
Sylvius, aqueduct of, 10-13, 46-47
Sympathetic trunk, 174-177, 180-181
Symphysis, pubic, 150-155, 204-207

Talocalcaneal joint cavity, 252-255
Talocalcaneal ligaments, 254-255
Talofibular ligament, posterior, 256-257
Talonavicular joint cavity, 252-253
Talus
   body of, 254-257
   head of, 252-253
   lateral process of, 252-253
   posterior process of, 254-257
   trochlea of, 256-257
Temporal bone
   mastoid portion of, 4-9, 40-45, 66-73
   petrous portion of, 4-9, 40-45, 72-73
      in *in vivo* studies using metrizamide,
      32, 35
   squamous portion of, 42-45
   styloid process of, 66-69
Temporal gyrus
   inferior, 10-17, 46-47
   middle, 10-17, 46-47
   superior, 10-17, 46-47
Temporal horn of lateral ventricle, 10-13, 46-47
   in *in vivo* studies, 24
Temporal lobe, 6-17, 40-47
   uncus of, in *in vivo* studies using
      metrizamide, 30
Temporalis muscle, 4-7, 40-45, 70-73
Temporalis tendon, 70-73
Tendon(s)
   abductor pollicis longus, 232-235
   Achilles, 256-261
   adductor magnus
      in knee, 272-277
      in thigh, 278-279
   biceps brachii
      in elbow, 238-241
      in shoulder, 246-251
   biceps femoris, 264-269
   brachioradialis, 232-235
   common extensor, 238-239
   extensor carpi radialis brevis, 228-235
   extensor carpi radialis longus, 228-235
   extensor carpi ulnaris, 228-235
   extensor digiti minimi, 228-235
   extensor digitorum, 228-235
   extensor hallucis brevis, 252-253
   extensor hallucis longus, 252-261
   extensor indicis, 228-233
   extensor pollicis brevis, 228-229, 232-235
   extensor pollicis longus, 228-235

Tendon(s) (*continued*)
   flexor carpi radialis, 228-235
   flexor carpi ulnaris, 230-231
   flexor digitorum longus, 252-259
   flexor digitorum profundus, 228-233
   flexor digitorum superficialis, 228-233
   flexor hallucis longus, 252-257
   flexor pollicis longus, 228-231
   gastrocnemius, 270-271
   gracilis, 266-275
   latissimus dorsi, 246-247
   masseter, 64-71
   obturator internus, 208-209
   palmaris longus, 234-235
   peroneus brevis, 252-257
   peroneus longus, 252-261
   plantaris, 256-261
   popliteus, 266-267
   quadriceps, 272-275
   of rectus abdominis muscle, 206-207
   rectus femoris
      in abdomen and pelvis, 162-163
      in knee, 276-277
   sartorius, 264-265
   semimembranosus
      in abdomen and pelvis, 148-149
      in knee, 264-271
   semitendinosus
      in abdomen and pelvis, 146-149
      in knee, 264-275
   subscapularis, 250-251
   temporalis, 70-73
   tibialis anterior, 252-261
   tibialis posterior, 252-261
   triceps brachii
      in elbow, 240-243
      in upper arm, 244-245
   vastus intermedius, 276-277
   vastus lateralis, 272-273
Tensor fasciae latae muscle, 146-167,
   202-207
Tentorium cerebelli, 8-13
   in *in vivo* studies, 26
Teres major muscle, 120-127
   in chest, 120-127
   in shoulder, 246-247
Teres minor muscle, 248-249
Thalamus, 12-13
   in *in vivo* studies using metrizamide, 30
Thigh, computed tomography of, 278-279
Thoracic aorta, 88-89
   ascending
      in chest, 118-125
      in *in vivo* studies, 138-139
   descending
      in abdomen and pelvis, 214-217
      in chest, 104-125
      in *in vivo* studies, 138-139
Thoracic duct, 112-123, 126-127, 134-137,
   198-201
Thoracic ribs, 246-251
Thoracic spinal cord in *in vivo* studies using
   metrizamide, 98-99
Thoracic subarachnoid space in *in vivo*
   studies using metrizamide,
   98-99
Thoracic vertebra
   eighth
      inferior articular process of, 88-89
      pedicle of, 88-89
      spinous process of, 212-213

Thoracic vertebra, eighth (continued)
  superior articular process of, 88-89
  eleventh
    body of, 194-197
    spinous process of, 192-197
  first
    body of, 54-55
    lamina of, 54-55
    spinous process of, 54-55
  seventh
    inferior articular process of, 88-89
    lamina of, 88-89
    spinous process of, 88-89
    transverse process of, 88-89
  tenth
    body of, 198-201
    spinous process of, 198-201
    transverse process of, 200-201
  twelfth
    body of, 188-193
      in *in vivo* studies using metrizamide, 98-99
    inferior articular facet of, 86-87
    lamina of, 86-87
      in *in vivo* studies using metrizamide, 98-99
    spinous process of, 86-87, 186-191
    transverse process of, 188-189
Thyrohyoid muscle, 58-59
Thyroid cartilage
  lamina of, 56-59
  superior cornu of, 90-91
Thyroid gland, lateral lobe of, 54-59
Tibia, 256-265
  lateral condyle of, 264-267
  medial condyle of, 264-267
  tuberosity of, 264-265
Tibial artery
  anterior
    in ankle, 256-261
    in lower leg, 262-263
  posterior
    in ankle, 256-261
    in lower leg, 262-263
Tibial collateral ligament, 268-269
Tibial nerve
  in ankle, 256-261
  in knee, 264-277
  in lower leg, 262-263
Tibial vein
  anterior
    in ankle, 256-259
    in lower leg, 262-263
  posterior
    in ankle, 256-261
    in lower leg, 262-263
Tibialis anterior muscle, 262-263
Tibialis anterior tendon, 252-261
Tibialis posterior muscle in ankle, 260-261
Tibialis posterior tendon, 252-261
Tibiofibular joint cavity, 264-265
Tibiofibular ligament, posterior, 256-259
Tomography, computed. *See* Computed tomography
Tongue, 62-67, 94-97
Tonsil
  cerebellar
    in skull and brain, 6-7
    in *in vivo* studies using metrizamide, 32, 34
    in spine, 92-93

Tonsil, cerebellar, in spine (continued)
    in *in vivo* studies using metrizamide, 100
  palatine, 66-67
Torcular Herophili, 12-13
Torus tubarius, 68-69
Trachea, 54-57, 126-137
  bifurcation of, 124-125
  carina of, in *in vivo* studies, 139
  in *in vivo* studies, 139-140
Tract, optic, 10-11
Transversalis fascia, 174-183, 186-187, 208-209
Transverse colon, 174-185, 208-211, 216
  distal, 186-189
Transverse odontoid ligament, 92-93
Transverse pericardial sinus, 120-121
Transverse process
  of first cervical vertebra, 92-93
  of first lumbar vertebra, 86-87, 180-183
  of fourth cervical vertebra, 90-91
  of lumbar vertebra, 210-211, 216-217
  of second lumbar vertebra, 176-179
  of seventh thoracic vertebra, 88-89
  of tenth thoracic vertebra, 200-201
  of third cervical vertebra, 94-95
  of twelfth thoracic vertebra, 188-189
Transverse sinus, 70-73
Transversus abdominis muscle, 166-183, 186-193, 208-213, 216-219
Trapezium (greater multangular), 228-229
Trapezius, muscle
  in abdomen and pelvis, 200-201
  in chest, 122-127
  in neck and face, 54-61
  in shoulder, 246-251
Trapezoid (lesser multangular), 228-229
Triceps brachii muscle
  in elbow, 242-243
  in shoulder, 246-249
  in upper arm, 244-245
Triceps brachii tendon in elbow, 240-243
Tricuspid valve, 108-113
Trigeminal nerve (V), 8-9
Trigone, parietal
  definition of, 102
  in *in vivo* studies, 140
Triquetrum, 228-231
Trochanter of femur
  greater, 156-161, 204-205
  lesser, 146-149, 202-203
Trochanteric bursa, 156-159
Trochlea, 46-47
  of humerus, 240-241
  of talus, 256-257
Truncus anterior of right pulmonary artery, 124-125
Trunk, sympathetic, 174-177, 180-181
Tubercles of humerus, 250-251
Tuberosity
  calcaneal, 254-255
  ischial, 148-153
  tibial, 264-265
Tympanic cavity, 40-41, 72-73
Tympanic membrane, 40-41

Ulna, 232-237
  coronoid process of, 240-241

Ulna (continued)
  olecranon process of, 238-241
Ulnar artery
  in forearm, 236-237
  in wrist, 228-235
Ulnar collateral ligament, 238-239
Ulnar nerve
  in elbow, 238-243
  in forearm, 236-237
  in upper arm, 244-245
  in wrist, 232-235
Umbilical artery, 172-173
Umbilical ligament
  medial, 172-173
  median, 172-173
Umbilical vein, 188-193
Uncus of temporal lobe, 10-11, 46-47
  in *in vivo* studies using metrizamide, 30
Urachus, 172-173
Ureter, 156-157, 162-165, 168-177
Urethra, 146-149, 206-207, 214-215
  prostatic, 204-205
Uterovaginal vascular plexus, 156-163
Uterus, 160-165, 214
  broad ligament of, 162-165
Uvula, 66-67

Vagina, 148-159, 214-215
  introitus, 146-147
  posterior fornix of, 158-159
Vallecula
  of cisterna magna in *in vivo* studies using metrizamide, 34
  of larynx, 60-61
Valve
  aortic, 114-117
  iliocecal, 168-169
  mitral, 110-113
  pulmonary, 118-119
  tricuspid, 108-113
Vastus intermedius muscle
  in abdomen and pelvis, 146-155, 202-203
  in thigh, 278-279
Vastus intermedius tendon, 276-277
Vastus lateralis muscle
  in abdomen and pelvis, 146-153, 202-207
  in knee, 270-277
  in thigh, 278-279
Vastus lateralis tendon, 272-273
Vastus medialis muscle
  in abdomen and pelvis, 146-147
  in knee, 272-277
  in thigh, 278-279
Vein(s)
  axillary, 246-249
    left, 132-133
    right, 132-135
  azygos
    in abdomen and pelvis, 194-201
    arch of
      anterior portion of, 124-125
      in *in vivo* studies, 139
      posterior portion of, 124-125
    in chest, 106-123
    in spine, 86-89

Vein(s) (continued)
  basilic
    in elbow, 238–243
    in forearm, 236–237
    in upper arm, 244–245
    in wrist, 232–233
  brachiocephalic, 130–135
    left, 132–135
      in in vivo studies, 141
    right, in in vivo studies, 141
  cardiac
    great, 108–109, 114–115
    middle, 106–109
  cephalic
    in elbow, 238–241
    in forearm, 236–237
    in upper arm, 244–245
  condylar, 4–7
  diploic, 22–23
  emissary, 4–7
  femoral
    in abdomen and pelvis, 146–161, 202–207
    in knee, 276–277
    in thigh, 278–279
  gastric
    left, 192–197
    short, 196–197
  hemiazygos
    in abdomen and pelvis, 196–201
    accessory, 110–113, 124–127
    in chest, 106–109
  hepatic, 198–201, 208–213
    in chest entering inferior vena cava, 104–105
  humeral, posterior circumflex, 246–247
  iliac
    common, 80–83, 170–171, 212–217
    external, 78–79, 162–169, 210–211, 218–219
    internal, 166–169, 210–211, 216–217
  innominate, 130–135
    left, 132–135
      in in vivo studies, 141
    right, in in vivo studies, 141
  intercostal
    entering azygos vein, 106–107
    left superior, 134–135
  jugular
    external, branches of, 60–61
    internal
      in neck and face, 54–69
      in skull and brain, 4–7
      in spine, 90–97
    left internal, in chest, 136–137
    right internal, in chest, 136–137
  mammary, internal, 126–127
  mesenteric
    inferior, 174–187
    superior, 178–185, 188–189, 212–215
      in in vivo studies, 220–223
      and superior splenic vein, confluence of, 186–187
  peroneal
    in ankle, 258–261
    in lower leg, 262–263
  phrenic, inferior, 190–191, 216–217
  plantar
    lateral, 252–255
    medial, 252–253
  popliteal, 264–275

Vein(s) (continued)
  portal
    in abdomen and pelvis, 184–185, 188–197, 208–213
    in in vivo studies, 221–222
    right branch of, in in vivo studies, 220–223
  pulmonary, 212–213
    left inferior, 116–119
      in in vivo studies, 138
    left superior, 122–123
    right inferior, 114–117
      in in vivo studies, 138
    right superior, 116–121
  renal, 180–181, 186–187, 210–211, 216–217
    left, 178–179, 182–185
      in in vivo studies, 223
    right, 176–179
  saphenous
    in abdomen and pelvis, 146–153
    greater
      in ankle, 252–261
      in knee, 264–277
      in lower leg, 262–263
      in pelvis, 202–203
      in thigh, 278–279
    small
      in ankle, 260–261
      in knee, 272–275
      in lower leg, 262–263
  splenic
    in abdomen and pelvis, 184–197, 214–219
    in in vivo studies, 222–223
    superior, and superior mesenteric vein, confluence of, 186–187
  subclavian
    left, 134–137
    right, 136–137
  suprascapular, 250–251
  tibial
    anterior
      in ankle, 256–259
      in lower leg, 262–263
    posterior
      in ankle, 256–261
      in lower leg, 262–263
  umbilical, 188–193
  vertebral, 90–91, 94–95
Velum interpositum, cistern of, in in vivo studies, 25, 28
  using metrizamide, 31
Vena cava
  inferior
    in abdomen and pelvis, 172–201, 212–213
    in in vivo studies, 220–223
    in chest, 104–109
      entering right atrium, 110–113
  superior, 116–129
    in in vivo studies, 138–140
Venous plexus, epidural, spinal, 94–95
Ventricle(s)
  of brain
    enlarged, in vivo studies of, 24–25
    fourth, 8–9
      lateral recess of, in in vivo studies using metrizamide, 32, 35
      in in vivo studies of, 24, 26, 29
      in in vivo studies using metrizamide, 33, 35
    lateral

Ventricle(s), of brain, lateral (continued)
  atrium of, 12–15
    in in vivo studies, 25
  body of, 14–17
    in in vivo studies, 25
    posterior portion of, in in vivo studies using metrizamide, 31
  choroid plexus of, glomus of, 14–15
  horns of
    frontal, 10–13
      in in vivo studies, 24, 25, 26, 28
      in in vivo studies using metrizamide, 30
    occipital, 14–15
      in in vivo studies, 28
    temporal, 10–13, 46–47
      in in vivo studies, 24
  third, 10–13
    inferior recesses of, in in vivo studies using metrizamide, 30
    in in vivo studies, 24, 29
    using metrizamide, 30
  of heart
    left, 106–113, 218–219
    right, 106–117, 216–217
Ventricular outflow tract, right, in in vivo studies, 138
Ventricular wall, left, 114–117
Vermis, cerebellar, 8–13
Vertebra
  cervical
    fifth, body of, 60–61
    first
      anterior arch of, 66–71, 92–93
        in in vivo studies using metrizamide, 100
      inferior articular facet of, in in vivo studies using metrizamide, 100
      posterior arch of, 66–67, 92–93
        in in vivo studies using metrizamide, 100
      superior articular facet of, 92–93
      transverse process of, 92–93
    fourth
      body of, 62–63, 90–91
      lamina of, 90–91
      lateral mass of, 90–91
      pedicle of, 90–91
      spinous process of, 90–91
      superior articular facet of, 96–97
    second
      body of, 64–67
      lamina of, 64–65
      odontoid process of, 66–69, 92–93
        in in vivo studies using metrizamide, 100
      spinous process of, 64–65
    seventh
      body of, 56–57
      lamina of, 56–57
      spinous process of, 56–57
    sixth
      body of, 58–59
        in in vivo studies using metrizamide, 98–99
      spinous process of, 58–59
    third
      body of, 94–95, 96–97
        in in vivo studies using metrizamide, 98–99

Vertebra, cervical (*continued*)
    inferior articular facet of, 96–97
    lamina of, 94–95, 96–97
    lateral mass of, 94–95
    pedicle of, 94–95
    spinous process of, 94–95, 96–97
    transverse process of, 94–95
  lumbar
    body of, in *in vivo* studies, 220–223
    fifth
      body of, 80–83, 172–173
      inferior articular facet of, 82–82
      inferior articular process of, 212–213
      lamina of, 82–83
      spinous process of, 82–83
    first
      body of, 86–87, 180–187
      pedicle of, 86–87, 182–183
      spinous process of, 178–181
      superior articular facet of, 86–87
      transverse process of, 86–87, 180–183
    fourth
      body of, in *in vivo* studies using metrizamide, 98–99
      spinous process of, 172–173
    second
      body of, 176–179, 212–213
      inferior articular facet of, 84–85
      lamina of, 84–85
      pedicle of, 214–215
      spinous process of, 84–85, 174–177
      superior articular facet of, 178–179
      superior articular process of, 212–213
      transverse process of, 176–179
    third
      body of, 84–85, 174–175, 214–215
      lamina of, 214–215
      superior articular facet of, 84–85, 174–175
    transverse process of, 210–211, 216–217
  sacral
    first
      body of, 78–81, 170–171
      lamina of, 80–81
      spinous process of, 80–81
      superior articular facet of, 82–83
    second, 168–169
      body of, 78–79
      lamina of, 78–79
      spinous process of, 78–79

Vertebra (*continued*)
  thoracic
    eighth
      inferior articular process of, 88–89
      pedicle of, 88–89
      spinous process of, 212–213
      superior articular process of, 88–89
    eleventh
      body of, 194–197
      spinous process of, 192–197
    first
      body of, 54–55
      lamina of, 54–55
      spinous process of, 54–55
    seventh
      inferior articular process of, 88–89
      lamina of, 88–89
      spinous process of, 88–89
      transverse process of, 88–89
    tenth
      body of, 198–201
      spinous process of, 198–201
      transverse process of, 200–201
    twelfth
      body of, 188–193
        in *in vivo* studies using metrizamide, 98–99
      inferior articular facet of, 86–87
      lamina of, 86–87
        in *in vivo* studies using metrizamide, 98–99
      spinous process of, 86–87, 186–191
      transverse process of, 188–189
Vertebral artery
  in chest, 136–137
  in neck and face, 54–57, 60–61, 64–67
  in skull and brain, 4–5
  in spine, 90–97
    in *in vivo* studies using metrizamide, 100
Vertebral column, computed tomography of, 77–100
Vertebral vein, 90–91, 94–95
Vessels
  femoral, circumflex, 146–153, 204–205
  gluteal
    inferior, 164–165, 202–207
    superior, 166–169, 208–211, 218–219
  hemorrhoidal
    inferior, 214–215
    superior, 154–161, 166–167

Vessels (*continued*)
  iliac, circumflex, deep, 166–171
  iliolumbar, branches of, 208–209
  intercostal, 198–201, 216–219
  internal mammary, 198–201
  obturator, 204–207
  pancreaticoduodenal, posterior superior, 186–187
  pudendal, internal, 152–153, 202–207
Visceral pleura, 128–129
Vocal cord, 56–59
Vomer, 68–73

Window, aortic-pulmonic, 126–127
  definition of, 102
  lateral aspect of, lymph nodes at, 126–127
  medial aspect of, lymph nodes at, 124–127
  posterior aspect of, left lower lobe of lung in, in *in vivo* studies, 139
Window settings for computed tomography
  of abdomen and pelvis, 145
  of chest, 102
  of extremities, 227
  of neck and face, 53
  of orbit, 39
  of skull and brain, 3
  of spine, 77
Wrist, computed tomography of, 227–235

Xiphoid process, 198–201, 214–215

Zygoma, 40–43, 68–73
  frontal process of, 44–45
  in *in vivo* studies, 48–49
Zygomatic process of frontal bone, 46–47